AF134048

Computational Approaches in Discovery & Design of Antimicrobial Peptides

Computational Approaches in Discovery & Design of Antimicrobial Peptides

Editors

Agostinho Antunes
Guillermin Agüero-Chapin
Yovani Marrero-Ponce

MDPI • Basel • Beijing • Wuhan • Barcelona • Belgrade • Manchester • Tokyo • Cluj • Tianjin

Editors
Agostinho Antunes
CIIMAR- Centro Interdisciplinar de Investigação Marinha e Ambiental
Universidade do Porto
Porto
Portugal

Guillermin Agüero-Chapin
CIIMAR- Centro Interdisciplinar de Investigação Marinha e Ambiental
Universidade do Porto
Porto
Portugal

Yovani Marrero-Ponce
Grupo de Medicina Molecular y Traslacional (MeM&T)
Universidad San Francisco de Quito
Quito
Ecuador

Editorial Office
MDPI
St. Alban-Anlage 66
4052 Basel, Switzerland

This is a reprint of articles from the Special Issue published online in the open access journal *Antibiotics* (ISSN 2079-6382) (available at: www.mdpi.com/journal/antibiotics/special_issues/Peptides_Discovery).

For citation purposes, cite each article independently as indicated on the article page online and as indicated below:

LastName, A.A.; LastName, B.B.; LastName, C.C. Article Title. *Journal Name* **Year**, *Volume Number*, Page Range.

ISBN 978-3-0365-7961-0 (Hbk)
ISBN 978-3-0365-7960-3 (PDF)

© 2023 by the authors. Articles in this book are Open Access and distributed under the Creative Commons Attribution (CC BY) license, which allows users to download, copy and build upon published articles, as long as the author and publisher are properly credited, which ensures maximum dissemination and a wider impact of our publications.
The book as a whole is distributed by MDPI under the terms and conditions of the Creative Commons license CC BY-NC-ND.

Contents

About the Editors vii

Preface to "Computational Approaches in Discovery & Design of Antimicrobial Peptides" . . ix

Guillermin Agüero-Chapin, Agostinho Antunes and Yovani Marrero-Ponce
A 2022 Update on Computational Approaches to the Discovery and Design of Antimicrobial Peptides
Reprinted from: *Antibiotics* **2023**, *12*, 1011, doi:10.3390/antibiotics12061011 . . . . **1**

Guillermin Agüero-Chapin, Deborah Galpert-Cañizares, Dany Domínguez-Pérez, Yovani Marrero-Ponce, Gisselle Pérez-Machado and Marta Teijeira et al.
Emerging Computational Approaches for Antimicrobial Peptide Discovery
Reprinted from: *Antibiotics* **2022**, *11*, 936, doi:10.3390/antibiotics11070936 . . . . **5**

Yasser B. Ruiz-Blanco, Guillermin Agüero-Chapin, Sandra Romero-Molina, Agostinho Antunes, Lia-Raluca Olari and Barbara Spellerberg et al.
ABP-Finder: A Tool to Identify Antibacterial Peptides and the Gram-Staining Type of Targeted Bacteria
Reprinted from: *Antibiotics* **2022**, *11*, 1708, doi:10.3390/antibiotics11121708 . . . . **37**

Luis Pablo Avila-Barrientos, Luis Fernando Cofas-Vargas, Guillermin Agüero-Chapin, Enrique Hernández-García, Sergio Ruiz-Carmona and Norma A. Valdez-Cruz et al.
Computational Design of Inhibitors Targeting the Catalytic Subunit of *Escherichia coli* F_OF_1-ATP Synthase
Reprinted from: *Antibiotics* **2022**, *11*, 557, doi:10.3390/antibiotics11050557 . . . . **55**

Maylin Romero, Yovani Marrero-Ponce, Hortensia Rodríguez, Guillermin Agüero-Chapin, Agostinho Antunes and Longendri Aguilera-Mendoza et al.
A Novel Network Science and Similarity-Searching-Based Approach for Discovering Potential Tumor-Homing Peptides from Antimicrobials
Reprinted from: *Antibiotics* **2022**, *11*, 401, doi:10.3390/antibiotics11030401 . . . . **75**

Diana Lin, Darcy Sutherland, Sambina Islam Aninta, Nathan Louie, Ka Ming Nip and Chenkai Li et al.
Mining Amphibian and Insect Transcriptomes for Antimicrobial Peptide Sequences with rAMPage
Reprinted from: *Antibiotics* **2022**, *11*, 952, doi:10.3390/antibiotics11070952 . . . . **97**

Felix L. Santana, Karel Estrada, Morgan A. Alford, Bing C. Wu, Melanie Dostert and Lucas Pedraz et al.
Novel Alligator Cathelicidin As-CATH8 Demonstrates Anti-Infective Activity against Clinically Relevant and Crocodylian Bacterial Pathogens
Reprinted from: *Antibiotics* **2022**, *11*, 1603, doi:10.3390/antibiotics11111603 . . . . **115**

Neelma Ashraf, Sana Zafar, Roman Makitrynskyy, Andreas Bechthold, Dieter Spiteller and Lijiang Song et al.
Revealing Genome-Based Biosynthetic Potential of *Streptomyces* sp. BR123 Isolated from Sunflower Rhizosphere with Broad Spectrum Antimicrobial Activity
Reprinted from: *Antibiotics* **2022**, *11*, 1057, doi:10.3390/antibiotics11081057 . . . . **137**

Norma Rivera-Fernández, Jhony Anacleto-Santos, Brenda Casarrubias-Tabarez, Teresa de Jesús López-Pérez, Marcela Rojas-Lemus and Nelly López-Valdez et al.
Bioactive Peptides against Human Apicomplexan Parasites
Reprinted from: *Antibiotics* **2022**, *11*, 1658, doi:10.3390/antibiotics11111658 . . . . **149**

Davor Juretić
Designed Multifunctional Peptides for Intracellular Targets
Reprinted from: *Antibiotics* **2022**, *11*, 1196, doi:10.3390/antibiotics11091196 . . . . **169**

Tawanny K. B. Aguiar, Nilton A. S. Neto, Romério R. S. Silva, Cleverson D. T. Freitas, Felipe P. Mesquita and Luciana M. R. Alencar et al.
Behind the Curtain: In Silico and In Vitro Experiments Brought to Light New Insights into the Anticryptococcal Action of Synthetic Peptides
Reprinted from: *Antibiotics* **2023**, *12*, 153, doi:10.3390/antibiotics12010153 . . . . **229**

About the Editors

Agostinho Antunes

Prof. Agostinho Antunes is the Head of Evolutionary Genomics and Bioinformatics in the CIIMAR, Interdisciplinary Centre of Marine and Environmental Research, University of Porto, and he is a Professor at the Department of Biology at the University of Porto, Portugal. His major research interests include genomics and blue biotechnology of natural resources, from microorganisms to animals, and their environmental interactions, disease, and health.

Guillermin Agüero-Chapin

He is an auxiliary researcher (PhD) at CIIMAR, Centro Interdisciplinar de Investigação Marinha e Ambiental, Universidade do Porto (UP), Portugal. He majored in Pharmaceutical Sciences (1998) at the Universidad Central de Las Villas (UCLV), Cuba, and holds a Master's degree in biochemistry (2009) from the Medical School "Dr. Zerafin de Zarate Ruiz", Cuba. PhD in biology awarded with honors by UP, Portugal (2009). His overall research expertise has been related to genetic engineering applied to plant and microbial biotechnology and, later, in the chemo-bio-informatics field applied to drug discovery. He also worked in algorithm development to address functional and comparative genomics, molecular evolution, and peptide drug search and design. Recently, he has been dedicated to applying complex networks for visualizing and analyzing functional classes of antimicrobial peptides (AMPs) and for multi-reference similarity-based searches. The research in these areas, along with internal and external collaborators, has allowed him to register 43 publications in the WoS (17 in the last 5 years), 5 book chapters, and 1 book with recognized publishers. In the last 5 years, he has participated in 4 projects funded by the Foundation for Science and Technology (FCT) of Portugal, acting as co-PI and PI in two of them. He has been a member of academic boards in Portugal (Master, 2021), Spain, and Italy (PhD, 2022–2023), as well as a member of the Research Topic and Reviewer Boards in Marine Drugs and Antibiotics Journals (2020–2022). He is also a reviewer of prestigious journals and an evaluator of national projects in Ecuador and Chile. His current research interest is in the field of discovery and design of peptide drugs from AMPs, assisted by classical and emerging computational tools from marine sources.

Yovani Marrero-Ponce

He is a full professor and principal researcher at the University of San Francisco de Quito, leading the "Grupo de Medicina Molecular y Traslacional (MeM&T)". He holds a degree in pharmaceutical sciences and a Master's degree in biochemistry, followed by a PhD in chemistry from Havana University, Cuba. He has expertise in chemo-bio-med-informatics, medicinal chemistry, pharmacogenomics, computational biology, mathematical chemistry, and peptide drug design. He has developed 11 multiplatform software products and published over 170 papers in ISI journals (more than 120 as first, last, or corresponding author, h-index = 47). He has directed numerous graduate and undergraduate theses, participated in 14 R&D projects, and won several prestigious awards, such as the Cuban Academy of Sciences Award, the TWAS Award, and the Royal Spanish Academy of Pharmacy Award. Prof. Marrero-Ponce has also been included in the list of the top 2% of world researchers in all 22 fields of science.

Preface to "Computational Approaches in Discovery & Design of Antimicrobial Peptides"

Antimicrobial resistance continues to be a pressing concern in the field of medicine, especially during the COVID-19 pandemic, where microbial infections were frequently observed as side-complications. To combat antibiotic-resistant pathogens, there has been a renewed interest in the use of antimicrobial peptides (AMPs). The naturally occurring AMPs have shown great promise in the search for new antibiotics. To this end, various computational approaches have been developed to assist in the search for and design of new AMPs. These computational methods range from classical homology-based and machine-learning prediction algorithms to complex similarity networks and evolutionary algorithms that use models of sequence evolution. Moreover, the improvement of high-throughput screening techniques in the discovery of AMPs from biological samples has also led to the evolution of computational approaches that aid in this biodiscovery process. This reprint is aimed at disclosing original research and review papers on in silico approaches used for the rational discovery and design of AMPs, addressed to the problem of antimicrobial resistance. The reprinted content will serve as a reference for researchers dedicated to peptide drug development.

Agostinho Antunes, Guillermin Agüero-Chapin, and Yovani Marrero-Ponce
Editors

antibiotics

MDPI

Editorial

A 2022 Update on Computational Approaches to the Discovery and Design of Antimicrobial Peptides

Guillermin Agüero-Chapin [1,2,*], Agostinho Antunes [1,2] and Yovani Marrero-Ponce [3,4,*]

1 CIIMAR/CIMAR, Interdisciplinary Centre of Marine and Environmental Research, University of Porto, 4450-208 Porto, Portugal
2 Department of Biology, Faculty of Sciences, University of Porto, 4169-007 Porto, Portugal
3 Universidad San Francisco de Quito (USFQ), Grupo de Medicina Molecular y Traslacional (MeM&T), Colegio de Ciencias de la Salud (COCSA), Escuela de Medicina, Edificio de Especialidades Médicas, Diego de Robles y vía Interoceánica, Quito 170157, Pichincha, Ecuador
4 Departamento de Ciencias de la Computación, Centro de Investigación Científica y de Educación Superior de Ensenada (CICESE), Ensenada 22860, Baja California, Mexico
* Correspondence: gchapin@ciimar.up.pt (G.A.-C.); ymarrero@usfq.edu.ec (Y.M.-P.)

The antimicrobial resistance process has been accelerated by the over-prescription and misuse of antibiotics. The World Health Organization (WHO) has listed it as one of the top 10 global public health threats. This worrisome situation has encouraged the search for new classes of antimicrobial agents, leveraging the ability of antimicrobial peptides (AMPs) to overcome resistance, mainly due to their versatile mode of action and multifunctionalities. However, the discovery of promising AMPs with relevant biological activities is a real challenge, considering the great structural diversity of the AMP class and their under-representation in terms of non-bioactive peptides. Consequently, several databases and computational approaches have been developed for over two decades to assist in the long development process of peptide-based drugs.

This Special Issue, entitled "*Computational Approaches to the Discovery & Design of Antimicrobial Peptides*," is mainly dedicated to state-of-the-art in silico approaches applied to the discovery and design of AMPs for therapeutic purposes. In this sense, Agüero-Chapin et al. published a comprehensive review article on emerging in silico approaches to the search for/design of bioactive peptides, from new machine learning (ML) algorithms to other non-conventional methodologies, such as complex networks and algorithms simulating peptide sequence evolution. New considerations incorporated into the biodiscovery workflow for unravelling AMPs from omics data were also analyzed [1].

Aligning with the previously mentioned review, Ruiz-Blanco et al. developed a new machine learning (ML)-based classifier for the detection of antibacterial peptides (ABPs) and their putative targets, including multi-drug-resistant (MDR) bacterial strains. The ML model was implemented in a web server called "ABP-Finder", which is one of the most state-of-the-art ABP predictors, with a proven high precision when detecting a promising peptide hit against *P. aeruginosa* during the screening of large databases such as the human urine peptidome [2]. The revision also comprised non-conventional methodologies applied to the field of AMPs. For example, García-Hernández et al. repurposed ROSE (Random Model of Sequence Evolution), an algorithm simulating sequence evolution, to generate diversity-oriented libraries of peptides as one of the steps for the de novo design/optimization of antibacterial peptides (ABPs) by inhibiting the E. coli FoF1-ATP synthase [3].

On the other hand, Marrero-Ponce et al. applied network science to study the chemical space of tumor-homing peptides (THPs) by using alignment-free similarity networks and centrality measures to identify the most relevant and non-redundant THPs within the network. Such THPs, representing the original TH chemical space, were considered as references for multi-query similarity searches that apply a group fusion (MAX-SIM rule) model. The resulting multi-query similarity searching models outperformed state-of-the-art

Citation: Agüero-Chapin, G.; Antunes, A.; Marrero-Ponce, Y. A 2022 Update on Computational Approaches to the Discovery and Design of Antimicrobial Peptides. *Antibiotics* **2023**, *12*, 1011. https://doi.org/10.3390/antibiotics12061011

Received: 16 May 2023
Accepted: 30 May 2023
Published: 5 June 2023

Copyright: © 2023 by the authors. Licensee MDPI, Basel, Switzerland. This article is an open access article distributed under the terms and conditions of the Creative Commons Attribution (CC BY) license (https://creativecommons.org/licenses/by/4.0/).

predictors in the detection of THPs in benchmark datasets. This approach also served to search for THP leads and to discover TH motifs [4].

Related to the previously discussed on the new considerations and tools incorporated into the workflow for AMP biodiscovery [1], Birol et al. developed rAMPage, a scalable bioinformatics tool for identifying AMP sequences from RNA sequencing (RNA-seq) datasets. rAMPage was extensively evaluated on publicly available RNA-seq datasets from amphibian and insect species. It identified 1137 putative AMPs, of which 1024 were considered novel by homology criteria. From these, 21 peptides were tested for antimicrobial susceptibility against two bacteria species, *E. coli* and *S. aureus*, and 7 showed high activity. Thus, rAMPage can be integrated into the workflow for AMP biodiscovery to accelerate the process of antimicrobial drug development [5].

Although transcriptomic and proteomic analyses can streamline the biodiscovery workflow of AMPs by focusing on gene coding and protein expression, such high-throughput screening can be performed at the genomic level to unravel both encoded and cryptic AMPs. Hancock et al. proposed profile hidden Markov models to screen the genomes of four crocodilian species for identifying encoded cathelicidin sequences. Cathelicidins are one of the largest family of host defense peptides, showing a broad-spectrum activity against planktonic bacteria and some biofilm, as well as other beneficial features such as anti-inflammatory properties. Eighteen novel cathelicidin sequences were identified and subsequently synthetized and evaluated in vitro against planktonic and biofilm bacteria. Among the cathelicidins which displayed a broad-spectrum antimicrobial and antibiofilm activity against a range of antibiotic-resistant bacteria, As-CATH8 was highlighted because of its similar profile to the last-resort antibiotics vancomycin and polymyxin B [6]. An alternative method of searching for AMPs at the genomic level involves the in silico detection of corresponding biosynthetic gene clusters (BGCs). Ashraf et al. sequenced the genome of the Streptomyces sp. isolate BR123 and used the online antiSMASH (antibiotics & Secondary Metabolite Analysis Shell) platform to analyze the resulting assembled regions. Multiple BGCs were detected that were involved in the production of antimicrobial, antiparasitic, and anticancer compounds [7].

Two additional review papers were published in this Special Issue. Rivera-Fernández et al. examined the experimental effects of various bioactive peptides on Apicomplexan parasites, which are responsible for a range of dangerous diseases, such as toxoplasmosis, cryptosporidiosis, and malaria. They also discussed some biological and metabolomic generalities of the parasites to explain the mechanisms of action of the peptides on the Apicomplexan targets [8]. The other review paper was written by Prof. Juretić, which emphasizes the importance of designing multi-functional peptides that can reach intracellular targets in order to develop more effective peptide drugs. The review ranked known and novel peptides based on their predicted low toxicity to mammalian cells and broad-spectrum activity. The 20 most promising candidates that exhibited optimized cell-penetrating, antimicrobial, anticancer, anti-viral, antifungal, and anti-inflammatory activities were identified. These peptides also have the ability to form an amphipathic structure upon contact with membranes or nucleic acids [9].

Prof. Juretić's work also mentioned the urgent need to develop antifungal compounds that target intracellular molecules as a strategy to combat multidrug-resistant (MDR) pathogens such as *Cryptococcus neoformans*, which pose a threat to immunocompromised patients. Consequently, the study by Souza et al. designed and tested anticryptococcal AMPs and provided further information on their mechanism of action against *C. neoformans* using computational and experimental analyses [10].

Author Contributions: All authors wrote and reviewed the manuscript. All authors have read and agreed to the published version of the manuscript.

Funding: This work was financially supported by national funds through FCT—Foundation for Science and Technology of Portugal within the scope of UIDB/04423/2020 and UIDP/04423/2020 and by the USFQ Collaboration Grant (Project ID16911).

Conflicts of Interest: The authors declare no conflict of interest.

References

1. Aguero-Chapin, G.; Galpert-Canizares, D.; Dominguez-Perez, D.; Marrero-Ponce, Y.; Perez-Machado, G.; Teijeira, M.; Antunes, A. Emerging Computational Approaches for Antimicrobial Peptide Discovery. *Antibiotics* **2022**, *11*, 936. [CrossRef] [PubMed]
2. Ruiz-Blanco, Y.B.; Aguero-Chapin, G.; Romero-Molina, S.; Antunes, A.; Olari, L.R.; Spellerberg, B.; Munch, J.; Sanchez-Garcia, E. ABP-Finder: A Tool to Identify Antibacterial Peptides and the Gram-Staining Type of Targeted Bacteria. *Antibiotics* **2022**, *11*, 1708. [CrossRef] [PubMed]
3. Avila-Barrientos, L.P.; Cofas-Vargas, L.F.; Aguero-Chapin, G.; Hernandez-Garcia, E.; Ruiz-Carmona, S.; Valdez-Cruz, N.A.; Trujillo-Roldan, M.; Weber, J.; Ruiz-Blanco, Y.B.; Barril, X.; et al. Computational Design of Inhibitors Targeting the Catalytic beta Subunit of Escherichia coli F(O)F(1)-ATP Synthase. *Antibiotics* **2022**, *11*, 557. [CrossRef] [PubMed]
4. Romero, M.; Marrero-Ponce, Y.; Rodriguez, H.; Aguero-Chapin, G.; Antunes, A.; Aguilera-Mendoza, L.; Martinez-Rios, F. A Novel Network Science and Similarity-Searching-Based Approach for Discovering Potential Tumor-Homing Peptides from Antimicrobials. *Antibiotics* **2022**, *11*, 401. [CrossRef] [PubMed]
5. Lin, D.; Sutherland, D.; Aninta, S.I.; Louie, N.; Nip, K.M.; Li, C.; Yanai, A.; Coombe, L.; Warren, R.L.; Helbing, C.C.; et al. Mining Amphibian and Insect Transcriptomes for Antimicrobial Peptide Sequences with rAMPage. *Antibiotics* **2022**, *11*, 952. [CrossRef] [PubMed]
6. Santana, F.L.; Estrada, K.; Alford, M.A.; Wu, B.C.; Dostert, M.; Pedraz, L.; Akhoundsadegh, N.; Kalsi, P.; Haney, E.F.; Straus, S.K.; et al. Novel Alligator Cathelicidin As-CATH8 Demonstrates Anti-Infective Activity against Clinically Relevant and Crocodylian Bacterial Pathogens. *Antibiotics* **2022**, *11*, 1603. [CrossRef] [PubMed]
7. Ashraf, N.; Zafar, S.; Makitrynskyy, R.; Bechthold, A.; Spiteller, D.; Song, L.; Anwar, M.A.; Luzhetskyy, A.; Khan, A.N.; Akhtar, K.; et al. Revealing Genome-Based Biosynthetic Potential of Streptomyces sp. BR123 Isolated from Sunflower Rhizosphere with Broad Spectrum Antimicrobial Activity. *Antibiotics* **2022**, *11*, 1057. [CrossRef] [PubMed]
8. Rivera-Fernandez, N.; Anacleto-Santos, J.; Casarrubias-Tabarez, B.; Lopez-Perez, T.J.; Rojas-Lemus, M.; Lopez-Valdez, N.; Fortoul, T.I. Bioactive Peptides against Human Apicomplexan Parasites. *Antibiotics* **2022**, *11*, 1658. [CrossRef] [PubMed]
9. Juretic, D. Designed Multifunctional Peptides for Intracellular Targets. *Antibiotics* **2022**, *11*, 1196. [CrossRef] [PubMed]
10. Aguiar, T.K.B.; Neto, N.A.S.; Silva, R.R.S.; Freitas, C.D.T.; Mesquita, F.P.; Alencar, L.M.R.; Santos-Oliveira, R.; Goldman, G.H.; Souza, P.F.N. Behind the Curtain: In Silico and In Vitro Experiments Brought to Light New Insights into the Anticryptococcal Action of Synthetic Peptides. *Antibiotics* **2023**, *12*, 153. [CrossRef] [PubMed]

Disclaimer/Publisher's Note: The statements, opinions and data contained in all publications are solely those of the individual author(s) and contributor(s) and not of MDPI and/or the editor(s). MDPI and/or the editor(s) disclaim responsibility for any injury to people or property resulting from any ideas, methods, instructions or products referred to in the content.

antibiotics

MDPI

Review

Emerging Computational Approaches for Antimicrobial Peptide Discovery

Guillermin Agüero-Chapin [1,2,*], Deborah Galpert-Cañizares [3], Dany Domínguez-Pérez [1,4], Yovani Marrero-Ponce [5], Gisselle Pérez-Machado [6], Marta Teijeira [7,8] and Agostinho Antunes [1,2,*]

1 CIIMAR—Centro Interdisciplinar de Investigação Marinha e Ambiental, Universidade do Porto, Terminal de Cruzeiros do Porto de Leixões, Av. General Norton de Matos, s/n, 4450-208 Porto, Portugal; dany.perez@ciimar.up.pt
2 Departamento de Biologia, Faculdade de Ciências, Universidade do Porto, Rua do Campo Alegre, 4169-007 Porto, Portugal
3 Departamento de Ciencia de la Computación, Universidad Central Marta Abreu de Las Villas (UCLV), Santa Clara 54830, Cuba; deborah@uclv.edu.cu
4 Proquinorte, Unipessoal, Lda, Avenida 5 de Outubro, 124, 7° Piso, Avenidas Novas, 1050-061 Lisboa, Portugal
5 Universidad San Francisco de Quito (USFQ), Grupo de Medicina Molecular y Translacional (MeM&T), Colegio de Ciencias de la Salud (COCSA), Escuela de Medicina, Edificio de Especialidades Médicas and Instituto de Simulación Computacional (ISC-USFQ), Diego de Robles y vía Interoceánica, Quito 170157, Ecuador; ymarrero@usfq.edu.ec
6 EpiDisease S.L—Spin-Off of Centro de Investigación Biomédica en Red de Enfermedades Raras (CIBERER), 46980 Valencia, Spain; giselle.perez@epidisease.com
7 Departamento de Química Orgánica, Facultade de Química, Universidade de Vigo, 36310 Vigo, Spain; qomaca@uvigo.es
8 Instituto de Investigación Sanitaria Galicia Sur, Hospital Álvaro Cunqueiro, 36213 Vigo, Spain
* Correspondence: gchapin@ciimar.up.pt (G.A.-C.); aantunes@ciimar.up.pt (A.A.); Tel.: +351-22-340-1813 (G.A.-C. & A.A.)

Citation: Agüero-Chapin, G.; Galpert-Cañizares, D.; Domínguez-Pérez, D.; Marrero-Ponce, Y.; Pérez-Machado, G.; Teijeira, M.; Antunes, A. Emerging Computational Approaches for Antimicrobial Peptide Discovery. *Antibiotics* **2022**, *11*, 936. https://doi.org/10.3390/antibiotics11070936

Academic Editor: Mire Zloh

Received: 14 June 2022
Accepted: 8 July 2022
Published: 13 July 2022

Publisher's Note: MDPI stays neutral with regard to jurisdictional claims in published maps and institutional affiliations.

Copyright: © 2022 by the authors. Licensee MDPI, Basel, Switzerland. This article is an open access article distributed under the terms and conditions of the Creative Commons Attribution (CC BY) license (https://creativecommons.org/licenses/by/4.0/).

Abstract: In the last two decades many reports have addressed the application of artificial intelligence (AI) in the search and design of antimicrobial peptides (AMPs). AI has been represented by machine learning (ML) algorithms that use sequence-based features for the discovery of new peptidic scaffolds with promising biological activity. From AI perspective, evolutionary algorithms have been also applied to the rational generation of peptide libraries aimed at the optimization/design of AMPs. However, the literature has scarcely dedicated to other emerging non-conventional in silico approaches for the search/design of such bioactive peptides. Thus, the first motivation here is to bring up some non-standard peptide features that have been used to build classical ML predictive models. Secondly, it is valuable to highlight emerging ML algorithms and alternative computational tools to predict/design AMPs as well as to explore their chemical space. Another point worthy of mention is the recent application of evolutionary algorithms that actually simulate sequence evolution to both the generation of diversity-oriented peptide libraries and the optimization of hit peptides. Last but not least, included here some new considerations in proteogenomic analyses currently incorporated into the computational workflow for unravelling AMPs in natural sources.

Keywords: artificial intelligence; machine learning; AMPs; evolutionary algorithms; molecular descriptors; complex networks; proteogenomics

1. Introduction

The rise of resistance to antimicrobial agents evidenced in the last decades have caused excess healthcare costs worldwide [1]. The microbial natural resistance process, moved by evolutionary events, has been accelerated by the over-prescription and misuse of antibiotics [2]. This worrying situation has encouraged the search of new antibiotics from antimicrobial peptides (AMPs) with the ability to overcome resistance, mainly given by their versatile mode of action [3].Indeed, AMPs are not only considered for the development of antibiotics to treat multi-resistant bacterial strains [4,5], but also they are promising for the developing of antitumoral [6], antiviral [7], antifungal agents [8] and so on.

The discovery of peptides with relevant biological activities is a real challenge considering the great diversity of AMPs in terms of origin, structure, mode of action, activity, and, on the other hand by considering the overabundance of natural-occurring non-bioactive peptides [8]. Thus, several AMP databases with associated machine learning (ML)-based classifiers have been developed for over one decade, in order to assist wet-lab researchers in the long development process of peptide-based drugs [9]. AMP databases such as DAMPD [10], CAMPR3 [11], LAMP [12], DRAMP [13], ADAM [14], DBAASP [15] have incorporated ML predictors trained with alignment-free (AF) protein features such as amino acid (aa) and pseudo-aa composition, structural features, word frequency-based features, physicochemical aa properties with influence on the AMP activity, and some others [16,17] (Table 1). Figure 1 illustrates how databases and ML algorithms have been integrated to assist the discovery/design of AMPs for the developing of peptide drugs.

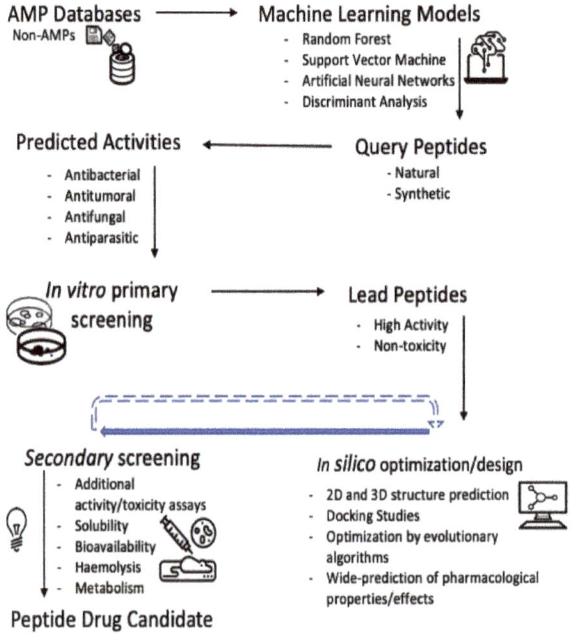

Figure 1. Workflow illustrating peptide drug discovery. The strategy involves the screening of query peptides from either natural or synthetic sources by applying ML models trained with the information stored in AMP databases. ML algorithms also assist the optimization/design step of lead peptides by means of a fitness/selection criterion [18,19].

The prediction tools built up with Support Vector Machine (SVM) and Random Forest (RF) based classifiers have been widely applied, but hardly considered the natural imbalance between the AMPs and non-AMPs [18]. On the other hand, emerging ML techniques such as Deep-Learning Neural Networks [18–21] and those based on the Rough Set Theory [22,23] have been applied to improve certain classification pitfalls like the quality in the learning phase and the classification boundaries between AMPs and non-AMPs, respectively. Although most of the classical predictive tools have focused on if a query peptide is an AMP or not, without targeting a specific biological activity among the reported for the AMPs [24], the current tendency is to address a hierarchical multi-level classification by downstream considering the specific biological activities of the AMPs as labels e.g., the antibacterial, antifungal, antiviral and antitumoral among others.

The most popular hierarchical multi-label classifiers, also listed in Table 1, are the following: (i) the iAMP-2L, a two-level classifier trained with Chou's pseudo amino acid composition (PseACC) [25], aimed at identifying AMPs and their five functional types [26], (ii) the iAMPpred predictor that combines compositional, physicochemical, and structural features into Chou's general PseACC for training a SVM multi-classifier [16], (iii) the MLAMP, a RF-based classifier built up with a non-classical PseACC sequence formulation incorporating a Grey Model that firstly discriminates AMP from non-AMPs, and then subclassify their biological activities into antibacterial, anti-cancer, antifungal, antiviral, and anti-HIV [27], (iv) the Antimicrobial Activity Predictor (AMAP) [28], a hierarchical multi-label classifier targeting 14 biological activities that is built up with SVM and XGboost tree [29] algorithms trained with amino acid composition (ACC) features, (v) the AMPfun webserver containing RF-based models that firstly classify AMPs and non-AMPs and afterwards address the prediction of AMPs functional activities including their possible target types [30], and more recently, the (vi) AMPDiscover [31] and the (vii) ABPFinder webservers (https://protdcal.zmb.uni-due.de/ABP-Finder/index.php; accessed on 7 March 2022) containing hierarchical RF-based classifiers built up with protein descriptors from the ProtDCal software [32] to firstly detect AMPs and antibacterial peptides (ABPs), respectively. While the AMPDiscover uses several downstream RF models to predict AMPs specific functions (antibacterial, antifungal, antiparasitic and antiviral), the ABP-Finder sub-classifies ABPs according to the Gram staining type of the potential targets (Gram-positive, Gram-negative bacteria, or broad-spectrum peptides with expected activity against both types of bacteria) by using a multi-classifier. The high success classification rates of both tools stems from considering the StarPep database [33] which is probably the most comprehensive curated repository of AMPs so far, and from performing an applicability domain (AD) analysis for the proposed ML models [31]. Both, AMPDiscover and ABP-Finder defined ADs for their corresponding RF-based models, however, AMPDiscover perform a rigours AD analysis at applying a consensus-based decision from five different approaches [31].

Despite the great number of reported ML-based tools for AMPs prediction, only few ones have considered the lack of balance among either the specific activities of AMPs or among their putative targets, as well as the AD of their corresponding models. The imbalance among AMPs and non-AMPs as well as the existing one among AMP activities was addressed by applying the synthetic minority over-sampling technique (SMOTE) during the IAMPE and MLAMP building [27,34] while the ABP-Finder addressed the imbalance among the bacterial target types of the ABPs (Gram+, Gram- and Gram+/- bacteria) by training a RF multi-classifier with a cost matrix weighting the different types of misclassified cases according to the imbalance ratio between the two classes (https://protdcal.zmb.uni-due.de/ABP-Finder/index.php; accessed on 7 March 2022).

On the other side, artificial intelligence (AI)-derived approaches like evolutionary algorithms have been applied to optimize lead candidates retrieved from the high-throughput screening in drug discovery. Evolutionary algorithms are inspired on several evolutionary events occurring in nature; they generally start with a small population of peptides identified as putative leads due to its relevant biological activities. The optimization is carried out by the generation of offspring peptides from these initial peptides by applying several operators simulating natural evolutionary process like cross-over and mutation operators, a parent and survival selection algorithms [40,41]. A parent selection algorithm is firstly applied on the initial peptide population to select the best parent peptides for the offspring generation. The survival aims at selecting a subset of good individuals (new population) from the generated offspring peptides. Then, the new peptide population will be iteratively subjected to the parent selection algorithm, evolutionary operators and the survival selection until finding an offspring peptide meeting a termination condition (selection criteria in Figure 2). The selection criteria can be represented by a fitness function which can be a ML model scoring peptide bioactivity. This selection process may be accompanied to experimental evaluations against the desired biological activities [42] (Figure 2).

Table 1. Summary of the most relevant ML approaches, from the classical to the emerging ones, for assisting the discovery of bioactive peptides from AMPs.

Classical AMP Prediction Tools				
Integrated to Database	**ML Algorithm**	**Peptide features**	**Implementation**	**Ref.**
$CAMP_{R3}$	RF, SVM, ANN, DA	AAC, net charge, hydrophobicity	http://www.camp3.bicnirrh.res.in/prediction.php	[11]
DRAMP 3.0	ANN, SVM, RF	Secondary structure features	http://shicrazy.pythonanywhere.com/	[13]
ADAM	SVM	AAC	http://bioinformatics.cs.ntou.edu.tw/adam/tool.html	[14]
DBAASPv3.0	Threshold value-based discrimination	Physicochemical properties acconuting for the interaction with membrane	https://dbaasp.org/tools?page=general-prediction	[15]
Independent Tools				
ClasssAMP *	RF, SVM	Sequence-based features	http://www.bicnirrh.res.in/classamp/predict.php	[35]
iAMPpred *	SVM	compositional, physicochemical, and structural features	http://cabgrid.res.in:8080/amppred/server.php	[16]
iAMP-2L **	k-NN	PseAAC	http://www.jci-bioinfo.cn/iAMP-2L	[25]
AmPEP	RF	Sequence-based features	https://cbbio.online/software/AmPEP/	[36]
amPEPpy	RF	Global protein sequence descriptors	https://github.com/tlawrence3/amPEPpy	[37]
AMPScannerv1 **	RF	Physicochemical features	https://www.dveltri.com/ascan/v1/index.html	[38]
AMPfun **	RF	AAC-based features, physicochemical features and word frequency-based features	http://fdblab.csie.ncu.edu.tw/AMPfun/index.html	[30]
AMAP **	SVM and XGboost tree	AAC-based features	http://amap.pythonanywhere.com/	[28]
Emerging AMP prediction tools				
MLAMP **	RF	Non-classical PSeAAC	http://www.jci-bioinfo.cn/MLAMP	[27]
IAMPE	RF, k-NN, SVM, XGboost	NMR-based features	http://cbb1.ut.ac.ir/AMPClassifier/Index	[34]
AMPDiscover **	RF/DNN	Non-classical protein features (ProtDCal)	https://biocom-ampdiscover.cicese.mx/	[31,39]
ABP-Finder **	RF	Non-classical protein features (ProtDCal)	https://protdcal.zmb.uni-due.de/ABP-Finder/index.php	[Unpub]
AMPScannerv2	DNN	AA alphabet	https://www.dveltri.com/ascan/v2/ascan.html	[19]
ACP-DL	DNN	Binary profile feature and K-mer sparce matrix	https://github.com/haichengyi/ACP-DL (Standalone)	[20]
xDeep-AcPEP *	DNN	Physicochemical, biochemical, evolutionary and positional	https://app.cbbio.online/acpep/home	[21]

Methods listed in Table 1 are currently active (Accessed on 7 March 2022) * Multi-label classifiers allowing the prediction of specific biological activities (antibacterial, antifungal, antiviral, antitumoral and others) from AMPs ** Hierarchical multi-label classifiers addressing firstly AMPs detection and in the second level their specific biological activities. ACC: amino acid composition, ANN: artificial neural networks, DA: discriminant analysis, DNN: deep neural networks, k-NN: k- nearest neighbours, NMR: nuclear magnetic resonance, PseAAC: pseudo amino acid composition, RF: random forest, SVM: support vector machine.

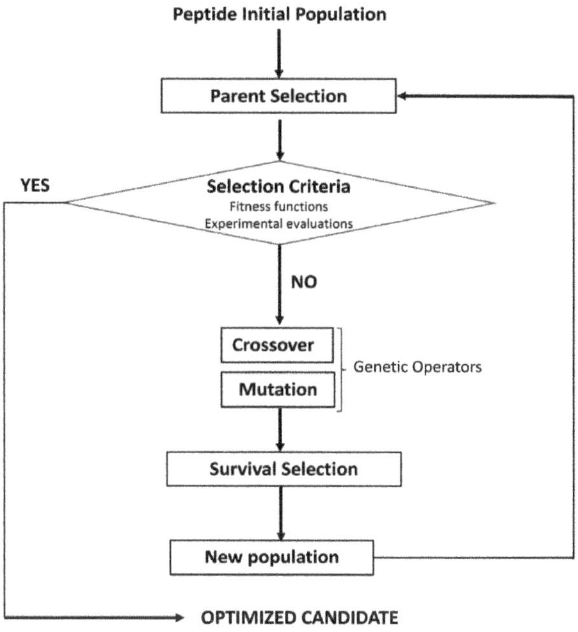

Figure 2. Workflow illustrating the main steps of evolutionary and genetic algorithms. Both approaches are very similar, in fact the use of evolutionary and genetic terms have been interchangeable. Genetic algorithms particularly use a fixed-length binary array to represent peptides as genes into a chromosome-like structure.

The genetic algorithm is the most popular technique among the evolutionary approaches where the peptides with promising biological properties (initial solution) are encoded as binary strings into chromosome-like structures, called genotypes. The optimization process is performed by evolving each chromosome toward optimized solutions by iteratively applying genetic recombination (crossover) operators and survival fitness functions that is somehow similar to the parent selection mechanism [40,42–44]. Optimized solutions in the case of peptides consist in generating structural entities with optimized biological properties e.g., peptides showing a trade-off among their pharmaceutical potency, solubility, haemolytic and toxicity properties [42] (Figure 2).

Despite AI-derived approaches have been largely applied to the rational search and design of bioactive peptides; most of them are represented by classical ML and evolutionary algorithms that frequently also use canonical sequence-based features as peptide descriptors and therefore have been documented in literature [18,45,46]. However, there is a growing number of emerging computational approaches effectively applied to the search/design of bioactive peptides that are comprehensively revisited here (Table 1).

Most of the non-standard approaches are represented by classical ML algorithms which are either trained with non-conventional peptide features [31] or combined with sequence alignment methods [47]. In addition to the singularity of these predictors; preprocessing steps managing the natural imbalance between bioactive and inactive peptides have been hardly applied to the AMPs predictions [27,34] as well as no big data solutions have been implemented yet to address scalability problems. As mentioned before, other less-known ML algorithms in the field of protein/peptide science like those based on the Rough Sets Theory (RST) are being currently intended for peptide classification/design [22,48]. Moreover, a non-conventional methodology that analyses the known chemical space of bioactive peptides by similarity networks was developed to identify the most relevant ones for each specific biological activity [33]. Such representative peptides were recently used in multi-query similarity searches against the StarPep database to repurpose AMPs for specific activities such as antiparasitic and tumour homing [49,50].

By other side, evolutionary algorithms that simulate sequence evolution have been recently applied to design/optimize peptides having a pharmaceutical activity [51,52]. Last but not least, computational tools used in proteogenomic analyses are being modified for uncovering cryptic peptides with biological activities in natural sources [53,54]. From now on we go deeper into these emerging approaches in peptide search and design

2. Non-Classical Peptide Features for Bioactivity Prediction

2.1. Peptide Features Inspired in Molecular Descriptors Used in Cheminformatics

There is a set of chemoinformatics-derived peptide features considered as "non-conventional" because of its in-house development; however, have been successfully applied in the recognition of bioactive peptides by ML-based classifiers [31,55–58]. The definition of these peptide/protein features is generally inspired on the mathematical formalisms applied to the calculation of molecular descriptors for small organic molecules [59,60], which have been traditionally used to Quantitative-Structure-Activity Relationship (QSAR) studies for drug design/search. Most of them are classified as topological descriptors since they consider the connectivity either between adjacent amino acids (aas) or between aa groups by using both algebraic and statistic invariants [32,61,62].

Those based on algebraic forms express protein/peptide structural topology through the definition of connectivity or adjacency matrices. The elements of these matrices (n_{ij} or e_{ij}) reflect topological relationships between the aas or aa groups, they are equal to 1 if i and j are adjacent otherwise take the value of 0. Topological indices (TIs) are estimated by applying several algorithms on the connectivity/adjacency matrix. The most common algorithms for the TIs calculation involve the powers of the topological matrix, the multiplication of a property vector by the topological matrix and the multiplication of vector-matrix-vector (Figure 3). Many of the most popular TIs within the cheminformatic have been defined by these algebraic formalisms, such as the Winner index (W) [63], the Randić invariant (χ) [64], Broto–Moreau autocorrelation (ATSd) [65], the Balaban index (J) [66], and the spectral moments introduced by Estrada [59]. Thus, many of them were reformulated to describe the spatial topology of aa sequences at different structural levels, e.g., linear sequences (1D), pseudo-secondary structure (2D) and the 3D-dimensional space [61,62] (Figure 3).

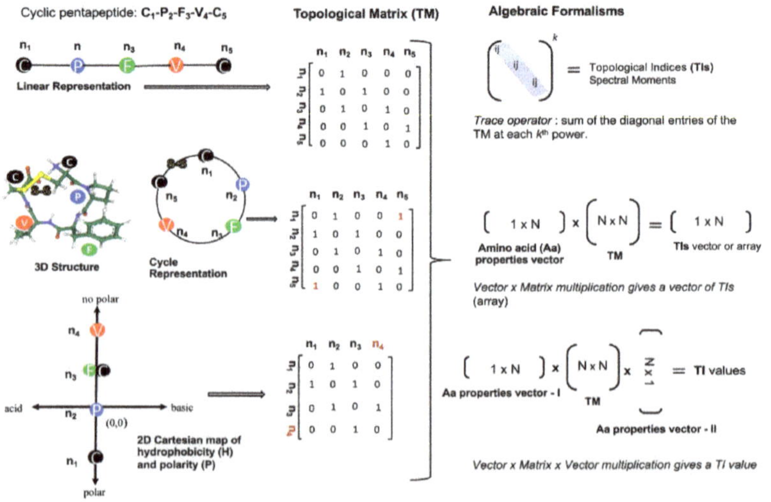

Figure 3. Workflow for the calculation of topological indices from several representation types of the cyclopentapeptide [CPFVC] with promising antiviral activity against the hantavirus cardiopulmonary

syndrome [67]. Each peptide representation defines a singular topological matrix (TM) encoding structural features at different degrees. In addition to the several ways to represent the topology of a peptide (linear, circular, 2D-Cartesian), several algebraic formalisms/operators can be applied on the TM to calculate different topological indices (TIs) types. n represents the nodes in the peptidic representations (linear, circular, and Cartesian) as well as in their corresponding TMs, which may contain some elements in red font (e.g., n_4 and 1) to highlight differences in structural encoding from the cyclopentapeptide. N indicates the number of rows and columns of matrices involved in TI calculation.

On the other hand, there is another set of topological descriptors that also comes from the chemoinformatic field that have been applied to the identification and design of AMPs [31,52,56,58]. They are not formulated by using algebraic forms but rather they rely on descriptive statistics as invariant operators on the aa properties either along the sequence or the 3D protein structure. In this case, the 1D or 3D topology is encoded by the application of classic cheminformatics algorithms that consider the neighborhood such as autocorrelation [65], Kier-Hall's electro-topological state [68], Ivanshiuc-Balaban [69], and Gravitational-like operators [70].

2.1.1. Topological Indices from Algebraic Forms

Among the TIs defined for small molecules, the spectral moments formalism probably is one of the most extended to characterize proteins and peptides structures [61,62,71,72]. The spectral moments may encode peptide structures through the definition of their corresponding topological matrixes and the application of the trace operator on the k-th power of such matrixes (Figure 3).

A sort of stochastic spectral moments applied to the electronic or charge delocalization of the aas within the peptide backbone and the entropy involved on such delocalization, were applied to model the bitter tasting threshold of dipeptides by linear discriminant and regression analyses [57]. These non-standard peptide features provided accuracies higher than 83% in the detection of bitter taste, and the regression models could explain the experimental variance of the bitter tasting threshold in more than 80%. It was shown the non-standard peptide descriptors correlate with the bitter taste as good as or even better than other well-known peptide features like the z-scale [73].

The spectral moments have been also applied to characterize bacteriocins. Bacteriocins are peptidic toxins produced and exported by bacteria as a defense mechanism to kill or inhibit the grow of other strains but the producer. The bacteriocins are very attractive for the development of new antibiotics and anticancer agents, however their high structural diversity represents a challenge for alignment-based predictive tools. Since the hydrophobicity and basicity of bacteriocins are relevant for their antibacterial activity, Agüero-Chapin et al. introduced the 2D-Hydrophobicity and Polarity (2D-HP) maps to pseudo-fold bacteriocin protein sequences in order to derive a set of spectral moments encoding information beyond the linear sequence [74] (Figure 4). These TIs are implemented in the Topological Indices to Biopolymers (TI2BioP) software [75] and were useful to build an AF model based on Linear Discriminant Analysis with a higher sensitivity (66.7%) than the attained by InterProScan (60.2%). In addition, they could detect cryptic bacteriocins, ignored by alignment methods [74].

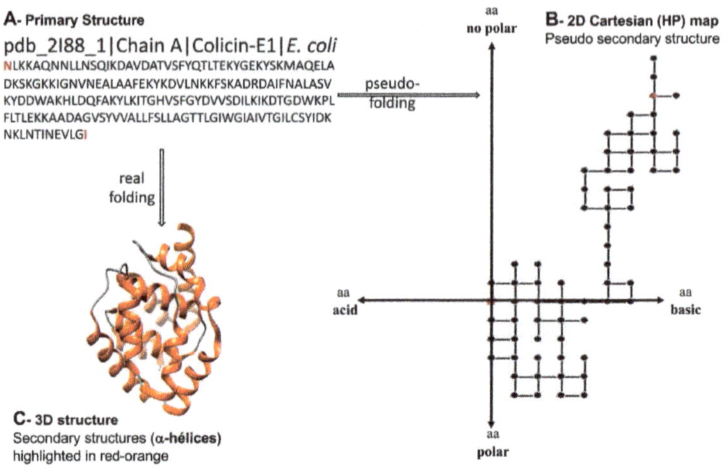

Figure 4. Different structural representations for the channel-forming domain of Colicin E1 (pdb 2I88). **A**—Primary structure, **B**—Pseudo secondary Cartesian map of hydrophobicity (H) and polarity (P) (2D Cartesian (HP) map), **C**—Three-dimensional structure. The 2D Cartesian protein map is an arbitrary bidimensional arrangement (pseudo-folding) of the protein/peptide sequences bearing higher-order useful patterns than contained in linear sequences.

2.1.2. Topological Indices from Descriptive Statistics

The cheminformatic-derived protein descriptors that have been widely applied to the prediction and design of bioactive peptides were developed and implemented by Ruiz-Blanco et al. in the ProtDCal software [32]. ProtDCal provides a great diversity of protein/peptide descriptors thanks to its divide-and-conquer methodology that considers both the aa properties and those estimated for groups, which can be modified by the neighbourhood through the application of classic previously-mentioned chemoinformatics algorithms. The modified properties of the aas or their resulting groups are later aggregated using statistical operators to estimate local or global descriptors either at sequence or 3D structural level. Although a more detailed description of ProtDCal's protein descriptors can be found in [32], the Figure 5 shows an schematic representation of the protein descriptor generation process of ProtDCal. The diversity of ProtDCal's protein descriptors represented by different families stems from combinatorically applying different aa properties, the ways to consider the vicinity to the target aa by several operators, the criteria used to group the aas as well as the invariant operator used for aggregating aa properties within the same array (Figure 5).

ProtDCal's descriptors have been involved in the discovery of antibacterial peptides by developing a non-conventional multi-target QSAR models [56]. Despite the AMPs selected for training were evaluated against multiple targets (Gram-positive bacterial strains), they could be integrated in the same model by modifying their ProtDCal's descriptors through the Box-Jenkins moving average operator. This operator allows modifying the sequence-based descriptors by subtracting the corresponding mean of the descriptors of all AMPs assayed against the same Gram-positive bacterial strain. This is a way to particularize a sequence-based descriptor by incorporating information about the experimental conditions or biological assays. With this kind of descriptors, the multi-target cheminformatic model displayed percentages of correct classification higher than 90.0% in both training and prediction (test) sets [56].

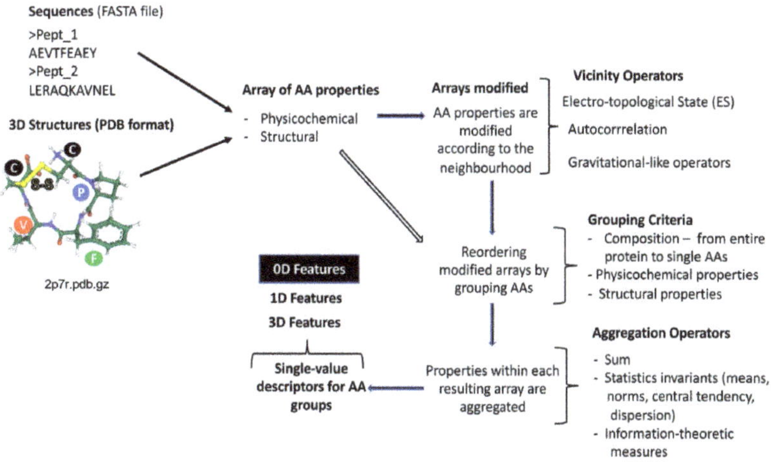

Figure 5. Schematic representation of ProtDCal's descriptors calculation. 1D and 3D protein features implies the application of vicinity operators to modify amino acid (aa) properties while 0D features estimation go straightforward to group the original aa properties according to several grouping criteria.

Similarly, the same authors also applied the Box-Jenkins moving average operator to develop non-conventional multi-task QSAR models able to predict simultaneously antibacterial activity and toxicity [58]. This time, the continuous response variables measured on AMPs such as minimum inhibitory concentration (MIC), cytotoxic concentration at 50% (CC50), and haemolytic concentration at 50% (HC50) were transformed in a binary variable labelled as (1) referred to high antibacterial activity/low cytotoxicity, and (−1) assigned to low antibacterial activity/high cytotoxicity. The ProtDCal's descriptors that usually encodes only peptide features were modified by the Box-Jenkins moving average operator in order to consider the variability implying the evaluation of the antimicrobial activity and toxicity on different biological systems. Thus, a multi-task QSAR model displayed an accuracy higher than 96% for classifying/predicting peptides was built by using LDA discriminant [58].

ProtDCal's descriptors have also been involved in the design of new peptides that inhibit the *E. coli* ATP synthase, as putative antibiotics [52,76]. ProtDCal's descriptors, implemented in PPI-Detect [77], were applied to predict interactions between peptides and the main subunits of *E. coli*'s (Ec) and human's (Hs) F1Fo-ATP synthase. Those peptide with a maximum and a minimum interaction likelihood with EcF1Fo and HsF1Fo were selected for in vitro assays. An overall of three peptides resulted attractive for further optimization steps in the design of new antibiotics [52,76].

More recently, ProtDCal's protein descriptors were successfully applied to improve the prediction performance of the existing alignment-free models by using the largest experimentally validated non-redundant peptide dataset reported to date, the StarPepDB [78], together with Random Forest (RF) classifiers [31]. Pinacho-Castellanos at al. not only built RF-based models for identifying AMPs, but also addressed the main biological activities reported for them (antibacterial, antifungal, antiparasitic, and antiviral) as endpoints. The specific functions of AMPs were either directly predicted or by a hierarchical classification that first consider the antimicrobial activity. RF-based models, developed with ProtDCal's descriptors aimed to predict specific activities of AMPs, showed a higher effectivity and reliability than 13 freely available prediction tools. The best reported models were implemented in the AMPDiscover tool [31], publicly available at https://biocom-ampdiscover.cicese.mx/ (accessed on 7 March 2022). Ruiz-Blanco et al. also applied successfully ProtDCal's descriptors to predict antibacterial peptides by using

RF-based models trained with StarPepDB instances and, in a second step they are predicted on what bacterial targets according to their Gram-staining classification could be active by using a multi-classifier. These two RF-based models were implemented in the web server ABP-Finder: https://protdcal.zmb.uni-due.de/ABP-Finder/ (accessed on 7 March 2022) which is freely available but unpublished yet.

2.2. Integration of Peptide Features from Heterogenous Sources

Considering previous experiences in protein functional classification where protein features from heterogeneous sources have been integrated to improve classification rates; we wonder if this strategy has been applied to peptide classification? In this sense, the integration/combination of alignment-based (AB) and alignment-free (AF) protein features in machine learning models have been evaluated for such purpose. For example, Galpert et al. improved orthologs classification at the twilight zone (<30% of identity) by combining AB and AF protein similarity measures in supervised big data classifiers [79]. It has also been shown that the integration of AB and AF methods gives the best exploration of highly diverse protein classes, such as the nonribosomal peptide synthases (NRPS) represented by their A-domains [80]. Other examples of feature integration methods for remote homology detection can be found in [81], and the one of Borozan's et al. [82], based on weighted aggregation which is a very inclusive approach avoiding the loss of information.

Regarding AMPs classification improvements by integrating AB and AF peptide features, an algorithm applying AB measures and the SVM algorithm trained with AF pairwise measures was published for increasing AMPs prediction sensitivity [47]. The algorithm consists in two stages. Firstly, AMPs are identified by Basic Local Alignment Search Tool (BLAST) scores, and those peptides that cannot be unequivocally identified by pairwise alignments were inputted in an SVM-based classifier built with AF pairwise similarity scores. The AF similarity scores were estimated with the Lempel–Ziv's complexity algorithm [83]. The integrative algorithm achieved higher sensitivity performance for AMPs prediction than the prediction tools implemented within the first version of CAMPR3 database [11] and the integrated method proposed by Wang et al. [84]. Wang and colleagues had previously proposed a similar algorithmic workflow where BLAST is used to firstly classify a query peptide against a training set made up by 870 AMPs and 8661 non-AMPs. Classification label is transferred to the query peptide from the matching with highest similarity score. Query peptides that did not match with any within the training set were encoded by protein features like ACC and PseACC and the aas by five of their physicochemical and biochemical properties. As the number of generated features were relatively high, a rigorous feature selection step was performed by applying both the Maximum Relevance, Minimum Redundancy (mRMR) method [85] and the Incremental Feature Selection method [86] before building a Nearest Neighbour (NN)-based predictor. The NN algorithm assign the label AMP or non-AMP to a query peptide according to the class of the nearest neighbour.

Despite the efforts for integrating AB and AF features in a classification peptide system; they have actually been combined through their corresponding algorithms and have not been included in the same model or function. In this sense, AB and AF similarity scores could be combined to build an unique classifier for AMP prediction, as Galpert et al. did it for ortholog detection [79].

2.3. NMR-Based Features for Peptides

In 2020, the IAMPE webserver (http://cbb1.ut.ac.ir/; accesed on 17 March 2022) was released for an accurate prediction of AMPs by using classical ML-based classifiers trained with both conventional and ^{13}CNMR-based features. The non-conventional ^{13}CNMR-based features for peptides were defined from the quantitative NMR spectra for ^{13}C isotope of the naturally-occurring aas. Firstly, ^{13}CNMR-based features for each aa were calculated using ^{13}CNMR spectra signals. Secondly the aas were grouped according to their ^{13}CNMR-based features by applying Fuzzy c-means clustering algorithm. The resulting aa clusters were used to extract feature vectors along the peptide sequences according to classical "composition", "transition" and "distribution" patterns. Despite the new information provided by such non-conventional peptide descriptors, authors suggested their combination with physicochemical features to yield higher accuracy for the prediction of active AMP sequences [34].

3. Breakthroughs of ML Algorithms in the AMP Prediction

3.1. Data Imbalance and Multi-Label Classification in the Prediction of AMPs—New Algorithm Approaches

As mentioned in the Introduction, data imbalance is an issue to tackle in the classification of potential peptide sequences. Here, we collected some other reported solutions combining two-level classifiers with imbalance management in both, the first level binary AMP/non-AMP problem, and the second level multi-label functional type problem. For example, the authors of MAMP-Pred [87] proposed two alternative imbalance management methods: (i) under-sampling of the non-AMP class, and (ii) weighting sequences according to the imbalance ratio; the second one being eligible after the experiment process. Then, they used pruned sets and label combinations, considering label correlations, to transform the RF binary classification. For the classification assessment, the Matthew's correlation coefficient was selected for the first level, and the multi-label metrics: Exact-Match Ratio (EMR), Hamming-Loss (H-Loss), Accuracy (Acc), Precision (Precision, Recall), Ranking-Loss (RL), Log-Loss, One-error (OE), F1-Measure (F1-Mic, F1-Mac), for the second level. As they assessed, MAMP-Pred outperformed iAMP-2L (proposed in 2013 as a two-level multi-label classifier) because of the feature extraction process involved ACC and its eight physicochemical selected properties, besides the classification process.

Another example of imbalance management can be found in [88] where the authors tried to identify peptides with dedicated anti-CoV antimicrobial function on an imbalanced dataset with relatively insufficient positive data. They used NearMiss under-sampling and balanced RF to build the classification model, and the sensitivity, specificity and geometric mean for the unbiased evaluation.

Ensemble learning has also been used to cope with class imbalance in the binary AMP/non-AMP prediction tool Ensemble-AMPPred [89]. The prediction model based on ensemble methods (RF, max probability voting, majority voting, adaptive boosting, or extreme gradient boosting) was combined with feature extraction (vectors of 517 numerical descriptors representing peptide sequences), feature engineering (hybrid feature generation by the fusion of various selected features using a logistic regression model) and feature selection to improve classification accuracy after the application of a balancing clustering-based proportionate stratified random sampling that selected peptide sequences representing the positive and negative data. Thus, representative sequences selected from each cluster were used as training data, while the other remaining sequences, as testing data.

A recent report in [90] presents a multi-label framework HMD-AMP to hierarchically annotate peptide sequences into AMP/non-AMP, and then, into eleven functional classes that can be small and extremely imbalanced classes. The classification framework includes an embedding layer of protein sequences, a protein language encoder, a feature transformer and a hierarchical deep forest model. An ablation study and a reduced feature test demonstrate the effectiveness of the framework based on the detailed structural information of AMPs to improve the accuracy of the prediction model and to manage data imbalance problem. At each function prediction level, the model demonstrates a cascade forest structure where each cascade level is an ensemble of decision tree forests, and different types of forests are included to make the model diverse. It's worth noting that deep forest does not rely on backpropagation, so it is suitable for training data with either imbalance labels or small sample sizes, hence preventing the model from overfitting.

3.2. Deep-Learning in the Recognition of AMPs

The lack of samples in the positive class, as well as, the ambiguity in the negative class are key issues concerning deep learning models in AMP prediction as stated in review [91]. The starting point for knowledge discovery in this rough scenario is the correct representation of raw data. Precisely, deep learning provides a solution to the human expert dependence problem of featurization, which is known as representation learning; but also allows the application of some widely-used features in peptide machine learning by means of unsupervised embeddings (pretrained representations that can be fine-tuned with specific downstream supervised tasks), learned embeddings (usually one-hot or one-letter encoding on the amino-acid level, producing a dimension-reduced dense vector for subsequent layers), or engineered features (physicochemical or evolution-based properties).

In generative approaches for AMP discovery, recently reviewed in [92], the reliance on expertise-engineered features may limit the generation of candidates qualitatively distinct from known AMPs, or the limited number of known structures of the annotated peptides may reduce the effectiveness of structured-based models [93]. On the contrary, those attribute-controlled models based on recurrent neural networks, variational autoencoders, adversarial autoencoders, generative adversarial networks may encourage novelty of designed sequences. That is the case of the specific bidirectional conditional generative adversarial network developed in AMPGAN v2 [94] that learns data driven priors through generator-discriminator dynamics and controls generation using conditioning variables. Thus, a learned encoder mapping data samples into the latent space of the generator implements the bidirectional component that aids iterative manipulation of novel, diverse, and application-tailored candidate peptides.

The diversity target in generative models has been also tackled with a semi-supervised learning approach combined with a variational autoencoder (VAE) that can simultaneously learn from the large unlabelled peptide sequence databases and a limited number of labelled sequences as in PepCVAE [95]. In this case, a controlled generative model is learned from large unlabelled peptide database for the encoder and decoder losses, together with a much smaller labelled dataset (peptides with reported antimicrobial annotation) for the classifier loss, that is, using a large unlabelled corpus to capture the distribution with VAE, and a small labelled corpus to learn a certain controlling attribute code.

Also with VAE generation, the report in [96] used the Giant Repository of AMP Activity (GRAMPA) [97] to apply an improved automated semi-supervised approach based on stochastic long short-term memory (LSTM) encoder-decoder networks for generating promising new sequences and an experimental investigation, resulting in low minimal inhibitory concentration (MIC) AMPs against *Escherichia coli*, *Staphylococcus aureus*, and *Pseudomonas aeruginosa*. In this approach, the decoding from the same point in the latent space may result in a different peptide being generated and is dependent on the random seed set prior to running. Thus, the VAE is trained on a curated AMP dataset followed by the development of a regression model for activity prediction and the subsequent development of the latent space. Then, new AMP sequences are identified from the latent space (by sampling) and, subsequently, the AMPs are produced and characterized with their corresponding MIC values. This method produces peptides with similar MICs as the input reference peptides, but with novel sequences not found in the training set; at the same time, without imposing thresholds on peptide characteristics or otherwise biasing output post-sequence generation. As a result, a list of newly generated active peptides includes non-canonical AMPs of low helicity and low net charge.

An alternative data augmentation method is presented in [98] to improve the recognition of neurotoxic peptides via a convolutional neural network model. Novel potential neurotoxic peptides were discovered from the best performed model in a simulation dataset among the transcriptome of an endemic spider of South Korea, *Callobius koreanus* (*C. koreanus*). The BLAST-based augmentation method was intended to improve the generalization property of the model.

Specifically, for candidate short peptide generation, the authors in [99] combined LSTM generation and bidirectional LSTM classification to design short novel AMP sequences with potential antibacterial activity against *E. coli*. The models were trained using sequences with proven low MICs and tuned with Bayesian hyperparameter optimization.

Some other deep learning methods are reviewed in [100] as a promising approach to meet short-length peptides requirements [101] where they combine deep convolutional neural network with reduced aa composition comprising clustered aas on the basis of evolutionary information, substitution score, hydrophobicity, and contact potential energy. As a result, a short peptide of 20 aa was selected by Deep-AmPEP30 from sequences extracted from the gut commensal fungus *C. glabrata* genome and experimentally validated to have antibacterial activities similar to ampicillin.

In a recent review [39], the authors presented some reasons to select ML approaches over deep learning ones in AMP prediction and design, when a fair balance is required among high accuracy and generalization capability, interpretability and low computational cost. However, some improvements like parameter tuning or model hybridization may lead to more robust deep learning classifiers in this field.

3.3. Rough Sets Theory in the Classification of AMPs

As an example of model hybridization, the authors in [48] presented a codon-based genetic algorithm combined with rough set theory methods to find a peptide active against *S. epidermidis*. Their rough set theory method provided explicit boundaries between physicochemical properties that active sequences possess and inactive sequences do not possess. Since this method produced explicit decision components, they could test sequences containing multiple components. They were inspired in their previous publication [22] where they tried to reduce false discovery rate with a rough set-based classification method generating similarity rule set boundaries between active and non-active peptides based on their physicochemical properties.

Another example of the rough set theory application can be found in [102] where they implemented a rough set classification framework together with a Rough Set Quick Reduct and Rough Set Relative Reduct based on an improved Harmony Search algorithm to classifyAnti-HIV-1 peptides. Specifically, they hybridized a rough set-based feature selection technique, with population-based meta-heuristic algorithms (Particle Swarm Optimization), to classify the peptide sequences and solve dimensionality problems. Besides, a fuzzy set classification framework [23] was also intended to cope with limited and severely skewed high-dimensional space for short (<30 aa) AMP activity prediction.

4. Other Methodologies Than Classical ML for Identifying and Modelling AMPs

4.1. Homology-Based Prediction and Modelling of AMPs

The most popular approaches in addition to classical machine learning algorithms for the identification of AMPs in databases are local alignments which are represented by BLAST and FASTA tools [103,104]. Although local alignments have been successfully applied by using iterative rounds and filters such as the presence of signal peptides, aa patterns and gene vicinity during AMP searches [105–107], they can fail in identifying some AMP sequences [55], if compared to pattern-matching searches [107,108]. There are two main ways for searching for sequences by patterns: hidden markov models (profile-HMM) [109] or regular expressions (REGEX) [110]. Both the REGEX and profile-HMM methodologies work similarly for the identification of AMPs. Firstly, a set of homologous sequences are aligned and the multiple sequence alignment (MSA) is inputted to a specific program such as Pratt [111] or HMMER [112] for the identification of REGEX patterns or profile-HMM, respectively. Currently, instead of building REGEX patterns and profile-HMMs, they are available for many protein families at the Prosite [113] and Pfam [114] databases where a query sequence/peptide can be identified. The pattern/profile-based searches for AMPs can be complemented with the identification of signal peptides and other structural filters. In fact, improved versions of databases have incorporated MSA, profiles-HMM and molecular modelling for AMPs detection [11,115,116]. Even so, when a query peptide could be high-scored against profile-HMMs from different peptide families, it is advisable to use a prediction tool combining different protein signature recognition methods such as InterProScan [117].

As we previously mentioned, the molecular modelling complements AMPs pattern-based searches by confirming expected three-dimensional (3D) structural features characterizing them. The 3D structure can be also integrated into homology-based searches to identify homologous sequences sharing low identity but retaining a great structural conservation. Such structural similarities have enabled the detection of AMPs in databases with higher accuracy [9]. When the structures of peptides are not experimentally elucidated, two modelling techniques are suggested: homology-based and *ab initio* modelling. The homology-based modelling uses the structure experimentally-determined from available homologous as template to infer the 3D structure of novel peptides, but rather using structural than sequence similarities, especially if the query and template are remote homologous [118]. By contrast, the *ab initio* method is used to predict the structures of peptides with yet unknown homologs. The prediction of the 3D protein structure starts from scratch requiring an energy model describing the main factors that contribute to the stability of the folding process and an efficient method for the conformational space exploration of the peptide chain [119]. However, homology-based approaches are more suitable for peptides when homologs are identified. In fact, the second release of BACTIBASE [115] incorporated the MODELLER program [120], as a tool for the 3D structure prediction of query peptides by homology to known bacteriocins [115]. Besides, the incorporation of 3D structure prediction tools to AMP databases provide another filter for an accurate identification of query AMPs, the 3D structure can be used for scoring peptide-cellular target interactions which is a crucial step for the *in-silico* design of novel AMPs [121].

Especially, since classical ML algorithms were recently reviewed in [18], we have addressed here, traditional homology-based approaches applied to the search and the modelling of AMPs, and will describe next, the most singular algorithms.

4.2. Emerging ML-Independent Methodologies for AMP Prediction/Design

In this section, we will address other emerging methodologies regardless of ML approaches and classical homology-based approaches for AMP discovery. Firstly, we want to highlight the AMPA webserver (http://tcoffee.crg.cat/apps/ampa, accessed on 7 March 2022), developed to detect antimicrobial stretches within the protein sequences. The antimicrobial regions detected in proteins can serve as new templates for AMP design, especially those uncovered within proteins no related with the defense function. AMPA algorithm does not depend on homology-based searches since it estimates an antimicrobial index (AI) to each aa, derived from half-maximal inhibitory concentration (IC_{50}) values in high-throughput screening experiments, encoding the propensity of each aa to be present in an AMP sequence. As low IC_{50} values correspond to high activity, aas with low AIs are more likely to be part of an AMP. By applying a sliding-windows analysis along the protein sequence, AMPA generates an antimicrobial profile based on the AIs. Those regions scored below certain threshold are considered putative antimicrobial domains [122]. The singularity of this approach is that it doesn't either rely on building machine learning models or similarity searches against AMP databases. However, potentially conserved antimicrobial regions can be checked in conjunction with the T-coffee alignment tool [123].

On the other hand, complex networks have been applied to explore the chemical space of AMPs aimed to discover structural entities with promising biological activities that also could serve as template for peptide drugs design/optimization. In this sense, Marrero-Ponce et al. were the pioneers on this topic by publishing a seminal of related works [33,78,124]. Firstly, Marrero-Ponce et al. analyzed both the diversity among 25 AMP databases and the showed within each one. The study revealed some AMP databases contained common sequences showing certain overlapping degree. After removing duplicates among AMP databases, a representative set of 16 990 non-redundant

AMPs was collected, which probably was the most comprehensive and exhaustively curated AMP dataset at that moment [124]. This relevant dataset was further enriched and structured in a graph database called StarPepDB (http://mobiosd-hub.com/starpep/; accessed on 17 March 2022) integrating 45 120 unique peptide sequences from 42 AMPs databases (Figure 6), with their metadata (origin organisms, function, biological target, source database, chemical modifications, cross-referenced entries to UniProt, PDB and PubMed) [78].

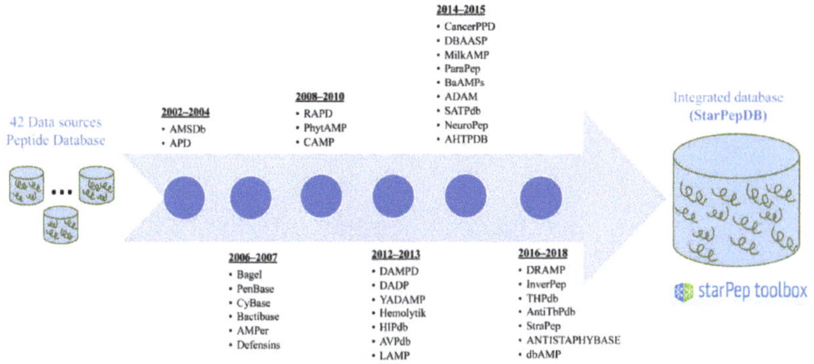

Figure 6. Chronological listing of AMP databases used in StarPep Database (StarPepDB) compilation. After collecting web pages from a large variety of bioactive peptide databases (see Table 1 in Ref. [78]), their contents were integrated into a graph database that holds total of 71.310 nodes and 348.505 relationships. In this graph structure, there are 45.120 nodes representing peptides (unique sequences) and the rest of the nodes are connected to peptides for the describing metadata.

StarPepDB has a star-like network architecture where a central node represents the peptide sequence and is connected to neighbour nodes labelled with the metadata. The edges depict a relational and unidirectional connection of the central node by a using a set of selection criteria "produced by", "assessed against", *"related to"*, *"compiled in"* with its corresponding metadata nodes such as the origin, target, function and database, respectively. Peptide nodes besides the sequence also contain peptide's ID and length, while the metadata nodes have the 'name' property and relationships have the 'db-ref' property (referred as source database) [78]. Finally, different network topologies can be visualized by applying filtering criteria on StarPepDB. For example, it is possible to display a network of those peptides (central nodes) *"related to"* (edges) function "antibacterial" (metadata node) and *"compiled in"* (edges) the ADP database (metadata node).

Thus, the StarPepDB structure together with the StarPep toolbox allows building customized networks and their visualization. The visual and analytics exploration of the network by extracting some centralities measures (e.g., weighted degree or harmonic centralities) allows identifying the most relevant bioactive peptides in the network (Figure 7). Furthermore, peptide subsets can be either retrieved from the graph database by sequence identity searches or by applying filtering criteria such as peptide length, sequence motifs/patterns, physicochemical properties, and other metadata.

More recently, the same research group encoded each peptide sequence with a set of molecular descriptors bearing non-redundant structural information to set alignment-free (AF) pairwise similarity/distance relationships among the peptide nodes of the network by using a general pipeline as show in Figure 7. The resulting chemical space represented by these AF similarity networks are explored by visual inspection in combination with clustering and network science techniques [49,50].

Here, we show the chemical space network (CSN) of 174 non-redundant Anti-Biofilm Peptides (ABPs) (Figure 8) by applying the StarPep Toolbox flowchart represented above. Networks become more interpretable through visual inspection if having a community structure. Note that communities of ABPs may represent some biologically relevant regions from the chemical space where bioactive compounds reside. Hence, we have explored the CSNs by varying the similarity threshold until a well-defined community structure emerged. In this way, a final CSN has been analyzed by adjusting the similarity threshold to 0.65, at network density of 0.0068, achieving 20 ABP outliers (singletons) with atypical or unique sequences (Figure 8). Also, for each peptide discovered to be a relevant node, additional information (metadata) is available in Supplementary Materials (File S1, SI1-A and B).

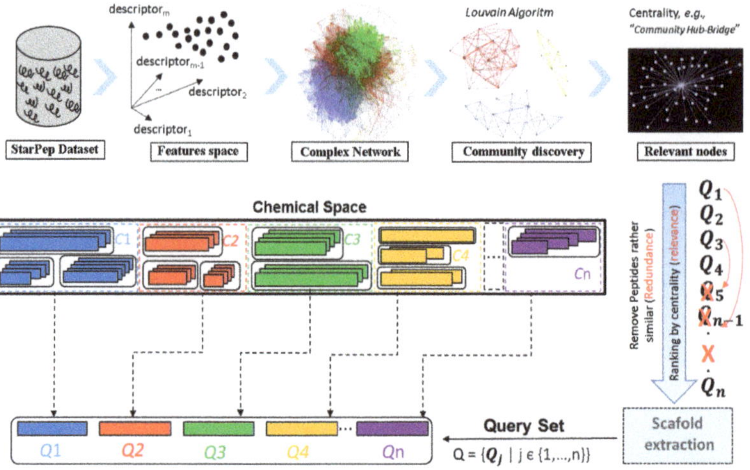

Figure 7. StarPep Toolbox flowchart. A flow diagram guiding the automatic construction and visual graph mining of similarity networks (see Figure 1 in Ref. [33]). Networks can be clustered, and communities are optimized using the Louvain method [125]. Moreover, the centrality of each node can be particularly measured by harmonic, community hub-bridge, betweenness, and weighted degree. Centrality is crucial to perform scaffold extractions because peptides are ranked according to their centrality score, and then redundant sequences are removed, prioritizing the most central. Thus, scaffold extractions depend on the type of centrality applied.

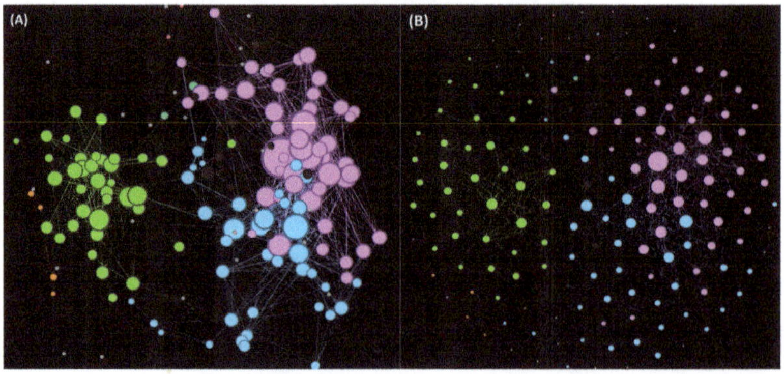

Figure 8. Visualizing the similarity network (Chemical Space Network, CSN) of a set of 174 non-redundant Anti-Biofilm Peptides (ABP_98% identity) at threshold t = 0.65 and density = 0.068, using the (**A**) three main PCAs as coordinated of each ABPs, and (**B**) Fruchtermann Reingold layout algorithm. Node colour represents the community (e.g., the biggest communities represented by cluster 3, 10 and 12 are in blue, purple and green colours, respectively), and node size symbolizes the centrality values. There are 20 ABP outliers (singletons). This figure has been created using the software starPep toolbox (version 0.8), available at http://mobiosd-hub.com/starpep; accessed on 17 March 2022.

Once a community structure is found, we rank nodes in decreasing order according to the community Harmonic centrality measure for retaining the top-k of the ranked list. Particularly, the top 10 exposes densely connected groups of nodes like cliques, which are defined to be complete subgraphs. These related sequences may be forming families in the chemical space of ABPs. These central peptides within each local leading community are given in SI1-B, and they may be representing sequence fragments or naturally occurring peptides that could be identified as starting structures for lead discovery. For instance, the peptide starpep_00000, starpep_05561, starpep_00361 are the most central nodes of the CSN (all in cluster 10). ABPs starpep_03668, starpep_04267, starpep_00004 and starpep_07895, starpep_12531, starpep_012529 are more central inside Communities 3 and 12, respectively (Figure 8 and SI1-C).

As can be observed in Table in SI1-C, some neighbor nodes within the communities may be representing a family of similar ABPs. Another example of closely related sequences can be seen in the 3 members of the Cluster 3 (see all ABPs in Community 3 in SI1-B). The peptides inside this cluster have the same length of 12 aas. So, it is expected that there are many ABPs with similar centrality values in the CSN, and it is advisable to extract some non-redundant ABPs from communities than just selecting the highest-ranked ones. To clearly extract central but non-redundant ABPs from each cluster (scaffold extraction, see Figure 7), we sort ABPs according to the decreasing order of their harmonic values. Then, the redundant sequences are removed at a given % of sequence identity. We have used an identity cutoff of > 35% to consider that a particular sequence is related to already-selected central ABPs and, as a consequence, removed from the CSN. Finally, the non-redundant 44 ABPs were ranked according to their decreasing values of Harmonic measure. The sorted list is given in SI1-D, and the top ranked peptides are those having relatively small similarity paths to all other nodes in the CSN.

This workflow allows the extraction of the most representative nodes/peptides describing the biologically-active chemical space (SI1-D). This representative subset can be used for multi-query similarity searches against peptide databases to retrieve all possible hits (Figure 9). The multi-query similarity search consists in using both the most central/representative nodes of the network communities and also the so-called singletons (isolated peptide nodes) as references/queries to retrieve the most similar peptides from databases by using local alignments. The best matches against the reference/query chemical space are determined by the maximum fusion rule by firstly ranking-down the similarity scores, to retrieve the best match between a query peptide and a target database and afterwards the best similarity scores are ranked for all reference peptides. Some studies have demonstrated that fusion by similarity scores and the maximum fusion rule are the best parameters for these models [126,127].

The integrated collection of 45 120 bioactive peptides registered in StarPepDB (http://mobiosd-hub.com/starpep/; accessed on 17 March 2022), that probably is the largest and most diverse bioactive peptide database to date, can be used for the discovering of central peptide nodes targeting an specific biological activity in the Chemical Space Networks (CSNs) and for taking advantage of them in multi-query similarity searches [33]. In this sense, Marrero-Ponce et al. explored different similarity networks of antiparasitic peptides (APPs) from StarPepDB to identify the most relevant and non-redundant APPs, that were later used as queries in similarity-based searches to identify potential APPs among non-labelled peptides as such in the StarPepDB. The proposed multi-query similarity search strategy outperformed state-of-the-art machine learning models aimed at APPs prediction like the AMPDiscover (https://biocom-ampdiscover.cicese.mx; accessed on 17 March 2022) and the AMPFun (http://fdblab.csie.ncu.edu.tw/AMPfun/index.html; accessed on 17 March 2022) webservers [30,31]. The methodology will also permit the design of new APPs by using the motifs found among the repurposed APPs [49]. More recently, a similar workflow using CSNs was applied to identify the most relevant tumor-homing peptides (THPs) within the StarPepDB. Such THPs were considered as queries (Qs) for multi-query similarity searches that apply a group fusion (MAX-SIM rule) model.

The resulting similarity searching models outperformed state-of-the-art tools for THPs detection, and the best one was applied to repurpose AMPs from the StarPepDB as THPs. Novel THP leads were identified as well as new motifs accounting for their TH activity [50].

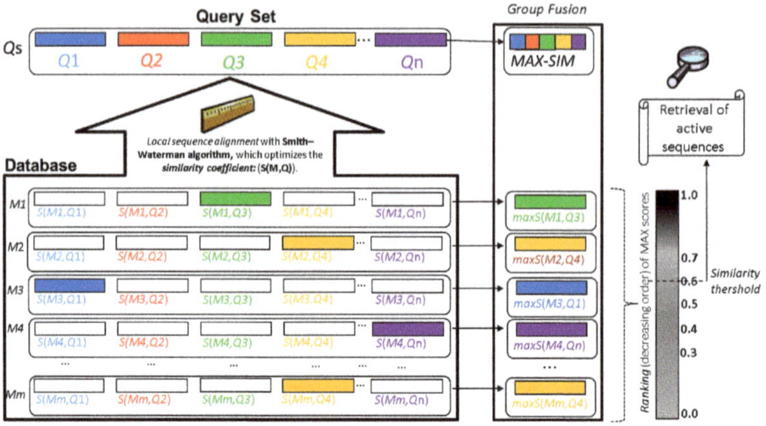

Figure 9. Schematic representation of the group fusion and similarity searching processes. Qi is a i peptide from a query/reference dataset, n is the number of peptides contained in a query dataset, S is identity coefficient between M and Q obtained by local alignment with Smith-Waterman algorithm, m is the number of peptides included in the target dataset. The similarity threshold is related to the percentage of identity.

5. Models of Sequence Evolution for the Design and Optimization of Bioactive Peptides

Several *in silico* computational approaches inspired in molecular evolution events have been applied to the design and optimization of a peptide with a promising biological activity, known in medicinal chemistry as a "leading compound". These algorithms are aimed to produce offspring peptides from a parent (hit peptide) until the "desired property" is meet according to selection criteria conducted either by ML prediction models or by biological assays (Figure 2). The offspring generation process can be iterated until reaching optimized peptidic scaffolds showing a trade-off between desirable/undesirable activities. The simulation process for generating offspring have evolved from inducing random mutations within the peptide sequence until guiding such aa substitutions under directed evolution concepts [41,128,129]. Although, algorithms inducing random mutations are commonly applied to generate sequence diversity in the peptide library, they could render unpredictable results that should be carefully analysed with selection algorithms. By contrast, computational algorithms inspired on directed mutagenesis have focused the design and optimization of "leading peptides" by guiding the generation of peptide offspring incorporating secondary structure features that influence positively on the antimicrobial activity such as amphipathic helices, kinked amphipathic helices, and other structures aimed to interact with lipid membranes [130].

Schneider et al. were the pioneers to apply simulated molecular evolution (SME) algorithms as a strategy for a rational peptide design by coupling the *in silico* generation of peptidases cleavage sites of 12 residues long to a selection mechanism represented by trained ANN [131,132]. The design was oriented to this region by generating offspring from a 12-residue sequence/peptide (parent sequence) which was iteratively mutated until meeting the best ANN quality classification metrics, used as a selection criterion of the design. The offspring sequence simulation was performed by introducing random mutations according to Gaussian-distributed probability values around the parent sequence. The mutation degree (small or large) is then conditioned by the estimation of position-specific mutability and the selected aa distance matrix [131,132]. As the position-specific mutability is averaged resulting the same for every position in the sequence; the aa mutation degree is determined by the aa substitution/scoring matrix type such the Grantham matrix [133], the Myata matrix [134], and the Risler matrix [135].

This SME approach was later applied by the same group to the optimization of anticancer peptides (ACP) aimed at improving their membranolytic activity and cell-type selectivity [51,136]. In [51], a known α-helical ACP served as the parent sequence for the generation of the offspring (ACP-derivatives). So that the generated offspring peptides retained similarity with the initial structural/property space and thus enabling a systematic optimization; the mutation function was controlled. This time the SME approach was accompanied with experimental measurements as a selection criteria or fitness objective within the optimization scheme. They used the half-effective concentration (EC_{50}) on the breast cancer cell line MCF7 and the secondary structure preferences by circular dichroism (CD) spectroscopy as experimental filters. A similar SME protocol was applied in [136] to optimize the cell-type selectivity of the highest-scored candidate toward non-cancer cells and human erythrocytes. This candidate termed AmphiArc2 peptide resulted from the screening of virtual libraries generated by more advanced algorithms incorporating secondary structures features (alpha and amphipathic helices) that influence positively on the membranolytic action [130]. AmphiArc2 was selected as a parent sequence in the SME algorithm in which the mutated sequences (offspring) are generated from it. The offspring was scored according to a fitness function, defined by the anticancer activity and selectivity with respect to non-transformed cells. The best offspring was selected as a parent for the following optimization iteration [136].

Although the SME approach and the generation of oriented libraries toward certain secondary structures, relevant for the interaction with lipid membranes, have represented a step forward in the design and optimization pipeline of AMPs and ACPs [130,136], there still room for improving the simulation of molecular evolution of the offspring peptides. In this sense, algorithms that traditionally have been used for simulating sequence evolution in the field of molecular phylogenetics were recently applied to provide more rationality to the peptide library generation [52]. These algorithms were initially developed to evaluate the accuracy of MSA and phylogenetic reconstruction tools by generating sets of related simulated protein sequences from known phylogenies. The most representative ones are: ROSE (Random Model of Sequence Evolution) [137], SIMPROT (Simulation Protein Evolution) [138], and INDELible (Insertions and Deletions Simulator) [139]. In general, they are controlled by several evolutionary parameters such as tree topology, evolutionary distance matrices, mutation rate, insertion and deletion probabilities to simulate the evolution of offspring from a parent sequence. Ruiz-Blanco et al. incorporated the ROSE algorithm into the *de novo* design pipeline of peptide inhibitors of *E. coli* ATP synthase [52,76]. As parent peptides, both the natural inhibitor (IF_1) of the mitochondrial ATP synthase and fragments of interfaces involved in protein—protein interactions between subunits of *E. coli* ATP synthase, were selected to generate peptide libraries. The residue conservation degree on these parent peptides was identified by MSAs within each class. A consensus parent peptide with its corresponding conservation scoring profile was estimated so different mutation rates to each position in the sequence could be assigned. This mutation probability vector together with a user-defined phylogenetic tree with a known topology and branch lengths guided the probabilistic function performing mutations, insertion and deletions on the parent peptide [52,76]. On the other hand, the sequence diversity of the offspring peptides in the library can be controlled by calibrating ROSE parameters against the pairwise identity [81]. A predefined binary phylogenetic tree with 1023 nodes and depth 9 implemented in ROSE was used in [52,76] for the generation of diversity-oriented libraries. The Figure 10 shows a schematic description of the ROSE algorithm.

Peptide libraries were screened by the PPI-Detect [77], an SVM-based model that predicts peptide interactions with both domains of the *E. coli* and human ATP synthases. As selection criterion, the high-scored interacting peptides with the *E. coli* ATP synthase but showing low values with the human's were subsequently evaluated by in vitro inhibition tests. At applying advanced SME algorithms involving more evolutionary models/parameters like ROSE makes easier subsequently screening steps to find lead peptides at high success rate.

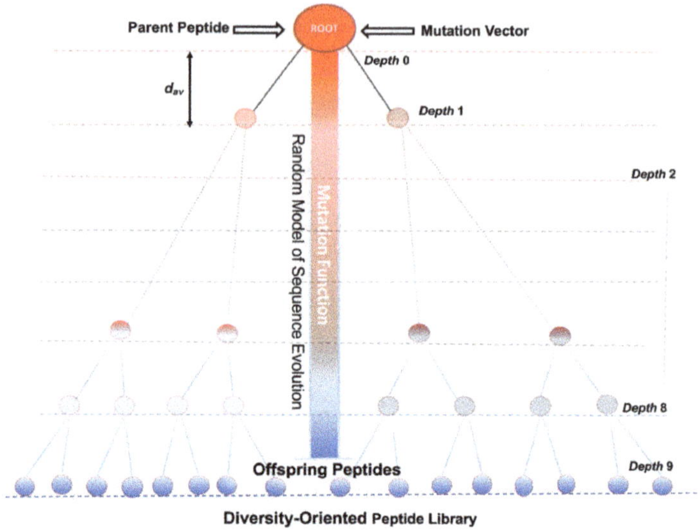

Figure 10. The binary mutation guide tree used by ROSE to mutate the parent/root peptide. The binary tree topology is determined by the number of nodes (1023), depth (9) and average distance (dav = 5–20 PAMs). Peptide library may be selected either from internal or terminal nodes of the tree. The identity percentage of the offspring peptides respect to the parent/root peptide is coloured-illustrated. Red colour means closely-related peptides to the parent while blue colour represents those distantly-related ones.

6. Considerations in the Workflow for the High-Throughput Discovering of Bioactive Peptides

6.1. *Brief Comparisons between High-Throughput (HT) and Classical Methods*

The classical approach for discovery of bioactive peptides has changed from analysing biological extracts/fluids to perform a wide-genomics and proteomics search. In this sense both next-generation sequencing (NGS) technologies and mass spectrometry (MS)–based proteomics combined with bioinformatic tools have provided suitable approaches for the large-scale identification of bioactive peptides outperforming the classical methods. These last ones usually include a purification step combined with bio-guided assays, which require higher amount of biomass from the subject organism. Although they can determine the biological activity of bioactive compounds relatively at high accuracy, are time-consuming and the yield of bioactive compounds is low as well as the coverage of the chemical space [140]. On the contrary, the HT analyses can be performed with around 1 cm^3 or 0.5–1 g of fresh or preserved tissues, for genomic/transcriptomic or proteomic purposes, respectively [53,141,142]. Generally, the HT methods allow covering the whole picture for potential bioactive compounds much faster. Despite HT methods usually require of powerful computational resources, both NGS and MS-based proteomics are becoming cheaper and their corresponding workflows are continuously optimized within the discovery process as well, resulting in a long-term sustainable approach [143,144]. Moreover, HT OMICs technologies yield a big amount of free public data, allowing the decentralization of the knowledge for the biodiscovery process.

Hence, the integration of OMICs approaches is more recommendable than the classical ones at the early stage of bioactive peptide discovery. However, bioassays-guided methods are still valid and complementary at advanced phases of the research [140,145].

6.2. Optimized Workflow for the Large-Scale AMPs Discovery from Profiled/Unexplored Organisms

Despite the advances in the discovery of bioactive peptides, improved protocols are still needed to increase the accuracy in both their large-scale identification and functional characterization, which is a major challenge, nowadays. Figure 11 illustrates the overall steps for the HT bioactive peptide discovery from model and unexplored organisms.

In order to analyze OMICs data released by NGS and MS-based HT proteomics, several computational/bioinformatic tools and platforms have been developed. Among them, for the *de novo* genome/transcriptome assembly we can mention, i.e., MIRA [146], Spades [147], CAP3 [148], OASES [149] and the Trinity package [150] including the *de novo* assembler and the TransDecoder for ORFs prediction (https://github.com/TransDecoder/TransDecoder/releases; accessed on 17 March 2022). Other ALL-IN-ONE licensed software like the toolbox CLC Genomic Workbench (CLC Bio-Qiagen, Aarhus, Denmark) [151] and OMICsBox (BioBam Bioinformatics, Valencia, Spain) [152], have integrated several tools for the complete workflow, including the *de novo* assemblers, custom/online/cloud functional annotation options with Blast+ [153], eggNOG [154], KEGG [155], providing as well as a set of functional analyses and statistical tests (i.e., Gene Ontology, deferential expression analyses and enrichment).

Among the NGS analyses, the RNA-seq has gained relevance because it can explore the coding regions of the genome by assembling, annotating and comparing expression profiles of the resulting transcripts [141,156]. Since elucidating the transcriptome demands lower computational cost than whole genome, and also provide useful information, its number has increasingly growth in databases. In this sense, transcriptomes from the same or related species are translated, usually with the TransDecoder or Six-Frame Translations Tool (S-FTT) (https://github.com/iracooke/protk; accessed on 17 March 2022), then annotated, and thus considered as reference database for improving protein identification in proteomics analyses from a target organism [157]. These are the grounds of proteogenomic analyses where genomic, transcriptomic and proteomic data are combined to assist the discovery of peptides from MS–based proteomic data, especially if they are not present in protein databases such as UniprotKB and other related ones (i.e, Swiss-Prot, TrEMBL and UniRef), the protein section of NCBI, Mendeley and ProteomExchange consortium [158]. On the other hand, the proteomic data can also be used to confirm gene expression [159].

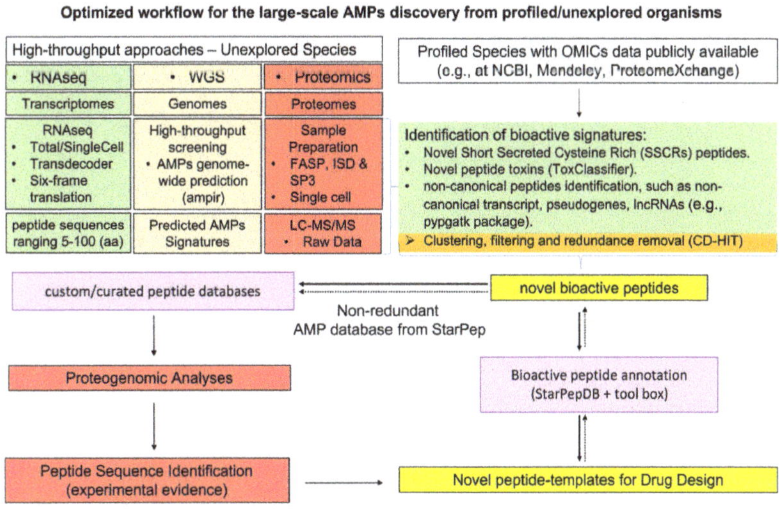

Figure 11. Optimized workflow for the high-throughput (HT) AMPs discovery from profiled and/or unexplored organisms. The figure summarizes the main phases in the AMPs discovery using genomic,

transcriptomic and proteomic data from profiled or underexplored organisms. The figure depicts the pipeline for de novo HT discovery from un(der)explored organisms using OMICs approaches (shown in the top-left panel), and from nucleotide and proteomic information available at public databases (top-right). Genomic information publicly available at NCBI (Genome database https://www.ncbi.nlm.nih.gov/genome/; accessed on 17 March 2022) and transcripts encoding protein sequences under 100 aa length provided by the Transcriptome Shotgun Assembly (TSA) database (https://www.ncbi.nlm.nih.gov/genbank/tsa/; accessed on 17 March 2022), can be screened with the computational tool ampir for fast genome-wide prediction of AMPs [160]. Likewise, the remaining transcripts encoding peptides sequences ranging 5-100 aas length, usually discarded in transcriptomic analyses, can be translated with the six-frame translations tool (S-FTT) [157,161] after ORFs prediction with the TransDecoder. Considering bioactive peptides include animal toxins which are usually rich in cysteine, the aa sequences obtained with S-FFT can be either analyzed by the Proteomic toolkit (https://github.com/iracooke/protk; accessed on 17 March 2022) to identify cysteine-rich regions to discover novel Short Secreted Cysteine Rich (SSCRs) peptides, or by the Machine Learning (ML) tool ToxClassifier, that enables a simple and consistent discrimination of toxins from non-toxin sequences [162]. In addition, new tools like the pypgatk package [163] can recover a significant number of cryptic peptides of biomedical interest from pseudogenes, long non-coding RNAs (lncRNAs) and other non-canonical coding transcripts produced by alternative splicing. These filtering tools can be applied together CD-HIT [164] to screen nucleotide databases before custom and non-redundant peptide databases building for proteogenomic analyses or HT annotation. Finally, the StarPepDB with its associated tools [33] may have several roles within the presented workflow by providing non-redundant bioactive databases and also at reducing custom peptide databases with the identification of the most relevant peptides for proteogenomic analyses. Moreover, bioactive peptides detected in HT screening can be classified and clustered with StarPep in different categories according to their biomedical potential (e.g., AMPs, antitumor, antibacterial, antiparasitic, etc.).

In general, the overall proteomic approach for the discovery of bioactive peptides includes the following steps: (*i*) protein digestion, (*ii*) peptide separation, (*iii*) peptide fragmentation and MS spectra acquisition, (*iv*) peptide identification using MS spectra database by similarity searches or by *de novo* sequencing. In this sense, steps (*i*) and (*ii*) are addressed by several sample preparation protocols which selection determine the best yields/results. Specifically, for bioactive peptide discovery, it is advisable the solid-phase-enhanced sample-preparation (SP3) protocol [165] since it reaches a wider coverage of peptides than the filter-aided sample preparation (FASP) [166]; moreover, is less complicated and faster than the in-solution digestion (ISD) [167].

Besides to protocol improvements in sample processing [161], there have been advances in the peptide identification step by applying several computational strategies that have also refined their bioactivity prediction [159]. In addition to use transcriptomic data to increase peptide detection accuracy, the inclusion of custom databases is being applied to characterize the part of the proteome that remains unannotated. In this sense, composite databases have been explored for a deeper proteomic characterization of the salivary glands from *Octupus vulgaris* looking for revealing underexplored bioactive peptides/toxins from previous studies [54,157,161]. The composite database comprised data from the UniProtKB, built from *de novo* transcriptome assembly of Anterior (ASGs) and Posterior Salivary Glands (PSGs), combined with those retrieved from all transcriptomes available from the cephalopods' PSGs. In addition, a comprehensive non-redundant AMPs database [124] was also included to provide additional insights about bioactive compounds such as putative AMPs [54]. In a previous work the same AMP subset was also considered as custom database to characterize the Ascidian tunic proteome by shotgun proteomics [53]. The computational analysis of the raw data implied searches against the Uniprot database (Bacteria and Metazoan section) and the AMP database. The Ascidian tunic revealed the presence of AMPs from both eukaryotes and prokaryotes and the "Biosynthesis of antibiotics" pathway was among the most significant ones, which support this tissue as an interesting reservoir of bioactive peptides/toxins and its role on the interactions Ascidians and their associated organisms. The AMP subset integrated in these previous analyses was published by Aguilera-Mendoza and probably was the most comprehensive and non-redundant AMP database reported so far [124], that later was updated in the StarPepDB (http://mobiosd-hub.com/starpep/; accessed on 17 March 2022) [78], as mentioned above.

Other important handicaps in the workflow of proteogenomic analysis are the False Discover Rate generated at analysing large protein/peptide databases [168–170] and the probable loss of information represented by small size transcripts encoding protein fragments < 100 aas that could be discarded by the TransDecoder [54,157,161], the tool dedicated to identify candidate coding regions within transcripts generated by *de novo* RNA-Seq, and such small-sized fragments could account for bioactive peptides. In order to perform a wider proteome analysis looking for uncovered AMPs and peptide toxins in the PSGs of *O. vulgaris*, contigs discarded in previous proteogenomic analyses (<100 aas) were translated with the S-FTT and then included in the protein database [54]. To optimize further proteogenomic analyses (i.e., time of analyses, FDR), or peptide annotation, sequences redundancy should be reduced with the CD-HIT [164] since the S-FTT generates many peptides sharing high similarities that could affect the overall peptide identification when increasing the FDR [170].

Other filters within the computational pipeline to process proteomic data have been applied to refine the search of peptide toxins against both canonical and custom databases. For example, the search can be framed against those toxins/peptides having signal peptides, responsible for their transport and secretion. Signal peptides have shown to contain common features across all life kingdoms [171]. In addition, cysteine-rich secretory proteins (CRISPs), small toxins (<100 aas) commonly found within the secretions of animal venoms, can be extracted from protein databases, to enrich reference databases for increasing proteomic toxin peptides detection [172]. Besides, the custom protein/peptide database can also be screened with ML-based tools e.g., ToxClassifier, that enables simple and consistent discrimination of toxins from non-toxin sequences [162], allowing the discovery of novel toxin-like bioactive peptides. Moreover, the fast genome-wide prediction of AMPs, using the ampir R package [160] can be used in the pipeline to retrieve novel peptides with antimicrobial signatures from public nucleotide databases, *de novo* transcriptomes/genomes assemblies, or as a filtering step before using S-FTT. More recently, new tools for the creation of proteogenomic databases considering the translation of pseudogenes, long non-coding RNAs (lncRNAs) and other non-canonical coding transcripts produced by alternative splicing, have allowed the identification of a significant number of cryptic peptides that may show interesting biological activities [163].

7. Concluding Remarks

Protein features inspired on molecular descriptors from chemoinformatics have emerged as successful predictors for AMPs activities. Particularly, ProtDCal's descriptors have been recently incorporated in two RF-based webservers (AMPDiscover and ABPFinder) targeting AMPs predictions as well as their specific activities and putative bacterial targets. Moreover, ProtDCal's descriptors have been involved in the design of antibiotic peptides by predicting their interaction to druggable targets from *E. coli*.

Among the recent ML approaches, undoubtedly DNNs have been the algorithm of choice for AMPs prediction in emerging tools. However, recently it has been shown that deep learning models' performance in AMP prediction is comparable to the one of classical ML algorithms being their use mostly advisable when the performance gains justify the associated computational cost.

Currently, the network science implemented in StarPep is being applied as one of the top emerging approaches, regardless of ML, to assist the search and design of bioactive peptides through the identification of lead peptides within the known chemical space. On the other hand, methodologies that simulate sequence evolution in the phylogenetics field have been repurposed to assist the optimization of such peptide leads by generating diversity-oriented libraries which are strictly controlled by evolutionary parameters.

New considerations in analysing genomic, transcriptomic and proteomic data for AMPs discovery from either profiled or underexplored organisms are being also applied. Several filtering steps have been proposed to reduce the FDR in AMPs detection when custom databases are included, but at the same time, to encompass the highest number and diversity of peptides as possible.

8. Future Research Directions

Despite a great diversity of peptide features (classical and non-classical) that has been used in AMPs prediction/design, most of those features are sequences- or property- based; however, the 3D structural information of AMPs has not been deeply exploited for such aims [173–175]. Although experimental determinate 3D structures of AMPs are used in minor proportion than their sequences, the 3D structure prediction tools are becoming more accessible and less computational demanding when considering new advances in both software and computer architectures [176,177]. These facts will ease the gradually inclusion of 3D structural features in the prediction models.

Another alternative for the inclusion of higher structural information in AMPs encoding is the use of artificial representations, which have been commonly used in comparative analyses of DNA and proteins and in QSAR-type modelling [81]. The integration of peptide features from heterogeneous sources e.g., from pairwise alignments and peptide sequences into the same classifier could be another outlook for improving the classification rates of AMPs. The main problem is to figure out a framework to integrate them (the resulting features, not the source methodologies) into ML models training. As a clue for future research directions, the alignment- based and -free similarity measures were successfully integrated for training bigdata ML-based classifiers for orthologs detection [79]. Bigdata solutions applied to the prediction/optimization of AMPs have not been explored yet in spite of the fact that the number of AMPs has grown in databases as well as the number of features/descriptors that can be derived from them. Bigdata platforms could be applied when performing virtual screening of millions of peptides, especially if they are described with computationally demanding structural descriptors. As previously mentioned, it would be advisable that future ML models for the AMP prediction could consider the natural imbalance ratio between AMPs and non-AMPs as well as the existing one among the AMPs activities. Moreover, the prediction of AMPs activities should be addressed with fuzzy-based models since they generally show overlapping activities which are not evenly-distributed within the AMP population [23]. Therefore, the resulting predictions for AMPs activities may be scored with probability values and not only treated as a binary value. On the other hand, for peptide leads optimization, the offspring generation step is crucial for the overall process. This step generally is carried out by evolutionary algorithms that introduce structural diversity among child peptides somewhat randomly. Although these AI-based algorithms have been continuously evolving to guide such diversity in order to gain optimization efficiency; there is still room for improvements in this direction. Thus, the algorithms commonly used in phylogenetics for simulating sequence evolution could provide more rationality to the generation of offspring peptides since they have been designed with more evolutionary parameters that can be strictly controlled [52,76].

Finally, StarPep is probably the most promising methodology regardless of ML approaches, that has been reported so far. The complex network theory implemented in this tool has provided a different outlook to address several steps in peptide drug discovery process. StarPep bears particular analysis tools that have not previously reported for peptides, such as (*i*) the chemical space analysis of AMP databases by similarity networks, (*ii*) the identification of the most representative and non-redundant subset of AMPs from the original chemical space, (*iii*) the mapping of unlabelled peptide datasets on similarity networks built with the representative AMPs (*iv*) the multi-query similarity searches using representative peptides against target databases. Consequently, StarPep is becoming in a competing tool to the existing ML-based methods since it has being giving clues of improved classification rates [49,50], and because of its great potentialities for the identification and optimization of new peptide leads from either in silico generated peptide libraries or released data by the Omics techniques (Figure 11).

The effort of StarPepDB developers to gather all AMP databases in a non-redundant database [124] has shown a direct impact for the AMPs prediction tools [31]. However, the annotation quality for the reported AMPs must still be improved as well as the information on their biological or molecular targets. It is urgent that AMPs activity evaluations can be harmonized under the same protocols to construct more reliable benchmark datasets for the accuracy sake of the computational analysis tools. The diverse computational methods available for AMPs discovery are a powerful tool for the accurate design of peptide drugs. The growing availability of 3D structural descriptors and scoring functions will allow developing more effective in silico peptide drug design technologies. The assembling of ML methods with peptide-protein docking and molecular dynamics seems to be an effective alternative as well [178]. If all these aspects were considered for the computational-assisted search/design of peptide drugs, the next-generation of AMP leads will be more valuable for developing therapeutic agents to face challenging health problems such as cancer, infectious diseases and more recently, COVID-19.

Supplementary Materials: The following are available online at https://www.mdpi.com/article/10.3390/antibiotics11070936/s1. File S1—Additional data relative to the analysis of the Chemical Space Network built with Anti-Biofilm Peptides (ABPs) from StarPepDB. File SI1-A—Metadata associated to ABPs. SI1-B—Node properties of the 174 ABPs embedded in the similarity network representing the ABPs chemical space. SI1-C—More central ABPs according to network centrality measures. SI1-D—ABPs selected as queries for multi-query similarity searches.

Author Contributions: G.A.-C. and A.A. designed and structured the overall review as well as drafted the initial manuscript. D.G.-C. analyzed emerging ML algorithms for the AMP prediction. D.D.-P. gathered the new considerations in OMICs analysis/workflow for the biodiscovery of AMPs. Y.M.-P. worked on the conceptualizing of the complex networks and similarity searching methods applied to AMPs discovery. G.P.-M. and M.T. looked for the non-standard peptide features used for AMPs prediction. G.A-C. reviewed the application of algorithms simulating sequence evolution to peptide drug design. G.A.-C., D.G.-C. and A.A. participated in the review-edition of the manuscript All authors have read and agreed to the published version of the manuscript.

Funding: Yovani Marero-Ponce was supported by the USFQ Collaboration Grant (Project ID16885). This research was supported in part by the Strategic Funding UIDB/04423/2020 and UIDP/04423/2020 through national funds provided by FCT and the European Regional Development Fund (ERDF) in the framework of the program PT2020, by the European Structural and Investment Funds (ESIF) through the Competitiveness and Internationalization Operational Program—COMPETE 2020 and by National Funds through the FCT under the project PTDC/CTA-AMB/31774/2017 (POCI-01-0145-FEDER/031774/2017).

Institutional Review Board Statement: Not applicable.

Informed Consent Statement: Not applicable.

Data Availability Statement: Not applicable.

Conflicts of Interest: The authors declare no conflict of interest. The funders had no role in the design of the study; in the collection, analyses, or interpretation of data; in the writing of the manuscript, or in the decision to publish the results.

References

1. Murray, C.J.; Ikuta, K.S.; Sharara, F.; Swetschinski, L.; Aguilar, G.R.; Gray, A.; Han, C.; Bisignano, C.; Rao, P.; Wool, E.; et al. Global burden of bacterial antimicrobial resistance in 2019: A systematic analysis. *Lancet* **2022**, *399*, 629–655. [CrossRef]
2. Fair, R.J.; Tor, Y. Antibiotics and Bacterial Resistance in the 21st Century. *Perspect. Med. Chem.* **2014**, *6*, S14459. [CrossRef] [PubMed]
3. Yeaman, M.R.; Yount, N.Y. Mechanisms of Antimicrobial Peptide Action and Resistance. *Pharmacol. Rev.* **2003**, *55*, 27–55. [CrossRef] [PubMed]
4. Guevara Agudelo, A.; Muñoz Molina, M.; Navarrete Ospina, J.; Salazar Pulido, L.; Castro-Cardozo, B. New Horizons to Survive in a Post-Antibiotics Era. *J. Trop Med. Health* **2018**, *10*, JTMH-130. [CrossRef]

5. Breijyeh, Z.; Jubeh, B.; Karaman, R. Resistance of Gram-Negative Bacteria to Current Antibacterial Agents and Approaches to Resolve It. *Molecules* **2020**, *25*, 1340. [CrossRef]
6. Gohel, V.; Kamal, A. Peptides as Potential Anticancer Agents. *Curr. Top. Med. Chem.* **2019**, *19*, 1491–1511. [CrossRef]
7. Schütz, D.; Ruiz-Blanco, Y.B.; Münch, J.; Kirchhoff, F.; Sanchez-Garcia, E.; Müller, J.A. Peptide and peptide-based inhibitors of SARS-CoV-2 entry. *Adv. Drug Deliv. Rev.* **2020**, *167*, 47–65. [CrossRef]
8. Zhang, L.-J.; Gallo, R.L. Antimicrobial peptides. *Curr. Biol.* **2016**, *26*, R14–R19. [CrossRef]
9. Porto, W.F.; Pires, A.S.; Franco, O.L. Computational tools for exploring sequence databases as a resource for antimicrobial peptides. *Biotechnol. Adv.* **2017**, *35*, 337–349. [CrossRef]
10. Sundararajan, V.S.; Gabere, M.N.; Pretorius, A.; Adam, S.; Christoffels, A.; Lehväslaiho, M.; Archer, J.A.C.; Bajic, V.B. DAMPD: A manually curated antimicrobial peptide database. *Nucleic Acids Res.* **2011**, *40*, D1108–D1112. [CrossRef]
11. Waghu, F.H.; Barai, R.S.; Gurung, P.; Idicula-Thomas, S. CAMP R3: A database on sequences, structures and signatures of antimicrobial peptides: Table 1. *Nucleic Acids Res.* **2016**, *44*, D1094–D1097. Available online: http://www.ncbi.nlm.nih.gov/pubmed/26467475 (accessed on 23 January 2019). [CrossRef] [PubMed]
12. Zhao, X.; Wu, H.; Lu, H.; Li, G.; Huang, Q. LAMP: A Database Linking Antimicrobial Peptides. *PLoS ONE* **2013**, *8*, e66557. [CrossRef] [PubMed]
13. Fan, L.; Sun, J.; Zhou, M.; Zhou, J.; Lao, X.; Zheng, H.; Xu, H. DRAMP: A comprehensive data repository of antimicrobial peptides. *Sci. Rep.* **2016**, *6*, 24482. [CrossRef] [PubMed]
14. Lee, H.-T.; Lee, C.-C.; Yang, J.-R.; Lai, J.Z.C.; Chang, K.Y. A Large-Scale Structural Classification of Antimicrobial Peptides. *BioMed Res. Int.* **2015**, *2015*, 1–6. [CrossRef]
15. Pirtskhalava, M.; Amstrong, A.A.; Grigolava, M.; Chubinidze, M.; Alimbarashvili, E.; Vishnepolsky, B.; Gabrielian, A.; Rosenthal, A.; Hurt, D.E.; Tartakovsky, M. DBAASP v3: Database of antimicrobial/cytotoxic activity and structure of peptides as a resource for development of new therapeutics. *Nucleic Acids Res.* **2021**, *49*, D288–D297. [CrossRef]
16. Meher, P.K.; Sahu, T.K.; Saini, V.; Rao, A.R. Predicting antimicrobial peptides with improved accuracy by incorporating the compositional, physico-chemical and structural features into Chou's general PseAAC. *Sci. Rep.* **2017**, *7*, srep42362. [CrossRef]
17. Spänig, S.; Heider, D. Encodings and models for antimicrobial peptide classification for multi-resistant pathogens. *BioData Min.* **2019**, *12*, 7. [CrossRef]
18. Xu, J.; Li, F.; Leier, A.; Xiang, D.; Shen, H.-H.; Lago, T.T.M.; Li, J.; Yu, D.-J.; Song, J. Comprehensive assessment of machine learning-based methods for predicting antimicrobial peptides. *Briefings Bioinform.* **2021**, *22*, bbab083. [CrossRef]
19. Veltri, D.; Kamath, U.; Shehu, A. Deep learning improves antimicrobial peptide recognition. *Bioinformatics* **2018**, *34*, 2740–2747. [CrossRef]
20. Yi, H.-C.; You, Z.-H.; Zhou, X.; Cheng, L.; Li, X.; Jiang, T.-H.; Chen, Z.-H. ACP-DL: A Deep Learning Long Short-Term Memory Model to Predict Anticancer Peptides Using High-Efficiency Feature Representation. *Mol. Ther.-Nucleic Acids* **2019**, *17*, 1–9. [CrossRef]
21. Chen, J.; Cheong, H.H.; Siu, S.W.I. xDeep-AcPEP: Deep Learning Method for Anticancer Peptide Activity Prediction Based on Convolutional Neural Network and Multitask Learning. *J. Chem. Inf. Model.* **2021**, *61*, 3789–3803. [CrossRef] [PubMed]
22. Boone, K.; Camarda, K.; Spencer, P.; Tamerler, C. Antimicrobial peptide similarity and classification through rough set theory using physicochemical boundaries. *BMC Bioinform.* **2018**, *19*, 1–10. [CrossRef] [PubMed]
23. Chharia, A.; Upadhyay, R.; Kumar, V. Novel fuzzy approach to Antimicrobial Peptide Activity Prediction: A tale of limited and imbalanced data that models won't hear; 2021. In Proceedings of the NeurIPS 2021 AI for Science Workshop, Vancouver, BC, Canada, 13 December 2021.
24. Wang, G.; Li, X.; Wang, Z. APD3: The antimicrobial peptide database as a tool for research and education. *Nucleic Acids Res.* **2016**, *44*, D1087–D1093. [CrossRef]
25. Chou, K.-C. Prediction of protein cellular attributes using pseudo-amino acid composition. *Proteins: Struct. Funct. Bioinform.* **2001**, *43*, 246–255. [CrossRef]
26. Xiao, X.; Wang, P.; Lin, W.-Z.; Jia, J.-H.; Chou, K.-C. iAMP-2L: A two-level multi-label classifier for identifying antimicrobial peptides and their functional types. *Anal. Biochem.* **2013**, *436*, 168–177. [CrossRef] [PubMed]
27. Lin, W.; Xu, D. Imbalanced multi-label learning for identifying antimicrobial peptides and their functional types. *Bioinformatics* **2016**, *32*, 3745–3752. [CrossRef]
28. Gull, S.; Shamim, N.; Minhas, F. AMAP: Hierarchical multi-label prediction of biologically active and antimicrobial peptides. *Comput. Biol. Med.* **2019**, *107*, 172–181. [CrossRef]
29. Chen, T.; Guestrin, C. XGBoost: A Scalable Tree Boosting System. In Proceedings of the 22nd ACM SIGKDD International Conference on Knowledge Discovery and Data Mining, San Francisco, CA, USA, 13–17 August 2016; pp. 785–794.
30. Chung, C.-R.; Kuo, T.-R.; Wu, L.-C.; Lee, T.-Y.; Horng, J.-T. Characterization and identification of antimicrobial peptides with different functional activities. *Brief. Bioinform.* **2019**, *21*, 1098–1114. [CrossRef]
31. Pinacho-Castellanos, S.A.; García-Jacas, C.R.; Gilson, M.K.; Brizuela, C.A. Alignment-Free Antimicrobial Peptide Predictors: Improving Performance by a Thorough Analysis of the Largest Available Data Set. *J. Chem. Inf. Model.* **2021**, *61*, 3141–3157. [CrossRef]
32. Ruiz-Blanco, Y.B.; Paz, W.; Green, J.; Marrero-Ponce, Y. ProtDCal: A program to compute general-purpose-numerical descriptors for sequences and 3D-structures of proteins. *BMC Bioinform.* **2015**, *16*, 162. [CrossRef]

33. Aguilera-Mendoza, L.; Marrero-Ponce, Y.; García-Jacas, C.R.; Chavez, E.; Beltran, J.A.; Guillen-Ramirez, H.A.; Brizuela, C.A. Automatic construction of molecular similarity networks for visual graph mining in chemical space of bioactive peptides: An unsupervised learning approach. *Sci. Rep.* **2020**, *10*, 1–23. [CrossRef]
34. Kavousi, K.; Bagheri, M.; Behrouzi, S.; Vafadar, S.; Atanaki, F.F.; Lotfabadi, B.T.; Ariaeenejad, S.; Shockravi, A.; Moosavi-Movahedi, A.A. IAMPE: NMR-Assisted Computational Prediction of Antimicrobial Peptides. *J. Chem. Inf. Model.* **2020**, *60*, 4691–4701. [CrossRef] [PubMed]
35. Joseph, S.; Karnik, S.; Nilawe, P.; Jayaraman, V.K.; Idicula-Thomas, S. ClassAMP: A Prediction Tool for Classification of Antimicrobial Peptides. *IEEE/ACM Trans. Comput. Biol. Bioinform.* **2012**, *9*, 1535–1538. [CrossRef]
36. Bhadra, P.; Yan, J.; Li, J.; Fong, S.; Siu, S.W.I. AmPEP: Sequence-based prediction of antimicrobial peptides using distribution patterns of amino acid properties and random forest. *Sci. Rep.* **2018**, *8*, 1–10. [CrossRef]
37. Lawrence, T.J.; Carper, D.L.; Spangler, M.K.; Carrell, A.A.; Rush, T.A.; Minter, S.J.; Weston, D.J.; Labbe, J.L. amPEPpy 1.0: A portable and accurate antimicrobial peptide prediction tool. *Bioinformatics* **2021**, *37*, 2058–2060. [CrossRef] [PubMed]
38. Veltri, D.P. A Computational and Statistical Framework for Screening Novel Antimicrobial Peptides. Ph.D. Thesis, George Mason University, Fairfax County, VA, USA, 2015.
39. García-Jacas, C.R.; Pinacho-Castellanos, S.A.; García-González, L.A.; Brizuela, C.A. Do deep learning models make a difference in the identification of antimicrobial peptides? *Brief. Bioinform.* **2022**, *23*, bbac094. [CrossRef]
40. Wong, K.-C. Evolutionary algorithms: Concepts, designs, and applications in bioinformatics. In *Nature-Inspired Computing: Concepts, Methodologies, Tools, and Applications*; IGI Global: Hershey, PA, USA, 2017; pp. 111–137.
41. Bozovičar, K.; Bratkovič, T. Evolving a Peptide: Library Platforms and Diversification Strategies. *Int. J. Mol. Sci.* **2019**, *21*, 215. [CrossRef]
42. Yoshida, M.; Hinkley, T.; Tsuda, S.; Abul-Haija, Y.; McBurney, R.T.; Kulikov, V.; Mathieson, J.S.; Reyes, S.G.; Castro, M.D.; Cronin, L. Using Evolutionary Algorithms and Machine Learning to Explore Sequence Space for the Discovery of Antimicrobial Peptides. *Chem* **2018**, *4*, 533–543. [CrossRef]
43. Barigye, S.J.; Garcia de la Vega, J.M.; Perez-Castillo, Y.; Castillo-Garit, J.A. Evolutionary algorithm-based generation of optimum peptide sequences with dengue virus inhibitory activity. *Future Med. Chem.* **2021**, *13*, 993–1000. [CrossRef]
44. Fjell, C.D.; Jenssen, H.; Cheung, W.; Hancock, R.; Cherkasov, A. Optimization of Antibacterial Peptides by Genetic Algorithms and Cheminformatics. *Chem. Biol. Drug Des.* **2010**, *77*, 48–56. [CrossRef]
45. Fjell, C.D.; Hiss, J.A.; Hancock, R.E.W.; Schneider, G. Designing antimicrobial peptides: Form follows function. *Nat. Rev. Drug Discov.* **2011**, *11*, 37–51. [CrossRef]
46. Aronica, P.G.; Reid, L.M.; Desai, N.; Li, J.; Fox, S.J.; Yadahalli, S.; Essex, J.W.; Verma, C.S. Computational Methods and Tools in Antimicrobial Peptide Research. *J. Chem. Inf. Model.* **2021**, *61*, 3172–3196. [CrossRef]
47. Ng, X.Y.; Rosdi, B.A.; Shahrudin, S. Prediction of Antimicrobial Peptides Based on Sequence Alignment and Support Vector Machine-Pairwise Algorithm Utilizing LZ-Complexity. *BioMed Res. Int.* **2015**, *2015*, 1–13. [CrossRef]
48. Boone, K.; Wisdom, C.; Camarda, K.; Spencer, P.; Tamerler, C. Combining genetic algorithm with machine learning strategies for designing potent antimicrobial peptides. *BMC Bioinform.* **2021**, *22*, 1–17. [CrossRef]
49. Ayala-Ruano, S.; Marrero-Ponce, Y.; Aguilera-Mendoza, L.; Pérez, N.; Agüero-Chapin, G.; Antunes, A.; Aguilar, A.C. Exploring the Chemical Space of Antiparasitic Peptides and Discovery of New Promising Leads through a Novel Approach based on Network Science and Similarity Searching. *ChemRxiv* **2021**. [CrossRef]
50. Romero, M.; Marrero-Ponce, Y.; Rodríguez, H.; Agüero-Chapin, G.; Antunes, A.; Aguilera-Mendoza, L.; Martinez-Rios, F. A Novel Network Science and Similarity-Searching-Based Approach for Discovering Potential Tumor-Homing Peptides from Antimicrobials. *Antibiotics* **2022**, *11*, 401. [CrossRef]
51. Neuhaus, C.S.; Gabernet, G.; Steuer, C.; Root, K.; Hiss, J.A.; Zenobi, R.; Schneider, G. Simulated Molecular Evolution for Anticancer Peptide Design. *Angew. Chem. Int. Ed.* **2018**, *58*, 1674–1678. [CrossRef]
52. Ruiz-Blanco, Y.B.; Ávila-Barrientos, L.P.; Hernández-García, E.; Antunes, A.; Agüero-Chapin, G.; García-Hernández, E. Engineering protein fragments via evolutionary and protein–protein interaction algorithms: De novo design of peptide inhibitors for $F_O F_1$-ATP synthase. *FEBS Lett.* **2020**, *595*, 183–194. [CrossRef]
53. Matos, A.; Domínguez-Pérez, D.; Almeida, D.; Agüero-Chapin, G.; Campos, A.; Osório, H.; Vasconcelos, V.; Antunes, A. Shotgun Proteomics of Ascidians Tunic Gives New Insights on Host–Microbe Interactions by Revealing Diverse Antimicrobial Peptides. *Mar. Drugs* **2020**, *18*, 362. [CrossRef] [PubMed]
54. Almeida, D.; Domínguez-Pérez, D.; Matos, A.; Agüero-Chapin, G.; Osório, H.; Vasconcelos, V.; Campos, A.; Antunes, A. Putative Antimicrobial Peptides of the Posterior Salivary Glands from the Cephalopod *Octopus vulgaris* Revealed by Exploring a Composite Protein Database. *Antibiotics* **2020**, *9*, 757. [CrossRef]
55. Agüero-Chapin, G.; Pérez-Machado, G.; Molina-Ruiz, R.; Pérez-Castillo, Y.; Morales-Helguera, A.; Vasconcelos, V.; Antunes, A. TI2BioP: Topological Indices to BioPolymers. Its practical use to unravel cryptic bacteriocin-like domains. *Amino Acids* **2010**, *40*, 431–442. [CrossRef] [PubMed]
56. Speck-Planche, A.; Kleandrova, V.V.; Ruso, J.M.; Cordeiro, M.N.D.S. First Multitarget Chemo-Bioinformatic Model To Enable the Discovery of Antibacterial Peptides against Multiple Gram-Positive Pathogens. *J. Chem. Inf. Model.* **2016**, *56*, 588–598. [CrossRef] [PubMed]

57. De Armas, R.R.; Díaz, H.G.; Molina, R.; González, M.P.; Uriarte, E. Stochastic-based descriptors studying peptides biological properties: Modeling the bitter tasting threshold of dipeptides. *Bioorganic Med. Chem.* **2004**, *12*, 4815–4822. [CrossRef] [PubMed]
58. Kleandrova, V.V.; Ruso, J.M.; Speck-Planche, A.; Cordeiro, M.N.D.S. Enabling the Discovery and Virtual Screening of Potent and Safe Antimicrobial Peptides. Simultaneous Prediction of Antibacterial Activity and Cytotoxicity. *ACS Comb. Sci.* **2016**, *18*, 490–498. [CrossRef]
59. Estrada, E. Spectral Moments of the Edge Adjacency Matrix in Molecular Graphs. 1. Definition and Applications to the Prediction of Physical Properties of Alkanes. *J. Chem. Inf. Comput. Sci.* **1996**, *36*, 844–849. [CrossRef]
60. Mauri, A.; Consonni, V.; Pavan, M.; Todeschini, R. Dragon software: An easy approach to molecular descriptor calculations. *Match* **2006**, *56*, 237–248.
61. Agüero-Chapin, G.; Molina-Ruiz, R.; Pérez-Machado, G.; Vasconcelos, V.; Rodríguez-Negrin, Z.; Antunes, A. TI2BioP—Topological Indices to BioPolymers. A Graphical–Numerical Approach for Bioinformatics. In *Recent Advances in Biopolymers*; IntechOpen: Zagreb, Croatia, 2016.
62. González-Díaz, H.; González-Díaz, Y.; Santana, L.; Ubeira, F.M.; Uriarte, E.; González-Díaz, H. Proteomics, networks and connectivity indices. *Proteomics* **2008**, *8*, 750–778. [CrossRef]
63. Wiener, H. Structural Determination of Paraffin Boiling Points. *J. Am. Chem. Soc.* **1947**, *69*, 17–20. [CrossRef]
64. Randić, M. Graph theoretical approach to structure-activity studies: Search for optimal antitumor compounds. *Prog. Clin. Biol. Res.* **1985**, *172*, 309–318.
65. Moreau, G.; Broto, P. The Autocorrelation of a topological structure. A new molecular descriptor. *Nouv. J. Chim.* **1980**, *4*, 359–360.
66. Balaban, A.T.; Beteringhe, A.; Constantinescu, T.; Filip, P.A.; Ivanciuc, O. Four New Topological Indices Based on the Molecular Path Code. *J. Chem. Inf. Model.* **2007**, *47*, 716–731. [CrossRef]
67. Hall, P.R.; Malone, L.; Sillerud, L.O.; Ye, C.; Hjelle, B.L.; Larson, R.S. Characterization and NMR Solution Structure of a Novel Cyclic Pentapeptide Inhibitor of Pathogenic Hantaviruses. *Chem. Biol. Drug Des.* **2007**, *69*, 180–190. [CrossRef]
68. Kier, L.B.; Hall, L.H. An Electrotopological-State Index for Atoms in Molecules. *Pharm. Res.* **1990**, *07*, 801–807. [CrossRef]
69. Ivanciuc, O. Building–Block Computation of the Ivanciuc–Balaban Indices for the Virtual Screening of Combinatorial Libraries. *Internet Electron. J. Mol. Des.* **2002**, *1*, 1–9.
70. Todeschini, R.; Consonni, V. *Handbook of Molecular Descriptors*, 1st ed.; Wiley-VCH: Mannheim, Germany, 2000; Volume 1, p. 667.
71. Estrada, E. Characterization of the folding degree of proteins. *Bioinformatics* **2002**, *18*, 697–704. [CrossRef]
72. Estrada, E. Characterization of the amino acid contribution to the folding degree of proteins. *Proteins: Struct. Funct. Bioinform.* **2004**, *54*, 727–737. [CrossRef]
73. Sandberg, M.; Eriksson, L.; Jonsson, J.; Sjöström, A.M.; Wold, S. New Chemical Descriptors Relevant for the Design of Biologically Active Peptides. A Multivariate Characterization of 87 Amino Acids. *J. Med. Chem.* **1998**, *41*, 2481–2491. [CrossRef]
74. Quevillon, E.; Silventoinen, V.; Pillai, S.; Harte, N.; Mulder, N.; Apweiler, R.; Lopez, R. InterProScan: Protein domains identifier. *Nucleic Acids Res.* **2005**, *33*, W116–W120. [CrossRef]
75. Molina, R.; Agüero-Chapin, G.; Pérez-González, M. *TI2BioP (Topological Indices to BioPolymers) Version 2.0*; Molecular Simulation and Drug Design (MSDD): Chemical Bioactives Center, Central University of Las Villas, Santa Clara, Cuba, 2011.
76. Avila-Barrientos, L.P.; Cofas-Vargas, L.F.; Agüero-Chapin, G.; Hernández-García, E.; Ruiz-Carmona, S.; Valdez-Cruz, N.A.; Trujillo-Roldán, M.; Weber, J.; Ruiz-Blanco, Y.B.; Barril, X.; et al. Computational Design of Inhibitors Targeting the Catalytic β Subunit of Escherichia coli FOF1-ATP Synthase. *Antibiotics* **2022**, *11*, 557. [CrossRef]
77. Romero-Molina, S.; Ruiz-Blanco, Y.B.; Harms, M.; Münch, J.; Sanchez-Garcia, E. PPI-Detect: A support vector machine model for sequence-based prediction of protein-protein interactions. *J. Comput. Chem.* **2019**, *40*, 1233–1242. [CrossRef]
78. Aguilera-Mendoza, L.; Marrero-Ponce, Y.; Beltran, J.A.; Tellez Ibarra, R.; Guillen-Ramirez, H.A.; Brizuela, C.A. Graph-based data integration from bioactive peptide databases of pharmaceutical interest: Toward an organized collection enabling visual network analysis. *Bioinformatics* **2019**, *35*, 4739–4747. [CrossRef]
79. Galpert, D.; Fernández, A.; Herrera, F.; Antunes, A.; Molina-Ruiz, R.; Agüero-Chapin, G. Surveying alignment-free features for Ortholog detection in related yeast proteomes by using supervised big data classifiers. *BMC Bioinform.* **2018**, *19*, 166. [CrossRef]
80. Agüero-Chapin, G.; Molina-Ruiz, R.; Maldonado, E.; de la Riva, G.; Sánchez-Rodríguez, A.; Vasconcelos, V.; Antunes, A. Exploring the adenylation domain repertoire of nonribosomal peptide synthetases using an ensemble of sequence-search methods. *PLoS ONE* **2013**, *8*, e65926. [CrossRef]
81. Agüero-Chapin, G.; Galpert, D.; Molina-Ruiz, R.; Ancede-Gallardo, E.; Pérez-Machado, G.; De la Riva, G.A.; Antunes, A. Graph Theory-Based Sequence Descriptors as Remote Homology Predictors. *Biomolecules* **2019**, *10*, 26. [CrossRef]
82. Borozan, I.; Watt, S.; Ferretti, V. Integrating alignment-based and alignment-free sequence similarity measures for biological sequence classification. *Bioinformatics* **2015**, *31*, 1396–1404. [CrossRef]
83. Empel, A.; Ziv, J. On the complexity of finite sequences. *IEEE Trans. Inf. Theory* **1976**, *22*, 75–81. [CrossRef]
84. Wang, P.; Hu, L.; Liu, G.; Jiang, N.; Chen, X.; Xu, J.; Zheng, W.; Li, L.; Tan, M.; Chen, Z.; et al. Prediction of Antimicrobial Peptides Based on Sequence Alignment and Feature Selection Methods. *PLoS ONE* **2011**, *6*, e18476. [CrossRef]
85. Peng, H.; Long, F.; Ding, C. Feature selection based on mutual information criteria of max-dependency, max-relevance, and min-redundancy. *IEEE Trans. Pattern Anal. Mach. Intell.* **2005**, *27*, 1226–1238. [CrossRef]
86. Kohavi, R.; John, G.H. Wrappers for feature subset selection. *Artif. Intell.* **1997**, *97*, 273–324. [CrossRef]

87. Lin, Y.; Cai, Y.; Liu, J.; Lin, C.; Liu, X. An advanced approach to identify antimicrobial peptides and their function types for penaeus through machine learning strategies. *BMC Bioinform.* **2019**, *20*, 1–10. [CrossRef]
88. Pang, Y.; Wang, Z.; Jhong, J.-H.; Lee, T.-Y. Identifying anti-coronavirus peptides by incorporating different negative datasets and imbalanced learning strategies. *Brief. Bioinform.* **2021**, *22*, 1085–1095. [CrossRef]
89. Lertampaiporn, S.; Vorapreeda, T.; Hongsthong, A.; Thammarongtham, C. Ensemble-AMPPred: Robust AMP Prediction and Recognition Using the Ensemble Learning Method with a New Hybrid Feature for Differentiating AMPs. *Genes* **2021**, *12*, 137. [CrossRef]
90. Yu, Q.; Dong, Z.; Fan, X.; Zong, L.; Li, Y. HMD-AMP: Protein Language-Powered Hierarchical Multi-label Deep Forest for Annotating Antimicrobial Peptides. *bioRxiv* **2021**. [CrossRef]
91. Chen, X.; Li, C.; Bernards, M.T.; Shi, Y.; Shao, Q.; He, Y. Sequence-based peptide identification, generation, and property prediction with deep learning: A review. *Mol. Syst. Des. Eng.* **2021**, *6*, 406–428. [CrossRef]
92. Wan, F.; Kontogiorgos-Heintz, D.; de la Fuente-Nunez, C. Deep generative models for peptide design. *Digit. Discov.* **2022**, *1*, 195–208. [CrossRef]
93. Das, P.; Sercu, T.; Wadhawan, K.; Padhi, I.; Gehrmann, S.; Cipcigan, F.; Chenthamarakshan, V.; Strobelt, H.; dos Santos, C.; Chen, P.-Y.; et al. Accelerated antimicrobial discovery via deep generative models and molecular dynamics simulations. *Nat. Biomed. Eng.* **2021**, *5*, 613–623. [CrossRef]
94. Van Oort, C.M.; Ferrell, J.B.; Remington, J.M.; Wshah, S.; Li, J. AMPGAN v2: Machine Learning-Guided Design of Antimicrobial Peptides. *J. Chem. Inf. Model.* **2021**, *61*, 2198–2207. [CrossRef]
95. Das, P.; Wadhawan, K.; Chang, O.; Sercu, T.; Santos, C.N.D.; Riemer, M.; Padhi, I.; Chenthamarakshan, V.; Mojsilovic, A. PepCVAE: Semi-Supervised Targeted Design of Antimicrobial Peptide Sequences. *arXiv* **2018**, arXiv:1810.07743.
96. Dean, S.N. Variational Autoencoder for the Generation of New Antimicrobial Peptides. *ACS Omega* **2021**, *5*, 20746–20754. [CrossRef]
97. Witten, J.; Witten, Z. Deep learning regression model for antimicrobial peptide design. *bioRxiv* **2019**. [CrossRef]
98. Lee, B.; Shin, M.K.; Hwang, I.-W.; Jung, J.; Shim, Y.J.; Kim, G.W.; Kim, S.T.; Jang, W.; Sung, J.-S. A Deep Learning Approach with Data Augmentation to Predict Novel Spider Neurotoxic Peptides. *Int. J. Mol. Sci.* **2021**, *22*, 12291. [CrossRef]
99. Wang, C.; Garlick, S.; Zloh, M. Deep Learning for Novel Antimicrobial Peptide Design. *Biomolecules* **2021**, *11*, 471. [CrossRef] [PubMed]
100. Bin Hafeez, A.; Jiang, X.; Bergen, P.J.; Zhu, Y. Antimicrobial Peptides: An Update on Classifications and Databases. *Int. J. Mol. Sci.* **2021**, *22*, 11691. [CrossRef] [PubMed]
101. Yan, J.; Bhadra, P.; Li, A.; Sethiya, P.; Qin, L.; Tai, H.K.; Wong, K.H.; Siu, S.W. Deep-AmPEP30: Improve Short Antimicrobial Peptides Prediction with Deep Learning. *Mol. Ther.-Nucleic Acids* **2020**, *20*, 882–894. [CrossRef] [PubMed]
102. Babgi, B.A.; Alsayari, J.H.; Davaasuren, B.; Emwas, A.-H.; Jaremko, M.; Abdellattif, M.H.; Hussien, M.A. Synthesis, structural studies, and anticancer properties of [CuBr (PPh3) 2 (4,6-dimethyl-2-thiopyrimidine-S]. *Crystals* **2021**, *11*, 688. [CrossRef]
103. Altschul, S.F.; Madden, T.L.; Schäffer, A.A.; Zhang, J.; Zhang, Z.; Miller, W.; Lipman, D.J. Gapped BLAST and PSI-BLAST: A new generation of protein database search programs. *Nucleic Acids Res.* **1997**, *25*, 3389–3402. [CrossRef]
104. Pearson, W.R. Rapid and sensitive sequence comparison with FASTP and FASTA. *Methods Enzymol.* **1990**, *183*, 63–98. [CrossRef]
105. Hammami, R.; Zouhir, A.; Ben Hamida, J.; Fliss, I. BACTIBASE: A new web-accessible database for bacteriocin characterization. *BMC Microbiol.* **2007**, *7*, 89. [CrossRef]
106. De Jong, A.; Van Hijum, S.A.F.T.; Bijlsma, J.J.E.; Kok, J.; Kuipers, O.P. BAGEL: A web based bacteriocin genome mining tool. *Nucleic Acids Res.* **2006**, *34*, W273–W279. [CrossRef]
107. Mulvenna, J.; Mylne, J.; Bharathi, R.; Burton, R.; Shirley, N.; Fincher, G.B.; Anderson, M.; Craik, D.J. Discovery of Cyclotide-Like Protein Sequences in Graminaceous Crop Plants: Ancestral Precursors of Circular Proteins? *Plant Cell* **2006**, *18*, 2134–2144. [CrossRef]
108. Porto, W.F.; Silva, O.N.; Franco, O.L. Prediction and rational design of antimicrobial peptides. In *Protein Structure*; IntechOpen: Zagreb, Croatia, 2012.
109. Eddy, S.R. Profile hidden Markov models. *Bioinformatics* **1998**, *14*, 755–763. [CrossRef]
110. Thompson, K. Programming Techniques: Regular expression search algorithm. *Commun. ACM* **1968**, *11*, 419–422. [CrossRef]
111. Jonassen, I. Efficient discovery of conserved patterns using a pattern graph. *Comput. Appl. Biosci.* **1997**, *13*, 509–522. [CrossRef]
112. Finn, R.D.; Clements, J.; Eddy, S.R. HMMER web server: Interactive sequence similarity searching. *Nucleic Acids Res.* **2011**, *39*, W29–W37. [CrossRef]
113. Sigrist, C.J.A.; de Castro, E.; Cerutti, L.; Cuche, B.A.; Hulo, N.; Bridge, A.; Bougueleret, L.; Xenarios, I. New and continuing developments at PROSITE. *Nucleic Acids Res.* **2012**, *41*, D344–D347. [CrossRef]
114. El-Gebali, S.; Mistry, J.; Bateman, A.; Eddy, S.R.; Luciani, A.; Potter, S.C.; Qureshi, M.; Richardson, L.J.; Salazar, G.A.; Smart, A.; et al. The Pfam protein families database in 2019. *Nucleic Acids Res.* **2019**, *47*, D427–D432. [CrossRef]
115. Hammami, R.; Zouhir, A.; Le Lay, C.; Ben Hamida, J.; Fliss, I. BACTIBASE second release: A database and tool platform for bacteriocin characterization. *BMC Microbiol.* **2010**, *10*, 22. [CrossRef]
116. Fjell, C.D.; Hancock, R.E.W.; Cherkasov, A. AMPer: A database and an automated discovery tool for antimicrobial peptides. *Bioinformatics* **2007**, *23*, 1148–1155. [CrossRef]

117. Jones, P.; Binns, D.; Chang, H.-Y.; Fraser, M.; Li, W.; McAnulla, C.; McWilliam, H.; Maslen, J.; Mitchell, A.; Nuka, G.; et al. InterProScan 5: Genome-scale protein function classification. *Bioinformatics* **2014**, *30*, 1236–1240. [CrossRef]
118. Gille, C.; Goede, A.; Preißner, R.; Rother, K.; Frömmel, C. Conservation of substructures in proteins: Interfaces of secondary structural elements in proteasomal subunits. *J. Mol. Biol.* **2000**, *299*, 1147–1154. [CrossRef]
119. Lee, J.; Wu, S.; Zhang, Y. Ab Initio Protein Structure Prediction. In *From Protein Structure to Function with Bioinformatics*; Rigden, D.J., Ed.; Springer: Dordrecht, The Netherlands, 2009; pp. 3–25.
120. Eswar, N.; Webb, B.; Marti-Renom, M.A.; Madhusudhan, M.; Eramian, D.; Shen, M.y.; Pieper, U.; Sali, A. Comparative protein structure modeling using Modeller. *Curr. Protoc. Bioinform.* **2006**, *15*, 5–6. [CrossRef]
121. Hammami, R.; Fliss, I. Current trends in antimicrobial agent research: Chemo- and bioinformatics approaches. *Drug Discov. Today* **2010**, *15*, 540–546. [CrossRef]
122. Torrent, M.; Di Tommaso, P.; Pulido, D.; Nogués, M.V.; Notredame, C.; Boix, E.; Andreu, D. AMPA: An automated web server for prediction of protein antimicrobial regions. *Bioinformatics* **2011**, *28*, 130–131. [CrossRef]
123. Notredame, C.; Higgins, D.; Heringa, J. T-coffee: A novel method for fast and accurate multiple sequence alignment. *J. Mol. Biol.* **2000**, *302*, 205–217. [CrossRef]
124. Aguilera-Mendoza, L.; Marrero-Ponce, Y.; Tellez-Ibarra, R.; Llorente-Quesada, M.T.; Salgado, J.; Barigye, S.J.; Liu, J. Overlap and diversity in antimicrobial peptide databases: Compiling a non-redundant set of sequences. *Bioinformatics* **2015**, *31*, 2553–2559. [CrossRef]
125. Blondel, V.D.; Guillaume, J.-L.; Lambiotte, R.; Lefebvre, E. Fast unfolding of communities in large networks. *J. Stat. Mech. Theory Exp.* **2008**, *2008*, P10008. [CrossRef]
126. Willett, P. Similarity-based virtual screening using 2D fingerprints. *Drug Discov. Today* **2006**, *11*, 1046–1053. [CrossRef]
127. Hert, J.; Willett, P.; Wilton, D.J.; Acklin, P.; Azzaoui, K.; Jacoby, E.; Schuffenhauer, A. Comparison of Fingerprint-Based Methods for Virtual Screening Using Multiple Bioactive Reference Structures. *J. Chem. Inf. Comput. Sci.* **2004**, *44*, 1177–1185. [CrossRef]
128. Marasco, D.; Perretta, G.; Sabatella, M.; Ruvo, M. Past and future perspectives of synthetic peptide libraries. *Curr. Protein Pept. Sci.* **2008**, *9*, 447–467. [CrossRef]
129. Irving, M.B.; Pan, O.; Scott, J.K. Random-peptide libraries and antigen-fragment libraries for epitope mapping and the development of vaccines and diagnostics. *Curr. Opin. Chem. Biol.* **2001**, *5*, 314–324. [CrossRef]
130. Müller, A.; Gabernet, G.; Hiss, J.A.; Schneider, G. modlAMP: Python for antimicrobial peptides. *Bioinformatics* **2017**, *33*, 2753–2755. [CrossRef] [PubMed]
131. Schneider, G.; Wrede, P. The rational design of amino acid sequences by artificial neural networks and simulated molecular evolution: De novo design of an idealized leader peptidase cleavage site. *Biophys. J.* **1994**, *66*, 335–344. [CrossRef]
132. Schneider, G.; Schuchhardt, J.; Wrede, P. Peptide design in machina: Development of artificial mitochondrial protein precursor cleavage sites by simulated molecular evolution. *Biophys. J.* **1995**, *68*, 434–447. [CrossRef]
133. Grantham, R. Amino Acid Difference Formula to Help Explain Protein Evolution. *Science* **1974**, *185*, 862–864. [CrossRef]
134. Miyata, T.; Miyazawa, S.; Yasunaga, T. Two types of amino acid substitutions in protein evolution. *J. Mol. Evol.* **1979**, *12*, 219–236. [CrossRef] [PubMed]
135. Risler, J.; Delorme, M.; Delacroix, H.; Henaut, A. Amino acid substitutions in structurally related proteins a pattern recognition approach: Determination of a new and efficient scoring matrix. *J. Mol. Biol.* **1988**, *204*, 1019–1029. [CrossRef]
136. Gabernet, G.; Gautschi, D.; Müller, A.T.; Neuhaus, C.S.; Armbrecht, L.; Dittrich, P.S.; Hiss, J.A.; Schneider, G. In silico design and optimization of selective membranolytic anticancer peptides. *Sci. Rep.* **2019**, *9*, 1–11. [CrossRef]
137. Stoye, J.; Evers, D.; Meyer, F. Rose: Generating sequence families. *Bioinformatics* **1998**, *14*, 157–163. [CrossRef]
138. Pang, A.; Smith, A.D.; Nuin, P.A.; Tillier, E.R. SIMPROT: Using an empirically determined indel distribution in simulations of protein evolution. *BMC Bioinform.* **2005**, *6*, 236. [CrossRef]
139. Fletcher, W.; Yang, Z. INDELible: A Flexible Simulator of Biological Sequence Evolution. *Mol. Biol. Evol.* **2009**, *26*, 1879–1888. [CrossRef]
140. Bosso, M.; Ständker, L.; Kirchhoff, F.; Münch, J. Exploiting the human peptidome for novel antimicrobial and anticancer agents. *Bioorganic Med. Chem.* **2018**, *26*, 2719–2726. [CrossRef] [PubMed]
141. Domínguez-Pérez, D.; Durban, J.; Agüero-Chapin, G.; López, J.T.; Molina-Ruiz, R.; Almeida, D.; Calvete, J.J.; Vasconcelos, V.; Antunes, A. The Harderian gland transcriptomes of Caraiba andreae, Cubophis cantherigerus and Tretanorhinus variabilis, three colubroid snakes from Cuba. *Genomics* **2018**, *111*, 1720–1727. [CrossRef] [PubMed]
142. Mayr, L.M.; Bojanic, D. Novel trends in high-throughput screening. *Curr. Opin. Pharmacol.* **2009**, *9*, 580–588. [CrossRef] [PubMed]
143. Prentis, P.J.; Pavasovic, A.; Norton, R.S. Sea Anemones: Quiet Achievers in the Field of Peptide Toxins. *Toxins* **2018**, *10*, 36. [CrossRef] [PubMed]
144. Holford, M.; Daly, M.; King, G.F.; Norton, R.S. Venoms to the rescue. *Science* **2018**, *361*, 842–844. [CrossRef]
145. Rodríguez, A.A.; Otero-González, A.; Ghattas, M.; Ständker, L. Discovery, Optimization, and Clinical Application of Natural Antimicrobial Peptides. *Biomedicines* **2021**, *9*, 1381. [CrossRef]
146. Chevreux, B. MIRA: An Automated Genome and EST Assembler. Ph.D. Thesis, Ruprecht-Karls University, Heidelberg, Germany, 2007.
147. Bankevich, A.; Nurk, S.; Antipov, D.; Gurevich, A.A.; Dvorkin, M.; Kulikov, A.S.; Lesin, V.M.; Nikolenko, S.I.; Pham, S.; Prjibelski, A.D.; et al. SPAdes: A new genome assembly algorithm and its applications to single-cell sequencing. *J. Comput. Biol.* **2012**, *19*, 455–477. [CrossRef]

148. Huang, X.; Madan, A. CAP3: A DNA Sequence Assembly Program. *Genome Res.* **1999**, *9*, 868–877. [CrossRef]
149. Schulz, M.H.; Zerbino, D.R.; Vingron, M.; Birney, E. Oases: Robust de novo RNA-seq assembly across the dynamic range of expression levels. *Bioinformatics* **2012**, *28*, 1086–1092. [CrossRef]
150. Grabherr, M.G.; Haas, B.J.; Yassour, M.; Levin, J.Z.; Thompson, D.A.; Amit, I.; Adiconis, X.; Fan, L.; Raychowdhury, R.; Zeng, Q.D.; et al. Full-length transcriptome assembly from RNA-Seq data without a reference genome. *Nat. Biotechnol.* **2011**, *29*, 644–652. [CrossRef]
151. Sequencing, H. CLC Genomics Workbench. 2011. Available online: https://research.ncsu.edu/gsl/bioinformatic-resources/clc/ (accessed on 17 March 2022).
152. Bioinformatics, B.; Valencia, S. OmicsBox-Bioinformatics made easy. *March* **2019**, *3*, 2019.
153. Altschul, S.F.; Gish, W.; Miller, W.; Myers, E.W.; Lipman, D.J. Basic local alignment search tool. *J. Mol. Biol.* **1990**, *215*, 403–410. [CrossRef]
154. Huerta-Cepas, J.; Szklarczyk, D.; Heller, D.; Hernández-Plaza, A.; Forslund, S.K.; Cook, H.V.; Mende, D.R.; Letunic, I.; Rattei, T.; Jensen, L.J.; et al. eggNOG 5.0: A hierarchical, functionally and phylogenetically annotated orthology resource based on 5090 organisms and 2502 viruses. *Nucleic Acids Res.* **2018**, *47*, D309–D314. [CrossRef] [PubMed]
155. Mitchell, A.L.; Attwood, T.K.; Babbitt, P.C.; Blum, M.; Bork, P.; Bridge, A.; Brown, S.D.; Chang, H.-Y.; El-Gebali, S.; Fraser, M.I.; et al. InterPro in 2019: Improving coverage, classification and access to protein sequence annotations. *Nucleic Acids Res.* **2019**, *47*, D351–D360. [CrossRef] [PubMed]
156. Domínguez-Pérez, D.; Martins, J.C.; Almeida, D.; Costa, P.R.; Vasconcelos, V.; Campos, A. Transcriptomic Profile of the Cockle *Cerastoderma edule* Exposed to Seasonal Diarrhetic Shellfish Toxin Contamination. *Toxins* **2021**, *13*, 784. [CrossRef] [PubMed]
157. Fingerhut, L.C.H.W.; Strugnell, J.M.; Faou, P.; Labiaga, R.; Zhang, J.; Cooke, I.R. Shotgun Proteomics Analysis of Saliva and Salivary Gland Tissue from the Common Octopus Octopus vulgaris. *J. Proteome Res.* **2018**, *17*, 3866–3876. [CrossRef]
158. Deutsch, E.W.; Bandeira, N.; Sharma, V.; Perez-Riverol, Y.; Carver, J.J.; Kundu, D.J.; García-Seisdedos, D.; Jarnuczak, A.F.; Hewapathirana, S.; Pullman, B.S.; et al. The ProteomeXchange consortium in 2020: Enabling 'big data' approaches in proteomics. *Nucleic Acids Res.* **2020**, *48*, D1145–D1152. [CrossRef]
159. Nesvizhskii, A. Proteogenomics: Concepts, applications and computational strategies. *Nat. Methods* **2014**, *11*, 1114–1125. [CrossRef]
160. Fingerhut, L.C.H.W.; Miller, D.J.; Strugnell, J.M.; Daly, N.L.; Cooke, I.R. ampir: An R package for fast genome-wide prediction of antimicrobial peptides. *Bioinformatics* **2020**, *36*, 5262–5263. [CrossRef]
161. Almeida, D.; Domínguez-Pérez, D.; Matos, A.; Agüero-Chapin, G.; Castaño, Y.; Vasconcelos, V.; Campos, A.; Antunes, A. Data Employed in the Construction of a Composite Protein Database for Proteogenomic Analyses of Cephalopods Salivary Apparatus. *Data* **2020**, *5*, 110. [CrossRef]
162. Gacesa, R.; Barlow, D.; Long, P.F. Machine learning can differentiate venom toxins from other proteins having non-toxic physiological functions. *PeerJ Comput. Sci.* **2016**, *2*, e90. [CrossRef]
163. Umer, H.M.; Audain, E.; Zhu, Y.; Pfeuffer, J.; Sachsenberg, T.; Lehtiö, J.; Branca, R.M.; Perez-Riverol, Y. Generation of ENSEMBL-based proteogenomics databases boosts the identification of non-canonical peptides. *Bioinformatics* **2022**, *38*, 1470–1472. [CrossRef] [PubMed]
164. Fu, L.; Niu, B.; Zhu, Z.; Wu, S.; Li, W. CD-HIT: Accelerated for clustering the next-generation sequencing data. *Bioinformatics* **2012**, *28*, 3150–3152. [CrossRef]
165. Hughes, C.S.; Moggridge, S.; Müller, T.; Sorensen, P.H.; Morin, G.B.; Krijgsveld, J. Single-pot, solid-phase-enhanced sample preparation for proteomics experiments. *Nat. Protoc.* **2019**, *14*, 68–85. [CrossRef]
166. Wiśniewski, J.R.; Zougman, A.; Nagaraj, N.; Mann, M. Universal sample preparation method for proteome analysis. *Nat. Methods* **2009**, *6*, 359–362. [CrossRef] [PubMed]
167. León, I.R.; Schwämmle, V.; Jensen, O.N.; Sprenger, R.R. Quantitative Assessment of In-solution Digestion Efficiency Identifies Optimal Protocols for Unbiased Protein Analysis. *Mol. Cell. Proteom.* **2013**, *12*, 2992–3005. [CrossRef] [PubMed]
168. Jeong, K.; Kim, S.; Bandeira, N. False discovery rates in spectral identification. *BMC Bioinform.* **2012**, *13*, S2. [CrossRef]
169. The, M.; MacCoss, M.J.; Noble, W.S.; Käll, L. Fast and Accurate Protein False Discovery Rates on Large-Scale Proteomics Data Sets with Percolator 3.0. *J. Am. Soc. Mass Spectrom.* **2016**, *27*, 1719–1727. [CrossRef]
170. Käll, L.; Storey, J.D.; MacCoss, M.J.; Noble, W.S. Posterior Error Probabilities and False Discovery Rates: Two Sides of the Same Coin. *J. Proteome Res.* **2007**, *7*, 40–44. [CrossRef]
171. Bhandari, B.K.; Gardner, P.P.; Lim, C.S. Razor: Annotation of signal peptides from toxins. *bioRxiv* **2021**. [CrossRef]
172. Maxwell, M.; Undheim, E.A.B.; Mobli, M. Secreted Cysteine-Rich Repeat Proteins "SCREPs": A Novel Multi-Domain Architecture. *Front. Pharmacol.* **2018**, *9*, 1333. [CrossRef]
173. Liu, S.; Bao, J.; Lao, X.; Zheng, H. Novel 3D Structure Based Model for Activity Prediction and Design of Antimicrobial Peptides. *Sci. Rep.* **2018**, *8*, 1–12. [CrossRef] [PubMed]
174. Kumar, V.; Kumar, R.; Agrawal, P.; Patiyal, S.; Raghava, G.P. A Method for Predicting Hemolytic Potency of Chemically Modified Peptides From Its Structure. *Front. Pharmacol.* **2020**, *11*, 54. [CrossRef]
175. Zhao, Y.; Wang, S.; Fei, W.; Feng, Y.; Shen, L.; Yang, X.; Wang, M.; Wu, M. Prediction of Anticancer Peptides with High Efficacy and Low Toxicity by Hybrid Model Based on 3D Structure of Peptides. *Int. J. Mol. Sci.* **2021**, *22*, 5630. [CrossRef] [PubMed]

176. Zhong, B.; Su, X.; Wen, M.; Zuo, S.; Hong, L.; Lin, J. Parafold: Paralleling alphafold for large-scale predictions. In Proceedings of the International Conference on High Performance Computing in Asia-Pacific Region Workshops, Kobe, Japan & Online, 12–14 January 2022; pp. 1–9.
177. Contreras-Torres, E.; Marrero-Ponce, Y.; Terán, J.E.; García-Jacas, C.R.; Brizuela, C.A.; Sánchez-Rodríguez, J.C. *MuLiMs-MCoMPAs*: A Novel Multiplatform Framework to Compute Tensor Algebra-Based Three-Dimensional Protein Descriptors. *J. Chem. Inf. Model.* **2019**, *60*, 1042–1059. [CrossRef] [PubMed]
178. Torres, M.D.T.; de la Fuente-Nunez, C. Reprogramming biological peptides to combat infectious diseases. *Chem. Commun.* **2019**, *55*, 15020–15032. [CrossRef]

antibiotics

MDPI

Article

ABP-Finder: A Tool to Identify Antibacterial Peptides and the Gram-Staining Type of Targeted Bacteria

Yasser B. Ruiz-Blanco [1,*], Guillermin Agüero-Chapin [2,3], Sandra Romero-Molina [1], Agostinho Antunes [2,3], Lia-Raluca Olari [4], Barbara Spellerberg [5], Jan Münch [4] and Elsa Sanchez-Garcia [1,*]

1 Computational Biochemistry, Center of Medical Biotechnology, University of Duisburg-Essen, 45141 Essen, Germany
2 CIIMAR—Centro Interdisciplinar de Investigação Marinha e Ambiental, Universidade do Porto, Terminal de Cruzeiros do Porto de Leixões, Av. General Norton de Matos, s/n, 4450-208 Porto, Portugal
3 Departamento de Biologia, Faculdade de Ciências, Universidade do Porto, Rua do Campo Alegre, 4169-007 Porto, Portugal
4 Institute of Molecular Virology, University Hospital Ulm, 89081 Ulm, Germany
5 Institute of Medical Microbiology and Hygiene, University Hospital Ulm, 89081 Ulm, Germany
* Correspondence: ybruizblanco@gmail.com (Y.B.R.-B.); elsa.sanchez-garcia@uni-due.de (E.S.-G.)

Citation: Ruiz-Blanco, Y.B.; Agüero-Chapin, G.; Romero-Molina, S.; Antunes, A.; Olari, L.-R.; Spellerberg, B.; Münch, J.; Sanchez-Garcia, E. ABP-Finder: A Tool to Identify Antibacterial Peptides and the Gram-Staining Type of Targeted Bacteria. *Antibiotics* **2022**, *11*, 1708. https://doi.org/10.3390/antibiotics11121708

Academic Editor: Jean-Marc Sabatier

Received: 20 October 2022
Accepted: 17 November 2022
Published: 26 November 2022

Publisher's Note: MDPI stays neutral with regard to jurisdictional claims in published maps and institutional affiliations.

Copyright: © 2022 by the authors. Licensee MDPI, Basel, Switzerland. This article is an open access article distributed under the terms and conditions of the Creative Commons Attribution (CC BY) license (https://creativecommons.org/licenses/by/4.0/).

Abstract: Multi-drug resistance in bacteria is a major health problem worldwide. To overcome this issue, new approaches allowing for the identification and development of antibacterial agents are urgently needed. Peptides, due to their binding specificity and low expected side effects, are promising candidates for a new generation of antibiotics. For over two decades, a large diversity of antimicrobial peptides (AMPs) has been discovered and annotated in public databases. The AMP family encompasses nearly 20 biological functions, thus representing a potentially valuable resource for data mining analyses. Nonetheless, despite the availability of machine learning-based approaches focused on AMPs, these tools lack evidence of successful application for AMPs' discovery, and many are not designed to predict a specific function for putative AMPs, such as antibacterial activity. Consequently, among the apparent variety of data mining methods to screen peptide sequences for antibacterial activity, only few tools can deal with such task consistently, although with limited precision and generally no information about the possible targets. Here, we addressed this gap by introducing a tool specifically designed to identify antibacterial peptides (ABPs) with an estimation of which type of bacteria is susceptible to the action of these peptides, according to their response to the Gram-staining assay. Our tool is freely available via a web server named ABP-Finder. This new method ranks within the top state-of-the-art ABP predictors, particularly in terms of precision. Importantly, we showed the successful application of ABP-Finder for the screening of a large peptide library from the human urine peptidome and the identification of an antibacterial peptide.

Keywords: antibacterial peptide; machine learning; AMPs database; StarPep; Gram staining-based target; peptide library screening; human peptidome

1. Introduction

Antibiotic resistance is a life-threatening health problem worldwide, and one of the main causes of death in developing countries [1,2]. The potential capability of peptides to overcome resistance [3] has motivated the development of new antibiotics from antimicrobial peptides (AMPs) to combat multi-drug resistant pathogens and the threats of Gram-negative infections [4,5].

AMPs are oligopeptides produced by a great variety of organisms, from prokaryotes to eukaryotes, including humans. Due to their various functions, AMPs are considered a part of the innate immune system of higher eukaryotes. The structural diversity of AMPs allows them to display a broad range of antimicrobial activity against pathogenic agents, including viruses, Gram-positive and Gram-negative bacteria, as well as fungi. Besides, the bacterial selectivity of AMPs over eukaryotic cells and their different action modes make peptides excellent antibiotic candidates [3,4,6]. A widespread mechanism of antibacterial peptides (ABPs) is the destabilization and destruction of bacterial membranes. However, these peptides can also interfere with intracellular processes such as nucleic acid and protein synthesis, enzymatic modulation, and protein degradation [7–9], which is an advantage over traditional antibiotics [3,10].

Most AMPs are naturally occurring peptides that represent promising candidates for optimization in advanced steps of the drug design process [11]. AMP-based drugs have been clinically approved to treat both topical and systemic infections. For instance, polymyxins and gramicidin S were formulated for the prevention of topical infections caused by *Pseudomonas aeruginosa* and *Acinetobacter baumannii*. Colistin, a polymyxin derivative, is currently used for the systemic treatment of lung infections, especially those caused by *Pseudomonas aeruginosa* [12]. Due to its problematic resistance profile, *Pseudomonas aeruginosa* is often difficult to treat by antibiotics [13]. However, it can be targeted by a variety of different AMPs [13–15] that may be further developed into innovative therapeutics.

The specificity of peptides toward certain targets is usually highlighted as an important benefit for therapeutic intervention. Nonetheless, a downside of this feature is the associated challenge for the drug design process, given that small structural modifications can significantly influence both the activity and pharmacokinetic properties of the peptides. Consequently, optimizing the precision of tools for the screening of large datasets of peptides is of utmost relevance to improve efficiency at the early steps of drug design processes.

For over a decade, growth in the publicly available data of AMPs has been witnessed, with the subsequent development of several machine learning (ML)-based predictors integrated with AMP databases such as DAMP [16], APD3 [17], CAMP [18], $CAMP_{R3}$ [19], LAMP [20], DRAMP [21], ADAM [22], and DBAASP [23]. However, most of these prediction tools only discriminate between AMPs and non-AMPs. This is a highly ambiguous outcome given the broad scope of antimicrobial activity, which typically refers to more than 20 biological functions, such as the annotations in APD3 [17].

A group of predictors addressed this issue by applying a hierarchical classification scheme where first the peptides are classified as AMPs or not, and the positive cases are then sub-divided into a couple of classes based on selected AMP functions (e.g., antibacterial, antiviral, and antifungal peptides). Examples of such predictors, which include the antibacterial function are AntiBP2 [24], ClassAMP [25], MLAMP [26], *i*AMPpred [27], AMAP [28], AMP Scanner [29,30], and AMPDiscover [31]. However, of them, only AMP Scanner vr.1 predicts a type of bacterial target (*E. coli* or *S. aureus*) for the identified ABP [29].

In this context, we implemented a two-level predictor focused on antibacterial peptides (ABPs), named ABP-Finder, whose inner classifier estimates the Gram staining type of the putative targets. This tool leverages random forest (RF) classifiers trained with peptide data extracted from StarPep, the largest up to date public database of AMPs [32]. ABP-Finder categorizes ABPs and non-ABPs in the first classification level. Subsequently, the peptides identified as ABPs are sub-classified according to the Gram staining type of the potential targets i.e., exclusively Gram-positive, exclusively Gram-negative bacteria, or broad-spectrum peptides with expected activity against both types of bacteria. The ABPs used to develop this predictor show activity against at least one of nine representative bacterial targets (see Dataset section), among which are species with known multi-drug resistance such as *Acinetobacter baumannii*, *Enterococcus faecium*, *Klebsiella pneumonia*, *Pseudomonas aeruginosa*, and *Staphylococcus aureus*. With ABP-Finder, we weigh precision as the main performance feature of the prediction. In this way, we boost the efficiency of the screening step at the early stages of the drug design process aiming at the development of peptide-based antibiotics. Remarkably, we prove the efficacy of ABP-Finder for such screenings with the identification of a peptide from the human urine peptidome, displaying antimicrobial activity against *Pseudomonas aeruginosa*.

2. Materials and Methods

2.1. Data Collection and Pre-Processing

The models developed in this study were derived from the StarPep database [32,33]. This resource, as described by the authors, is a non-redundant compendium from 40 publicly available data sources, which encompasses annotations of more than 20 functions in approximately 45,000 AMPs, with nearly 8000 entries labelled as antibacterial peptides.

Before describing the construction of our training and test sets, we point out a shortcoming of several AMP-based predictors found in the literature [16–22], whose models do not obey the first principle dictated by the Organisation for Economic Co-operation and Development (OECD) to build reliable Quantitative Structure–Activity Relationship (QSAR)/ML-based models [34] (https://doi.org/10.1787/9789264085442-en (accessed on 16 November 2022)). This principle is stated as "a defined endpoint". Commonly, AMPs are annotated as such regardless of the target, mechanism, source, the method used to study the activity, to name some characteristics. The lack of such detailed information makes the discrimination between AMPs and non-AMPs a largely ambiguous endpoint for data analysis. In consequence, several criteria must be introduced to better define the modelled data and thus bring reliability to the predicted outcome. Notably, the most recent AMP predictors [24–29,31] have designed their modeling approaches to break down the AMP annotation into three classes (typically antibacterial, antifungal, and antiviral peptides). This strategy is a suitable approach to fulfil the need for a defined endpoint.

Our work focused on the identification of ABPs. To this end, we extracted peptides from the StarPep database ranging between 5 and 50 residues, and whose composition contains only the 20 standard amino acids. To further refine the selection of ABPs, we only extracted those peptides annotated as active against at least one of the following targets: *Acinetobacter baumannii, Bacillus subtilis, Enterococcus faecium, Escherichia coli, Klebsiella pneumonia, Listeria monocytogenes, Pseudomonas aeruginosa, Streptococcus agalactiae*, and *Staphylococcus aureus*. In this way, we discarded entries that are annotated as ABPs without information of their targets, and those exclusively reported with activity against underrepresented targets in the entire database. The selected species cover a set of both Gram-positive and Gram-negative bacteria and are examples of relevant targets for therapeutic applications. The peptides labeled as non-ABP for our learning process are not annotated as antibacterial, against any target, in StarPep, but with a different function such as antifungal or anticancer, among others. This approach clearly carries the risk of mislabeling non-ABP in our dataset, due to insufficient annotation of the peptide in the original source. The pseudo-negative cases in the training data lead to a more stringent prediction of positive cases, and consequently lower false-positive rate and higher precision. The downside is the expected lower recall as the true positives can be also diminished. Nonetheless, the favourable precision is aligned with our stated goal of boosting the precision of the classifier instead of its recall or a combined metric such as accuracy or AUC.

Hence, we extracted a total of 22,707 peptides to design our training and testing schemes. This collection was partitioned into four datasets: training, development, validation, and test sets. The two first are intended for the learning process, while the others are meant for testing the models with hold-out data. The development (Dev) set was used to monitor the generalization of the models built during the optimization of the hyperparameters in the learning algorithm. Usually, the terms development and validation set are applied indistinctively to a dataset used for the above-mentioned purpose. In this work, we made a distinction between these nomenclatures and reserved the term validation for a hold-out set, i.e., peptides that are not used in any step of the learning process. The difference between the validation and the strict test set is that we built the validation set in a way that its peptides share high similarity ($\geq$90% identity) with at least one peptide in the training set (excluding identical matches). In turn, the test set was built in a way that its peptides share less than 90% identity among them, and with any peptide in the training data. Consequently, the test set comprises non-redundant peptides that are also not closely represented in our training. Challenging a peptide predictor in both scenarios, one that closely resembles the training conditions (without strict superposition), and another more distant setup, is important to assess the biasing effect on the generalization of the model due to the characteristics of the training data.

Finally, a production dataset was generated by combining the training and the development sets. The purpose of this set is to perform a final re-training of the model with an augmented dataset, while keeping the selection of descriptors and configuration of hyper-parameters as optimized with the training and development sets. Figure 1 depicts the workflow followed to obtain the four datasets.

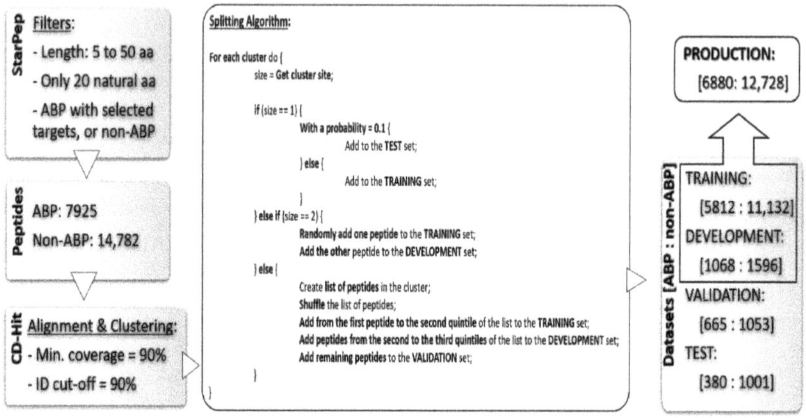

Figure 1. Workflow for the preparation of the datasets. The peptides extracted from StarPep were clustered with CD-Hit and subsequently distributed among the four sets used for training and testing the predictor. The final panel of the pipeline contains information about the number of peptides in every subset as well as their classification according to StarPep.

Together with the peptide sequences and their classification as ABP or non-ABP, we also extracted, from StarPep, the information about the Gram staining type of their known targets. Accordingly, we further categorized the ABPs into three activity classes: exclusively against Gram-positive targets (Gram+), exclusively against Gram-negative targets (Gram-), and broad-spectrum peptides. The four datasets resulting from the previous splitting were also used to train and assess the secondary classifier based on the Gram staining type of the targets. For this purpose, the non-ABP peptides were removed from such datasets. Table 1 summarizes the number of peptides per type of Gram staining class in the four datasets.

Table 1. Number of peptides per type of Gram staining class in the training, development, validation, and test datasets.

	Gram+	Gram−	Broad Spectrum
Training	351	478	4983
Development	52	105	911
Validation	37	82	546
Test	27	38	315

2.2. *Performance Measures*

In this section, we summarize the formulations of the performance measures used to assess the different models described here. The measures are sensitivity (Sn), precision (Pr), accuracy (Acc), F1 score, and the Mathew Correlation Coefficient (MCC) [35]. All of them are formulated in terms of the elements of a binary confusion matrix: true positives (TP), true negatives (TN), false positives (FP), and false negatives (FN).

$$\mathrm{Sn} = \frac{\mathrm{TP}}{\mathrm{TP} + \mathrm{FN}}$$

$$\mathrm{Pr} = \frac{\mathrm{TP}}{\mathrm{TP} + \mathrm{FP}}$$

$$\mathrm{Acc} = \frac{\mathrm{TP} + \mathrm{TN}}{\mathrm{TP} + \mathrm{TN} + \mathrm{FP} + \mathrm{FN}}$$

$$\mathrm{F1} = 2\frac{\mathrm{Sn} * \mathrm{Pr}}{\mathrm{Sn} + \mathrm{Pr}} = \frac{\mathrm{TP}}{\mathrm{TP} + \frac{1}{2}(\mathrm{FP} + \mathrm{FN})}$$

$$\mathrm{MCC} = \frac{\mathrm{TP} * \mathrm{TN} - \mathrm{FP} * \mathrm{FN}}{\sqrt{(\mathrm{TP} + \mathrm{FP})(\mathrm{TP} + \mathrm{FN})(\mathrm{TN} + \mathrm{FP})(\mathrm{TN} + \mathrm{FN})}}$$

Besides, we define an ad-hoc measure named Fitness–Robustness Score (FRS) that is specifically used as a scoring function to tune the values of the hyper-parameters of the learning technique.

$$\mathrm{FRS} = \left(\frac{\mathrm{R_T} + \mathrm{R_{CV}} + \mathrm{R_D}}{3}\right)^2 - (\mathrm{R_T} - \mathrm{R_{CV}})^2 - (\mathrm{R_T} - \mathrm{R_D})^2$$

The FRS is a quality measure that provides a consolidated value for the performance of a particular model considering its goodness-of-fit, generalization, and robustness. The first term corresponds to the average performance in the following assessments: re-substitution (RT, fitting the training data), 10-fold cross-validation (RCV, within the training data), and generalization (RD, using the development set). The other two terms weigh the robustness of the model by measuring the deviations from the performance in training samples when the model is evaluated in hold-out data (cross-validation and development set). We formulated this ad-hoc measure as a function of another base quality measure, labelled as R, which should be evaluated in the different assessment schemes. For this study, we selected the MCC as the base measure to evaluate our fitness-robustness score. In the case of the multi-classifier trained to distinguish between the Gram staining classes, the average MCC value among the three classes was used as the base measure. The average was weighted according to the number of peptides in each class.

The FRS, when computed as a function of the MCC, has an optimum maximum value of one. We leveraged this score to identify optimum values for the hyper-parameters of the random forest [36] algorithm used to develop our models.

2.3. Machine Learning Approach and Software

The classifiers developed in this work were random forest (RF) [36] predictors, based on the implementation of this technique in the WEKA environment [37]. RF belongs to the family of ensemble methods [38] with base classifiers formed by decision trees. Recently, RF has been compared with deep learning approaches showing comparable performance for modeling AMP datasets [39]. There, the authors conclude that no definitive evidence was found to support using deep-learning approaches for this problem, knowing the increased algorithmic complexity and computational cost of these methods.

Within RF, all the trees provide a prediction for every instance entering the forest, and the unified outcome is obtained as the majority vote among all the predictions. The hyper-parameters optimized during the learning process were the number of trees, the maximum number of descriptors used to build a tree (these descriptors are taken at the beginning of the training process from the global pool of attributes), and the maximum depth of the trees. In addition, the minimum number of instances in the final leaves of the trees was fixed to 10 in the case of the main classifier (ABPnon-ABP), and to five for the multi-classifier (Gram+/Gram−/broad spectrum).

The peptide descriptors fed to the learning algorithm were computed with the ProtDCal-Suite [40] using the configuration files enclosed in the Supplementary Material. The Prot-

DCal module [41] is intended for the calculation of general-purpose and alignment-free descriptors of amino acid sequences and protein structures. These features are descriptive statistics (such as the variance, average, maximum, minimum, percentiles, etc.) of the distribution of amino acid properties (such as hydrophobicity, isoelectric point, molar weight, among others), in multiple groups of residues extracted from a given protein or peptide. The program possesses additional procedures that modify the intrinsic properties of a residue according to its vicinity in the sequence, thus adding connectivity information in the descriptors. The features derived from ProtDCal have been used by us and other authors to develop machine-learning-based predictors of posttranslational modifications [42,43], protein–protein interaction [44], enzyme-like amino acid sequences [45], residues critical for protein functions [46], and antibacterial peptides [47,48], although with smaller databases. The project files enclosed in the Supplementary Material contain the setup used to compute all the descriptors employed in this work.

2.4. Web Servers Available for ABPs Predictions

In this section, we briefly describe the most relevant state-of-the-art ABP predictors that are available via web server tools. ClassAMP was among the first methods that broke down the AMP family thus allowing the prediction of ABPs specifically [25]. This tool was trained with peptides from the CAMP database [18] and used RF and support vector machine (SVM) [49] algorithms to identify antibacterial, antifungal, and antiviral peptides.

MLAMP, a multi-label classifier of AMPs was developed using a variant of Chou's pseudo amino acid composition (PseACC) features [50] to build an RF-based classifier that firstly distinguishes AMP from non-AMPs, and then subdivides the biological activity into antibacterial, anticancer, antifungal, antiviral, and anti-HIV [26].

Similarly, the *i*AMPpred predictor combines compositional, physicochemical, and structural features into Chou's general PseACC as input variables for an SVM multi-classifier [27]. This work reunited peptides from the databases CAMPR3 [19], APD3 [17], and AntiBP2 [24]. The multi-classifier uses three categories in the outcome variable: antibacterial, antifungal, and antiviral peptides [27].

The Antimicrobial Activity Predictor (AMAP) [28], with a hierarchical multi-label classification scheme, was trained with AMPs annotated with 14 biological activities in the APD3 database and a designed subset of non-AMP. The models used amino acid composition features to feed SVM and XGboost tree [51] algorithms.

The introduction of the AMP-Scanner webserver represented a significant improvement with respect to other predictors. AMP-Scanner vr.1 consists of two RF classifiers, trained with peptides selected from multiple sources [18,52,53]. The first output of the classifier is the identification of ABPs. The second is a classifier trained to distinguish between peptides with Gram-positive or Gram-negative targets, using data of *S. aureus* and *E. coli* as reference targets. The authors refer that peptides predicted with scores within the range [0.4–0.6] for both classes should be considered as active against both types of targets (broad-spectrum peptides) [29]. On the other hand, AMP-Scanner vr.2 is based on a Deep Neural Networks (DNN) classifier fed with ABP data only, obtained from the updated version of the ADP3 database [19,30].

Very recently, AMPDiscover [31] was developed by mining AMP data from StarPep [33]. AMPDiscover encompasses several binary (active/non-active) predictors of functions such as antibacterial, antiviral, antifungal, and antiparasitic peptides. The authors analyzed the performance of RF to model the antibacterial peptides data, which agrees with our choice of this learning scheme for our models.

2.5. Experimental Determination of Antibacterial Activity

Two batches of chemically synthetized peptides from different providers (KE Biochem and the U-PEP facility at Ulm University) were used to assess antimicrobial effects. Antibacterial activity was evaluated by agar diffusion as previously described [54]. Bacteria were cultured in liquid broth at 37 °C overnight, pelleted by centrifugation, and washed in

10 mM sodium phosphate buffer. Following resuspension, optical density was determined at 600 nm and 2×10^7 bacteria were seeded into a Petri dish in 1% agarose. After cooling at 4 °C for 30 min, 3–5 mm holes were placed into the 1% agarose. Peptides adjusted to the desired concentration in 10 µL of buffer were filled into the agar-holes. Following incubation at 37 °C in ambient air for 3 h, plates were overlaid with 1% agarose, tryptic soy solved in 10 mM phosphate buffer. Inhibition zones in cm were determined after 16–18 h incubation time at 37 °C in 5% CO_2. LL37 at a concentration of 100 µg/mL served as positive control. Antimicrobial activity was tested on the following bacterial strains: *Bacillus subtilis*, *Streptococcus agalactiae* ATCC 12403, *Staphylococcus aureus* MRSA ATCC 43300, *Klebsiella pneumoniae* Extended Spectrum β-Lactamase (ESBL) ATCC 700603, *Pseudomonas aeruginosa* (ATCC 27853) and *Listeria monocytogenes* (ATCC BAA-679/EGD-e).

3. Results and Discussion

Below, we summarize the characteristics of the ML-based models developed in this work, as well as their performance relative to the available state-of-the-art ABP predictors. We also introduce a web server, ABP-Finder, which permits the free and user-friendly screening of large peptide libraries. Finally, we present the application of ABP-Finder for the screening of peptides obtained from the human urine peptide. Notably, ABP-Finder permitted to screen and propose a reduced set of eight ABP candidates out of an initial pool of 4696 peptides. From them, one active hit was experimentally validated with activity against *Pseudomonas aeruginosa*.

3.1. Modeling Antibacterial Peptide Data

Feature selection: The feature selection process comprises three steps. (*i*) First, the Information Gain (IG) [55,56] of all the descriptors was calculated with WEKA, retaining only those descriptors whose IG is >5% of the information content of the class variable. This procedure reduced an initial set of 11,298 descriptors to 2746, whose information contents are the most closely related to our end point variable. (*ii*) Secondly, the redundancy in this subset of features was removed, by clustering the descriptors using a quality-threshold-based [57] clustering algorithm, which employs the Spearman correlation coefficient [58] as the similarity measure to group the descriptors. A correlation cut-off of 0.9 was used to form the clusters. The outcome of these steps is thus a non-redundant and smaller dataset that contains only the central attributes of the formed clusters. This step rendered 1242 attributes. (*iii*) Given the still large set of features, a last selection step was used by employing the Wrapper Evaluator and the Classifier Subset Evaluators of WEKA coupled with a genetic search algorithm [59]. The Wrapper Evaluator used five-fold cross validation on the training data to assess the models obtained from diverse subsets of descriptors. Such models were built with an RF whose number of trees was limited to 15. Next, the Classifier Subset Evaluator used the performance with the development set to identify the most suitable pool of descriptors to train the RF. For both evaluators, the F1 measure was used to score all the assessed subsets of attributes. The genetic search employed to explore the space of all possible combinations of attributes was configured with 20 chromosomes (subsets of attributes) per population, 500 generations, and probabilities of cross-over and mutation of 0.6 and 0.1 respectively. The optimal subset resulting from these selection steps comprised 281 descriptors. A project file type IDL (Individual Descriptor Labels) is enclosed in the Supplementary Material; this project file can be uploaded directly to ProtDCal-Suite to compute the selected 281 descriptors in new peptide datasets.

Tuning hyperparameters: The hyperparameters of the RF were explored using a grid search according to ranges and binning schemes summarized in the top-left panel of Figure 2. The ad hoc FRS function was used to determine the optimum combination of hyperparameters' values, which was obtained with 75 trees each one built from a pool of 40 descriptors and a maximum depth of 14 splits. Such combinations of values rendered the maximum FRS at 0.517.

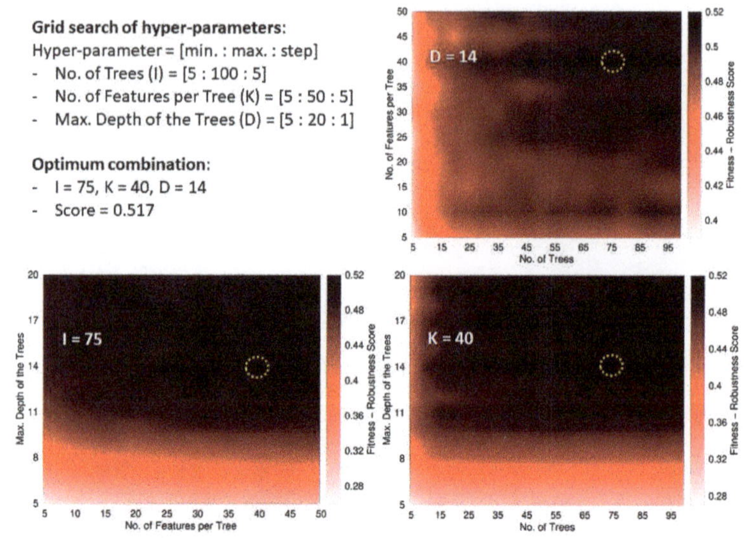

Figure 2. Tuning scheme of the RF's hyperparameters. The top-left panel summarizes the boundaries and binning of the grid search with the three hyper-parameters. This panel also shows the optimum value found for the FRS function and the values of the hyper-parameters in the corresponding solution. The remaining panels show surfaces plotted as heat maps keeping one of the hyper-parameters fixed at its optimum value. The dark regions indicate the best solutions. The optimum regions are highlighted with a dashed circle. The plots highlight that the most critical parameter is the depth of the trees, while high-scored models can be obtained with almost any value of the other hyper-parameters; solutions with a depth below 10 are poorly scored.

3.2. Modeling Data of Gram-Staining Types

This model was trained with the same set of 281 descriptors obtained from the feature selection procedure to discriminate between ABPs and non-ABPs. The training, development, validation, and test sets used for this model were obtained from the splitting described in the Methods section, by removing the non-ABP present in these datasets. The ABPs were then subdivided according to the Gram-staining type of their known targets.

Due to the imbalance in the number of instances from each class, the cost-sensitive RF multi-classifier was trained by applying a cost matrix in the training process with distinct weights for the different types of misclassified cases. The cost matrix takes the form shown in Figure 3.

Prediction

BS	G−	G+	Actual class
0	1	1	BS
10.425	0	1	G−
14.197	1.362	0	G+

Figure 3. Cost matrix applied during the training process of the multi-classifier based on the Gram-staining types of the targets.

The multi-class classifier was built with a cost-sensitive learning scheme, which aims to balance the effective error between pairs of classes considering their different prevalence in the training data. The costs were defined as the inverse ratio of the imbalance between the two classes involved in the matrix element, i.e., given the imbalance between Gram+ and broad-spectrum (BS) peptides in the training data is [1:14.197], then the cost of a Gram+ peptide classified as BS was fixed at 14.197 and the cost of a BS peptide classified as Gram+ remained at 1. This approach diminishes the trend towards BS predictions that originates due to the highest representation of this class in the training data.

The costs affect the training process by re-weighting the training samples in the calculation of the different misclassification errors during the training. No re-weighting is applied to the instances in the test datasets.

Tuning hyperparameters: Analogous to the previous model, the hyper-parameters of the RF were explored using a grid search with the ranges and binning schemes summarized in the top-left panel of Figure 4. The FRS function rendered a maximum value for a solution with 35 trees, 20 descriptors per tree, and a maximum depth of 7 splits. Such combinations of values rendered the maximum FRS at 0.185. The lower value of the optimum FRS value, compared with the ABP/non-ABP model, indicates the larger difficulty of discriminating between the three classes of Gram-staining types. Such difficulty is a natural consequence of the overlap between the classes, given that the peptides in the broad-spectrum category should gather intrinsic features of the other two classes.

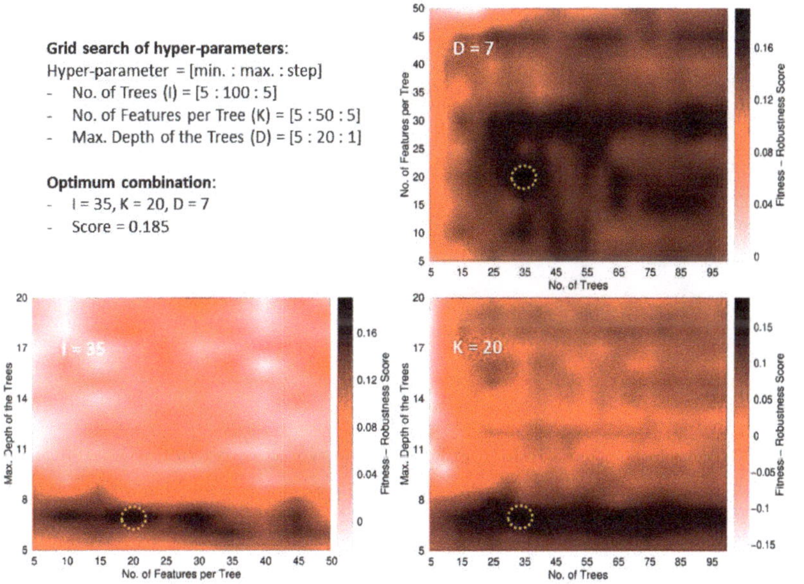

Figure 4. Tuning scheme of the RF's hyper-parameters. The top-left panel summarizes the boundaries and binning of the grid search with the three hyper-parameters. This panel also shows the optimum value found for the FRS function and the hyper-parameters' values of the corresponding solution. The remaining panels show surfaces plotted as heat maps keeping one of the hyper-parameters fixed at its optimum value. The dark regions indicate the best solutions. The optimum regions are highlighted with a dashed circle. As in the exploration for the model ABPs/non-ABPs, the plots show that the most critical parameter is the depth of the trees. Nonetheless, the opposite trend is observed because high-scored models are only obtained with low (<8) depth values. The smaller size of the dataset for this model, as compared with the previous one, leads to the occurrence of overfitting when deep trees are trained.

3.3. Applicability Domain

Following the regulatory principles for QSAR models established by the OECD, we discuss the applicability domain (AD) of our models. Both of our models were built using peptides with lengths between 5 and 50 residues and containing exclusively the 20 standard amino acids. Thus, these length and composition boundaries constitute soft limits of our applicability domain. A quantitative approach for the AD is provided via the range of the descriptors' values in the training or production dataset. In the Supplementary Material, we provide the minimum and maximum values of the descriptors in these datasets. As part of the implementation of these predictors, we automatically evaluate whether any new peptide is found within these ranges or not. If any of the descriptor values of a new peptide falls outside the training ranges, this peptide is labelled as an outlier and the corresponding information is given in the outcome of the program.

3.4. Performance of ABP-Finder in the Context of the State-of-the-Art

Predictors of antibacterial peptides: We compare the performance of our models to five ML-based ABP predictors by employing the hold-out validation and test sets, respectively (Tables 2 and 3). In addition, we employ an external test set originally used by Veltri et al. [30] to assess the performance of AMP-Scanner vr2 (Table 4). We present the performance of our models obtained with the training data only, and with the production dataset. Additionally, we show the performance of our tool considering only those instances that are within the AD of our models.

Table 2. Comparison with external predictors in the validation set. The values in bold denote the best performance for a given measure.

Webserver	Algorithm	Pr.	Sn.	Acc.
ClassAMP	SVM	0.46	0.33	0.59
MLAMP	RF	0.48	0.82	0.59
iAMPred	SVM	0.48	0.90	0.58
AMPScanner_v1 #	RF	0.50	0.98	0.61
AMPScanner_v2 *	DNN	0.48	0.97	0.58
AMPDiscover	RF	0.50	**0.99**	0.61
ABP-Finder (Training)	RF	0.72	0.95	0.84
ABP-Finder (Training, AD)	RF	0.70	0.95	0.83
ABP-Finder (Production)	RF	**0.75**	0.95	**0.85**
ABP-Finder (Production, AD)	RF	**0.75**	0.95	**0.85**

AD: only instances within our applicability domain are considered as valid predictions. # AMPScanner_v1 only considers peptides $\geq$ 10 AA for the predictions. * The method was updated on 20.02.2020.

Table 3. Comparison with external predictors in the test set. The values in bold denote the best performance for a given measure.

Webserver	Algorithm	Pr.	Sn.	Acc.
ClassAMP	SVM	0.34	0.41	0.61
MLAMP	RF	0.38	0.77	0.59
iAMPred	SVM	0.36	0.81	0.56
AMPScanner vr.1 #	RF	0.50	0.80	0.68
AMPScanner vr.2 *	DNN	0.37	0.84	0.57
AMPDiscover	RF	0.42	**0.94**	0.62
ABP-Finder (Training)	RF	0.77	0.68	0.86
ABP-Finder (Training, AD)	RF	0.78	0.67	0.86
ABP-Finder (Production)	RF	**0.80**	0.71	**0.87**
ABP-Finder (Production, AD)	RF	**0.80**	0.70	**0.87**

AD: only instances within our applicability domain are considered valid predictions. # AMPScanner_v1 only considers peptides $\geq$ 10 AA for the predictions. * The method was updated on 20 February 2020.

Table 4. Comparison with external predictors in the test set built by Veltri et al. [30]. Redundant instances with our training set were removed. The values in bold denote the best performance for a given measure.

Webserver	Algorithm	Pr.	Sn.	Acc.
ClassAMP	SVM	0.36	0.27	0.66
MLAMP	RF	0.51	0.65	0.72
*i*AMPred	SVM	0.74	**0.90**	0.88
AMPScanner vr.1 #	RF	0.64	0.77	0.81
AMPScanner vr.2 *	DNN	0.82	0.89	**0.91**
AMPDiscover	RF	0.83	0.84	**0.91**
ABP-Finder (Training)	RF	0.83	0.43	0.81
ABP-Finder (Training, AD)	RF	0.83	0.51	0.86
ABP-Finder (Production)	RF	**0.84**	0.48	0.83
ABP-Finder (Production, AD)	RF	**0.84**	0.57	0.86

AD: only instances within our applicability domain are considered valid predictions. # AMPScanner_v1 only considers peptides $\geq$ 10 AA for the prediction. * Performance based on the model from the original training in Veltri et al. [30], where the cases in this test set are held out of the training process.

Tables 2 and 3 show that our models achieved the best precision and global accuracy in the test and validation sets. Particularly, the precision was significantly higher with ABP-Finder with respect to the other methods. This is a key feature to be leveraged when filtering large peptide libraries because the main aim during the screenings for new hits is to avoid false-positive predictions.

We also challenged our models with an external test set designed by Veltri et al. [30] (Table 4) to further assess the robustness of our predictions. This dataset is qualitatively different from our test set since it is not derived from the StarPep database as all our data, and therefore it was not subjected to any of the curation procedures carried out by the StarPep's developers.

These comparisons confirm that our RF-based models render the most precise predictions, although the sensitivity (and consequently the global accuracy) decays in this case compared with other ABP predictors. Nevertheless, we note the importance of a low false-positive rate in virtual screening analyses, which highlights the higher practical value of our predictors.

Predictors of Gram-staining types: Our antibacterial predictor was designed to provide an estimation of against which type of bacteria are the peptides active. Therefore, we tested how our multi-classifier performs for the Gram+, Gram−, and Broad-Spectrum classes compared to AMP-Scanner vr.1. Tables 5 and 6 summarize the comparison with respect to precision and sensitivity of our models and AMP-Scanner vr.1 on the validation and test sets, respectively. The performance measures were computed for the three classes (Gram+, Gram−, and Broad Spectrum).

Table 5. Comparison of ABP-Finder with AMP-Scanner_v1 in the discrimination between Gram-staining classes within the validation set. The values in bold denote the best performance for a given measure.

Method	Gram+		Gram−		Broad Spectrum	
	Pr	Sn	Pr	Sn	Pr	Sn
AMPScanner vr.1 #	0.04	0.19	0.16	0.42	0.81	0.27
ABP-Finder (Training *)	**0.63**	**0.73**	**0.91**	0.38	0.90	**0.97**
ABP-Finder (Production *)	0.62	0.70	0.85	**0.48**	**0.91**	0.96

AD: only instances within our applicability domain are considered valid predictions. # AMPScanner_v1 only considers peptides $\geq$ 10 AA for the predictions. * There are no instances outside the AD of the model.

Table 6. Comparison of ABP-Finder with AMP-Scanner_v1 in the discrimination between Gram-staining classes within the test set. The values in bold denote the best performance for a given measure.

Method	Gram+		Gram−		Broad Spectrum	
	Pr	Sn	Pr	Sn	Pr	Sn
AMPScanner vr.1 #	0.08	**0.42**	0.13	**0.33**	**0.88**	0.23
ABP-Finder (Training)	**0.44**	0.41	**0.90**	0.24	0.87	**0.96**
ABP-Finder (Training, AD)	**0.44**	0.39	**0.90**	0.24	0.87	**0.96**
ABP-Finder (Production)	**0.44**	0.41	0.82	0.24	**0.88**	**0.96**
ABP-Finder (Production, AD)	**0.44**	0.39	0.82	0.24	**0.88**	**0.96**

AMPScanner_v1 only considers peptides $\geq$ 10 AA for the predictions.

Our models largely outperformed AMP-Scanner vr.1, particularly in terms of precision when detecting the specific types of Gram-staining types (Gram+ and Gram−). Regarding the prediction of broad-spectrum peptides, both methodologies delivered the same precision. However, in this case we greatly surpassed the sensitivity of AMP-Scanner vr.1, thus making more accurate predictions overall. Notably, our multi-classifier showed the best performance for the three classes of Gram-staining types, thus providing a valuable complement to the identification of antibacterial peptides.

The comparison with the state-of-the-art tools showed that, together with ABP-Finder, the top-ranked methods in our tests were *i*AMPred, AMP-Scanner vr2, and AMPDiscover. These approaches were thus confirmed as suitable tools for ABP identification. Nonetheless, ABP-Finder outperformed these predictors, particularly in terms of precision. Importantly, as a distinctive feature, we complement our outcome with an estimation of the Gram-staining type of the putative targets, which can be further pinned down to specific bacterial species by considering that our models were trained with data from nine representative targets (see Dataset section). Furthermore, unlike previously published tools [24–30], we provide an estimation of our applicability domain, which delivers reliability to the predicted outcome.

3.5. *ABP-Finder Web Server*

Our emphasis in the application of regulatory principles to the development of ML-based predictors relies on our commitment to offer a freely accessible and well-maintained tool to reliably screen peptide libraries. To this end, we implemented our models in a user-friendly web server named ABP-Finder (https://protdcal.zmb.uni-due.de/ABP-Finder/ (accessed on 16 November 2022)). This tool allows screening seamlessly thousands of peptides with a single submission job. The ABP-Finder server delivers for each entry a prediction of the antibacterial function, as well as whether each specific peptide is or not within the AD of our models. ABP predictions are also accompanied by a Gram-staining-based estimation of the putative targets of the antibacterial peptides. Furthermore, the web server offers the functionality of screening regions within a long amino acid sequence to identify promising antibacterial fragments. This application of ABP-Finder's models was recently leveraged by us for the identification of antibacterial motifs within β2-microglobulin [60].

3.6. *Virtual Screening of the Human Urine Peptidome*

In this section, we describe the successful application of ABP-Finder to screen a peptide library obtained from the human urine peptidome. The library contains 4696 endogenous peptide fragments, detected in the Core Facility Functional Peptidomics at the University Hospital in Ulm, Germany. The peptide library was screened for antibacterial activity following the workflow depicted in Figure 5.

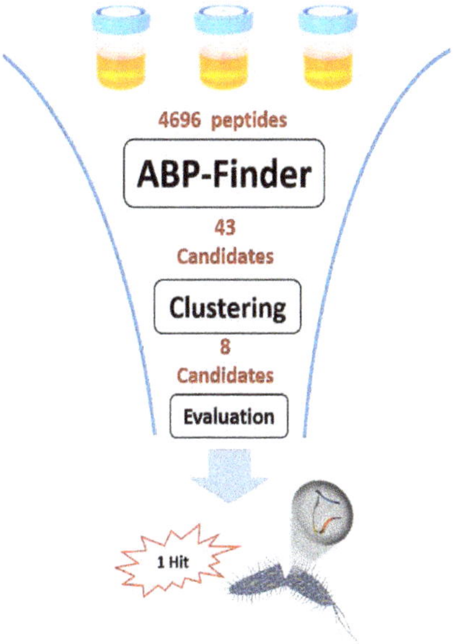

Figure 5. Schematic representation of the virtual screening process carried out on a library of peptides from the human urine peptidome.

ABP-Finder was used to score the original 4696 peptides of the library, obtaining 43 candidates with a probability score larger than 0.6, and within the applicability domain of the model. Subsequently, Blastp [61] was used to cross-align these peptides with known ABPs of our training samples. From there, we excluded two hits that showed 100% identity and coverage in the alignment with previously reported ABPs and therefore did not have value as newly identified peptides. Afterward, we clustered the peptide sequences using CD-Hit [62] with a cut-off of 90% of identity, and minimum coverage of the shortest sequence in the alignment of 90%. From this analysis, eleven clusters were obtained, from which we extracted the shortest sequence as representative of each cluster. Three polyproline peptides, containing none or only one residue other than proline were finally discarded because we considered them unsuitable as candidates for possible lead compounds due to synthetic unfeasibility and the highly homogenous character of their sequences. The final eight candidates (Table 7) were experimentally evaluated using an agar diffusion assay, leading to one active hit, Urine-3462, against *Pseudomonas aeruginosa*.

Table 7. The resulting eight ABP candidates from the virtual human urine peptidome screening and some of its global sequence descriptors. Global peptide descriptors were calculated using the Peptide Design and Analysis Under Galaxy (PDAUG) package [63].

Peptide	Sequence	Length	pI	Total Charge #	Global Hydrophobicity *	GRAVY Index &
U2162	KKVLGAFSDGLAHLDNLKGT	20	10.42	1.09	0.08	−0.12
U687	DKTNVKAAWGKVGAHAGEYGAE	22	9.53	0.10	0.01	−0.73
U4507	WLKEGVLGLVHEF	13	7.70	−0.90	0.39	0.52
U3462	RVDPVNFKLLSHCLLVT	17	10.03	1.03	0.18	0.67
U2125	KAVGKVIPELNGKLTGM	17	10.99	1.99	0.15	0.12
U1930	IAGVGAEILNVAKGIRSF	18	11.40	0.99	0.35	0.92
U1982	IFVKTLTGKTI	11	13.0	1.99	0.32	0.86
U2273	KVVAGVANALAHK	13	13.0	2.09	0.24	0.67

Total Molecular Charge given at pH = 7. * Eisenberg scale. & GRAVY (Grand Average of Hydropathy) is calculated as the sum of hydropathy values of all the amino acids, divided by the number of residues in the sequence [64]. Positive GRAVY values indicate hydrophobic; negative values mean hydrophilic.

3.7. Experimental Evaluation of the Reduced Set of Peptides from the Human Urine Peptidome

To test the antimicrobial potential of the eight candidate peptides identified with ABP-Finder, a radial diffusion assay was carried out, allowing the sensitive detection of antibacterial activity. Activity was determined against various Gram-positive and Gram-negative bacteria species, including *Bacillus subtilis*, *Streptococcus agalactiae*, *Staphylococcus aureus* (MRSA), *Escherichia coli*, *Pseudomonas aeruginosa*, *Klebsiella pneumoniae* (ESBL). While the peptide Urine-3462 was active against *Pseudomonas aeruginosa*, no relevant antibacterial activity could be detected at concentrations of 100 μg/mL and 1 mg/mL of the other peptides. Urine-3462 exhibited a dose-dependent growth of inhibition of *Pseudomonas aeruginosa*, comparable to the inhibitory activity observed for the well described antimicrobial peptide LL37 [54,65], which served as a positive control (Figure 6).

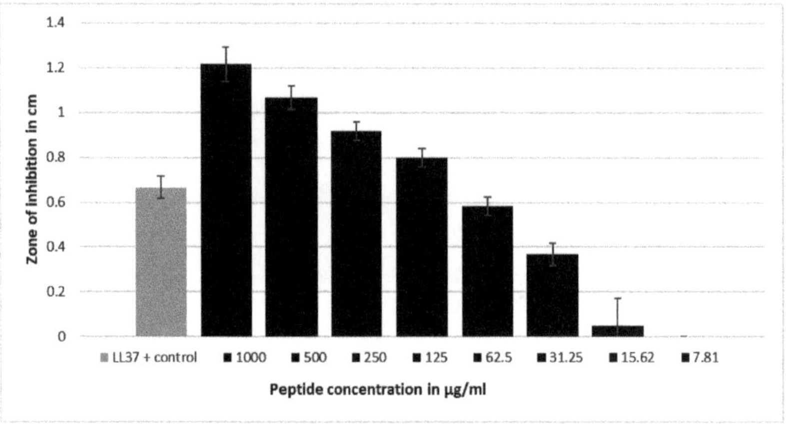

Figure 6. A radial diffusion assay indicated that the peptide Urine-3462 is active against the *Pseudomonas aeruginosa* strain ATCC 27853. Inhibition zones are quantified in cm. The mean values and standard deviations of six independent experiments are shown. LL37 at 100 μg/mL was used as positive control (see Table S3 for exact values).

4. Conclusions

Antibacterial peptides are promising candidates for a new generation of antibiotics designed to address the challenging problem of drug resistance in bacteria. With ABP-Finder we provide a tool that delivers top-ranked predictions as established by several comparisons with prominent examples of the state-of-the-art ABP predictors. Remarkably, ABP-Finder produces the most precise predictions in validation tests with known data. Furthermore, unlike other tools of the state-of-the-art that were used for comparison in this work, we present a successful application of the method in a real-life scenario dealing with the massive screening of unlabeled peptides from the human urine peptidome.

We implemented this RF-based predictor in the user-friendly and freely accessible web server ABP-Finder, which was also leveraged in the identification of the new ABP hit from a large library of peptides derived from the human peptidome.

In this way, the combination of in silico screening and experiments confirmed the applicability of ABP-Finder as a screening tool for the early steps of the design of peptide-based antibiotics. To the best of our knowledge, no other publicly available ABP predictor has delivered a similar study leading to the successful identification of an active hit from tens of thousands of unlabeled peptides. Further developments of our predictor will include its combination with target-specific models. This will allow improving the design of broad-spectrum candidates, as well as to orient the selection of targets in massive screenings of bioactive peptides.

Supplementary Materials: The following supporting information can be downloaded at: https://www.mdpi.com/article/10.3390/antibiotics11121708/s1, The Supporting Information is available free of charge and includes the project files containing the setup used to compute all the descriptors employed in this work, and the AD of the datasets.

Author Contributions: Y.B.R.-B. worked on the conceptualization, data curation, formal analysis, methodology, project administration, validation, visualization and writing of the manuscript. G.A.-C. and A.A. worked mainly on the conceptualization, formal analysis, funding acquisition, supervision, validation, writing and reviewing the manuscript. S.R.-M. carried out the software development. L.-R.O., B.S. and J.M. were responsible for experimental investigation, resources, supervision, validation and revision of the manuscript. E.S.-G. was responsible for the conceptualization, funding acquisition, resources, supervision, writing and reviewing the manuscript. All authors have read and agreed to the published version of the manuscript.

Funding: This work was funded by the German Research Foundation (DFG) through the CRC 1279-Project number 316249678 to E.S-G., J.M. and B.-S., E.S.-G. was also supported by the DFG under Germany´s Excellence Strategy—EXC 2033—390677874—RESOLV, by the DFG—Project-ID: 436586093 and by the CRC 1430—Project-ID: 424228829. GACh and AA were supported by the Strategic Funding UIDB/04423/2020 and UIDP/04423/2020 through national funds provided by the Portuguese Foundation for Science and Technology (Fundação para a Ciência e a Tecnologia—FCT).

Data Availability Statement: The web server presented in this manuscript, which evaluates the described models for ABP prediction and Gram staining type classification, is freely accessible at: https://protdcal.zmb.uni-due.de/ABP-Finder/index.php (accessed on 16 November 2022). The StarPep database, which was the source for all the in-silico data used to train and validate our models is accessible at: http://mobiosd-hub.com/starpep (accessed on 4 February 2020). WEKA was the machine-learning framework used for feature selection, hyper-parameters optimization, model training and validation steps. This program can be downloaded and installed following the guidelines at: https://waikato.github.io/weka-wiki/downloading_weka/ (accessed on 16 November 2022). ProtDCal descriptors, used to encode the peptide sequences into numeric vectors, can be computed directly from the web server: https://protdcal.zmb.uni-due.de/pages/form.php (accessed on 16 November 2022), using the project files given as Supplementary Material of this manuscript. The project files gather all the configuration of parameters used to obtain the initial set of descriptors screened in this work. The training, development, validation, and test datasets, as well as the boundaries of the applicability domains for the training and production models are included as part of the Supplementary Material of this work. The assessment of the applicability domain is also a feature implemented in our web server (ABP-Finder), therefore it is automatically done and reported by the server for any evaluated peptide.

Acknowledgments: Y-B.R.-B. acknowledges the CRC 1279 of the University Hospital Ulm for a Creative Young Researcher Award for the development of algorithms to identify bioactive peptides. L.-R.O. is part of and would like to acknowledge the International Graduate School in Molecular Medicine Ulm (IGradU).

Conflicts of Interest: The authors declare no conflict of interest.

References

1. Talebi Bezmin Abadi, A.; Rizvanov, A.A.; Haertlé, T.; Blatt, N.L. World Health Organization Report: Current Crisis of Antibiotic Resistance. *BioNanoScience* **2019**, *9*, 778–788. [CrossRef]
2. Antimicrobial Resistance, C. Global burden of bacterial antimicrobial resistance in 2019: A systematic analysis. *Lancet* **2022**, *399*, 629–655. [CrossRef]
3. Yeaman, M.R.; Yount, N.Y. Mechanisms of antimicrobial peptide action and resistance. *Pharmacol. Rev.* **2003**, *55*, 27–55. [CrossRef] [PubMed]
4. Guevara Agudelo, A.; Muñoz Molina, M.; Navarrete Ospina, J.; Salazar Pulido, L.; Castro-Cardozo, B. New Horizons to Survive in a Post-Antibiotics Era. *J. Trop. Med. Health* **2018**, *10*, JTMH-130. [CrossRef]
5. Breijyeh, Z.; Jubeh, B.; Karaman, R. Resistance of Gram-Negative Bacteria to Current Antibacterial Agents and Approaches to Resolve It. *Molecules* **2020**, *25*, 1340. [CrossRef] [PubMed]
6. Bahar, A.; Ren, D. Antimicrobial peptides. *Pharmaceuticals* **2013**, *6*, 1543–1575. [CrossRef]
7. Benfield, A.H.; Henriques, S.T. Mode-of-Action of Antimicrobial Peptides: Membrane Disruption vs. Intracellular Mechanisms. *Front. Med. Technol.* **2020**, *2*, 610997. [CrossRef]

8. Le, C.F.; Fang, C.M.; Sekaran, S.D. Intracellular Targeting Mechanisms by Antimicrobial Peptides. *Antimicrob. Agents Chemother.* **2017**, *61*, e02340-16. [CrossRef]
9. Cudic, M.; Otvos, L., Jr. Intracellular targets of antibacterial peptides. *Curr. Drug Targets* **2002**, *3*, 101–106. [CrossRef]
10. Cruz, J.; Ortiz, C.; Guzman, F.; Fernandez-Lafuente, R.; Torres, R. Antimicrobial peptides: Promising compounds against pathogenic microorganisms. *Curr. Med. Chem.* **2014**, *21*, 2299–2321. [CrossRef]
11. Henninot, A.; Collins, J.C.; Nuss, J.M. The Current State of Peptide Drug Discovery: Back to the Future? *J. Med. Chem.* **2018**, *61*, 1382–1414. [CrossRef]
12. Marr, A.K.; Gooderham, W.J.; Hancock, R.E. Antibacterial peptides for therapeutic use: Obstacles and realistic outlook. *Curr. Opin. Pharmacol.* **2006**, *6*, 468–472. [CrossRef]
13. Horcajada, J.P.; Montero, M.; Oliver, A.; Sorli, L.; Luque, S.; Gomez-Zorrilla, S.; Benito, N.; Grau, S. Epidemiology and Treatment of Multidrug-Resistant and Extensively Drug-Resistant Pseudomonas aeruginosa Infections. *Clin. Microbiol. Rev.* **2019**, *32*, e00031-19. [CrossRef]
14. Gonzalez-Garcia, M.; Morales-Vicente, F.; Pico, E.D.; Garay, H.; Rivera, D.G.; Grieshober, M.; Raluca Olari, L.; Gross, R.; Conzelmann, C.; Kruger, F.; et al. Antimicrobial Activity of Cyclic-Monomeric and Dimeric Derivatives of the Snail-Derived Peptide Cm-p5 against Viral and Multidrug-Resistant Bacterial Strains. *Biomolecules* **2021**, *11*, 745. [CrossRef]
15. Mahlapuu, M.; Bjorn, C.; Ekblom, J. Antimicrobial peptides as therapeutic agents: Opportunities and challenges. *Crit. Rev. Biotechnol.* **2020**, *40*, 978–992. [CrossRef]
16. Seshadri Sundararajan, V.; Gabere, M.N.; Pretorius, A.; Adam, S.; Christoffels, A.; Lehvaslaiho, M.; Archer, J.A.; Bajic, V.B. DAMPD: A manually curated antimicrobial peptide database. *Nucleic Acids Res.* **2012**, *40*, D1108–D1112. [CrossRef]
17. Wang, G.; Li, X.; Wang, Z. APD3: The antimicrobial peptide database as a tool for research and education. *Nucleic Acids Res.* **2016**, *44*, D1087–D1093. [CrossRef]
18. Thomas, S.; Karnik, S.; Barai, R.S.; Jayaraman, V.K.; Idicula-Thomas, S. CAMP: A useful resource for research on antimicrobial peptides. *Nucleic Acids Res.* **2010**, *38*, D774–D780. [CrossRef]
19. Waghu, F.H.; Barai, R.S.; Gurung, P.; Idicula-Thomas, S. CAMPR3: A database on sequences, structures and signatures of antimicrobial peptides. *Nucleic Acids Res.* **2016**, *44*, D1094–D1097. [CrossRef]
20. Zhao, X.; Wu, H.; Lu, H.; Li, G.; Huang, Q. LAMP: A Database Linking Antimicrobial Peptides. *PLoS ONE* **2013**, *8*, e66557. [CrossRef]
21. Fan, L.; Sun, J.; Zhou, M.; Zhou, J.; Lao, X.; Zheng, H.; Xu, H. DRAMP: A comprehensive data repository of antimicrobial peptides. *Sci. Rep.* **2016**, *6*, 24482. [CrossRef] [PubMed]
22. Lee, H.T.; Lee, C.C.; Yang, J.R.; Lai, J.Z.; Chang, K.Y. A large-scale structural classification of antimicrobial peptides. *BioMed Res. Int.* **2015**, *2015*, 475062. [CrossRef] [PubMed]
23. Pirtskhalava, M.; Amstrong, A.A.; Grigolava, M.; Chubinidze, M.; Alimbarashvili, E.; Vishnepolsky, B.; Gabrielian, A.; Rosenthal, A.; Hurt, D.E.; Tartakovsky, M. DBAASP v3: Database of antimicrobial/cytotoxic activity and structure of peptides as a resource for development of new therapeutics. *Nucleic Acids Res.* **2021**, *49*, D288–D297. [CrossRef]
24. Lata, S.; Mishra, N.K.; Raghava, G.P. AntiBP2: Improved version of antibacterial peptide prediction. *BMC Bioinform.* **2010**, *11* (Suppl. 1), S19. [CrossRef] [PubMed]
25. Joseph, S.; Karnik, S.; Nilawe, P.; Jayaraman, V.K.; Idicula-Thomas, S. ClassAMP: A prediction tool for classification of antimicrobial peptides. *IEEE/ACM Trans. Comput. Biol. Bioinform.* **2012**, *9*, 1535–1538. [CrossRef]
26. Lin, W.; Xu, D. Imbalanced multi-label learning for identifying antimicrobial peptides and their functional types. *Bioinformatics* **2016**, *32*, 3745–3752. [CrossRef]
27. Meher, P.K.; Sahu, T.K.; Saini, V.; Rao, A.R. Predicting antimicrobial peptides with improved accuracy by incorporating the compositional, physico-chemical and structural features into Chou's general PseAAC. *Sci. Rep.* **2017**, *7*, 42362. [CrossRef]
28. Gull, S.; Shamim, N.; Minhas, F. AMAP: Hierarchical multi-label prediction of biologically active and antimicrobial peptides. *Comput. Biol. Med.* **2019**, *107*, 172–181. [CrossRef]
29. Veltri, D.P. *A Computational and Statistical Framework for Screening Novel Antimicrobial Peptides*; George Mason University: Fairfax, VA, USA, 2015.
30. Veltri, D.; Kamath, U.; Shehu, A. Deep learning improves antimicrobial peptide recognition. *Bioinformatics* **2018**, *34*, 2740–2747. [CrossRef]
31. Pinacho-Castellanos, S.A.; García-Jacas, C.R.; Gilson, M.K.; Brizuela, C.A. Alignment-Free Antimicrobial Peptide Predictors: Improving Performance by a Thorough Analysis of the Largest Available Data Set. *J. Chem. Inf. Model.* **2021**, *61*, 3141–3157. [CrossRef]
32. Aguilera-Mendoza, L.; Marrero-Ponce, Y.; Garcia-Jacas, C.R.; Chavez, E.; Beltran, J.A.; Guillen-Ramirez, H.A.; Brizuela, C.A. Automatic construction of molecular similarity networks for visual graph mining in chemical space of bioactive peptides: An unsupervised learning approach. *Sci. Rep.* **2020**, *10*, 18074. [CrossRef]
33. Aguilera-Mendoza, L.; Marrero-Ponce, Y.; Beltran, J.A.; Tellez Ibarra, R.; Guillen-Ramirez, H.A.; Brizuela, C.A. Graph-based data integration from bioactive peptide databases of pharmaceutical interest: Toward an organized collection enabling visual network analysis. *Bioinformatics* **2019**, *35*, 4739–4747. [CrossRef]

34. OECD. *Guidance Document on the Validation of (Quantitative) Structure-Activity Relationship [(Q)SAR] Models*; OECD: Paris, France, 2014.
35. Chicco, D.; Jurman, G. The advantages of the Matthews correlation coefficient (MCC) over F1 score and accuracy in binary classification evaluation. *BMC Genom.* **2020**, *21*, 6. [CrossRef]
36. Breiman, L. Random Forests. *Mach. Learn.* **2001**, *45*, 5–32. [CrossRef]
37. Witten, I.H.; Frank, E.; Hall, M.A.; Pal, C.J. *Data Mining, Fourth Edition: Practical Machine Learning Tools and Techniques*, 4th ed.; Morgan Kaufmann Publishers Inc.: San Francisco, CA, USA, 2016.
38. Dietterich, T.G. *Ensemble Methods in Machine Learning*; Springer: Berlin/Heidelberg, Germany, 2000; pp. 1–15.
39. Garcia-Jacas, C.R.; Pinacho-Castellanos, S.A.; Garcia-Gonzalez, L.A.; Brizuela, C.A. Do deep learning models make a difference in the identification of antimicrobial peptides? *Brief. Bioinform.* **2022**, *23*, bbac094. [CrossRef]
40. Romero-Molina, S.; Ruiz-Blanco, Y.B.; Green, J.R.; Sanchez-Garcia, E. ProtDCal-Suite: A web server for the numerical codification and functional analysis of proteins. *Protein Sci.* **2019**, *28*, 1734–1743. [CrossRef]
41. Ruiz-Blanco, Y.B.; Paz, W.; Green, J.; Marrero-Ponce, Y. ProtDCal: A program to compute general-purpose-numerical descriptors for sequences and 3D-structures of proteins. *BMC Bioinform.* **2015**, *16*, 162. [CrossRef]
42. Biggar, K.K.; Charih, F.; Liu, H.; Ruiz-Blanco, Y.B.; Stalker, L.; Chopra, A.; Connolly, J.; Adhikary, H.; Frensemier, K.; Hoekstra, M.; et al. Proteome-wide Prediction of Lysine Methylation Leads to Identification of H2BK43 Methylation and Outlines the Potential Methyllysine Proteome. *Cell Rep.* **2020**, *32*, 107896. [CrossRef] [PubMed]
43. Ruiz-Blanco, Y.B.; Marrero-Ponce, Y.; García-Hernández, E.; Green, J. Novel "extended sequons" of human N-glycosylation sites improve the precision of qualitative predictions: An alignment-free study of pattern recognition using ProtDCal protein features. *Amino Acids* **2017**, *49*, 317–325. [CrossRef]
44. Romero-Molina, S.; Ruiz-Blanco, Y.B.; Harms, M.; Münch, J.; Sanchez-Garcia, E. PPI-Detect: A support vector machine model for sequence-based prediction of protein–protein interactions. *J. Comput. Chem.* **2019**, *40*, 1233–1242. [CrossRef]
45. Ruiz-Blanco, Y.B.; Agüero-Chapin, G.; García-Hernández, E.; Álvarez, O.; Antunes, A.; Green, J. Exploring general-purpose protein features for distinguishing enzymes and non-enzymes within the twilight zone. *BMC Bioinform.* **2017**, *18*, 349. [CrossRef] [PubMed]
46. Corral-Corral, R.; Beltrán, J.A.; Brizuela, C.A.; Del Rio, G. Systematic Identification of Machine-Learning Models Aimed to Classify Critical Residues for Protein Function from Protein Structure. *Molecules* **2017**, *22*, 1673. [CrossRef]
47. Kleandrova, V.V.; Ruso, J.M.; Speck-Planche, A.; Cordeiro, M.N.D.S. Enabling the Discovery and Virtual Screening of Potent and Safe Antimicrobial Peptides. Simultaneous Prediction of Antibacterial Activity and Cytotoxicity. *ACS Comb. Sci.* **2016**, *18*, 490–498. [CrossRef] [PubMed]
48. Speck-Planche, A.; Kleandrova, V.V.; Ruso, J.M.; Cordeiro, M.N.D.S. First Multitarget Chemo-Bioinformatic Model to Enable the Discovery of Antibacterial Peptides against Multiple Gram-Positive Pathogens. *J. Chem. Inf. Model.* **2016**, *56*, 588–598. [CrossRef]
49. Hearst, M.A. Support Vector Machines. *IEEE Intell. Syst.* **1998**, *13*, 18–28. [CrossRef]
50. Chou, K.C. Prediction of protein cellular attributes using pseudo-amino acid composition. *Proteins Struct. Funct. Bioinform.* **2001**, *43*, 246–255. [CrossRef]
51. Chen, T.; Guestrin, C. XGBoost: A Scalable Tree Boosting System. In Proceedings of the 22nd ACM SIGKDD International Conference on Knowledge Discovery and Data Mining, San Francisco, CA, USA, 13–17 August 2016; pp. 785–794.
52. Xiao, X.; Wang, P.; Lin, W.Z.; Jia, J.H.; Chou, K.C. iAMP-2L: A two-level multi-label classifier for identifying antimicrobial peptides and their functional types. *Anal. Biochem.* **2013**, *436*, 168–177. [CrossRef]
53. Fernandes, F.C.; Rigden, D.J.; Franco, O.L. Prediction of antimicrobial peptides based on the adaptive neuro-fuzzy inference system application. *Biopolymers* **2012**, *98*, 280–287. [CrossRef]
54. Vicente, F.E.M.; Gonzalez-Garcia, M.; Diaz Pico, E.; Moreno-Castillo, E.; Garay, H.E.; Rosi, P.E.; Jimenez, A.M.; Campos-Delgado, J.A.; Rivera, D.G.; Chinea, G.; et al. Design of a Helical-Stabilized, Cyclic, and Nontoxic Analogue of the Peptide Cm-p5 with Improved Antifungal Activity. *ACS Omega* **2019**, *4*, 19081–19095. [CrossRef]
55. Kent, J.T. Information gain and a general measure of correlation. *Biometrika* **1983**, *70*, 163–173. [CrossRef]
56. Lee, C.; Lee, G.G. Information gain and divergence-based feature selection for machine learning-based text categorization. *Inf. Process. Manag.* **2006**, *42*, 155–165. [CrossRef]
57. Heyer, L.J.; Kruglyak, S.; Yooseph, S. Exploring Expression Data: Identification and Analysis of Coexpressed Genes. *Genome Res.* **1999**, *9*, 1106–1115. [CrossRef]
58. Spearman Rank Correlation Coefficient. In *The Concise Encyclopedia of Statistics*; Springer: New York, NY, USA, 2008; pp. 502–505.
59. Goldberg, D.E. *Genetic Algorithms in Search, Optimization and Machine Learning*, 1st ed.; Addison-Wesley Longman Publishing Co. Inc.: Boston, MA, USA, 1989.
60. Holch, A.; Bauer, R.; Olari, L.-R.; Rodriguez, A.A.; Ständker, L.; Preising, N.; Karacan, M.; Wiese, S.; Walther, P.; Ruiz-Blanco, Y.B.; et al. Respiratory β-2-Microglobulin exerts pH dependent antimicrobial activity. *Virulence* **2020**, *11*, 1402–1414. [CrossRef]
61. Altschul, S.F.; Gish, W.; Miller, W.; Myers, E.W.; Lipman, D.J. Basic local alignment search tool. *J. Mol. Biol.* **1990**, *215*, 403–410. [CrossRef]
62. Li, W.; Godzik, A. Cd-hit: A fast program for clustering and comparing large sets of protein or nucleotide sequences. *Bioinformatics* **2006**, *22*, 1658–1659. [CrossRef]

63. Joshi, J.; Blankenberg, D. PDAUG: A Galaxy based toolset for peptide library analysis, visualization, and machine learning modeling. *BMC Bioinform.* **2022**, *23*, 197. [CrossRef]
64. Kyte, J.; Doolittle, R.F. A simple method for displaying the hydropathic character of a protein. *J. Mol. Biol.* **1982**, *157*, 105–132. [CrossRef]
65. Overhage, J.; Campisano, A.; Bains, M.; Torfs, E.C.; Rehm, B.H.; Hancock, R.E. Human host defense peptide LL-37 prevents bacterial biofilm formation. *Infect. Immun.* **2008**, *76*, 4176–4182. [CrossRef]

antibiotics

MDPI

Article

Computational Design of Inhibitors Targeting the Catalytic β Subunit of *Escherichia coli* F_OF_1-ATP Synthase

Luis Pablo Avila-Barrientos [1,†], Luis Fernando Cofas-Vargas [1,†], Guillermin Agüero-Chapin [2,3], Enrique Hernández-García [1], Sergio Ruiz-Carmona [4,‡], Norma A. Valdez-Cruz [5], Mauricio Trujillo-Roldán [5], Joachim Weber [6], Yasser B. Ruiz-Blanco [1,7,*], Xavier Barril [8,9] and Enrique García-Hernández [1,*]

1 Instituto de Química, Universidad Nacional Autónoma de México, Ciudad Universitaria, Ciudad de México 04510, Mexico; lpablo@comunidad.unam.mx (L.P.A.-B.); fcofas@comunidad.unam.mx (L.F.C.-V.); enrique.hernandez@iquimica.unam.mx (E.H.-G.)
2 CIMAR/CIIMAR, Centro Interdisciplinar de Investigação Marinha e Ambiental, Universidade do Porto, Terminal de Cruzeiros do Porto de Leixões, Av. General Norton de Matos, s/n, 4450-208 Porto, Portugal; gchapin@ciimar.up.pt
3 Departamento de Biologia, Faculdade de Ciências, Universidade do Porto, Rua do Campo Alegre, 4169-007 Porto, Portugal
4 Institut de Biomedicina de la Universitat de Barcelona (IBUB) and Facultat de Farmàcia, Universitat de Barcelona, Av. Joan XXIII s/n, 08028 Barcelona, Spain; sruizcarmona@gmail.com
5 Programa de Investigación de Producción de Biomoléculas, Departamento de Biología Molecular y Biotecnología, Instituto de Investigaciones Biomédicas, Universidad Nacional Autónoma de México, Cd. Universitaria, Ciudad de México 04510, Mexico; adri@biomedicas.unam.mx (N.A.V.-C.); maurotru@biomedicas.unam.mx (M.T.-R.)
6 Department of Chemistry and Biochemistry, Texas Tech University, Lubbock, TX 79409, USA; joachim.weber@ttu.edu
7 Center of Medical Biotechnology, Faculty of Biology, University of Duisburg-Essen, 45127 Essen, Germany
8 Departament de Farmacia i Tecnología Farmacèutica, i Fisicoquímica, Institut de Biomedicina (IBUB), Universitat de Barcelona, Av. Joan XXIII, 27-31, 08028 Barcelona, Spain; xbarril@ub.edu
9 Catalan Institution for Research and Advanced Studies (ICREA), 08010 Barcelona, Spain
* Correspondence: yasser.ruizblanco@uni-due.de (Y.B.R.-B.); egarciah@unam.mx (E.G.-H.)
† These authors contributed equally to this work.
‡ Current address: Cambridge Baker Systems Genomics Initiative, Baker Heart and Diabetes Institute, Melbourne, VIC 3004, Australia.

Citation: Avila-Barrientos, L.P.; Cofas-Vargas, L.F.; Agüero-Chapin, G.; Hernández-García, E.; Ruiz-Carmona, S.; Valdez-Cruz, N.A.; Trujillo-Roldán, M.; Weber, J.; Ruiz-Blanco, Y.B.; Barril, X.; et al. Computational Design of Inhibitors Targeting the Catalytic β Subunit of *Escherichia coli* F_OF_1-ATP Synthase. *Antibiotics* **2022**, *11*, 557. https://doi.org/10.3390/antibiotics11050557

Academic Editor: Jean-Marc Sabatier

Received: 7 March 2022
Accepted: 25 March 2022
Published: 22 April 2022

Publisher's Note: MDPI stays neutral with regard to jurisdictional claims in published maps and institutional affiliations.

Copyright: © 2022 by the authors. Licensee MDPI, Basel, Switzerland. This article is an open access article distributed under the terms and conditions of the Creative Commons Attribution (CC BY) license (https://creativecommons.org/licenses/by/4.0/).

Abstract: With the uncontrolled growth of multidrug-resistant bacteria, there is an urgent need to search for new therapeutic targets, to develop drugs with novel modes of bactericidal action. FoF1-ATP synthase plays a crucial role in bacterial bioenergetic processes, and it has emerged as an attractive antimicrobial target, validated by the pharmaceutical approval of an inhibitor to treat multidrug-resistant tuberculosis. In this work, we aimed to design, through two types of in silico strategies, new allosteric inhibitors of the ATP synthase, by targeting the catalytic β subunit, a centerpiece in communication between rotor subunits and catalytic sites, to drive the rotary mechanism. As a model system, we used the F1 sector of Escherichia coli, a bacterium included in the priority list of multidrug-resistant pathogens. Drug-like molecules and an IF1-derived peptide, designed through molecular dynamics simulations and sequence mining approaches, respectively, exhibited in vitro micromolar inhibitor potency against F1. An analysis of bacterial and Mammalia sequences of the key structural helix-turn-turn motif of the C-terminal domain of the β subunit revealed highly and moderately conserved positions that could be exploited for the development of new species-specific allosteric inhibitors. To our knowledge, these inhibitors are the first binders computationally designed against the catalytic subunit of FOF1-ATP synthase.

Keywords: F_OF_1-ATP synthase; allosteric inhibition; structure-based drug design; evolutionary and PPI algorithms; peptide design

1. Introduction

At the end of the last century, there were already alarming signs of a growing health crisis because of the emergence of antimicrobial resistance (AMR) [1], which, if left unattended, would cause worldwide mass fatalities and colossal financial burden [2,3]. As it was feared, the decline in investment in the development of novel antibiotics has aggravated this crisis, reflected in the decrease in newly approved antibiotics, although a slight change in this trend was recently reported [4]. AMR microorganisms have developed effective antibiotic evasion mechanisms [5]. The need to circumvent those mechanisms prompts the search for novel pharmacological targets [4]. Bacterial bioenergetic pathways have recently unveiled a new Achilles heel to combat AMR [6], as evidenced by bedaquiline, the first approved anti-tuberculosis drug in 40 years, which targets *Mycobacterium tuberculosis* ATP synthase [7]. Furthermore, mounting evidence supports that blocking the catalytic activity of this enzyme sensitizes AMR facultative anaerobic microorganisms (*v. gr.*, *Staphylococcus aureus* and *Escherichia coli*) to the action of other antimicrobial agents [8–10]. Therefore, ATP synthase appears as a momentous pharmacological target to broaden the battlefront against the pathogens of major concern.

ATP synthase is a sophisticated molecular motor, with an efficiency of ~100% [11], made up of two functionally coupled subcomplexes: a membrane embedded proton channel, F_O, and a soluble catalytic subcomplex, F_1. Together, F_O and F_1 harvest electrochemical gradient potential energy to produce rotational energy that is eventually converted into chemical energy as a phosphodiester bond [12,13]. The enzyme also catalyzes, with high efficiency, the hydrolysis of ATP, being able to restore the proton gradient under physiological demand (v.gr., to generate membrane potential in bacteria under anaerobic conditions) [14]. The minimal architecture of this enzyme is found in bacteria (Figure 1), composed of eight types of subunits, with F_O:$ab_2c_{10\text{-}17}$ and F_1:$\alpha_3\beta_3\gamma\delta\varepsilon$ stoichiometries [12,15]. Proton translocation (or sodium ions, in some species) drives the rotation of the transmembrane ring of *c* subunits relative to the *a* subunit. This rotation drives the torque of the asymmetric γ subunit, which is partially embedded in the catalytic $\alpha_3\beta_3$ ring. $\alpha_3\beta_3$ is stabilized against rotation by the stator stalk, composed of δ, *b*, and *a* subunits in bacteria [16], and by a larger number of different subunits in mitochondria [17]. ATP synthase operates under a mechanism dubbed as the binding change mechanism [18]. Each of the three catalytic sites, composed mainly of residues of the β subunit and some of the α subunit, transits through three alternating affinity states, corresponding to three different conformational states. According to the nucleotide occupancy exhibited in the first experimental F_1 structure from *Bos taurus* (BsF_1) [19], these states are usually termed as β_E (empty binding site), β_{TP} (ATP bound), and β_{DP} (ADP bound). When the enzyme acts as a hydrolase, in an alternate progression, each β subunit goes in the order $\beta_E \rightarrow \beta_{TP} \rightarrow \beta_{DP}$ as the catalytic cycle progresses. The conformational changes in the β subunits are coupled to the formation and breakdown of contacts with the asymmetric α-helices of the γ subunit and the adjacent α subunits. In this rotary mechanism, the helix-turn-helix (HTH) motif of the β-subunit C-terminal domain (βCterm) plays a central role in the communication with the other subunits and has been described as a pushrod, pushed by the γ subunit (or which sets the γ subunit in motion in the hydrolysis direction) [20,21]. βCterm is in an open conformation in β_E, with minimal intercatenary interactions. After 120° rotation of the γ subunit, driven by ATP binding, βCterm transits into a closed conformation in β_{TP}, contacting to the γ subunit and one of the adjacent α subunits (α_{TP}). A further 120° γ-subunit rotation leads to β_{DP}, a conformation very similar to β_{TP}, except for tighter packing of its βCterm against the γ subunit and the adjacent α subunit (α_{DP}). ATP hydrolysis and ADP release occur within $0° \rightarrow \sim 90°$ and $\sim 90° \rightarrow 120°$ rotation substeps in the $\beta_{TP} \rightarrow \beta_{DP}$ and $\beta_{DP} \rightarrow \beta_E$ transitions, respectively [13]. In the self-inhibited conformation of the *Escherichia coli's* F_1 (EcF_1), the β subunits β_2 and β_3 exhibit β_E- and β_{TP}-like conformations, respectively, while β_1 adopts a half-closed conformation because of a steric hindrance of the C-terminal domain of the ε subunit in an extended conformation (Figure 1) [16,22].

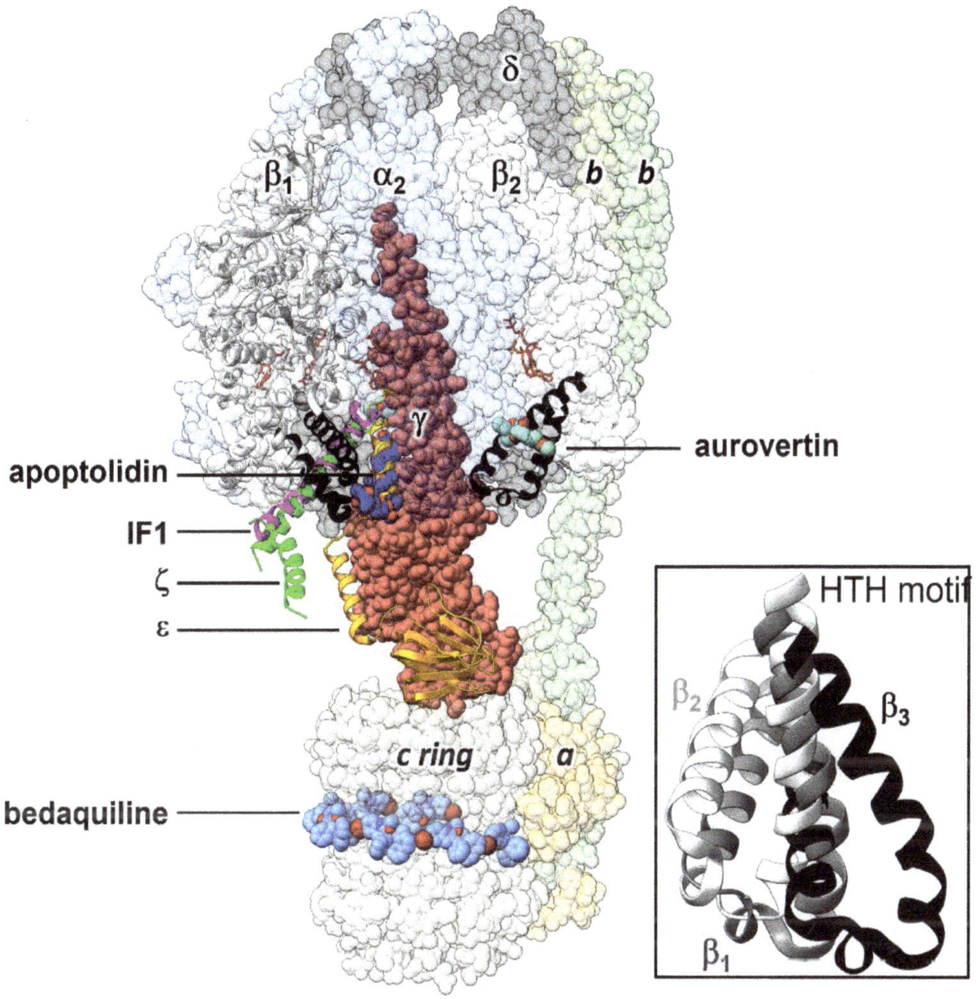

Figure 1. Schematic representation of the 3D structure of *E. coli* F_OF_1-ATP synthase, showing the binding sites of allosteric inhibitors that interact with the C-terminal domain of the β subunit. Inhibitors whose 3D structure in complex with the enzyme has been experimentally solved were docked by alignment on the cryoEM structure of the *E. coli* enzyme in an inhibited conformation by the ε subunit (PDB ID 6oqr [16]). HTH motifs of β_1 and β_2 are in black ribbons. The F_1 and F_O subcomplexes are composed of the $\alpha_3\beta_3\gamma\delta\varepsilon$ and ab_2c_{10} subunits, respectively. The endogenous inhibitory ε (PDB ID 6oqr [16]), ζ (PDB ID 5dn6 [23]) and IF1 (PDB ID 1ohh [24]) subunits are shown in ribbons. The exogenous inhibitors aurovertin B (PDB ID 1cow [25]) and the glycomacrolide apoptolidin A (PDB ID 7md3 [26]) are shown in spheres. Here, also shown is the position of the anti-tuberculosis drug bedaquiline (PDB ID 7jg8 [27]), which occupies sites equivalent to those of oligomycin in the *c* ring. Nucleotides are shown in sticks. **Inset:** Alignment of the HTH motifs of the three β subunits observed in the self-inhibited structure of *EcF1* [16,22]. In this conformation, the ε subunit hampers the closing of one β subunit, adopting a half-closed conformation (β_1). A β_1-like conformation is also observed in the complexes with the glycomacrolides apoptolidin A and ammocidin A [26].

A wealth of exogenous and endogenous ATP synthase inhibitors has been described [28,29]. Structural studies have identified several binding sites along the ATP synthase architecture for these inhibitors, revealing the existence of a diversity of allosteric mechanisms to inhibit the enzyme (Figure 1). Many of these inhibitors bind to sites involving βCterm. The eukaryotic inhibitor IF1 [30], and the prokaryotic ε and ζ subunits insert an α-helix motif into a pocket formed by the $\alpha_3\beta_3$ ring and the γ subunit, near the C-terminal domains of α_{DP} and β_{DP}, thus, stopping rotational catalysis and preventing wasteful ATP consumption [31–33]. Recently, the binding site of a family of glycomacrolide inhibitors was identified, in a region involving the HTH motif of a β_1-like subunit [26]. In addition, aurovertins, antibiotics produced by the fungus *Calcarisporium arbuscula,* target equivalent sites in the bovine β_E and β_{TP} subunits between βCterm and the nucleotide binding domain [25]. Taken together, the existence of these non-orthosteric inhibitors indicates that βCterm is a suitable target for the development of allosteric pharmacological modulators. Because of a less stringent evolutionary pressure, allosteric sites tend to be less conserved than catalytic sites [34–36]. This aspect is relevant to design specific ATP synthase inhibitors, since some regions of the active site of this enzyme are highly conserved across P-loop NTPases [37,38]. Furthermore, allosteric inhibitors do not compete with the substrate, so they do not require reaching an extremely high binding potency to exert an effective pharmacological action [39]. Target-based allosteric inhibitor design on ATP synthase has been limited. GaMF1 [40] and epigallocatechin gallate [41] are a notable exception. These compounds, which inhibit mycobacterial ATP synthase by binding to γ and ε subunits, respectively, have been obtained through pharmacophoric-restraints filtered docking studies.

Given the crucial role played by the βCterm in driving the rotational mechanism of F_OF_1-ATP synthase, in this work, we set out to design, through two types of in silico strategies, new allosteric inhibitors, by targeting the HTH motif of the *Escherichia coli* F_1 (EcF_1), a bacterium included in the ESKAPEE (*Enterococcus faecium, Staphylococcus aureus, Klebsiella pneumoniae, Acinetobacter baumannii, Pseudomonas aeruginosa, Enterobacter spp*, and *Escherichia coli*) list of the most threatening AMR microbes [42]. The underlying idea was that the engineered binders, by interfering with the conformational transitions of this motif, will exert an allosteric effect, leading to the blocking of the enzyme's rotation. On the one hand, through a molecular dynamics (MD) simulation approach with solvent mixtures (MDmix), we identified solvent sites (SS) on the HTH motif that helped guide the high-throughput virtual screening (HTVS) of drug-like molecules [43,44]. The best hits were further filtered using the dynamic undocking method (DUck), an orthogonal technique that evaluates the work developed upon pulling the ligand out from the binding site [45]. Using a new in silico strategy, guided by evolutionary and machine learning-based methods [46], we derived peptides from IF1, based on the observation that the residues that bind this inhibitor in BsF_1 are highly conserved in EcF_1. Both approaches led to the identification of drug-like and peptide hits that inhibited the hydrolytic activity of EcF_1 with micromolar potency. Remarkably, given the different nature of the identified hits and the distinct modeling approaches, we proved the feasibility of the in silico design of ATPase inhibitors, targeting the catalytic subunit. These molecules could serve as leading scaffolds for the development of novel drugs to combat AMR bacterial strains.

2. Results

2.1. Structure-Based Design of Small Organic Inhibitors

For the design of drug-like molecules, based on the structure of ATP synthase, we performed MD simulations using the crystallographic structure of EcF_1, self-inhibited by the ε subunit and MgADP (Figure 1, PDB ID 3oaa), a distinctive conformational state of the enzyme in bacteria and chloroplasts [16,22]. In this structure, β_2 and β_3 show conformations very close to bovine β_E and β_{TP}, respectively. In contrast, β_1 adopts an intermediate conformation, since the ε subunit impedes the total closure of βCterm (Figure 1 inset), a mechanism hypothesized to prevent the enzyme from falling to a low-energy state, inhibited by MgADP [47]. To sample the conformational space neighboring, the crystal structure of EcF_1, unrestrained 20-ns simulations were performed. Judging by the time evolution of the RMSD (Figure 2A), the HTH of β_1 converged to the same conformation in all solvent and pure water replicas, except for one trajectory in ethanol, in which a slightly more open conformation of the DELSEED motif was observed (Figure 2B). The analysis of this trajectory revealed the well-defined presence ($\Delta G_{SS} \leq -1$ kcal/mol) of a solvent site cluster, in an area close to the DELSEED region and intermediate between the two HTH helices. The cluster was composed of a site for the hydroxyl's oxygen (SS_{OH}) and three sites for the methyl carbon (SS_{CT}) of ethanol (Figure 2C). The carbonyl group of G^{378} stabilized the unique SS_{OH}, while the side chains of R^{366}, Y^{367}, I^{373}, V^{389}, and A^{393} were involved in the stabilization of the SS_{CT}. Consistently, the four solvent sites were closely reproduced in three MD replicas, in which harmonic constraints (k = 0.5 kcal/molÅ^2) were imposed on the heavy atoms of the protein to keep the HTH in open conformation (data not shown). Therefore, this open conformation of HTH, which was also significantly, albeit to a lesser degree, populated in pure water replicas, was apparently stabilized by the organic solvent.

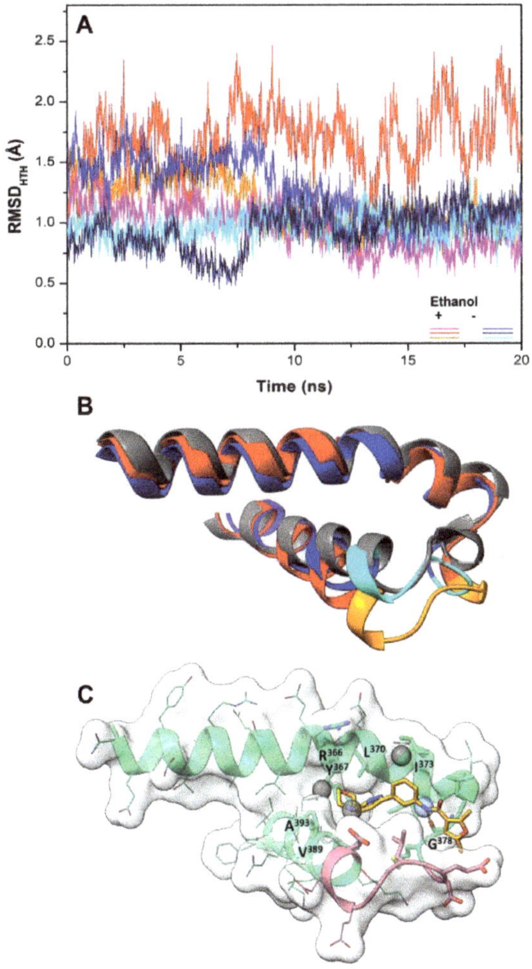

Figure 2. HTH dynamics and solvent sites determined from MD simulations. (**A**) RMSD was calculated using backbone atoms of the β_1 HTH motif. Values from three MD simulations in

pure water (blue colors) and three in water-ethanol mixture (red colors) are shown. (**B**) Average conformations of the HTH motif calculated over the last 10 ns of simulation. The open conformation obtained in one trajectory in a solvent mixture is shown in orange, while a closed conformation from one of the replicas in pure water is shown in blue. The DELSEED motif is in lighter color. The starting crystal conformation is in gray (PDB ID 3oaa, [22]). (**C**) Solvent sites for ethanol's methyl (gray spheres) and hydroxyl (blue sphere) groups determined from one trajectory in ethanol/water mixture. One of the ligands (Compd-5) obtained in this work by HTVS (vide infra) is shown in sticks, forming a hydrogen bond with the carbonyl group of G^{378}. The DELSEED motif is in pink.

The four solvent sites observed in β_1 were used as pharmacophoric restraints to guide HTVS of ~8×10^6 molecules from eight different commercial chemical libraries, using the rDock software [44]. After removing molecules with very similar chemical structures by visual inspection, the 100 top-ranked molecules, ordered according to the docking score, were additionally filtered using steering dynamics, with the DUck method [45]. The work required (W_{QB}) to move away the hydrogen donor atom of the docked molecule to 5 Å (quasi-bound state) from the carbonyl group of G^{378} was determined, discarding those molecules with W_{QB} < 6 kcal/mol. As a result, 27 potential ligands were selected and purchased (Table S1). The inhibitory potency of these compounds was assayed against purified EcF_1, using the malachite green method. As shown in Table 1, five compounds displayed significant inhibition of ATPase activity at 100 μM of inhibitor concentration. Measurements performed using the NADH-linked ATP regeneration system yielded similar inhibition values. According to the Chemaxon solubility predictor server [48], the five compounds are soluble in the micromolar range (Table 1). It is also worth mentioning that, according to the MOE software, the five hit molecules are not pan-assay interference compounds (PAINS). Only compound 18 and 26 contained a PAINS warning.

Table 1. Summary of the final active compounds designed against the HTH motif structure of EcF_1.

	Structure [a]	ΔG_{rDock} [b] (kcal/mol)	W_{QB} [c] (kcal/mol)	ΔG_{PB} [d] (kcal/mol)	Residual ATPase Activity (%) [e]	logS [f]
Compd-5	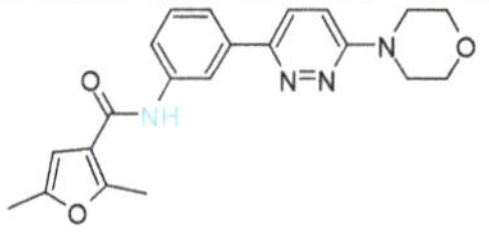	−6.0	8.7	−29	43 ± 6 (50 ± 5%)	−4.7
Compd-7	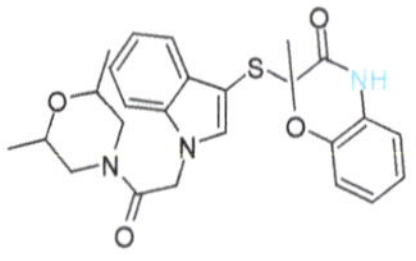	−5.5	6.0	−30	64 ± 12 (70 ± 10%)	−5.1
Compd-14	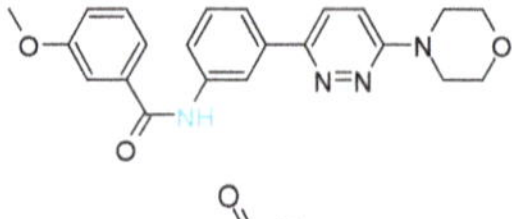	−4.5	6.7	−25	75 ± 8 (73 ± 2%)	−5.3
Compd-15	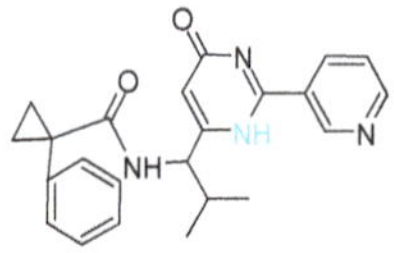	−4.3	6.0	−24	67 ± 5 (ND)	−4.9
Compd-19	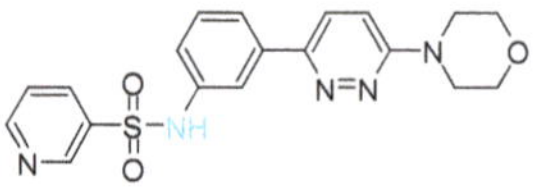	−4.0	6.0	−29	77 ± 7 (70 ± 10%)	−2.8

[a] NH atoms that established hydrogen bonds with the G^{378} backbone oxygen are in blue. [b] rDock score, a weighted sum of intermolecular, ligand intramolecular, site intramolecular and pharmacophoric restraints [44].

[c] Work needed to separate the ligand's atom forming a hydrogen bond with the protein to a 5 Å distance, calculated with DUck [45]. [d] Molecular mechanics Poisson–Boltzmann surface area (MM-PBSA) calculated free energy [49,50]. [e] Residual ATPase activity of EcF_1 determined by the malachite method (and the ATP regenerating system, values in parentheses), incubated with 100 µM of the indicated compound, in a 50 mM Tris-SO_4 buffer solution with 1% DMSO (pH 8.0), 25 °C. Data represent the average ± standard deviation of at least 3 independent experiments. ND, not determined. [f] Predicted aqueous solubility determined with the Chemaxon solubility predictor server.

To further characterize the inhibitory effect of Compd-5, the ligand that exhibited the most potent activity, dose-response measurements were performed (Figure 3). Nonlinear analysis of the data, using the Hill equation, yielded an IC_{50} value of 62 ± 5 µM and a Hill coefficient of 0.86 ± 0.02, suggesting that there is no cooperativity between the three β subunits. The fitting showed a residual enzyme activity of 9 ± 1% under saturation conditions, showing that Compd-5 nearly acts as a dead-end inhibitor.

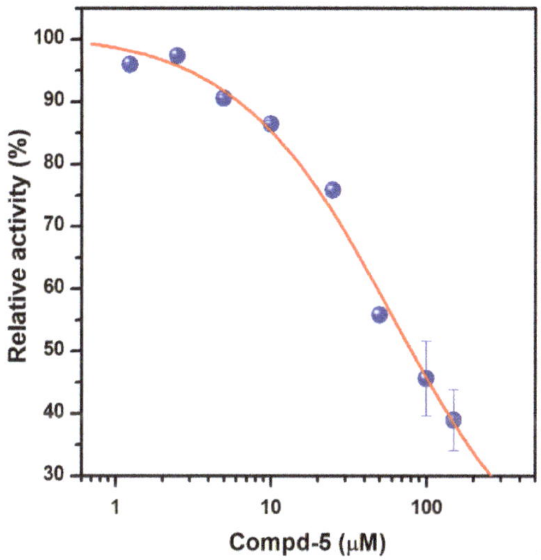

Figure 3. Dose-response plot of the inhibitory effect of Compd-5 on EcF_1. Residual ATPase activity was measured using compound concentrations in the 1.25–150 µM range, in a 100 mM Tris-SO_4 buffer solution with 1% DMSO (pH 8.0), 25 °C. The Hill equation was fitted to the experimental data, obtaining $IC_{50} = 62 \pm 5$ µM, $h = 0.86 \pm 0.02$, $v_r = 9 \pm 1\%$. Data shown represent the average ± standard deviation of 3 independent experiments.

All the active compounds had an NH group, serving as a hydrogen donor to the G^{378} carbonyl moiety. As an example, the predicted binding pose of Compd-5 is shown in Figure 2C. It is worth mentioning that Compd-5, Compd-14 and Compd-19 all come from the same family, being the only compounds in the tested set with the 4-(6-phenylpyridazin-3-yl)morpholine substructure (Simplified Molecular Input Line Entry System, SMILES, "[NH]c1cc(-c2nnc(N3CCOCC3)cc2)ccc1"). The binding energy (ΔG_{PB}) of the positive inhibitors was computed on the corresponding docked poses, using the molecular mechanics Poisson–Boltzmann surface area (MM-PBSA) method [49,50] and compared against the rDock scores (ΔG_{rDock}) in Table 1. Clearly, there is a better correlation of the degree of experimental inhibition with the energies calculated with rDock (r^2 = 0.77) than with the MM-PBSA method (r^2 = 0.12), which highlights the good performance of the HTVS method [43]. Finally, we computationally explored the possibility that the engineered inhibitors could also bind to the HTH motif of the other two β subunits. The pose of Compd-5 in β_1 was used to dock the ligand on the other two subunits to perform unrestrained MD simulations. Like β_1, β_3 kept the inhibitor bound for up to 50 ns in two replicas, a suitable time to consider the interaction as stable [51]. In contrast, the compound was consistently released from β_2 within the first nanoseconds of simulation (Figure S1).

2.2. De Novo Design of Peptide Inhibitors of EcF$_1$ Targeting the βCterm

In a previous report, we introduced a de novo design method of EcF$_1$ peptide inhibitors [46]. The new inhibitors were designed in silico from the interfaces connecting F$_O$F$_1$-ATP synthase subunits, thus, proving the suitability of these scaffolds for the generation of a new family of inhibitors. Peptide libraries were built by applying simulated molecular evolution approaches, represented by the ROSE (random model of sequence evolution) algorithm [52], and later screened using PPI-Detect, a protein–protein interaction predictor [53], to score the binding likelihood of the peptides and EcF$_1$. This new in silico strategy, guided by evolutionary and machine-learning-based methods, allowed widening and exploring the relevant structural space from natural peptide fragments to generate novel protein binders [46]. Here, we leveraged this approach for the de novo design of EcF$_1$ peptide inhibitors, specifically targeting the βCterm. The fourteen IF1 sequences registered in the UniProt database [54], ranging from 42 to 50 aa length, were aligned to identify conserved regions. Two conserved regions were identified in the multiple sequence alignment (MSA), resulting in two consensus regions that were considered root or parent peptides (Figure 4).

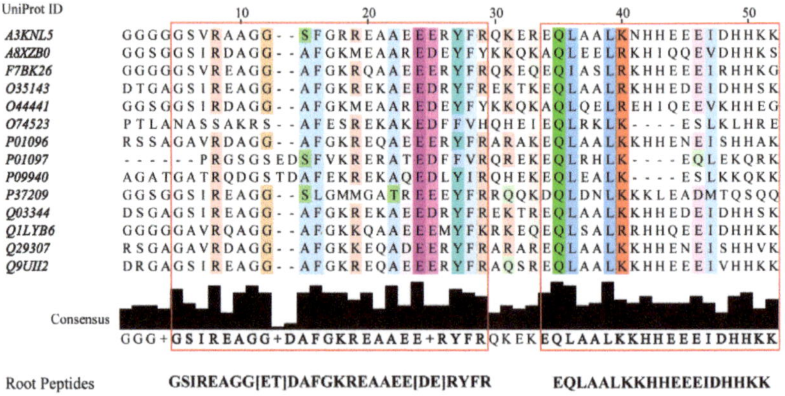

Figure 4. Multiple Sequence Alignment (MSA) performed with Multiple Alignment using Fast Fourier Transform, MAFFT, [55] for IF1 inhibitors deposited in the UniProt database. Consensus regions are identified at >40% of identity threshold at each position of the MSA. The resulting consensus regions are framed in a rectangular box. From them two root peptides were estimated IF1 sources: A3RKNL5, zebrafish. A8XZB0, Caenorhabditis briggsae. F7BK26, western clawed frog. O35143, mouse. O44441, Caenorhabditis elegans. 074523, fission yeast. P01096, bovine. P01097, baker's yeast. P09940, torula yeast. P37209, Caenorhabditis elegans. Q03344, rat. Q1LYB06, zebrafish. Q29307, pig. Q9UII2, human. Jalview ver: 2.11.1.4 was used to visualize the MSA and determine the consensus.

ROSE operates by introducing stochastic point mutations into the root amino acid sequence, which is guided by a binary phylogenetic tree and a mutability vector, representing the conservation degree of each position in the sequence. Both the root peptide and the mutability vector are obtained by multiple sequence alignment of the selected set of peptides, carried out with Multiple Alignment, using Fast Fourier Transform, MAFFT, [55] (Table S2). The obtained library was then screened using PPI-Detect, which classifies and ranks the peptides as putative binders of the targeted site [46,53]. This strategy allowed us the rational exploration of the sequence space around the selected templates. From the root peptides, 385 unique mutants were generated. These peptides have a minimum identity, relative to their root sequence, of 70 %. Using PPI-Detect [53], these candidates were screened based on their interaction likelihood with the subunit β of EcF_1 and the human sector (HsF_1). Selected candidates had to meet the following criteria: (a) Peptides with maximum interaction likelihood with HsF_1 below 0.5. (b) Peptides with maximum interaction likelihood with EcF_1 above 0.5. (c) The difference between the interaction probabilities with *E. coli* and human enzymes is at least 0.1. After applying these selection criteria, three peptides were filtered out (Table 2). Surprisingly, the selected peptides showed the highest interaction score and score difference with the central domain of the β subunit ('smart00382' domain), while a score value of ~0.32 was obtained for the HTH motifs of both EcF_1 and HsF_1.

Table 2. Interaction scores and chemical–physical properties of the selected peptide candidates.

Peptide	Sequence	Score [a] (EcF_1)	Score [a] (HsF_1)	Charge (pI) [b]	GRAVY [b]
Pept1-IF1	GSIREAGGTHAFGKRESAEEERYFR	0.512	0.402	0 (6.78)	−1.292
Pept2-IF1	GSIREAGGTDGFGKREAAEEEKYGR	0.561	0.420	−1 (5.11)	−1.392
Pept3-IF1	GSVREAGGTGAFGKRESAEEERYFR	0.580	0.479	0 (6.34)	−1.192

[a] The domain 'smart00382' was mapped on the β subunits of EcF_1 and HsF_1 using the NCBI tool CD-Search [56] to identify conserved domains. The extracted fragments of the subunits were used to compute the interaction scores with the peptides. [b] Values calculated with ProtParam [57].

The negative GRAVY index evidences the polar features of these peptides and their potentially good solubility. From them, the candidate termed as Pept1-IF1 was selected for synthesis because of its neutral charge and isoelectric point value, close to 7.0. This peptide (sequence: Ac-GSIREAGGTHAFGKRESAEEERYFR-NH_2) showed inhibitory activity against EcF_1, with IC_{50} = 155 ± 14 μM, h = 1.1 ± 0.1, and v_r = −1 ± 3% (Figure 5).

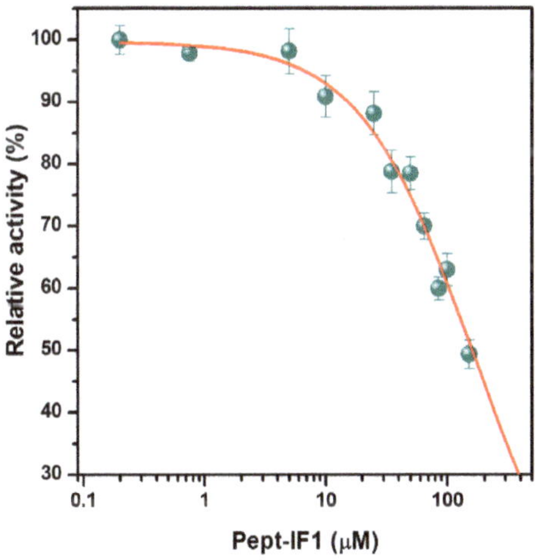

Figure 5. Dose-response plot of the inhibitory effect of Pept-IF1 on EcF_1. Residual ATPase activity was measured using peptide concentration in the 1.25–150 μM range, in a 100 mM Tris-SO_4 buffer solution with 1% DMSO (pH 8.0), 25 °C. The Hill equation was fitted to the experimental data, obtaining IC_{50} = 155 ± 14 μM, h = 1.1 ± 0.1, v_r = −1 ± 3%. Data represent the average ± standard deviation of 3 independent experiments.

2.3. Sequence Conservation of the HTH Motif in Bacteria

Given the observed inhibition results and the functional relevance of the HTH motif, we set out to explore the sequence conservation of this motif in bacterial species. From the UniProt database, 23,125 b-subunit sequences, from all bacterial F_OF_1-ATP synthases, were retrieved [54]. The dataset was aligned to generate sequence logos of the HTH motif [58,59]. As previously observed in less comprehensive sequence analysis [60,61], the HTH motif is significantly conserved among bacteria (Figure 6), and even more conserved among Mammalia (Figure S2). The HTH motif comprises the α-helix 1 (H1: R^{351}-I^{376}), the turn (T: L^{377}-S^{383}), and the α-helix 2 (H2: E^{384}-R^{399}) segments (*E. coli* numbering). The ^{380}DELSEED^{386} motif is within the C-terminal and N-terminal regions of T and H2, respectively. The most conserved regions encompass the central region D^{370}-K^{387} (or HTH tip, which besides the DELSEED, also includes the largely conserved ^{372}DIIAILG^{378} segment), the C-terminal segment ^{392}RARKI^{396}, plus some scattered, mostly hydrophobic residues, in H1 and H2. An analysis of the experimental 3D structures of F_1 reveals that, with few exceptions, the most conserved residues in the HTH motif also form interactions with highly conserved residues, located either in the same subunit (mostly in the HTH motif itself) or in the adjacent α, β, or γ subunits (Figure S3). Further, 18 out of 45 residues of the HTH motif show significant variability. The most variable segment is in H1, while the most conserved is in T. Importantly, the binding site of the compounds, designed herein, includes portions of the conserved DIIAIL and DELSEED segments, as well as some moderately conserved residues. In particular, the Bacilli class shows the most contrasting differences regarding the human enzyme (Figure S4), a characteristic that could be exploitable to optimize molecules capable of selectively recognizing pathogens of this taxonomic group, and that do not bind to the human enzyme.

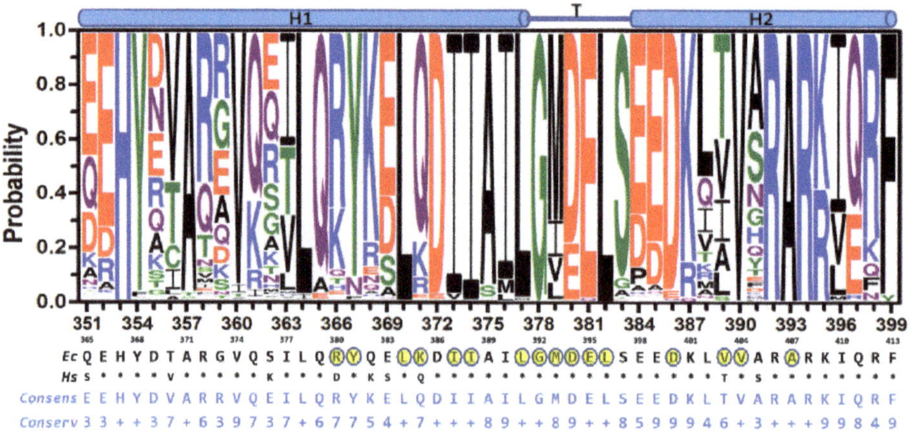

Figure 6. Conservation of the HTH motif in bacteria. Residue numbering in the up and down rows corresponds to the *E. coli* and human sequences, respectively. Multiple sequence alignment of 23,125 entries was performed with Clustal Omega [59]. Logos were generated using the Weblogo3 server [58]. Consensus, *E. coli* (*Ec*) and human (*Hs*) sequences are shown in the x-axis for comparison. Human residues identical to *E. coli* residues are shown with asterisks. The *Conserv* row corresponds to a conservation scale ranging from 0 (null conservation) to 10 (= +, complete conservation of physicochemical properties of the amino acid group) as defined in [62]. Residues within 5 Å of Compd-5 are highlighted in yellow.

3. Discussion

Although the declining trend of newly approved antibiotics has recently reversed, infections caused by AMR bacteria are still an alarming threat to global public health [4]. Interfering bioenergetic pathways is an emerging strategy to combat pathogens [6]. Indeed, pharmacological-approved bedaquiline has attested that ATP synthase inhibition can be successfully harnessed to target aerobic organisms, such as *M. tuberculosis* [63]. In addition, AMR facultative anaerobes, including the ESKAPEE pathogens *S. aureus* and *E. coli*, lose resistance towards antibiotics upon ATP synthase inhibition [64,65]. Given the major role played by βCterm in inter-subunit communication, orchestrating the rotary mechanism of ATP synthase, we strived to design molecules capable of selectively targeting the HTH motif. Inspired by the effect that endogenous regulatory subunits [66–68], and some peptide venoms [69] and other exogenous inhibitors [26] have on the F_1 subcomplex, the underlying idea was that by interfering with the conformational changes that the HTH motif undergoes, an inhibitory effect on the enzymatic activity can be achieved. To do this, we used two widely different in silico design strategies, one based on target 3D structure [70] and the other on peptide sequence data mining [46], obtaining organic molecules and an IF1-derived peptide, whose inhibitory potencies against EcF_1 were in the micromolar range, comparable to those of known natural inhibitors, such as polyphenols and venom peptides, among others [28,29,71].

It has been shown, for an increasing number of proteins, that solvent site clusters map both orthosteric and allosteric sites [43,72]. Thus, besides identifying critical interaction points with substrates or natural ligands, MDmix-determined solvent sites have proved valuable as pharmacophoric restraints in HTVS [44,73], improving the rate of true-positive hits and the discovery of new kinds of inhibitors and binding probes [74,75]. Furthermore, by relying exclusively on the interactions determined by the force field and the kinetic energy of the atoms in the system, MDmix unbiasedly maps entire protein surfaces, opening a window of opportunity to identify potential allosteric sites that may be difficult to detect experimentally or by knowledge-based potential methods [76,77]. In this work, MD-determined solvent sites were used to guide the docking of drug-like molecules on the HTH motif. The best-ranked hits obtained from our HTVS were further filtered by steering MD, a technique that has been used to develop new kinds of inhibitors against HSP90 [45] and several oncogenic tyrosine-kinases [78]. The combined use of these orthogonal approaches that evaluate equilibrium- and trajectory-derived energies, respectively, allowed us to identify and experimentally validate novel inhibitors of EcF_1.

The five inhibitory compounds (Table 1) showed a nitrogen atom that hydrogen bonded to, the carbonyl oxygen of the completely conserved G^{378} at the beginning of the HTH turn. In addition, hydrophobic contacts were established with H1 and H2 residues. Taken together, Compd-5, Compd-14 and Compd-19, the three 4-(6-phenylpyridazin-3-yl)morpholine-containing compounds, suggest the amide/sulfonamide position is amenable to a broad range of substituents and could be used to increase potency and modulate physicochemical properties. It is worth mentioning that Compd-5, our most potent inhibitor, is a relatively small molecule (MW = 378.2 Da), providing the opportunity to add chemical groups to it, to obtain more potent molecules. To our knowledge, no other activity for this compound has been reported so far [79]. Compd-7, our second-best inhibitor, with an overall different chemical structure, has a dimethylmorpholine moiety and, like Compd-14, a methoxyphenyl group. Compd-19 has no morpholine moiety, and the nitrogen with which it would hydrogen bond to, G^{378}, is within a hydroxypyrimidine. To our knowledge, these are the first reported inhibitors designed to bind to a site formed within the HTH motif of the ATP-synthase β subunit.

In a previous report, we introduced a de novo design method of EcF_1 peptide inhibitors [46]. The new inhibitors were designed in silico from the interfaces connecting F_OF_1-ATP synthase subunits, through a combination of simulated molecular evolution [52] and protein–protein interaction prediction [53] algorithms. The in vitro inhibitory capacity of the designed peptides proved the suitability of these scaffolds and the strategy for the generation of new inhibitor families. In this work, we derived new peptide sequences from known IF1 sequences. In contrast to the root IF1 peptides, which are incapable of inhibition of bacterial F_1 ATPase [24,80], Pept-IF1 inhibited EcF_1 with micromolar potency. However, to verify whether Pept-IF1 exhibits species discrimination and to determine its actual binding site on the β subunit, further experimental characterization is needed.

Antibiotics require tuned selectivity to achieve reliable discrimination between the pathogen target and the human or animal ortholog. Bedaquiline was initially proposed as a specific antibiotic for some species of the *Mycobacterium* genus. However, recent evidence has shown that the human enzyme is also susceptible to this antibiotic [81]. In addition, the *c* subunit, the binding target of bedaquiline, shows a low conservation among bacterial ATP synthases (e.g., mean identity of 33 $\pm$ 9 vs. 62 $\pm$ 8% of β subunits). Thus, unsurprisingly, bacteria can also evade this antibiotic, through mutations in the *c*-subunit-encoding *uncE* gene [82]. In contrast to the bedaquiline-binding site (mean identity 39 $\pm$ 20% in all bacteria), the HTH motif encompasses highly conserved sequence segments intercalated with variable positions (mean identity 69 $\pm$ 10% among bacteria). Furthermore, many of the HTH-conserved residues establish inter/intracatenary contacts with other highly conserved residues (Figure S3). Therefore, the HTH motif may offer a suitable target for allosteric drug discovery [83], as recently epitomized by the design of allosteric inhibitors against bacterial and viral enzymes, using conserved residues as binding anchors [84,85].

Site-directed mutagenic studies have unveiled that the rotary mechanism withstands severe changes in the HTH sequence [20,61,86–92]. Indeed, this rotational robustness is rooted in the fact that the γ-less $\alpha_3\beta_3$ subcomplex, although in a largely decreased way, exhibits catalysis and alternating conformational changes [93], while isolated α and β subunits also undergo nucleotide-induced rearrangements that resemble those observed in the F_1 subcomplex [21,94]. *Bacillus* PS3 enzymes, with deletions of up to 9 or 13 residues in HTH, keep catalytic activity in the synthesis or hydrolysis direction, respectively [20,61,90]. These results, together with point mutations in the HTH tip, led to the proposal that "... the physical length, rather than residue-specific interactions, of helix-1 is important for torque generation" [20], while the high conservation of some residues is due to the interaction that they establish with the regulatory subunits of the enzyme [88]. However, it has been repeatedly observed that in vitro mutations of the HTH sequence led to modifications of highly variable magnitude in the catalytic activity of the enzyme. The effects of these perturbations on oxidative phosphorylation and other ATP synthase-coupled processes on metabolic homeostasis have been scarcely studied [95,96]. Although it remains to be validated whether the inhibition of ATP synthase through molecules that bind the HTH motif is a feasible route for the development of new antibiotics, the most relevant finding of our study is the possibility of computationally predicting and validating novel sites of allosteric modulation, as biological evolution has repeatedly proved, with multiple sites for endogenous and exogenous inhibitors of this enzyme. This opens the door to the search for new pharmacological strategies, not only to attack infectious agents, but also to develop ATP synthase pharmacological modulators in metabolic and cellular contexts, where this enzyme plays a relevant role in the progression and establishment of pathologies [97,98].

4. Materials and Methods

4.1. Molecular Dynamics Simulations

MD trajectories were performed with the AMBER 14 suite using the FF99SB force field [99]. All simulations were carried out using the crystal structure of EcF_1 (PDB ID 3oaa [22]). Modeling of protein missing atoms, N- and C-termini capping, and protonation at pH 7.4 were carried out with the Molecular Operating Environment (MOE, [100]). Using AMBER's tLeap, the protein was placed in a truncated octahedral box spanning 18.0 Å further from the solute in each direction and solvated using a preequilibrated box of solvent containing pure water or 20% v/v ethanol/water. TIP3P water model was used. The system was first geometrically optimized (5000 cycles) to adjust the solvent orientation and eliminate local clashes, using the steepest descent algorithm. Initial velocities were assigned to get a 150 K distribution. The temperature was slowly raised to 300 K in 0.8 ns keeping the volume constant. The system was further equilibrated for one ns at 300 K in the NPT ensemble. The production was run in the NPT ensemble, using periodic boundary conditions. Temperature and pressure control were achieved using the Langevin thermostat and Berendsen barostat, respectively. Long-range electrostatic interactions were accounted for using the particle-mesh Ewald summation method as implemented in the PMEMD module of the AMBER suite, with a cut-off value of 9.0 Å to split direct electrostatics and Ewald summation [101,102]. The SHAKE algorithm was enabled and the integration timestep was 2fs. Running scripts were set up with the help of the pyMDMix software [43,103]. Trajectory analysis was performed with CPPTRAJ [104] and Chimera UCSF v14.1 [105]. Trajectories were run in triplicate. All the structure drawings were generated with ChimeraX [106].

4.2. Identification of Solvent Sites, Guided Docking, and Dynamic Undocking

Solvent sites were determined using the MDmix method as described elsewhere [43]. After trajectories were aligned, density maps for probe atoms were obtained by building a static mesh of grids over the entire simulation box and counting appearance of probe atoms in each grid during the trajectory. The observed appearance was converted into binding free energy (ΔG_{SS}) applying the Boltzmann relationship, considering the observed probe atom distribution with an expected distribution in bulk solvent at 1.0 M. Solvent sites were filtered imposing an energy threshold of –1 kcal/mol. Compound libraries from Specs, Asinex, Enamine, Vitas M, ChemBridge, Key Organics, Princeton Biomolecular Research, and Life Chemicals, with a total of ~8×10^6 molecules, were docked using rDock [44]. Solvent sites were used as pharmacophores to filter compound libraries. A penalty score that increased proportionally to the square of the distance to the required solvent sites was applied when the distance was larger than 2 Å. Best ranked ligands were further filtered using steered molecular dynamics (SMD) simulations using the dynamic undocking method DUck as described elsewhere [45]. A total of 100 SMD simulations yielding 50 ns per ligand were run, imposing harmonic restraints with a force constant of 1.0 kcal/molÅ^2 on all receptor non-hydrogen atoms to preserve the protein conformation. Compounds were filtered out according to the work (ΔG_{QB}) needed to separate the ligand's atom forming a hydrogen bond with the β-subunit G^{378} carbonyl oxygen to a 5.0 Å distance, using a cutoff value of 6.0 kcal/mol. A workflow illustrating the process from the identification of solvent sites to dynamic undocking has been published elsewhere [78].

4.3. Engineering Peptide Inhibitors via Evolutionary and Protein–Protein Interaction Algorithms

IF1-based peptide inhibitors were derived as recently described elsewhere [46]. IF1 sequences retrieved from the UniProt database [54] were used to estimate consensus sequences that served as the root peptide to generate offspring candidates (peptide library) by applying simulated molecular evolution approaches, represented by the ROSE (random model of sequence evolution) algorithm [52] (Figure 7). The structural diversity generated by ROSE is guided by evolutionary parameters, which were tuned to develop a diversity-oriented sampling around the root sequence. The library was subsequently screened using PPI-Detect, a protein–protein interaction predictor [53,107], to score the binding likelihood of the peptides and EcF_1.

4.4. Protein Production and Purification

Unless stated otherwise, all the chemicals were from FORMEDIUM (Norfolk, UK). EcF_1 was recombinantly expressed in *E. coli* strain DK8 using the pBWU13.4 plasmid containing the *unc* operon [108]. Briefly, *E. coli* membranes carrying EcF_1 were first washed in the presence of protease inhibitors 6-aminohexanoic acid and p-aminobenzamidine, and finally in the presence of the former to solubilize the enzyme. The subcomplex was then purified by ion exchange and size exclusion chromatography using Whatman DE52 Cellulose and Sephacryl S-300 resin columns. Protein concentrations were determined using the Pierce BCA Protein Assay Kit (Thermo-Fisher, Waltham, MA, USA).

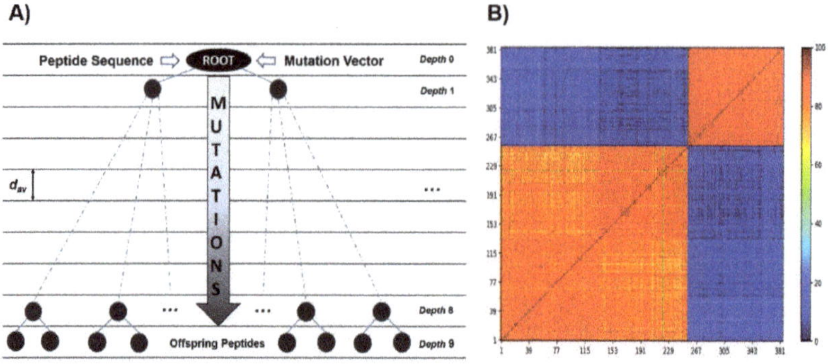

Figure 7. In silico design of a diversity-oriented peptide library. (**A**) Workflow illustrating the application of ROSE algorithm (https://bibiserv.cebitec.uni-bielefeld.de/rose, accessed on 12 March 2019). Root peptides and their corresponding mutation vectors are the input data. Besides the mutation vectors, ROSE also uses a binary tree to guide the stochastic point mutations on the root peptides. The binary tree topology is determined by the number of nodes (1023), depth (9) and average distance (dav = 5–20 PAMs). ROSE was calibrated to keep a minimum identity of ~70% of the generated peptides with the corresponding root sequence. The obtained library was composed of 385 unique peptides. (**B**) Heatmap showing the identity matrix among the generated peptides. Two blocks are distinguished, which corresponds to the root peptides selected from different fragments of IF1.

4.5. ATPase Activity Assays

The malachite green assay was used to determine ATPase activities as previously described [109]. All compounds were assayed in a concentration range spanning 0.05–150 µM, incubated with 10 nM (0.5 pmol) *Ec*F_1 (50 mM Tris-SO_4 pH 8.0, 1% DMSO) for 1 h at 30 °C in a total volume of 30 µL in 96-well microplates. Reactions were started by adding 20 µL 1 mM MgATP, incubated at 25 °C for 2 min and then stopped with 200 µL of 3.28 M H_2SO_4 and 15 mM $(NH_4)Mo_7O_{24}$ solution. Absorbance was read at 610 nm using a microplate reader (Biotek). The ATP regenerating system [110] was also used to determine ATPase activities. Experiments were carried out in a 50 mM KCl, 3 mM $MgCl_2$, 1.5 mM phosphoenolpyruvate, 300 mM NADH, 50 mM Tris pH 8.0, buffered solution incubating 3 U of rabbit pyruvate kinase (Merck Inc., Kenilworth, NJ, USA), 4.2 U of rabbit lactic dehydrogenase (Merck Inc.), 5.2 nM EcF_1 with 100 µM of assayed compounds, for 1 h at 30 °C in 120 mL per well in 96-well microplates. Reactions were started by adding 30 mL of a 50 mM KCl, 3 mM $MgCl_2$, 1.5 mM phosphoenolpyruvate, 300 mM NADH, 50 mM Tris pH 8.0 solution, including 1 mM ATP. ATPase activity was monitored through absorbance changes at 340 nm for 2 min in a microplate reader (Biotek, Winooski, VT, USA).

The concentration of inhibitor required to achieve a 50% reduction in enzymatic activity, IC_{50}, was obtained using the Hill equation:

$$\frac{v_i}{v_0} = \frac{[Inh]^h}{IC_{50}{}^h + [Inh]^h} + v_r$$

where v_0 and v_i are the initial catalytic velocities in absence and in presence of a given concentration of the inhibitor molecule, $[Inh]$, h is the Hill coefficient and v_r is the residual velocity under saturation conditions by the inhibitor.

4.6. Sequence Analysis of the HTH Motif

ATP synthase b subunits sequences from bacteria and Mammalia taxa were retrieved from the UniProt database [54]. Jalview2 [111] was used to curate the database, excluding redundant sequences (identity < 100%), yielding 23,125 and 142 sequences for bacteria and

Mammalia groups, respectively. The curated database was used to generate a multiple sequence alignment with Clustal Omega [59]. Sequence logos of the HTH motif were generated using the Weblogo3 server [58]. Very similar logo results were obtained for both taxonomic groups using a redundancy sequence identity cutoff of <98% or <99%.

Supplementary Materials: The following supporting information can be downloaded at: https://www.mdpi.com/article/10.3390/antibiotics11050557/s1, Table S1: Docked organic molecules on the HTH with best scores according to rDock and DUck methods; Table S2: Root peptides and mutation vectors for each peptide inhibitor family (IF1 and Heterogeneous Set); Figure S1: Distance between the carbonyl oxygen of G378 and the amino nitrogen of Compd-5 as a function of time. Figure S2: Conservation of the HTH motif in Mammalia class. Figure S3: Conserved contacts between residues of the HTH motif and neighboring subunits [112]. Figure S4: Conservation of the HTH motif in Bacilli class. [58,59,62,112] are cited in Supplementary Materials.

Author Contributions: Conceptualization, E.G.-H. and Y.B.R.-B.; methodology, X.B., S.R.-C., E.H.-G., N.A.V.-C., M.T.-R. and J.W.; formal analysis, L.P.A.-B., L.F.C.-V., G.A.-C., Y.B.R.-B. and E.G.-H.; investigation, L.P.A.-B. and L.F.C.-V.; writing—original draft preparation, L.P.A.-B., L.F.C.-V., G.A.-C., Y.B.R.-B. and E.G.-H.; writing—review and editing, all authors; funding acquisition, E.G.-H. and G.A.-C. All authors have read and agreed to the published version of the manuscript.

Funding: Luis Pablo Avila-Barrientos and Luis Fernando Cofas-Vargas are students from Programa de Doctorado en Ciencias Bioquímicas, Universidad Nacional Autónoma de México (UNAM), and received fellowships No. 275485 and 508395, respectively, from CONACyT, México. This work was financed, in part, by DGAPA, UNAM [PAPIIT IN206221]. G.A-C. was supported by national funds through FCT—Foundation for Science and Technology—within the scope of UIDB/04423/2020 and UIDP/04423/2020. We would like to thank Programa de Apoyo a los Estudios de Posgrado (PAEP) from Universidad Nacional Autónoma de México for the stipend awarded to LPAB for a research stay at Texas Tech University under guidance of JW.

Institutional Review Board Statement: Not applicable.

Informed Consent Statement: Not applicable.

Data Availability Statement: Not applicable.

Conflicts of Interest: The authors declare no conflict of interest. The funders had no role in the design of the study; in the collection, analyses, or interpretation of data; in the writing of the manuscript, or in the decision to publish the results.

References

1. Casadevall, A. Crisis in infectious diseases: 2 decades later. *Clin. Infect. Dis.* **2017**, *64*, 823–828. [CrossRef]
2. Taylor, J.; Hafner, M.; Yerushalmi, E.; Smith, R.; Bellasio, J.; Vardavas, R.; Bienkowska-gibbs, T.; Rubin, J. *Estimating the Economic Costs of Antimicrobial Resistance: Model and Results*; RAND Corporation: Cambridge, UK, 2014.
3. Review on Antimicrobial Resistance (London), & Grande-Bretagne. Antimicrobial Resistance: Tackling a Crisis for the Health and Wealth of Nations: December 2014. Available online: https://www.naturallivestockfarming.com/wp-content/uploads/2015/09/Antibiotics-UK-dec-2014-Review-paper-on-health-wealth1.pdf (accessed on 6 March 2022).
4. Talbot, G.H.; Jezek, A.; Murray, B.E.; Jones, R.N.; Ebright, R.H.; Nau, G.J.; Rodvold, K.A.; Newland, J.G.; Boucher, H.W. Infectious Diseases Society of America The Infectious Diseases Society of America's 10 × '20 Initiative (10 New Systemic Antibacterial Agents US Food and Drug Administration Approved by 2020): Is 20 × '20 a Possibility? *Clin. Infect. Dis.* **2019**, *69*, 1–11. [CrossRef]
5. Varela, M.F.; Stephen, J.; Lekshmi, M.; Ojha, M.; Wenzel, N.; Sanford, L.M.; Hernandez, A.J.; Parvathi, A.; Kumar, S.H. Bacterial resistance to antimicrobial agents. *Antibiotics* **2021**, *10*, 593. [CrossRef]
6. Hards, K.; Cook, G.M. Targeting bacterial energetics to produce new antimicrobials. *Drug Resist. Updat.* **2018**, *36*, 1–12. [CrossRef]
7. Diacon, A.; Pym, A.; Grobusch, M.; Patientia, R.; Rustomjee, R.; Page-Shipp, L.; Pistorius, C.; Krause, R.; Bogoshi, M.; Churchyard, G.; et al. The diarylquinoline TMC207 for Multidrug-Resistant Tuberculosis. *N. Engl. J. Med.* **2009**, *360*, 2397–2405. [CrossRef]
8. Vestergaard, M.; Nøhr-Meldgaard, K.; Bojer, M.S.; Krogsgård Nielsen, C.; Meyer, R.L.; Slavetinsky, C.; Peschel, A.; Ingmer, H. Inhibition of the ATP Synthase Eliminates the Intrinsic Resistance of Staphylococcus aureus towards Polymyxins. *MBio* **2017**, *8*, e01114–e01117. [CrossRef]
9. Liu, L.; Beck, C.; Nøhr-Meldgaard, K.; Peschel, A.; Kretschmer, D.; Ingmer, H.; Vestergaard, M. Inhibition of the ATP synthase sensitizes Staphylococcus aureus towards human antimicrobial peptides. *Sci. Rep.* **2020**, *10*, 11391. [CrossRef]

10. Liu, A.; Tran, L.; Becket, E.; Lee, K.; Chinn, L.; Park, E.; Tran, K.; Miller, J.H. Antibiotic Sensitivity Profiles Determined with an Escherichia coli Gene Knockout Collection: Generating an Antibiotic Bar Code. *Antimicrob. Agents Chemother.* **2010**, *54*, 1393–1403. [CrossRef]
11. Kinosita, K.; Yasuda, R.; Noji, H.; Adachi, K. A rotary molecular motor that can work at near 100% efficiency. *Philos. Trans. R. Soc. London. Ser. B Biol. Sci.* **2000**, *355*, 473–489. [CrossRef]
12. Kühlbrandt, W. Structure and Mechanisms of F-Type ATP Synthases. *Annu. Rev. Biochem.* **2019**, *88*, 515–549. [CrossRef] [PubMed]
13. Murphy, B.J.; Klusch, N.; Langer, J.; Mills, D.J.; Yildiz, Ö.; Kühlbrandt, W. Rotary substates of mitochondrial ATP synthase reveal the basis of flexible F1-Fo coupling. *Science* **2019**, *364*, eaaw9128. [CrossRef] [PubMed]
14. Rees, D.M.; Montgomery, M.G.; Leslie, A.G.W.; Walker, J.E. Structural evidence of a new catalytic intermediate in the pathway of ATP hydrolysis by F1-ATPase from bovine heart mitochondria. *Proc. Natl. Acad. Sci. USA* **2012**, *109*, 11139–11143. [CrossRef] [PubMed]
15. Schulz, S.; Wilkes, M.; Mills, D.J.; Kühlbrandt, W.; Meier, T. Molecular architecture of the N-type ATP ase rotor ring from *Burkholderia pseudomallei*. *EMBO Rep.* **2017**, *18*, 526–535. [CrossRef] [PubMed]
16. Sobti, M.; Walshe, J.L.; Wu, D.; Ishmukhametov, R.; Zeng, Y.C.; Robinson, C.V.; Berry, R.M.; Stewart, A.G. Cryo-EM structures provide insight into how E. coli F1Fo ATP synthase accommodates symmetry mismatch. *Nat. Commun.* **2020**, *11*, 2615. [CrossRef]
17. Gu, J.; Zhang, L.; Zong, S.; Guo, R.; Liu, T.; Yi, J.; Wang, P.; Zhuo, W.; Yang, M. Cryo-EM structure of the mammalian ATP synthase tetramer bound with inhibitory protein IF1. *Science* **2019**, *364*, 1068–1075. [CrossRef]
18. Boyer, P.D. The binding change mechanism for ATP synthase—Some probabilities and possibilities. *BBA—Bioenerg.* **1993**, *1140*, 215–250. [CrossRef]
19. Abrahams, J.P.; Leslie, A.G.W.; Lutter, R.; Walker, J.E. Structure at 2.8 Å resolution of F1-ATPase from bovine heart-mitochondria. *Nature* **1994**, *370*, 621–628. [CrossRef]
20. Usukura, E.; Suzuki, T.; Furuike, S.; Soga, N.; Saita, E.-I.; Hisabori, T.; Kinosita, K.; Yoshida, M.; Yoshida, M. Torque generation and utilization in motor enzyme F0F1-ATP synthase: Half-torque F1 with short-sized pushrod helix and reduced ATP Synthesis by half-torque F0F1. *J. Biol. Chem.* **2012**, *287*, 1884–1891. [CrossRef]
21. Pulido, N.O.; Salcedo, G.; Pérez-Hernández, G.; José-Núñez, C.; Velázquez-Campoy, A.; García-Hernández, E. Energetic effects of magnesium in the recognition of adenosine nucleotides by the F1-ATPase β subunit. *Biochemistry* **2010**, *49*, 5258–5268. [CrossRef] [PubMed]
22. Cingolani, G.; Duncan, T.M. Structure of the ATP synthase catalytic complex (F1) from Escherichia coli in an autoinhibited conformation. *Nat. Struct. Mol. Biol.* **2011**, *18*, 701–707. [CrossRef]
23. Morales-Rios, E.; Montgomery, M.G.; Leslie, A.G.W.; Walker, J.E. Structure of ATP synthase from Paracoccus denitrificans determined by X-ray crystallography at 4.0 Å resolution. *Proc. Natl. Acad. Sci. USA* **2015**, *112*, 13231–13236. [CrossRef] [PubMed]
24. Cabezón, E.; Montgomery, M.G.; Leslie, A.G.W.; Walker, J.E. The structure of bovine F1-ATPase in complex with its regulatory protein IF1. *Nat. Struct. Biol.* **2003**, *10*, 744–750. [CrossRef] [PubMed]
25. Van Raaij, M.J.; Abrahams, J.P.; Leslie, A.G.W.; Walker, J.E. The structure of bovine F1-ATPase complexed with the antibiotic inhibitor aurovertin B. *Proc. Natl. Acad. Sci. USA* **1996**, *93*, 6913–6917. [CrossRef] [PubMed]
26. Reisman, B.J.; Guo, H.; Ramsey, H.E.; Wright, M.T.; Reinfeld, B.I.; Ferrell, P.B.; Sulikowski, G.A.; Rathmell, W.K.; Savona, M.R.; Plate, L.; et al. Apoptolidin family glycomacrolides target leukemia through inhibition of ATP synthase. *Nat. Chem. Biol.* **2021**, *11*, 909. [CrossRef] [PubMed]
27. Guo, H.; Courbon, G.M.; Bueler, S.A.; Mai, J.; Liu, J.; Rubinstein, J.L. Structure of mycobacterial ATP synthase bound to the tuberculosis drug bedaquiline. *Nature* **2021**, *589*, 143–147. [CrossRef] [PubMed]
28. Hong, S.; Pedersen, P.L. ATP synthase and the actions of inhibitors utilized to study its roles in human health, disease, and other scientific areas. *Microbiol. Mol. Biol. Rev.* **2008**, *72*, 590–641, Table of Contents. [CrossRef]
29. Patel, B.A.; D'Amico, T.L.; Blagg, B.S.J. Natural products and other inhibitors of F1FO ATP synthase. *Eur. J. Med. Chem.* **2020**, *207*, 112779. [CrossRef]
30. Gledhill, J.R.; Walker, J.E. Inhibition sites in F1-ATPase from bovine heart mitochondria. *Biochem. J.* **2005**, *386*, 591–598. [CrossRef]
31. Feniouk, B.A.; Suzuki, T.; Yoshida, M. The role of subunit epsilon in the catalysis and regulation of FOF1-ATP synthase. *Biochim. Biophys. Acta Bioenerg.* **2006**, *1757*, 326–338. [CrossRef]
32. Sielaff, H.; Duncan, T.M.; Börsch, M. The regulatory subunit ε in Escherichia coli FOF1-ATP synthase. *Biochim. Biophys. Acta Bioenerg.* **2018**, *1859*, 775–788. [CrossRef]
33. Zarco-Zavala, M.; Mendoza-Hoffmann, F.; García-Trejo, J.J. Unidirectional regulation of the F1FO-ATP synthase nanomotor by the ζ pawl-ratchet inhibitor protein of Paracoccus denitrificans and related α-proteobacteria. *Biochim. Biophys. Acta Bioenerg.* **2018**, *1859*, 762–774. [CrossRef] [PubMed]
34. Bhat, A.S.; Dustin Schaeffer, R.; Kinch, L.; Medvedev, K.E.; Grishin, N.V. Recent advances suggest increased influence of selective pressure in allostery. *Curr. Opin. Struct. Biol.* **2020**, *62*, 183–188. [CrossRef] [PubMed]
35. Lu, S.; Shen, Q.; Zhang, J. Allosteric Methods and Their Applications: Facilitating the Discovery of Allosteric Drugs and the Investigation of Allosteric Mechanisms. *Acc. Chem. Res.* **2019**, *52*, 492–500. [CrossRef] [PubMed]
36. Chatzigoulas, A.; Cournia, Z. Rational design of allosteric modulators: Challenges and successes. *WIREs Comput. Mol. Sci.* **2021**, *11*, e1529. [CrossRef]

37. Walker, J.E.; Saraste, M.; Runswick, M.J.; Gay, N.J. Distantly related sequences in the α- and—subunits of ATP synthase, myosin, kinases and other ATP-rquiring enzymes and a common nucleotide binding fold. *EMBO J.* **1982**, *1*, 945–951. [CrossRef]
38. Leipe, D.D.; Koonin, E.V.; Aravind, L. Evolution and classification of P-loop kinases and related proteins. *J. Mol. Biol.* **2003**, *333*, 781–815. [CrossRef]
39. Nussinov, R.; Tsai, C.-J. The Different Ways through Which Specificity Works in Orthosteric and Allosteric Drugs. *Curr. Pharm. Des.* **2012**, *18*, 1311–1316. [CrossRef]
40. Hotra, A.; Ragunathan, P.; Shuyi-Ng, P.; Seankongsuk, P.; Harikishore, A.; Sarathy, J.-P.; Saw, W.-G.; Lakshmanan, U.; Sae-Lao, P.; Kalia, N.-P.; et al. Discovery of a novel Mycobacterial F-ATP synthase inhibitor and its potency in combination with diarylquinolines. *Angew. Chemie—Int. Ed.* **2020**, *59*, 13295–13304. [CrossRef]
41. Saw, W.G.; Wu, M.L.; Ragunathan, P.; Biuković, G.; Lau, A.M.; Shin, J.; Harikishore, A.; Cheung, C.Y.; Hards, K.; Sarathy, J.P.; et al. Disrupting coupling within mycobacterial F-ATP synthases subunit ε causes dysregulated energy production and cell wall biosynthesis. *Sci. Rep.* **2019**, *9*, 1–15. [CrossRef]
42. Ma, Y.-X.; Wang, C.-Y.; Li, Y.-Y.; Li, J.; Wan, Q.-Q.; Chen, J.-H.; Tay, F.R.; Niu, L.-N. Considerations and Caveats in Combating ESKAPE Pathogens against Nosocomial Infections. *Adv. Sci.* **2020**, *7*, 1901872. [CrossRef]
43. Alvarez-Garcia, D.; Barril, X. Molecular simulations with solvent competition quantify water displaceability and provide accurate interaction maps of protein binding sites. *J. Med. Chem.* **2014**, *57*, 8530–8539. [CrossRef]
44. Ruiz-Carmona, S.; Alvarez-Garcia, D.; Foloppe, N.; Garmendia-Doval, A.B.; Juhos, S.; Schmidtke, P.; Barril, X.; Hubbard, R.E.; Morley, S.D. rDock: A Fast, Versatile and Open Source Program for Docking Ligands to Proteins and Nucleic Acids. *PLoS Comput. Biol.* **2014**, *10*, e1003571. [CrossRef] [PubMed]
45. Ruiz-Carmona, S.; Schmidtke, P.; Luque, F.J.; Baker, L.; Matassova, N.; Davis, B.; Roughley, S.; Murray, J.; Hubbard, R.; Barril, X. Dynamic undocking and the quasi-bound state as tools for drug discovery. *Nat. Chem.* **2017**, *9*, 201–206. [CrossRef] [PubMed]
46. Ruiz-Blanco, Y.B.; Ávila-Barrientos, L.P.; Hernández-García, E.; Antunes, A.; Agüero-Chapin, G.; García-Hernández, E. Engineering protein fragments via evolutionary and protein–protein interaction algorithms: De novo design of peptide inhibitors for FOF1-ATP synthase. *FEBS Lett.* **2021**, *595*, 183–194. [CrossRef]
47. Krah, A.; Zarco-Zavala, M.; McMillan, D.G.G. Insights into the regulatory function of the ε subunit from bacterial F-type ATP synthases: A comparison of structural, biochemical and biophysical data. *Open Biol.* **2018**, *8*, 170275. [CrossRef] [PubMed]
48. Shoghi, E.; Fuguet, E.; Bosch, E.; Ràfols, C. Solubility-pH profiles of some acidic, basic and amphoteric drugs. *Eur. J. Pharm. Sci.* **2013**, *48*, 291–300. [CrossRef] [PubMed]
49. Miller, B.R.; McGee, T.D.; Swails, J.M.; Homeyer, N.; Gohlke, H.; Roitberg, A.E. *MMPBSA.py*: An Efficient Program for End-State Free Energy Calculations. *J. Chem. Theory Comput.* **2012**, *8*, 3314–3321. [CrossRef] [PubMed]
50. Wang, E.; Sun, H.; Wang, J.; Wang, Z.; Liu, H.; Zhang, J.Z.H.; Hou, T. End-Point Binding Free Energy Calculation with MM/PBSA and MM/GBSA: Strategies and Applications in Drug Design. *Chem. Rev.* **2019**, *119*, 9478–9508. [CrossRef] [PubMed]
51. Liu, K.; Kokubo, H. Exploring the Stability of Ligand Binding Modes to Proteins by Molecular Dynamics Simulations: A Cross-docking Study. *J. Chem. Inf. Model.* **2017**, *57*, 2514–2522. [CrossRef]
52. Stoye, J.; Evers, D.; Meyer, F. Rose: Generating sequence families. *Bioinformatics* **1998**, *14*, 157–163. [CrossRef]
53. Romero-Molina, S.; Ruiz-Blanco, Y.B.; Harms, M.; Münch, J.; Sanchez-Garcia, E. PPI-Detect: A support vector machine model for sequence-based prediction of protein-protein interactions. *J. Comput. Chem.* **2019**, *40*, 1233–1242. [CrossRef]
54. Bateman, A.; Martin, M.-J.; Orchard, S.; Magrane, M.; Agivetova, R.; Ahmad, S.; Alpi, E.; Bowler-Barnett, E.H.; Britto, R.; Bursteinas, B.; et al. UniProt: The universal protein knowledgebase in 2021. *Nucleic Acids Res.* **2021**, *49*, D480–D489. [CrossRef]
55. Katoh, K. MAFFT: A novel method for rapid multiple sequence alignment based on fast Fourier transform. *Nucleic Acids Res.* **2002**, *30*, 3059–3066. [CrossRef]
56. Lu, S.; Wang, J.; Chitsaz, F.; Derbyshire, M.K.; Geer, R.C.; Gonzales, N.R.; Gwadz, M.; Hurwitz, D.I.; Marchler, G.H.; Song, J.S.; et al. CDD/SPARCLE: The conserved domain database in 2020. *Nucleic Acids Res.* **2020**, *48*, D265–D268. [CrossRef] [PubMed]
57. Gasteiger, E.; Hoogland, C.; Gattiker, A.; Duvaud, S.; Wilkins, M.R.; Appel, R.D.; Bairoch, A. Protein Identification and Analysis Tools on the ExPASy Server. In *The Proteomics Protocols Handbook*; Humana Press: Totowa, NJ, USA, 2005; pp. 571–607.
58. Crooks, G.E.; Hon, G.; Chandonia, J.-M.; Brenner, S.E. WebLogo: A Sequence Logo Generator. *Genome Res.* **2004**, *14*, 1188–1190. [CrossRef]
59. Sievers, F.; Wilm, A.; Dineen, D.; Gibson, T.J.; Karplus, K.; Li, W.; Lopez, R.; McWilliam, H.; Remmert, M.; Söding, J.; et al. Fast, scalable generation of high-quality protein multiple sequence alignments using Clustal Omega. *Mol. Syst. Biol.* **2011**, *7*, 539. [CrossRef] [PubMed]
60. Mao, H.Z.; Abraham, C.G.; Krishnakumar, A.M.; Weber, J. A functionally important hydrogen-bonding network at the betaDP/alphaDP interface of ATP synthase. *J. Biol. Chem.* **2008**, *283*, 24781–24788. [CrossRef] [PubMed]
61. Mnatsakanyan, N.; Krishnakumar, A.M.; Suzuki, T.; Weber, J. The role of the betaDELSEED-loop of ATP synthase. *J. Biol. Chem.* **2009**, *284*, 11336–11345. [CrossRef]
62. Livingstone, C.D.; Barton, G.J. Protein sequence alignments: A strategy for the hierarchical analysis of residue conservation. *Comput. Appl. Biosci.* **1993**, *9*, 745–756. [CrossRef]
63. Diacon, A.H.; Donald, P.R.; Pym, A.; Grobusch, M.; Patientia, R.F.; Mahanyele, R.; Bantubani, N.; Narasimooloo, R.; De Marez, T.; van Heeswijk, R.; et al. Randomized pilot trial of eight weeks of bedaquiline (TMC207) treatment for multidrug-resistant

tuberculosis: Long-term outcome, tolerability, and effect on emergence of drug resistance. *Antimicrob. Agents Chemother.* **2012**, *56*, 3271–3276. [CrossRef]

64. Langlois, J.-P.; Millete, G.; Guay, I.; Dubé-Duquette, A.; Chamberland, S.; Jacques, P.-É.; Rodrigue, S.; Bourab, K.; Marsault, É. Malo Bactericidal Activity of the Bacterial ATP Synthase Inhibitor Tomatidine and the Combination of Tomatidine and Aminoglycoside Against Persistent and Virulent Forms of Staphylococcus aureus. *Front. Microbiol.* **2020**, *11*, 1–14. [CrossRef] [PubMed]
65. Vestergaard, M.; Roshanak, S.; Ingmer, H. Targeting the ATP Synthase in Staphylococcus aureus Small Colony Variants, Streptococcus pyogenes and Pathogenic Fungi. *Antibiotics* **2021**, *10*, 376. [CrossRef] [PubMed]
66. Milgrom, Y.M.; Duncan, T.M. F-ATP-ase of Escherichia coli membranes: The ubiquitous MgADP-inhibited state and the inhibited state induced by the ε–subunit's C-terminal domain are mutually exclusive. *Biochim. Biophys. Acta Bioenerg.* **2020**, *1861*, 148189. [CrossRef] [PubMed]
67. García-Aguilar, A.; Cuezva, J.M. A Review of the Inhibition of the Mitochondrial ATP Synthase by IF1 in vivo: Reprogramming Energy Metabolism and Inducing Mitohormesis. *Front. Physiol.* **2018**, *9*, 1322. [CrossRef] [PubMed]
68. Miranda-Astudillo, H.; Zarco-Zavala, M.; García-Trejo, J.J.; González-Halphen, D. Regulation of bacterial ATP synthase activity: A gear-shifting or a pawl–ratchet mechanism? *FEBS J.* **2021**, *288*, 3159–3163. [CrossRef]
69. Syed, H.; Tauseef, M.; Ahmad, Z. A connection between antimicrobial properties of venom peptides and microbial ATP synthase. *Int. J. Biol. Macromol.* **2018**, *119*, 23–31. [CrossRef]
70. Alvarez-Garcia, D.; Barril, X. Relationship between Protein Flexibility and Binding: Lessons for Structure-Based Drug Design. *J. Chem. Theory Comput.* **2014**, *10*, 2608–2614. [CrossRef] [PubMed]
71. Ahmad, Z.; Okafor, F.; Azim, S.; Laughlin, T.F. ATP synthase: A molecular therapeutic drug target for antimicrobial and antitumor peptides. *Curr. Med. Chem.* **2013**, *20*, 1956–1973. [CrossRef] [PubMed]
72. Talibov, V.O.; Fabini, E.; FitzGerald, E.A.; Tedesco, D.; Cederfeldt, D.; Talu, M.J.; Rachman, M.M.; Mihalic, F.; Manoni, E.; Naldi, M.; et al. Discovery of an Allosteric Ligand Binding Site in SMYD3 Lysine Methyltransferase. *ChemBioChem* **2021**, *22*, 1597–1608. [CrossRef]
73. Arcon, J.P.; Defelipe, L.A.; Lopez, E.D.; Burastero, O.; Modenutti, C.P.; Barril, X.; Marti, M.A.; Turjanski, A.G. Cosolvent-Based Protein Pharmacophore for Ligand Enrichment in Virtual Screening. *J. Chem. Inf. Model.* **2019**, *59*, 3572–3583. [CrossRef] [PubMed]
74. Ge, X.; Oliveira, A.; Hjort, K.; Bergfors, T.; Gutiérrez-de-Terán, H.; Andersson, D.I.; Sanyal, S.; Åqvist, J. Inhibition of translation termination by small molecules targeting ribosomal release factors. *Sci. Rep.* **2019**, *9*, 15424. [CrossRef] [PubMed]
75. Subiros-Funosas, R.; Ho, V.C.L.; Barth, N.D.; Mendive-Tapia, L.; Pappalardo, M.; Barril, X.; Ma, R.; Zhang, C.-B.; Qian, B.-Z.; Sintes, M.; et al. Fluorogenic Trp(redBODIPY) cyclopeptide targeting keratin 1 for imaging of aggressive carcinomas. *Chem. Sci.* **2020**, *11*, 1368–1374. [CrossRef] [PubMed]
76. Defelipe, L.; Arcon, J.; Modenutti, C.; Marti, M.; Turjanski, A.; Barril, X. Solvents to Fragments to Drugs: MD Applications in Drug Design. *Molecules* **2018**, *23*, 3269. [CrossRef] [PubMed]
77. Barril, X. Computer-aided drug design: Time to play with novel chemical matter. *Expert Opin. Drug Discov.* **2017**, *12*, 977–980. [CrossRef] [PubMed]
78. Rachman, M.; Bajusz, D.; Hetényi, A.; Scarpino, A.; Merő, B.; Egyed, A.; Buday, L.; Barril, X.; Keserű, G.M. Discovery of a novel kinase hinge binder fragment by dynamic undocking. *RSC Med. Chem.* **2020**, *11*, 552–558. [CrossRef] [PubMed]
79. Wang, Y.; Xiao, J.; Suzek, T.O.; Zhang, J.; Wang, J.; Zhou, Z.; Han, L.; Karapetyan, K.; Dracheva, S.; Shoemaker, B.A.; et al. PubChem's BioAssay Database. *Nucleic Acids Res.* **2012**, *40*, D400. [CrossRef]
80. Gledhill, J.R.; Montgomery, M.G.; Leslie, A.G.W.; Walker, J.E. Mechanism of inhibition of bovine F1-ATPase by resveratrol and related polyphenols. *Proc. Natl. Acad. Sci. USA* **2007**, *104*, 13632–13637. [CrossRef]
81. Luo, M.; Zhou, W.; Patel, H.; Srivastava, A.P.; Symersky, J.; Bonar, M.M.; Faraldo-Gómez, J.D.; Liao, M.; Mueller, D.M. Bedaquiline inhibits the yeast and human mitochondrial ATP synthases. *Commun. Biol.* **2020**, *3*, 452. [CrossRef]
82. Degiacomi, G.; Sammartino, J.C.; Sinigiani, V.; Marra, P.; Urbani, A.; Pasca, M.R. In vitro Study of Bedaquiline Resistance in Mycobacterium tuberculosis Multi-Drug Resistant Clinical Isolates. *Front. Microbiol.* **2020**, *11*, 2290. [CrossRef]
83. Lu, S.; Qiu, Y.; Ni, D.; He, X.; Pu, J.; Zhang, J. Emergence of allosteric drug-resistance mutations: New challenges for allosteric drug discovery. *Drug Discov. Today* **2020**, *25*, 177–184. [CrossRef] [PubMed]
84. Vella, P.; Rudraraju, R.S.; Lundbäck, T.; Axelsson, H.; Almqvist, H.; Vallin, M.; Schneider, G.; Schnell, R. A FabG inhibitor targeting an allosteric binding site inhibits several orthologs from Gram-negative ESKAPE pathogens. *Bioorg. Med. Chem.* **2021**, *30*, 115898. [CrossRef] [PubMed]
85. Cox, R.M.; Sourimant, J.; Toots, M.; Yoon, J.-J.; Ikegame, S.; Govindarajan, M.; Watkinson, R.E.; Thibault, P.; Makhsous, N.; Lin, M.J.; et al. Orally efficacious broad-spectrum allosteric inhibitor of paramyxovirus polymerase. *Nat. Microbiol.* **2020**, *5*, 1232–1246. [CrossRef]
86. Ketchum, C.J.; Al-Shawi, M.K.; Nakamoto, R.K. Intergenic suppression of the gammaM23K uncoupling mutation in F0F1 ATP synthase by betaGlu-381 substitutions: The role of the beta380DELSEED386 segment in energy coupling. *Biochem. J.* **1998**, *330*, 707–712. [CrossRef]
87. Hara, K.Y.; Noji, H.; Bald, D.; Yasuda, R.; Kinosita, K.; Yoshida, M. The role of the DELSEED motif of the beta subunit in rotation of F1-ATPase. *J. Biol. Chem.* **2000**, *275*, 14260–14263. [CrossRef] [PubMed]
88. Hara, K.Y.; Kato-Yamada, Y.; Kikuchi, Y.; Hisabori, T.; Yoshida, M. The role of the betaDELSEED motif of F1-ATPase: Propagation of the inhibitory effect of the epsilon subunit. *J. Biol. Chem.* **2001**, *276*, 23969–23973. [CrossRef]

89. Scanlon, J.A.B.; Al-Shawi, M.K.; Nakamoto, R.K. A rotor-stator cross-link in the F1-ATPase blocks the rate-limiting step of rotational catalysis. *J. Biol. Chem.* **2008**, *283*, 26228–26240. [CrossRef] [PubMed]
90. Mnatsakanyan, N.; Kemboi, S.K.; Salas, J.; Weber, J. The beta subunit loop that couples catalysis and rotation in ATP synthase has a critical length. *J. Biol. Chem.* **2011**, *286*, 29788–29796. [CrossRef] [PubMed]
91. Tanigawara, M.; Tabata, K.V.; Ito, Y.; Ito, J.; Watanabe, R.; Ueno, H.; Ikeguchi, M.; Noji, H. Role of the DELSEED loop in torque transmission of F1-ATPase. *Biophys. J.* **2012**, *103*, 970–978. [CrossRef] [PubMed]
92. Watanabe, R.; Koyasu, K.; You, H.; Tanigawara, M.; Noji, H. Torque transmission mechanism via DELSEED loop of F1-ATPase. *Biophys. J.* **2015**, *108*, 1144–1152. [CrossRef] [PubMed]
93. La, T.; Clark-Walker, G.D.; Wang, X.; Wilkens, S.; Chen, X.J. Mutations on the N-terminal edge of the DELSEED loop in either the α or β subunit of the mitochondrial F1-ATPase enhance ATP hydrolysis in the absence of the central γ rotor. *Eukaryot. Cell* **2013**, *12*, 1451–1461. [CrossRef] [PubMed]
94. Salcedo, G.; Cano-Sánchez, P.; De Gómez-Puyou, M.T.M.T.; Velázquez-Campoy, A.; García-Hernández, E. Isolated noncatalytic and catalytic subunits of F1-ATPase exhibit similar, albeit not identical, energetic strategies for recognizing adenosine nucleotides. *Biochim. Biophys. Acta Bioenerg.* **2014**, *1837*, 44–50. [CrossRef] [PubMed]
95. Rao, S.P.S.; Alonso, S.; Rand, L.; Dick, T.; Pethe, K. The protonmotive force is required for maintaining ATP homeostasis and viability of hypoxic, nonreplicating Mycobacterium tuberculosis. *Proc. Natl. Acad. Sci. USA* **2008**, *105*, 11945–11950. [CrossRef] [PubMed]
96. Nuskova, H.; Mikesova, J.; Efimova, I.; Pecinova, A.; Pecina, P.; Drahota, Z.; Houstek, J.; Mracek, T. Biochemical thresholds for pathological presentation of ATP synthase deficiencies. *Biochem. Biophys. Res. Commun.* **2020**, *521*, 1036–1041. [CrossRef] [PubMed]
97. Nesci, S.; Trombetti, F.; Algieri, C.; Pagliarani, A. A Therapeutic Role for the F1FO-ATP Synthase. *SLAS DISCOVERY: Adv. Sci. Drug Discov.* **2019**, *24*, 893–903. [CrossRef] [PubMed]
98. Fiorillo, M.; Ózsvári, B.; Sotgia, F.; Lisanti, M.P. High ATP Production Fuels Cancer Drug Resistance and Metastasis: Implications for Mitochondrial ATP Depletion Therapy. *Front. Oncol.* **2021**, *11*, 3875. [CrossRef] [PubMed]
99. Case, D.A.; Berryman, J.T.; Betz, R.M.; Cerutti, D.S.; Cheatham, T.E., III; Darden, T.A.; Duke, R.E.; Giese, T.J.; Gohlke, H.; Goetz, A.W.; et al. *AMBER 2014*; University of California: San Francisco, CA, USA, 2014.
100. *Molecular Operating Environment (MOE), 2014.09*; Chemical Computing Group ULC: Montreal, QC, Canada, 2015.
101. Götz, A.W.; Williamson, M.J.; Xu, D.; Poole, D.; Le Grand, S.; Walker, R.C. Routine Microsecond Molecular Dynamics Simulations with AMBER on GPUs. 1. Generalized Born. *J. Chem. Theory Comput.* **2012**, *8*, 1542–1555. [CrossRef] [PubMed]
102. Salomon-Ferrer, R.; Götz, A.W.; Poole, D.; Le Grand, S.; Walker, R.C. Routine Microsecond Molecular Dynamics Simulations with AMBER on GPUs. 2. Explicit Solvent Particle Mesh Ewald. *J. Chem. Theory Comput.* **2013**, *9*, 3878–3888. [CrossRef]
103. Hahn-Herrera, O.; Salcedo, G.; Barril, X.; García-Hernández, E. Inherent conformational flexibility of F1-ATPase α-subunit. *Biochim. Biophys. Acta Bioenerg.* **2016**, *1857*, 1392–1402. [CrossRef]
104. Roe, D.R.; Cheatham, T.E. PTRAJ and CPPTRAJ: Software for processing and analysis of molecular dynamics trajectory data. *J. Chem. Theory Comput.* **2013**, *9*, 3084–3095. [CrossRef]
105. Pettersen, E.F.; Goddard, T.D.; Huang, C.C.; Couch, G.S.; Greenblatt, D.M.; Meng, E.C.; Ferrin, T.E. UCSF Chimera—A visualization system for exploratory research and analysis. *J. Comput. Chem.* **2004**, *25*, 1605–1612. [CrossRef]
106. Pettersen, E.F.; Goddard, T.D.; Huang, C.C.; Meng, E.C.; Couch, G.S.; Croll, T.I.; Morris, J.H.; Ferrin, T.E. UCSF ChimeraX: Structure visualization for researchers, educators, and developers. *Protein Sci.* **2020**, *30*, 70–82. [CrossRef]
107. Romero-Molina, S.; Ruiz-Blanco, Y.B.; Green, J.R.; Sanchez-Garcia, E. *ProtDCal-Suite*: A web server for the numerical codification and functional analysis of proteins. *Protein Sci.* **2019**, *28*, 1734–1743. [CrossRef]
108. Senior, A.E.; Lee, R.S.F.; Al-shawi, M.K.; Weber, J. Catalytic properties of Escherichia coli F1-ATPase depleted of endogenous nucleotides. *Arch. Biochem. Biophys.* **1992**, *297*, 340–344. [CrossRef]
109. Van Veldhoven, P.P.; Mannaerts, G.P. Inorganic and organic phosphate measurements in the nanomolar range. *Anal. Biochem.* **1987**, *161*, 45–48. [CrossRef]
110. Kornberg, A.; Pricer, W.E. Enzymatic Phosphorylation of Adenosine and 2,6-Diaminopurine Riboside. *J. Biol. Chem.* **1951**, *193*, 481–495. [CrossRef]
111. Waterhouse, A.M.; Procter, J.B.; Martin, D.M.A.; Clamp, M.; Barton, G.J. Jalview Version 2—A multiple sequence alignment editor and analysis workbench. *Bioinformatics* **2009**, *25*, 1189–1191. [CrossRef]
112. Bowler, M.W.; Montgomery, M.G.; Leslie, A.G.W.; Walker, J.E. Ground state structure of F_1-ATPase from bovine heart mitochondria at 1.9 Å resolution. *J. Biol. Chem.* **2007**, *282*, 14238–14242. [CrossRef] [PubMed]

antibiotics

Article

A Novel Network Science and Similarity-Searching-Based Approach for Discovering Potential Tumor-Homing Peptides from Antimicrobials

Maylin Romero [1], Yovani Marrero-Ponce [2,*], Hortensia Rodríguez [1], Guillermin Agüero-Chapin [3,4], Agostinho Antunes [3,4], Longendri Aguilera-Mendoza [5] and Felix Martinez-Rios [6]

1 School of Chemical Sciences and Engineering, Yachay Tech University, Hda. San Jose s/n y Proyecto Yachay, Urcuqui 100119, Ecuador; maylin.romeroh@gmail.com (M.R.); hmrodriguez@yachaytech.edu.ec (H.R.)
2 Universidad San Francisco de Quito (USFQ), Grupo de Medicina Molecular y Traslacional (MeM&T), Colegio de Ciencias de la Salud (COCSA), Escuela de Medicina, Edificio de Especialidades Médicas, Diego de Robles y vía Interoceánica, Pichincha, Quito 170157, Ecuador
3 CIIMAR/CIMAR, Centro Interdisciplinar de Investigação Marinha e Ambiental, Universidade do Porto, Terminal de Cruzeiros do Porto de Leixões, Av. General Norton de Matos, s/n, 4450-208 Porto, Portugal; gchapin@ciimar.up.pt (G.A.-C.); aantunes@ciimar.up.pt (A.A.)
4 Departamento de Biologia, Faculdade de Ciências, Universidade do Porto, Rua do Campo Alegre, 4169-007 Porto, Portugal
5 Departamento de Ciencias de la Computación, Centro de Investigación Científica y de Educación Superior de Ensenada (CICESE), Ensenada 22860, Baja California, Mexico; longendri@gmail.com
6 Facultad de Ingeniería, Universidad Panamericana, Augusto Rodin No. 498, Insurgentes Mixcoac, Benito Juárez, Ciudad de México 03920, Mexico; felix.martinez@up.edu.mx
* Correspondence: ymarrero@usfq.edu.ec or ymarrero77@yahoo.es; Tel.: +593-2-297-1700 (ext. 4021)

Citation: Romero, M.; Marrero-Ponce, Y.; Rodríguez, H.; Agüero-Chapin, G.; Antunes, A.; Aguilera-Mendoza, L.; Martinez-Rios, F. A Novel Network Science and Similarity-Searching-Based Approach for Discovering Potential Tumor-Homing Peptides from Antimicrobials. *Antibiotics* **2022**, *11*, 401. https://doi.org/10.3390/antibiotics11030401

Academic Editor: Mire Zloh

Received: 1 February 2022
Accepted: 15 March 2022
Published: 17 March 2022

Publisher's Note: MDPI stays neutral with regard to jurisdictional claims in published maps and institutional affiliations.

Copyright: © 2022 by the authors. Licensee MDPI, Basel, Switzerland. This article is an open access article distributed under the terms and conditions of the Creative Commons Attribution (CC BY) license (https://creativecommons.org/licenses/by/4.0/).

Abstract: Peptide-based drugs are promising anticancer candidates due to their biocompatibility and low toxicity. In particular, tumor-homing peptides (THPs) have the ability to bind specifically to cancer cell receptors and tumor vasculature. Despite their potential to develop antitumor drugs, there are few available prediction tools to assist the discovery of new THPs. Two webservers based on machine learning models are currently active, the TumorHPD and the THPep, and more recently the SCMTHP. Herein, a novel method based on network science and similarity searching implemented in the starPep toolbox is presented for THP discovery. The approach leverages from exploring the structural space of THPs with Chemical Space Networks (CSNs) and from applying centrality measures to identify the most relevant and non-redundant THP sequences within the CSN. Such THPs were considered as queries (Qs) for multi-query similarity searches that apply a group fusion (MAX-SIM rule) model. The resulting multi-query similarity searching models (SSMs) were validated with three benchmarking datasets of THPs/non-THPs. The predictions achieved accuracies that ranged from 92.64 to 99.18% and Matthews Correlation Coefficients between 0.894–0.98, outperforming state-of-the-art predictors. The best model was applied to repurpose AMPs from the starPep database as THPs, which were subsequently optimized for the TH activity. Finally, 54 promising THP leads were discovered, and their sequences were analyzed to encounter novel motifs. These results demonstrate the potential of CSNs and multi-query similarity searching for the rapid and accurate identification of THPs.

Keywords: cancer; tumor-homing peptide; in silico drug discovery; complex network; chemical space network; centrality measure; similarity searching; group fusion; motif discovery; starPep toolbox software

1. Introduction

Cancer is a group of diseases developed in different cell and tissue types, and corresponds to the second leading cause of death globally [1]. It is based on the abnormal growth of cells due to an inherited genetic mutation or induced by the environment [2].

Despite novel therapy development for cancer treatment, improving chemotherapeutic drugs' specificity towards cancer cells remains a challenge [2,3]. Additionally, cancer cells are generating multi-drug resistance (MDR) [4]. Consequently, in the pharmaceutical industry, there is a need to develop new anticancer agents with a different mode of action to tackle the current drug resistance of cancer cells without being cytotoxic to healthy ones [2]. To fill this gap, peptides have emerged as a potential therapeutic alternative against cancer. From 2015 to 2019, 15 peptides or peptide-containing molecules were approved by the FDA as drugs, demonstrating the growing interest of the scientific community [5].

Peptides have different biochemical and therapeutic properties than small molecules and proteins, making them attractive to the pharmaceutical and biotechnological industry [6,7]. Being smaller than proteins allows peptides to penetrate tissues more easily, have low cost, more accessible synthesis, and do not require folding to be biologically active [8]. In contrast to small molecules, they have a higher specificity and efficacy due to representing the smallest functional part of a protein [9]. Moreover, they are not supposed to interact with the immune system, are biocompatible, have tunable bioactivity, and have low cytotoxicity due to their degradation products being amino acids [10–14]. Hence, peptide-based drugs open a new door to an improved cancer diagnosis and treatment.

Tumor blood and lymphatic vasculature differ molecularly and morphologically from normal lymphatic and blood vessels [15]. Tumor-homing peptides (THPs) take advantage of this peculiarity. Thus, they are widely investigated as drug carriers and for imaging purposes on oncology treatments and diagnosis [16]. The first-generation of THPs have RGD (Arg-Gly-Asp) and NGR (Asn-Gly-Arg) motifs. RGD peptides have the characteristic of selectively binding to α integrins expressed in vascular endothelial cells of the tumor and metastatic tumor cells, and NGR to aminopeptidase N (APN) receptors [17,18]. Although, there are neither non-RGD nor NGR peptides that home tumor blood vasculature and cancer cells by interactions with other receptors, such as the endothelial growth factor receptor (EGFR) [19–23].

THPs are discovered by using in vitro and ex vivo/in vivo phage display technology, which is time-consuming, expensive, and may not translate to humans due to differences between the animal models and humans [24–26]. For these reasons, bioinformatics tools such as databases and webservers are being employed for the accurate prediction of novel THPs [26–28]. In this way, short sets of the most promising THPs become the candidates for posterior experimental verification.

To date, the databases available for experimentally validated THPs are TumorHoPe (includes 744 THPs) [27] and starPepDB (includes 659 THPs) [29], and the available TH activity predictors are TumorHPD (https://webs.iiitd.edu.in/raghava/tumorhpd) (accessed on 1 May 2021) [26], THPep (http://codes.bio/thpep) (accessed on 1 May 2021) [28], and SCMTHP (SCMTHP (pmlabstack.pythonanywhere.com) (accessed on 5 January 2022) [30]. TumorHPD uses the supervised ML method Support Vector Machine (SVM) as a classifier with three features: amino acid composition, dipeptide composition, and binary profile patterns, achieving 86.56% as the highest accuracy [26]. The second ML method, THPep, has a Random Forest (RF) classifier with three features: amino acid composition, dipeptide composition, and pseudo amino acid composition, resulting in 90.13% of maximum overall accuracy [28]. However, the datasets used for training and testing both ML models contain peptides with highly similar sequences. On the other hand, SCMTHP is the most recently reported method based on the scoring card method (SCM) [30]. It determines the propensity scores for the amino acids' and dipeptides' composition accounting for THP sequences and applies a threshold value to discriminate between THP and non-THPs. Nonetheless, the performance of SCMTHP is similar to ML-based predictors, achieving a maximum accuracy of 82.7%.

Recently, Marrero-Ponce et al. published a new software named starPep toolbox (http://mobiosd-hub.com/starpep/) (accessed on 2 February 2021), which is aimed to perform network analyses on the integrated graph database called starPepDB, which include the most comprehensive and non-redundant database of antimicrobial peptides

(AMPs) [29,31]. Here, we propose an alternative methodology to identify potential THPs by combining network science with multi-query similarity searching against the AMPs of starPepDB. We used the starPep toolbox software as the main bioinformatics tool and the Chemical Space Network (CSN) to represent the chemical space of peptides as a coordinate-free system. To the best of our knowledge, there are no reported studies where data mining and screening is supported by network science to discover peptides for pharmaceutical purposes [29]. Firstly, we built models of representative and non-redundant THPs using centrality analysis and supervised retrospective similarity searching to perform the TH activity prediction. The outstanding model, named THP1, predicted the TH activity of three benchmarking datasets of THPs/non-THPs achieving accuracies between 92.64–99.18% and Matthews Correlation Coefficient (MCC) between 0.894–0.98, demonstrating the feasibility of this new methodology. Then, we performed a hierarchical screening for drug repurposing using network-based algorithms implemented in the starPep toolbox, the best model THP1, local alignments, and webservers to predict relevant activities related to the TH. Their TH activity was optimized by generating random libraries, where the peptide undergoes amino acid's stochastic substitutions at different positions. Finally, a set of 54 potential THPs from AMPs was proposed, where common motifs were identified.

2. Materials and Methods

The overall workflow of this report, shown in Figure 1, was based on two steps: (i) generation/selection of the model of representative THPs from starPepDB in starPep toolbox, and (ii) prediction of potential new THPs from AMPs. In the first step, some models of representative THPs from starPepDB were built using different centrality measures to rank the nodes and extract the representative and less similar sequences by applying local alignment. Then, the best multi-query similarity searching model (SSM) was selected by the classification performance and its ability to correctly retrieve THPs from benchmark THPs databases by using group fusion (MAX-SIM rule) similarity searching.

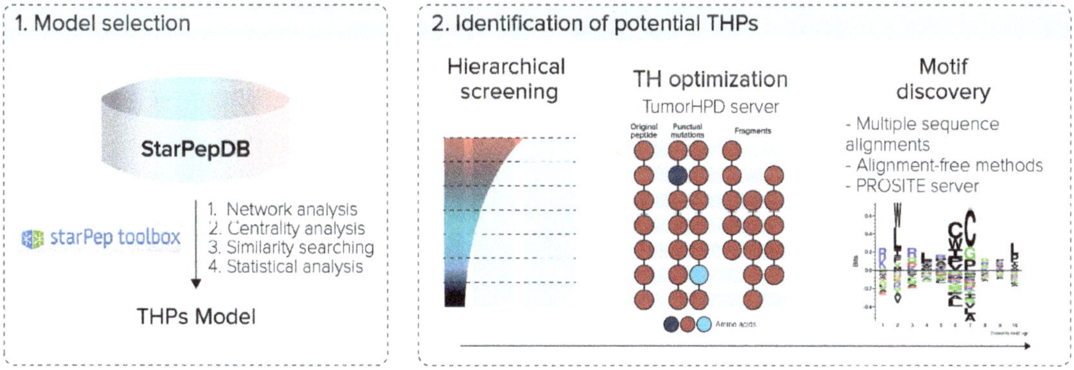

Figure 1. General overview of the experimental procedure.

In the second step, the model was used to perform similarity searching to repurpose AMPs as THPs from starPepDB, and their TH activity was optimized using the TumorHPD server. Additionally, sequence motifs were found from the set of potential THPs using multiple sequence alignments [32–35], alignment-free methods [36], and PROSITE server (https://www.genome.jp/tools/motif) (accessed on 15 July 2021).

2.1. StarPep Toolbox Software

The starPep toolbox uses FASTA files as inputs and includes the starPepDB. Peptides are represented as nodes connected by an edge if they have any relationship. It can perform querying, filtering, visualization of networks, scaffold extractions, single or multiple queries similarity searching, and analysis of peptides by graph networks [29,31].

Networks can be built based on the metadata of peptides or based on the pairwise similarity measures calculated for their respective sequence. In metadata networks, nodes are connected by a specific parameter in common, such as origin; the target against which they are assessed; functionality; the database where they come from; the cross-reference; N-terminus; C-terminus; or amino acid composition. In similarity networks, peptides are codified by descriptors, such as length, net charge, isoelectric point, molecular weight, Boman index, indices based on aggregation operators, hydrophobic moment, average hydrophilicity, hydrophobic periodicity, aliphatic index, and instability index [29,31,37]. Moreover, networks are visualized using different layouts, such as Fruchterman–Reingold [38].

Networks can be clustered, and communities are optimized using the Louvain method [39]. Moreover, the centrality of each node can be particularly measured by harmonic, community hub-bridge, betweenness, and weighted degree. Centrality is crucial to perform scaffold extractions because peptides are ranked according to their centrality score, and then redundant sequences are removed, prioritizing the most central. Thus, scaffold extractions depend on the type of centrality applied.

On the other hand, similarity searching, which is the basis of this study, is performed using a set of queries against a target dataset, where different percentages of identity (or similarity thresholds) can be applied. An identity score is a number between 0–1, and it is calculated using the Smith–Waterman local alignment with BLOSUM 62 substitution matrix [40]. Multiple queries similarity searching works using the group fusion model explained in the following section.

2.2. *Model Selection*

The dataset of reported THPs was extracted from starPepDB in the starPep toolbox. All 45120 peptides contained in starPepDB were filtered by the "Tumor Homing" query in the metadata function, where 659 entries were obtained (SI1-A).

2.2.1. Network Analysis

Similarity Threshold Analysis

Network analysis of peptides was performed by building the CSN of 659 THPs in the starPep toolbox. To choose the appropriate similarity threshold to build the network of THPs, CSNs were built by varying in 0.05 the cut-off value from 0.10 to 0.90 (17 CSNs in total). Some metrics were retrieved from each CSN using the starPep toolbox, such as density, number of communities, modularity, and number of singletons.

By default, when CSN was built, nodes with higher than 98% of similarity were removed using the local alignment Smith–Waterman algorithm. The similarity metric used to establish the pairwise similarity relationships between nodes was the min–max normalized Euclidean distance. Then, a centrality was calculated and those nodes with 0 as vertex degree were identified as outliers and then removed, leaving the giant (or connected) components of the CSN, i.e., subgraph where all nodes are connected. In this case, community hub-bridge centrality was calculated. However, any centrality measure could have been calculated since singletons always have zero centrality. After that, the network was clustered and the modularity optimized using the modularity optimization algorithm based on the Louvain method [39].

The network was saved as a Graph ML file to be opened in Gephi [41] for subsequent calculation of ACC. Finally, density, modularity, and ACC as a function of similarity threshold were graphed in Origin to decide what similarity threshold is the best.

Network Characterization

CSN of the giant components derived from the application of the best similarity threshold was characterized by the number of nodes, edges, outliers, density, number of communities, and modularity. These parameters were obtained from starPep toolbox while ACC, diameter (larger shortest path), average path length, and a total of triangles were drawn from Gephi. These parameters allow knowing the topology and structural patterns of the CSN.

For network visualization, Force Atlas 2 was used as a layout algorithm where colors represent different clusters, and node size means how central the node is according to the community hub-bridge centrality. Network visualization aims to obtain an aesthetically pleasing and understandable graph where nodes are not overlapped.

On the other hand, CSN of outliers was built with a cut-off of 0.30 to procure an appropriate density; then, it was clustered. Moreover, a subsequent scaffold extraction was applied based on hub-bridge centrality, and on 30% identity from local alignment.

The network of outliers was characterized according to the number of nodes, edges, communities, density, modularity, average degree, ACC, diameter obtained before scaffold extraction, and the number of nodes and edges obtained after scaffold extraction. For network visualization, Fruchterman–Reingold was used as a layout algorithm; colors represent different clusters while node size displays how central it is according to hub-bridge measure.

2.2.2. Centrality Analysis

The most influential nodes were used to find the new potential THPs, and centrality is the crucial parameter that provides this information. Thus, the four available centrality types in the starPep toolbox (weighted degree, community hub-bridge, betweenness, and harmonic) were calculated and normalized using the min–max method. Then, redundant peptides were removed by applying the scaffold extraction procedure that is described as follows: peptides were ranked based on the scores obtained after centrality calculation and we used 30% similarity cut-off of local identity from the Smith–Waterman algorithm to retrieve sets of sequences with a maximum of 30% similarity [40]. Subsequently, nodes with 10% lower centrality than the most central node were removed in each metric. The sets obtained after applying this process were named as 30 + 10%.

On the other hand, harmonic and weighted degree were calculated and normalized, and redundant peptides were removed by applying the scaffold extraction procedure using four different similarity cut-offs of local identity: 30, 40, 50, and 60%.

2.2.3. Similarity Searching Model for THPs Prediction

This study's proposed method for discovering potential THPs was based on similarity searching. For that reason, multiple query similarity searching models (SSMs) composed of several queries representing the most important and less redundant nodes of CSN and a similarity threshold were tested against datasets that contain well-known THPs/non-THPs through similarity searching. The recoveries from the similarity searching were statistically evaluated to select the best model for identifying potential THPs within the AMPs.

Query Datasets (Reference Sequences)

The retrieved sets after applying scaffold extractions at each centrality measure; the two sets of outliers; combinations of outliers with sets obtained from centrality-based scaffold extractions; and combinations between sets obtained from scaffold extractions performed using different centrality metrics were used as queries (Qs). In total, we tested 22 sets of Qs, where twelve sets resulted from the application of the scaffold extraction procedures as well as two sets of outliers, and eight sets resulted from the combination between sets.

Target Databases

Three training datasets that consider well-known THPs and randomly generated non-THPs [42] were used as the target or calibration for the recovery. THPep, TumorHPD, and SCMTHP employed these datasets for training their methods [26,30,42].

- Main dataset: 651 experimentally validated THPs and 651 random non-THPs (SI1-B). They were collected from TumorHoPe [27] and the literature [26].

- Small dataset: 469 experimentally validated THPs and 469 random non-THPs (SI1-C). They are peptides derived from the Main dataset with 4 to 10 aa residues.
- Main90 dataset: 176 THPs and 443 non-THPs (SI1-D). They are peptides from the Main dataset with equal or lower than 90% of sequence similarity.
- Main and Small datasets were retrieved from Ref. [26], while Main90 from Ref. [27].

Group fusion

Group fusion is based on the variation in the query (reference peptide), but keeping constant the identity measure [43]. Each peptide's identity score is calculated from the target dataset varying the Qs. The fusion group's algorithm associates a fused score to each target peptide, i.e., the maximum similarity (MAX-SIM) scores from all resulting identity scores against the Qs. Therefore, considering peptide S from the target dataset, reference peptide Q from the Qs, the identity score I(S,Q), and the MAX-SIM score obtained, the algorithm assigns I(S,Q) as the fused score to peptide S. The local identities were calculated with the Smith–Waterman, and is a number between 0–1, with 1 being the maximum identity. The procedure is illustrated in Figure 2.

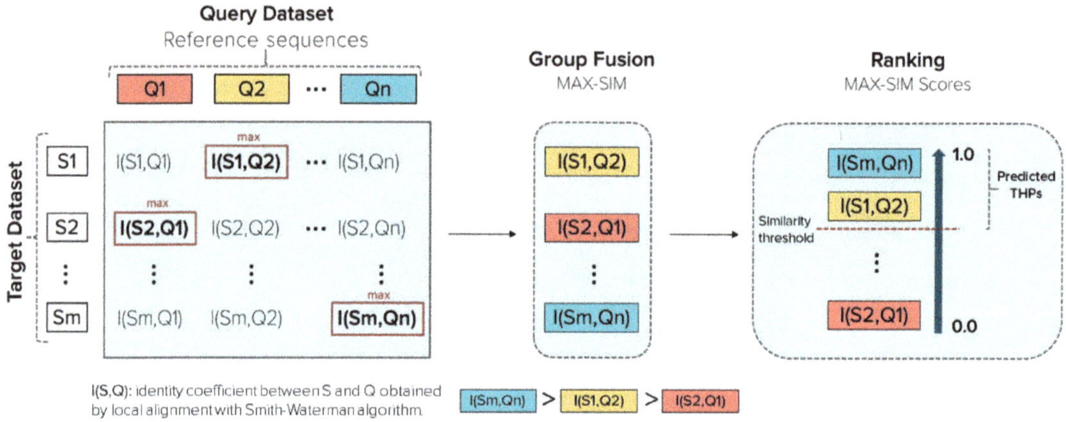

Figure 2. Schematic representation of the group fusion and similarity searching processes. Q is a peptide from a query dataset, n is the number of peptides contained in a query dataset, S is a peptide from the target dataset (Main, Small, or Main90 dataset), m is the number of peptides included in the target dataset (1302, 938, or 619, respectively). The similarity threshold is related to the percentage of identity.

Retrospective Similarity Searching

Main Dataset was imported to starPep toolbox. The similarity searching was performed using the "Multiple query sequences" option of the software and the Qs obtained from 30 + 10% similarity cut-offs of local alignment and outliers. The group fusion is applied by default during the similarity searching, and results were ranked according to the fused score (MAX-SIM value). Subsequently, seven different percentages of identity (similarity thresholds), 30, 40, 50, 60, 70, 80, and 90%, were tested, where peptides with identities equal to or higher than the applied threshold were retrieved as predicted THPs. Figure 2 illustrates how the similarity searching works.

The rescued nodes, i.e., predicted THPs, were statistically evaluated to validate the prediction. Thus, it is possible to identify the two centrality measures and percentages of sequence identity with the best performance.

Then, similarity searching was performed using only the sets of the best two centrality measures as Qs: harmonic and weighted degree, and 30, 40, 50, 60, and 70% of identity. In Small and Main90 datasets, only the sets of harmonic and weighted degrees were used as Qs, applying 40, 50, and 60% of identity for recovery. In total, 98 different SSMs were evaluated.

2.2.4. Statistical Analysis

The ability of the SSMs to predict THPs was validated by the measurement of their accuracy (Ac), kappa (κ), sensitivity (Sn), specificity (Sp), the precision of positives and negatives (P_{pos} and P_{neg}, respectively), MCC, and false accept rate (FAR%) using the following formulas.

$$Ac = \frac{TP + TN}{TP + TN + FP + FN}, \tag{1}$$

$$\kappa = \frac{Po - Pc}{1 - Pc}, \tag{2}$$

$$Sn = \frac{TP}{TP + FN}, \tag{3}$$

$$Sp = \frac{TN}{TN + FP}, \tag{4}$$

$$P_{pos} = \frac{TP}{TP + FP}, \tag{5}$$

$$P_{neg} = \frac{TN}{TN + FN}, \tag{6}$$

$$MCC = \frac{TP \times TN - FP \times FN}{\sqrt{(TP + FP) \times (TP + FN) \times (TN + FP) \times (TN + FN)}}, \tag{7}$$

$$FAR\% = \frac{FP}{FP + TN} \times 100, \tag{8}$$

where, TP is the number of true positives, TN is the number of true negatives, FP is the number of false positives, FN is the number of false negatives, Po is the relative observed agreement between the observers equal to the Ac, and Pc is the expected chance agreement calculated by the formula $Pc = \frac{(TP+FP)\times(TP+FN)+(FN+TN)\times(FP+TN)}{(TP+TN+FP+FN)^2}$.

Finally, the best 9 SSMs were compared and ranked using the Friedman test-based analysis performed in KEEL [44]. The Friedman test identified the best model based on the statistical metrics previously shown [45]. Moreover, it allowed us to compare the models and determine if their difference was statistically significant and not due to chance. The confusion or classification matrix of the best model was constructed. The best models were compared with reported ML models used for THP prediction, TumorHPD, and THPep, using the same three calibration datasets.

2.3. Identification of Potential THPs

2.3.1. Hierarchical Screening

Drug repurposing is an alternative methodology widely applied to discover drugs because it reduces approval time for their clinical use [46,47]. Thus, firstly, we repurposed AMPs from starPepDB as THPs.

1. Pipeline Prospective Screening. First, AMPs without reported TH activity and toxicity with a sequence length between 3 and 25 residues were filtered from the chemical space of starPepDB. Secondly, the "Scaffold extraction" option removed AMPs with higher than 95% sequence similarity by local alignment. Thirdly, multiple query similarity searching was performed using the best SSM (THP1), obtained in the previous section, to explore the chemical space of non-THPs, non-toxic, and non-redundant peptides with a length of 3–25 aa, using 60% as similarity threshold. In the recovered set, peptides with a similarity score of 1 were removed.
2. Activity Prediction. Peptides with reported tumor-homing activity in the literature were removed since the main objective of this study was to identify novel THPs. Then,

theoretical activities of virtual hits were predicted using webservers TumorHPD [26], THPep [28], AntiCP [48], CellPPD [49], ToxinPred [50], and HemoPI [51], to corroborate their potential as THPs and prioritize those that do not harm healthy cells. The activities of interest were tumor homing, anticancer, cell-penetrating, toxicity, and hemolysis. The SVM thresholds used were 0.30 in servers TumorHPD, AntiCP, and CellPPD, and 0 in server ToxinPred.

3. Redundancy Reduction by Network Analysis. CSN of hits was built, clustered, and the modularity was optimized using the Louvain method in the starPep toolbox. Then, harmonic and weighted degree centralities were calculated to perform a scaffold extraction using a 60% identity as the threshold.
4. Visual Mining. The neighborhood of well-known THPs of each potential THP was visualized using the starPep toolbox. CSN of 659 THPs in starPepDB was built using 0.60 as cut-off, clustered, and optimized modularity. Hits obtained in the previous step after scaffold extraction were embedded into the CSN of 659 THPs to study the neighborhood of each peptide. Hence, the 3 nearest neighbors from 659 THPs directly attached to each hit were visualized. If 2 peptides shared the same 2 or 3-nearest neighbors, one of them was prioritized, choosing the one with better predicted activities.

2.3.2. Tumor-Homing Activity Optimization

Lead hits detected from hierarchical virtual screening were AMPs from starPepDB with a natural or designed activity different from tumor homing. That is the reason why their tumor-homing action should be enhanced. Lead hits were optimized by punctual amino acid mutations using the "Designing of Tumor Homing Peptides" module of TumorHPD (https://webs.iiitd.edu.in/raghava/tumorhpd/peptide.php) (accessed on 10 September 2021), and the procedure is shown in Figure 3. Both lead and mutated sequences were shortened into fragments of 5, 10, and 15 residues in length using the same server.

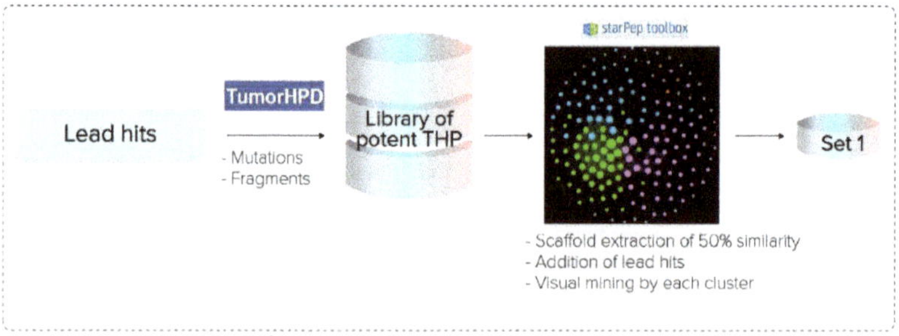

Figure 3. Procedure to optimize tumor-homing activity of lead hits.

The optimized sequences showing a higher tumor-homing activity score than parent hits were analyzed by CSN in the starPep toolbox using 0.60 as the similarity threshold to build the network. In addition, tumor homing, toxicity, hemolytic, anticancer, and cell penetrability were predicted using servers listed below: THPep (http://codes.bio/thpep), TumorHPD (https://webs.iiitd.edu.in/raghava/tumorhpd) (accessed on 25 September 2021), AntiCP (https://webs.iiitd.edu.in/raghava/anticp2) (accessed on 25 September 2021), CellPPD (https://webs.iiitd.edu.in/raghava/cppsite1) (accessed on 25 September 2021), ToxinPred https://webs.iiitd.edu.in/raghava/toxinpred (accessed on 25 September 2021), and HemoPI https://webs.iiitd.edu.in/raghava/hemopi (accessed on 25 September 2021). Redundant sequences with higher than 50% similarity were removed by scaffold extraction.

The optimized sequences and parent hits were merged, and the corresponding CSN was built using 0.50 of cut-off and clustered. Next, harmonic centrality was calculated. Each cluster was analyzed separately to prioritize the most central, potent, non-toxic, and non-hemolytic lead THPs. Finally, the heat map and histogram of pairwise sequence identity of lead compounds were constructed to explore their structural diversity.

2.3.3. Motif Discovery

Multiple Sequence Alignments

As the resulting potential THPs were hard-to-align sequences because of their short length and variability, they were grouped into seven clusters according to the neighborhood in the CSN. Given that two peptides underrepresented clusters 1 and 5, they were fused in a cluster labeled 1–5. Thus, peptide clusters (2–4, 1–5, and singletons) were aligned independently using multiple sequence alignments (MSA), publicly available at https://www.ebi.ac.uk/Tools/msa/ (accessed on 28 September 2021). Four different MSA algorithms were applied with their default parameters to determine consensus motifs within each cluster: (1) Clustal-Omega v 1.2.4 [32], (2) MAFFT (Multiple Alignment using Fast Fourier Transform) v7.487 with the iterative refinement FFT-NS-i option [33], (3) MUSCLE (Multiple Sequence Comparison by Log-Expectation) v3.8 [34], and T-Coffee (Tree-based Consistency Objective Function for Alignment Evaluation) v1.83 [35].

The resulting MSAs were employed to extract the conserved motifs by considering the consensus sequences estimation from the programs Jalview v2.11.1.4 [52], EMBOSS Cons v6.6.0 (https://www.ebi.ac.uk/Tools/msa/emboss_cons/) (accessed on 28 September 2021), and Seq2Logov2.1 (http://www.cbs.dtu.dk/biotools/Seq2Logo/) (accessed on 28 September 2021) [53].

Alignment-Free Method

Peptides were analyzed in STREME [36] (Sensitive, Thorough, Rapid, Enriched Motif Elicitation) to discover fixed-length patterns (ungapped motifs) that were enriched with respect to a control set generated by shuffling input peptides [52]. The analyses were performed via its webserver (https://meme-suite.org/meme/tools/streme) (accessed on 28 September 2021), by considering both total peptides and by each cluster. The motif width was set between 3–5 amino acids length. STREME applies a statistical test at p-value threshold = 0.05 to determine the enrichment of motifs in the input peptides compared to the control set.

Motif Search in PROSITE

Peptides were queried by the Motif Search tool (https://www.genome.jp/tools/motif/) (accessed on 28 September 2021) and integrated into the GenomeNet Suite (https://www.genome.jp/) (accessed on 28 September 2021). PROSITE Pattern and PROSITE Profile libraries were only considered for the motif search.

3. Results and Discussion

3.1. Model Selection

3.1.1. Network Analysis

Similarity Threshold Analysis

Out of the set of 659 THPs retrieved from starPepDB, 627 peptides (SI1-A-I) were filtered with lower than 98% similarity by local alignment. The adequate similarity threshold was chosen before building CSN with the 627 peptides. This step is non-trivial since it is the parameter that defines the topology and network features [54]. Hence, the appropriate cut-off for building the CSN was determined based on the variability of network parameters such as density, modularity, ACC, and singletons at different cut-off similarity values. Graphml files corresponding to the 17 CSNs are available at SI2. Table S1 shows the obtained parameters at each cut-off.

The graph of density, modularity, and ACC as a function of the similarity threshold is shown in Figure 4. The density is lower at a higher similarity threshold. ACC follows the same pattern until the 0.65 similarity threshold. By contrast, modularity increases as the similarity threshold increases, while the clustering is optimized.

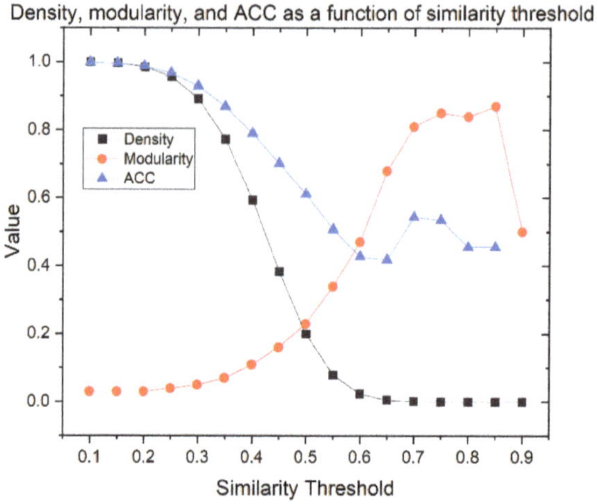

Figure 4. Density, modularity, and average clustering coefficient (ACC) as a function of similarity threshold of 627 THPs CSN.

A well-defined network needs a compromise among the density, modularity, and ACC parameters, but also accounts for the number of outlier nodes because they are atypical peptides with particular properties. Networks with very low density display too many outliers (see Table S1), while networks with very high density show a massive connection. In both cases, information is lost and interpretation becomes difficult. According to the literature, the best density percentages are generally around 1% or 2.5% because they generate high modularity but allow an adequate understanding of the network [54]. As modularity indicates the existence of community structures, the ideal value must show an equilibrium between a non-clustered network and an artificially clustered network due to the high modularity value. In this sense, the selected similarity threshold was 0.60, where CSN shows the best trade-off among network parameters and connectivity: 2.3% of density, 0.47 of modularity, 0.428 of ACC, and 99 outliers (15.8% of overall nodes). Therefore, the giant components of the network were 528 nodes (SI1-A-II).

Network Characterization

Some parameters such as density, number of clusters, modularity, average degree, ACC, and diameter were calculated and shown in Table 1 to get an overview on the giant component and outliers of the CSNs, which are represented in Figures 5 and 6, respectively.

Table 1. Global network properties of CSN of 528 nodes and outliers.

Set *	Nodes	Edges	Density	Clusters	Modularity	Average Degree	ACC	Diameter	Nodes after Sc. **	Edges after Sc. **
THPs	528	4452	0.023	10	0.47	16.864	0.428	8	-	-
Outliers	99	2691	0.891	3	0.13	54.364	0.733	3	34	384

* Density, number of clusters, and modularity were calculated in the starPep toolbox, while average degree, ACC, and diameter were calculated in Gephi. ** Sc.: Scaffold extraction.

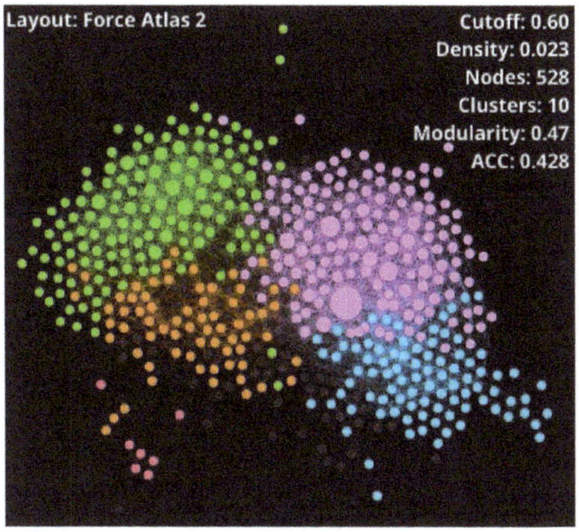

Figure 5. CSN of giant component conformed by 528 THPs retrieved from starPepDB. Node color represents the community (cluster), and node size symbolizes the centrality values.

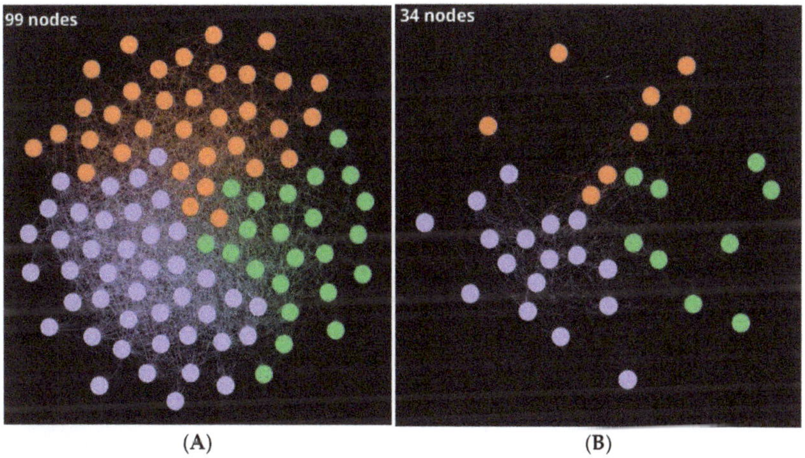

Figure 6. CSN of (**A**) 99 outliers with a density of 0.30 and (**B**) 34 remaining outliers resulting from 30% similarity extraction scaffold. *Layout: Fruchterman–Reingold.*

Additionally, the degree of distribution of the giant components is shown in Figure 7. It gives some information about the structure of the CSN. In this case, the distribution degree is concentrated in the nodes with low vertex degrees. However, it has a tail associated with the nodes with higher vertex degrees in a lower proportion. The nodes with higher degrees correspond to the most central nodes, which, as can be corroborated in Figure 5, are in the minority.

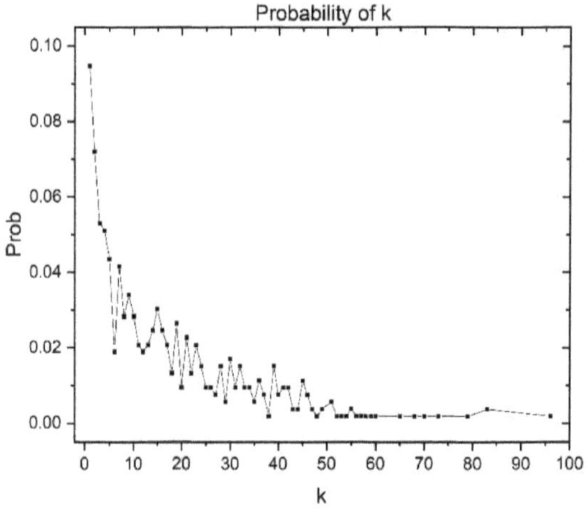

Figure 7. Degree distribution of the 528 giant components, where k is the vertex degree.

Outliers are relevant THPs because they present characteristics regarding 528 nodes that make up the giant component; so, they are unique or atypical sequences. CSN of the 99 singletons (SI1-E) was built using 0.30 of similarity threshold (Figure 6a). Then, sequences with higher similarity than 30% by local alignment were removed based on hub-bridge centrality ranking, where 34 outliers (SI1-E-I) with unique sequences were obtained (Figure 6b).

3.1.2. Centrality Analysis and Similarity Searching

Centrality is the crucial parameter to build the model that will be proposed to identify THPs. It allows the identification of the most influential sequences of the giant components. SI3 (Excel file) shows the normalized centrality measurements of 528 THPs. On the other hand, outliers are nodes with unique properties that enrich the influential sequences model. Therefore, both sets from centrality measurements and sets of outliers represent the chemical space of THPs and will be used as queries to perform the similarity searching against the target datasets. In total, 98 different SSMs were generated based on 22 query sets (FASTA files available at SI4) and similarity thresholds between 0.3 and 0.9.

The predictions and performance of the 98 SSMs are shown in SI5 and SI6-A, respectively, where active and inactive labels indicate predicted THPs and non-THPs, respectively. In general, it is observed that the performance of query datasets followed the following tendency of relevance: weighted degree > harmonic > hub-bridge > betweenness > singletons (outliers). However, the combination of query datasets from different centrality types overperforms the sets selected with only one centrality measure. The addition of the outliers set improved the performance of the combination sets since it generates the complete representation of the chemical space of THPs. Moreover, better performance was obtained using 40, 50, and 60% identity in the similarity searching.

The performance of the best nine SSMs to predict activity in Main, Small, and Main90 datasets are shown in Table 2, Table 3, and Table 4, respectively, where H is the set obtained when harmonic centrality was calculated, W is the set obtained when the weighted degree was calculated, and sing is the set of 99 outliers.

Table 2. Statistical analysis for the performance of the best 9 SSMs on the target Main dataset.

Query Set *	Nodes	% Id	Ac	Correct Class	Incorrect Class	κ	Sn	Sp	P_{pos}	P_{neg}
H + sing	467	40	0.933	1215	87	0.866	0.877	0.989	0.988	0.89
		50	0.935	1218	84	0.871	0.877	0.994	0.993	0.89
		60	0.935	1218	84	0.871	0.874	0.997	0.996	0.888
W + sing	469	40	0.934	1216	86	0.868	0.879	0.989	0.988	0.891
		50	0.936	1219	83	0.873	0.879	0.994	0.993	0.891
		60	0.937	1220	82	0.874	0.877	0.997	0.997	0.89
H + W + sing	479	40	0.942	1226	76	0.883	0.894	0.989	0.988	0.903
		50	0.944	1229	73	0.888	0.894	0.994	0.993	0.904
		60	0.945	1230	72	0.889	0.892	0.997	0.997	0.903

* H is the set obtained when harmonic centrality was calculated, W is the set obtained when the weighted degree was calculated, and sing is the set of 99 outliers.

Table 3. Statistical analysis for the performance of the best 9 SSMs on the target Small dataset.

Query Set *	Nodes	% Id	Ac	Correct Class	Incorrect Class	κ	Sn	Sp	P_{pos}	P_{neg}
H + sing	467	40	0.917	860	78	0.834	0.838	0.996	0.995	0.86
		50	0.916	859	79	0.832	0.836	0.996	0.995	0.858
		60	0.914	857	81	0.827	0.832	0.996	0.995	0.855
W + sing	469	40	0.92	863	75	0.84	0.844	0.996	0.995	0.865
		50	0.92	863	75	0.84	0.844	0.996	0.995	0.865
		60	0.919	862	76	0.838	0.842	0.996	0.995	0.863
H + W + sing	479	40	0.928	870	68	0.855	0.859	0.996	0.995	0.876
		50	0.928	870	68	0.855	0.859	0.996	0.995	0.876
		60	0.926	869	69	0.853	0.857	0.996	0.995	0.875

* H is the set obtained when harmonic centrality was calculated, W is the set obtained when the weighted degree was calculated, and sing is the set of 99 outliers.

Table 4. Statistical analysis for the performance of the best 9 SSMs on the target Main90 dataset.

Query Set *	Nodes	% Id	Ac	Correct Class	Incorrect Class	κ	Sn	Sp	P_{pos}	P_{neg}
H + sing	467	40	0.985	600	9	0.964	0.983	0.986	0.966	0.993
		50	0.99	603	6	0.976	0.983	0.993	0.983	0.993
		60	0.992	604	5	0.98	0.983	0.995	0.989	0.993
W + sing	469	40	0.98	597	12	0.952	0.966	0.986	0.966	0.986
		50	0.984	599	10	0.96	0.966	0.991	0.977	0.986
		60	0.987	601	8	0.968	0.966	0.995	0.988	0.986
H + W + sing	479	40	0.985	600	9	0.964	0.983	0.986	0.966	0.993
		50	0.989	602	7	0.972	0.983	0.991	0.977	0.993
		60	0.992	604	5	0.98	0.983	0.995	0.989	0.993

* H is the set obtained when harmonic centrality was calculated, W is the set obtained when the weighted degree was calculated, and sing is the set of 99 outliers.

It can be noticed that the best statistics were achieved using the query composed of the union of harmonic and weighted degree, both using 60% similarity cut-off of local alignment during scaffold extraction, and the 99 outliers sets, comprising in total 479 query sequences. Moreover, 60% was the best percentage of identity where there was a compromise for all statistical parameters. All statistical parameters showed values higher than 0.88.

The best nine SSMs were compared and ranked using the Friedman test by comparing multiple statistical metrics from each SSM on the three target datasets (details in SI6-B). The best SSM was the set **CSN-TH-0.60Sc-479-H+W+s-0.6-583 (479Q_0.6)**, named THP1, showing excellent statistical metrics (>0.85) for the model (shown in Tables 2–4). It is composed of the union of nodes with an identity lower than 60% from the global centrality harmonic with those obtained from applying weighted degree and the set of 99 outliers (479 nodes). The best percentage of identity used to search similarity was 60%. The confusion matrices of THP1 are shown in SI6-C. It can be seen that the prediction of the model was not at random as the MCC was much greater than zero [55].

Finally, the Friedman test of the THP1 versus the reported models used in TumorHPD [26] and THPep [28] servers revealed there is a significant difference between the models, being that the performance of the similarity searching methodology is superior (details in SI6-C and SI6-D). Figure 8 shows the ranking scores from the test, where THP1 is the first ranked method. Finally, Table 5 compares between the model on the three benchmarking datasets. The MCC of predictions using THP1 improved by an average of 28.76% over ML-based models.

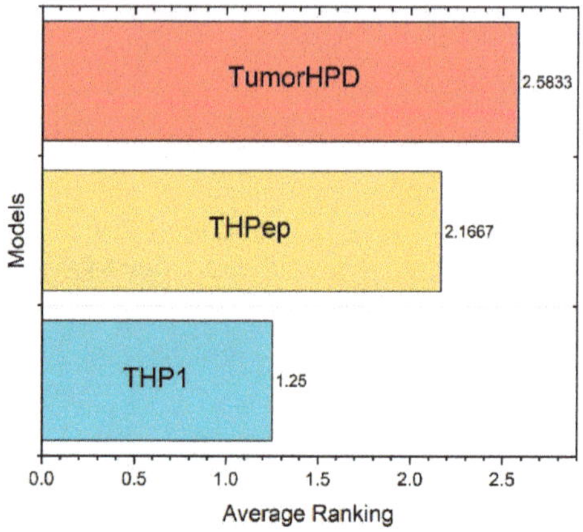

Figure 8. Ranking scores obtained in the Friedman Test. Friedman statistic (distributed according to chi-square with 2 degrees of freedom): 11.166667. P-value computed by Friedman Test: 0.00376.

Table 5. Comparison between the best SSM THP1 and the state-of-the-art ML model to predict tumor-homing activity of benchmarking datasets.

Dataset	Method	Ac (%)	Sn (%)	Sp (%)	MCC
	TumorHPD	86.56	80.63	89.71	0.7
Main	**THPep**	86.1	87.07	85.18	0.72
	THP1	***94.47***	***89.25***	***99.66***	***0.894***
	TumorHPD	81.88	73.13	90.92	0.65
Small	**THPep**	83.37	81.24	85.81	0.67
	THP1	*92.64*	*85.71*	*99.5*	*0.861*
	TumorHPD	89.66	83.64	80.68	0.74
Main90	**THPep**	90.8	91.8	87.97	0.77
	THP1	*99.18*	*98.3*	*99.54*	*0.98*

3.2. *Identification of Potential THPs*

3.2.1. Hierarchical Screening

Starting from the 45120 AMPs contained in starPepDB, and after applying the previously explained filters and performing the similarity searching, 43 lead hits were retrieved (SI7-A). Figure 9 shows the step-by-step hierarchical virtual screening. Until today, these repurposed sequences have not reported any tumor-homing activity.

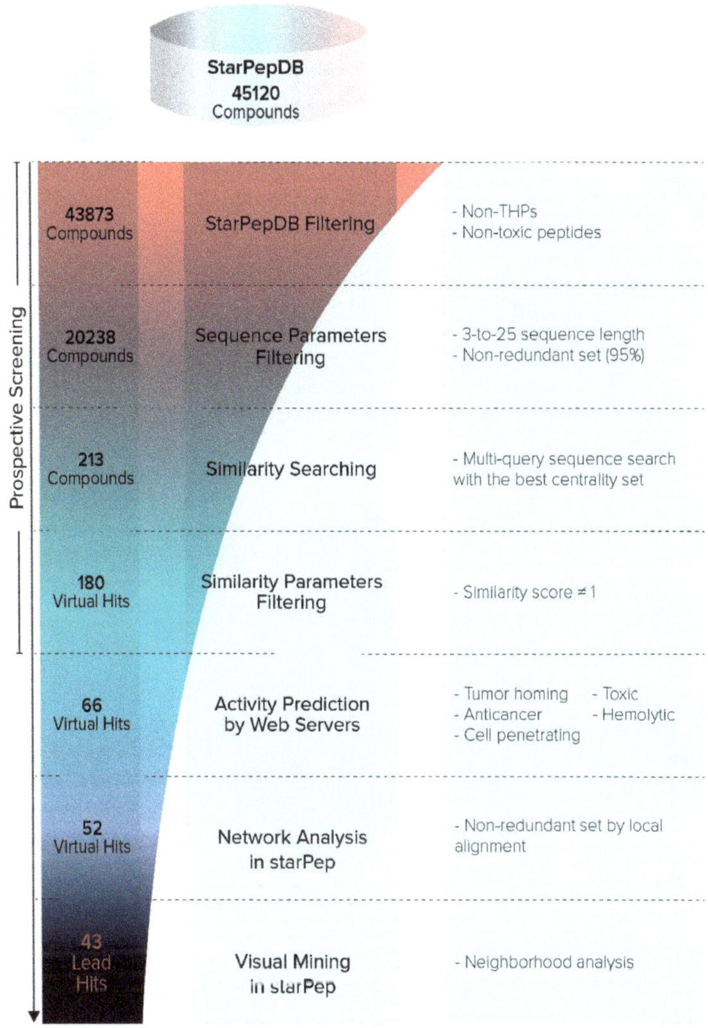

Figure 9. Hierarchical virtual screening for repurposing of peptides from starPepDB.

3.2.2. Tumor-Homing Activity Optimization

A library of 180 sequences (SI7-B) was obtained from the optimization of 43 hits in TumorHPD. They have a higher TH score, lower toxicity, and hemolytic activity than the originals. Mutations enriched the sequences with W and C residues. Mainly G and V residues from the originals were mutated to W, while R and K were to C. Studies report the presence of W contributes positively to the intracellular translocation of peptides [56]. Additionally, it was reported that W enhances the stability of peptides in serum and salt [57].

Forty-one peptides from the library were prioritized by studying their CSN, where 50% scaffold extraction by local alignment was accomplished. The sequences were clustered and ranked according to the global harmonic centrality to perform the scaffold extraction. Only the most central sequences with a similarity among them lower than 50% were kept. Forty-one sequences have higher predicted TH activity by TumorHPD than the original peptides, with scores between 0.39 and 1.92. Furthermore, they are anticancer and have less toxicity and hemolytic activity. 12 out of 41 sequences come from fragments of original sequences of 5, 10, and 15 lengths; 15 resulted from four punctual mutations from the originals; and 14 from fragments of mutated sequences of 5, 10, and 15 lengths. Two out of forty-one peptides, CNGRCGGKLA and WCAMS, are part of reported THPs, validating the novel methodology to discover potential THPs. CNGRCGGKLA is the *N*-end of the CNGRCGGKLAKLAKKLAKLAK peptide containing the NGR TH motif and a disulfide bridge that gives stability. CNGRCGGKLAKLAKKLAKLAK binds to CD13 of tumor cells acting as ACP and THP [58]. At the same time, WCAMS is the C-end of the KLWCAMS peptide that homes mouse B16B15b melanoma [59].

We selected the most promising 13 sequences from the 43 lead hits and these were combined with the 41 optimized hits. In total, we proposed 54 peptides (SET 1, FASTA file in SI7-C) with a diverse molecular structure, low toxicity, and hemolytic activity, with most of them also showing potential anticancer activity (SI7-D). Among the 54 lead hits, only one sequence has the well-known NGR motif. Therefore, SET 1 is composed of new structural entities within the known structural space of the THPs.

The sequence diversity of SET 1 was evaluated using all vs. all global alignment where pairwise sequence identities were explored. As shown in Figure 10, the 54 lead hits present a structure singularity sharing pairwise identities with 30%.

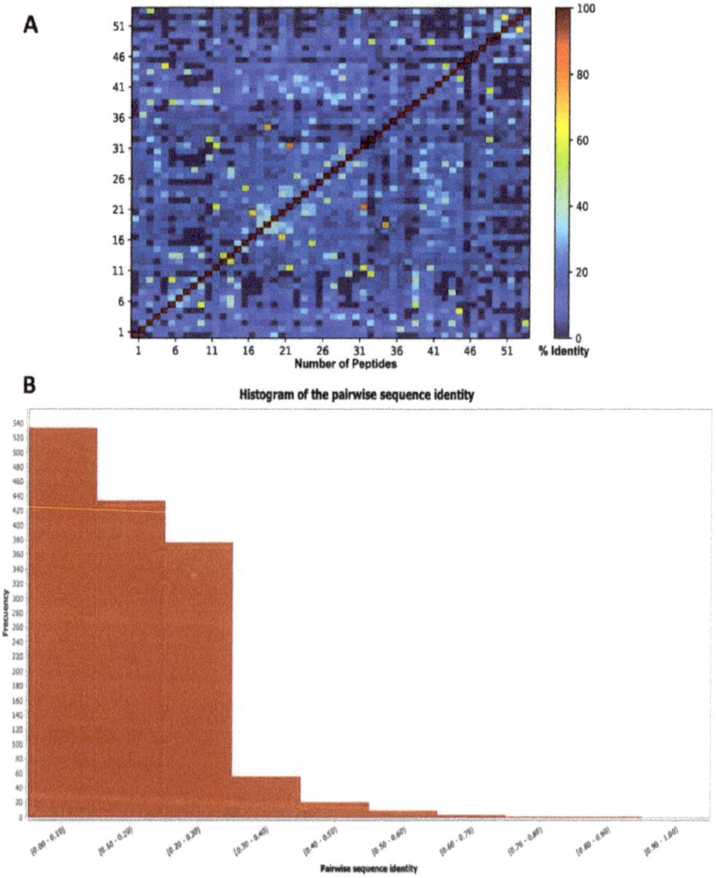

Figure 10. (**A**) Heat map and (**B**) histogram of pairwise sequence identity of SET 1 (54 lead compounds).

3.2.3. Motif Discovery

As a consequence of the structural diversity of SET 1, the discovery of motifs accounting for the TH activity is not a straightforward task. In this sense, sensitive multiple sequence alignment (MSA) tools and alignment-free (AF) approaches (e.g., STREME) were applied to unravel new TH motifs.

The resulting 54 lead THPs were mapped onto CSN space to identify putative communities and make possible the application of MSA algorithms for motif identification. These networks communities were considered clusters containing related peptides. Finally, six clusters were conformed with 14, 10, 8, 4, 10, and 8 members, respectively (SI7-E). The last cluster grouped the singletons (peptides identified as atypical in the CSN).

Clustal-Omega [32], MAFFT [33], MUSCLE [34], and T-Coffee [35], which are MSA algorithms developed after the classical ClustalW, were applied, so that they can deal with hard-to-align sequences shown in each cluster, and thus to detect any conserved signature or motif. Since each MSA has implemented a different algorithm to improve alignment quality, their consideration for the estimation of consensus regions helped us identify TH motifs by using the Jalview, EMBOSS Cons and Seq2Logo programs (SI8). As the EMBOSS Cons, gives a more legible output, only displaying high scored amino acids/positions (capital letters), less scored but positive residues (lower-case letters), and non-consensus positions (x), were selected as the primary source to set consensus/conserved regions. The non-consensus positions were estimated using default parameters by visual inspection of the corresponding positions in the Jalview program [52] and the Seq2Logo [53]. Table 6 depicts the consensus motifs, unraveled by each MSA algorithm.

Table 6. Discovered motifs by Multiple Sequence Alignment (MSA).

No	Motif	EMBOSS Consensus	Cluster	Cluster Size	Frequency *	MSA Method
1	wwW	wwW	2	14	1/(1)	CLUSTALW-O
		xxW				MAFFT
2	C[fl][rg][vl]rW	CxxxrW	3	10	0/(0)	MAFFT
3	C[gpi][gs]cR	CxxxR				MUSCLE
4	[rkl]GLC	RGlc	4	8	0/(0)	CLUSTALW-O
		kGLC				MAFFT
		xGLc				MUSCLE
5	c[wp]kG	cwkG	1+5	4	0/(0) 0/(0)	CLUSTALW-O MUSCLE
		cxkG			0/(1)	T-Coffee
6	Not Found	Non-consensus	6	10	0/(0)	CLUSTALW-O MUSCLE MAFFT T-Coffee
7	l[rp][cw]c	lxxc	Singletons	8	0/(0)	MUSCLE

* Taken from TumorHoPe (outside parenthesis), and starPepDB (inside parenthesis).

None of the motifs found by MSA have been reported as TH motifs (Table 6). However, one of the motifs from No. 3 CxxxR, CGGCR, contains the CXXC motif, which is the active site of thioredoxin (Trx), a relevant protein in mammalian cells that acts as an antioxidant and participates in programmed cell death inhibition and cell growth, commonly used as a target for cancer treatments [60,61]. Moreover, CWKG (No. 5) is contained in a nanoscale molecular platform used as a drug delivery system in chemotherapy to enhance the conjugation of mitomycin C to the carrier [62].

On the other hand, the AF approach STREME was used to find unaligned patterns ranging from 3–5 aa length within the overall 54 peptides and each peptide cluster. STREME has been recently reported as the most accurate and sensitive algorithm among its competing state-of-the-art partners [36]. Unlike previous algorithms [63–65], STREME uses a position weight matrix (PWM) to count position matches efficiently for a motif candidate against a Markov model built up from shuffling the same input set (control sequences).

Table 7 displays the enriched motifs, discriminating the 54 lead peptides against the control sequences. The same search was also performed by considering each cluster content. Motifs appearing in more than 20% of the query sequences are listed according to their statistical significance (score).

Table 7. Discovered Motifs by STREME.

No	Motif	Cluster	Cluster Size	Matches in Positive Seqs.	Matches in Control Seqs.	Sites (%)	Score	Frequency *
1	WRP	2	14	7	1	50	1.6×10^{-2}	5/(5)
2	WVL			5	1	35.7	8.2×10^{-2}	0/(0)
3	WS[YR]			3	0	21.4	1.1×10^{-1}	1/(1)Y
4	WWWM			3	0	21.4	1.1×10^{-1}	0/(0)
5	CFRV	3	10	3	0	30	1.1×10^{-1}	1/(1)
6	HWK			2	0	20	2.4×10^{-1}	0/(0)
7	PRW			2	0	20	2.4×10^{-1}	3/(3)
8	CN[WG]	4	8	3	0	37.5	1.0×10^{-1}	34/(32)G
9	WARG			3	0	37.5	1.0×10^{-1}	0/(0)
10	GIC			2	0	25.0	2.3×10^{-1}	5/(4)
11	WKG	1-5	4	3	1	75.0	2.4×10^{-1}	0/(0)
12	KNKHK	6	10	3	0	30.0	1.1×10^{-1}	0/(0)
13	PSHL			3	0	30.0	1.1×10^{-1}	0/(0)
14	LRLRI	Singletons	8	2	0	25.0	2.3×10^{-1}	1/(1)
15	CC[CQ]			3	1	37.5	2.8×10^{-1}	0/(0)
16	LSP	All sequences	54	11	1	20.4	3.4×10^{-3}	3/(3)
17	WSYG			7	0	13.0	8.2×10^{-3}	0/(0)
18	WRPW			5	0	9.3	3.2×10^{-2}	2/(2)

* Taken from TumorHoPe (outside parenthesis), and starPepDB (inside parenthesis).

One of the motifs discovered by STREME had been reported as tumor-homing, WRP interacting with VEGF-C [66,67]. Other found motifs have been reported but not as TH, such as WRPW, PRW, WKG, and PSHL. WRPW is the binding site of the 7 Enhancer of split E(spl) basic helix–loop–helix (bHLH) protein and the hairy protein to the corepressor protein Groucho-TLE via WD40 domain [68]. PRW is part of a biocatalyst, which is conjugated to a lipid by an ester or amide bond [69]. WKG is a ribosomally synthesized and post-translationally modified peptide [70] and PSHL is a tetrapeptide that affects HIV-1 protease (PR) [71].

Lastly, 54 lead THPs were queried against PROSITE's pattern and profile databases using the search engine Motif Search of the GenomeNet suite [72]. Only two query peptides, which are shown in Table 8, had significant matches with motifs found in gonadotropin-releasing hormones (GnRH) and bombesin-like peptides.

Table 8. Motifs found in PROSITE.

No	Motif Found	Hit Peptide	Accession	Match with	Signature	Related Seqs.	Frequency *
1	QHWSYGLRPG	starPep_07237	PS00473	Q[HY][FYW]Sx(4)PG	Gonadotropin-releasing hormones	67	1/(1)QHWSY
2	WARGHFM	starPep_10020	PS00257	WAxG[SH][LF]M	Bombesin-like peptides	36	0/(0)

* Taken from TumorHoPe (outside parenthesis), and starPepDB (inside parenthesis).

These two peptide signatures and their receptors are involved in neuroendocrine signaling pathways associated with physiological states and tumors. GnRH is the hypothalamic decapeptide that plays a crucial role controlling women's reproductive cycle. GnRH binds to specific receptors on the pituitary gonadotrophic cells, but it also is expressed in other reproductive organs, e.g., ovaries, and tumors derived from the ovaries. It has been shown GnRH is involved in ovarian cancer regulation proliferation and metastasis either by the indirect signaling pathway or direct interaction with the GnRH receptors placed at the surface of ovarian cancer cells [73].

Bombesin-like peptides were initially discovered from frog skin, where they are secreted from cutaneous glands as a means of communication and defense. They were later found to be widely distributed in mammalian neural and endocrine cells represented by the neuromedin B (NMB) and the gastrin-releasing peptide (GRP), respectively. Bombesin-like peptide receptors are G-protein-coupled and have seven membrane-spanning domains, so they are involved in signal transduction pathways [74]. Growing evidence shows that bombesin-like peptides and receptors play essential roles in physiological conditions and diseases. An abnormal expression of bombesin receptors has been observed in several types of tumors, which has motivated the development of more specific and safer bombesin derivatives for tumor diagnosis and therapy [75].

The motif search by using different approaches may render a diversity of outcomes. However, some hits shared by different search approaches can support the reliability of the findings. For example, one motif found by the PROSITE search, WSY, was also encountered by STREME, an algorithm that works regardless of database and sequence similarity. Some of the motifs estimated by MSA algorithms were also identified by the AF approach STREME, such as WWW and WKG. All motifs were searched against TH databases, TumorHoPe, and starPepDB to discriminate the possible new signatures from the existing ones. New motifs appear at very low frequency within THPs (last column of Table 6–8), except CNG found by STREME, which appears 34 times in TumorHoPe and 32 in starPepDB. However, CNG has not been reported as a TH motif.

4. Conclusions

In this study, a novel methodology based on network science and similarity searching was introduced to explore the chemical space of THPs and discover potential THPs from known AMPs. Statistically, the strategy's performance transcended current supervised ML approaches used in THP predictions, demonstrating the potential of this approach. Hence, in silico predictions using the model based on representative THPs, in conjunction with TumorHPD and THPep servers, gave a high reliability to discover potential THPs. As a result, 54 lead compounds were repurposed as potential from AMPs. In the set, novel motifs with promising tumor-homing activity were proposed.

The good performance of the methodology for predicting peptide activity based on similarity searching and network science suggests its application for the prediction of other endpoints in peptides, e.g., antibacterial activity, toxicity, hemolytic, or anticancer. Our models and pipeline are freely available through the starPep toolbox software at http://mobiosd-hub.com/starpep (accessed on 2 February 2021).

Supplementary Materials: The following are available online at https://www.mdpi.com/article/10.3390/antibiotics11030401/s1, Table S1. CSN parameters of similarity threshold analysis.

Author Contributions: M.R. worked on the datasets' extraction and curation, designed the experiments, performed SAR analysis, and performed the virtual screening, as well as drafted the initial manuscript. Y.M.-P. worked on the conceptualizing of the complex network and similarity searching methods, supervised the applications, and prepared the manuscript. H.R., G.A.-C., and A.A. worked mainly on the motif discovery analysis and drafted the initial manuscript. L.A.-M. and F.M.-R. worked primarily on the implementation of the complex network and similarity searching module and performed SAR and statistical analysis. All authors have read and agreed to the published version of the manuscript.

Funding: This research was funded by USFQ's Collaboration Grant 2019–2020 (Project ID16885), Yachay Tech grant number REG-INV-18-03244 and the APC was funded by Deanship of Research at USFQ.

Institutional Review Board Statement: Not applicable.

Informed Consent Statement: Not applicable.

Data Availability Statement: The starPep toolbox software and the respective user manual, as well as *SSMs*, are freely available online at http://mobiosd-hub.com/starpep (accessed on 2 February 2021).

Acknowledgments: Yovani Marrero-Ponce (Y.M.-P.) thanks the program *Profesor coinvitado* for a post-doctoral fellowship to work at Valencia University in 2020-21. Y.M.-P. acknowledges the support from Collaboration Grant 2019–2020 (Project ID16885). G.A.-C. and A.A. were supported by national funds through FCT—Foundation for Science and Technology—within the scope of UIDB/04423/2020 and UIDP/04423/2020. Hortensia Rodríguez (H.R.) and Maylin Romero (M.R.) acknowledge the support of Yachay Tech internal project "Therapeutic Peptides with biological activity" (REG-INV-18-03244).

Conflicts of Interest: The authors declare no conflict of interest.

References

1. World Health Organization. Cancer. Available online: https://www.who.int/health-topics/cancer#tab=tab_1 (accessed on 1 October 2021).
2. Hoskin, D.W.; Ramamoorthy, A. Studies on anticancer activities of antimicrobial peptides. *Biochim. Biophys. Acta Biomembr.* **2008**, *1778*, 357–375. [CrossRef]
3. Miller, K.D.; Nogueira, L.; Mariotto, A.B.; Rowland, J.H.; Yabroff, K.R.; Alfano, C.M.; Jemal, A.; Kramer, J.L.; Siegel, R.L. Cancer treatment and survivorship statistics, 2019. *CA Cancer J. Clin.* **2019**, *69*, 363–385. [CrossRef]
4. Gatti, L.; Zunino, F. Overview of Tumor Cell Chemoresistance Mechanisms. In *Chemosensitivity*; Humana Press: Clifton, NJ, USA, 2005; Volume 111, pp. 127–148.
5. de la Torre, B.G.; Albericio, F. Peptide therapeutics 2.0. *Molecules* **2020**, *25*, 2019–2021. [CrossRef]
6. Lau, J.L.; Dunn, M.K. Therapeutic peptides: Historical perspectives, current development trends, and future directions. *Bioorg. Med. Chem.* **2018**, *26*, 2700–2707. [CrossRef]
7. Albericio, F.; Kruger, H.G. Therapeutic peptides. *Future Med. Chem.* **2012**, *4*, 1527–1531. [CrossRef]
8. Ladner, R.C.; Sato, A.K.; Gorzelany, J.; De Souza, M. Phage display-derived peptides as therapeutic alternatives to antibodies. *Drug Discov. Today* **2004**, *9*, 525–529. [CrossRef]
9. Vlieghe, P.; Lisowski, V.; Martinez, J.; Khrestchatisky, M. Synthetic therapeutic peptides: Science and market. *Drug Discov. Today* **2010**, *15*, 40–56. [CrossRef]
10. Loffet, A. Peptides as drugs: Is there a market? *J. Pept. Sci.* **2002**, *8*, 1–7. [CrossRef]
11. Segura-Campos, M.; Chel-Guerrero, L.; Betancur-Ancona, D.; Hernandez-Escalante, V.M. Bioavailability of bioactive peptides. *Food Rev. Int.* **2011**, *27*, 213–226. [CrossRef]
12. Wu, D.; Gao, Y.; Qi, Y.; Chen, L.; Ma, Y.; Li, Y. Peptide-based cancer therapy: Opportunity and challenge. *Cancer Lett.* **2014**, *351*, 13–22. [CrossRef]
13. Wei, G.; Wang, Y.; Huang, X.; Hou, H.; Zhou, S. Peptide-Based Nanocarriers for Cancer Therapy. *Small Methods* **2018**, *2*, 1–16. [CrossRef]
14. Tesauro, D.; Accardo, A.; Diaferia, C.; Milano, V.; Guillon, J.; Ronga, L.; Rossi, F. Peptide-Based Drug-Delivery Systems in Biotechnological Applications: Recent Advances and Perspectives. *Molecules* **2019**, *24*, 351. [CrossRef] [PubMed]
15. Ruoslahti, E. Tumor penetrating peptides for improved drug delivery. *Adv. Drug Deliv. Rev.* **2017**, *110–111*, 3–12. [CrossRef] [PubMed]
16. Khandia, R.; Sachan, S.; Munjal, A.K.; Tiwari, R.; Dhama, K. Tumor Homing Peptides: Promising Futuristic Hope for Cancer Therapy. In *Topics in Anti-Cancer Research*; Bentham Science Publishers: Sharjah, United Arab Emirates, 2016; pp. 43–86.
17. Laakkonen, P.; Vuorinen, K. Homing peptides as targeted delivery vehicles. *Integr. Biol.* **2010**, *2*, 326–337. [CrossRef]
18. Elsabahy, M.; Shrestha, R.; Clark, C.; Taylor, S.; Leonard, J.; Wooley, K.L. Multifunctional hierarchically assembled nanostructures as complex stage-wise dual-delivery systems for coincidental yet differential trafficking of siRNA and paclitaxel. *Nano Lett.* **2013**, *13*, 2172–2181. [CrossRef]
19. Kolonin, M.G.; Bover, L.; Sun, J.; Zurita, A.J.; Do, K.A.; Lahdenranta, J.; Cardó-Vila, M.; Giordano, R.J.; Jaalouk, D.E.; Ozawa, M.G.; et al. Ligand-directed surface profiling of human cancer cells with combinatorial peptide libraries. *Cancer Res.* **2006**, *66*, 34–40. [CrossRef] [PubMed]
20. Peletskaya, E.N.; Glinsky, V.V.; Glinsky, G.V.; Deutscher, S.L.; Quinn, T.P. Characterization of peptides that bind the tumor-associated Thomsen-Friedenreich antigen selected from bacteriophage display libraries. *J. Mol. Biol.* **1997**, *270*, 374–384. [CrossRef]
21. Wang, F.; Li, Y.; Shen, Y.; Wang, A.; Wang, S.; Xie, T. The functions and applications of RGD in tumor therapy and tissue engineering. *Int. J. Mol. Sci.* **2013**, *14*, 13447–13462. [CrossRef]

22. He, X.; Na, M.; Kim, J.-S.; Lee, G.-Y.; Park, J.Y.; Hoffman, A.S.; Nam, J.; Han, S.; Sim, G.Y.; Oh, Y.; et al. A Novel Peptide Probe for Imaging and Targeted Delivery of Liposomal Doxorubicin to Lung Tumor. *Mol. Pharm.* **2011**, *8*, 430–438. [CrossRef]
23. Nazemian, M.; Hojati, V.; Zavareh, S.; Madanchi, H.; Hashemi-Moghaddam, H. Immobilized Peptide on the Surface of Poly l-DOPA/Silica for Targeted Delivery of 5-Fluorouracil to Breast Tumor. *Int. J. Pept. Res. Ther.* **2020**, *26*, 259–269. [CrossRef]
24. Wu, C.-H.; Liu, I.-J.; Lu, R.-M.; Wu, H.-C. Advancement and applications of peptide phage display technology in biomedical science. *J. Biomed. Sci.* **2016**, *23*, 8. [CrossRef]
25. Cui, W.; Aouidate, A.; Wang, S.; Yu, Q.; Li, Y.; Yuan, S. Discovering Anti-Cancer Drugs via Computational Methods. *Front. Pharmacol.* **2020**, *11*, 1–14. [CrossRef]
26. Sharma, A.; Kapoor, P.; Gautam, A.; Chaudhary, K.; Kumar, R.; Chauhan, J.S.; Tyagi, A.; Raghava, G.P.S. Computational approach for designing tumor homing peptides. *Sci. Rep.* **2013**, *3*, 1607. [CrossRef]
27. Kapoor, P.; Singh, H.; Gautam, A.; Chaudhary, K.; Kumar, R.; Raghava, G.P.S. TumorHoPe: A Database of Tumor Homing Peptides. *PLoS ONE* **2012**, *7*, e35187. [CrossRef]
28. Shoombuatong, W.; Schaduangrat, N.; Pratiwi, R.; Nantasenamat, C. THPep: A machine learning-based approach for predicting tumor homing peptides. *Comput. Biol. Chem.* **2019**, *80*, 441–451. [CrossRef] [PubMed]
29. Aguilera-Mendoza, L.; Marrero-Ponce, Y.; Beltran, J.A.; Tellez Ibarra, R.; Guillen-Ramirez, H.A.; Brizuela, C.A. Graph-based data integration from bioactive peptide databases of pharmaceutical interest: Toward an organized collection enabling visual network analysis. *Bioinformatics* **2019**, *35*, 4739–4747. [CrossRef]
30. Charoenkwan, P.; Chiangjong, W.; Nantasenamat, C.; Moni, M.A.; Lio', P.; Manavalan, B.; Shoombuatong, W. SCMTHP: A New Approach for Identifying and Characterizing of Tumor-Homing Peptides Using Estimated Propensity Scores of Amino Acids. *Pharmaceutics* **2022**, *14*, 122. [CrossRef] [PubMed]
31. Aguilera-Mendoza, L.; Marrero-Ponce, Y.; García-Jacas, C.R.; Chavez, E.; Beltran, J.A.; Guillen-Ramirez, H.A.; Brizuela, C.A. Automatic construction of molecular similarity networks for visual graph mining in chemical space of bioactive peptides: An unsupervised learning approach. *Sci. Rep.* **2020**, *10*, 18074. [CrossRef]
32. Sievers, F.; Wilm, A.; Dineen, D.; Gibson, T.J.; Karplus, K.; Li, W.; Lopez, R.; McWilliam, H.; Remmert, M.; Söding, J.; et al. Fast, scalable generation of high-quality protein multiple sequence alignments using Clustal Omega. *Mol. Syst. Biol.* **2011**, *7*, 539. [CrossRef]
33. Katoh, K.; Misawa, K.; Kuma, K.I.; Miyata, T. MAFFT: A novel method for rapid multiple sequence alignment based on fast Fourier transform. *Nucleic Acids Res.* **2002**, *30*, 3059–3066. [CrossRef]
34. Edgar, R.C. MUSCLE: Multiple sequence alignment with high accuracy and high throughput. *Nucleic Acids Res.* **2004**, *32*, 1792–1797. [CrossRef]
35. Notredame, C.; Higgins, D.G.; Heringa, J. T-coffee: A novel method for fast and accurate multiple sequence alignment. *J. Mol. Biol.* **2000**, *302*, 205–217. [CrossRef]
36. Bailey, T.L. STREME: Accurate and versatile sequence motif discovery. *Bioinformatics* **2021**, *37*, 2834–2840. [CrossRef]
37. Contreras-Torres, E.; Marrero-Ponce, Y.; Terán, J.E.; R. García-Jacas, C.; Brizuela, C.A.; Carlos Sánchez-Rodríguez, J. MuLiMs-MCoMPAs: A Novel Multiplatform Framework to Compute Tensor Algebra-Based Three-Dimensional Protein Descriptors. *J. Chem. Inf. Model.* **2020**, *60*, 1042–1059. [CrossRef]
38. Fruchterman, T.M.J.; Reingold, E.M. Graph Drawing by Force-Directed Placement. *Softw. Pract. Exp.* **1991**, *21*, 1129–1164. [CrossRef]
39. Blondel, V.D.; Guillaume, J.-L.; Lambiotte, R.; Lefebvre, E. Fast unfolding of communities in large networks. *J. Stat. Mech. Theory Exp.* **2008**, *2008*, P10008. [CrossRef]
40. Reigosa, M.J.; Gonzalez, L.; Sanches-Moreiras, A.; Duran, B.; Puime, D.; Fernadez, D.A.; Bolano, J.C. Comparison of physiological effects of allelochemicals and commercial herbicides. *Allelopath. J.* **2001**, *8*, 211–220.
41. Bastian, M.; Heymann, S.; Jacomy, M. Gephi: An open source software for exploring and manipulating networks. In Proceedings of the Third International Conference on Weblogs and Social Media, ICWSM 2009, San Jose, CA, USA, 17–20 May 2009; pp. 361–362.
42. Shoombuatong, W.; Schaduangrat, N.; Nantasenamat, C. Unraveling the bioactivity of anticancer peptides as deduced from machine learning. *EXCLI J.* **2018**, *17*, 734–752. [CrossRef] [PubMed]
43. Willett, P. Similarity-based virtual screening using 2D fingerprints. *Drug Discov. Today* **2006**, *11*, 1046–1053. [CrossRef] [PubMed]
44. Triguero, I.; González, S.; Moyano, J.M.; García, S.; Alcalá-Fdez, J.; Luengo, J.; Fernández, A.; del Jesús, M.J.; Sánchez, L.; Herrera, F. KEEL 3.0: An Open Source Software for Multi-Stage Analysis in Data Mining. *Int. J. Comput. Intell. Syst.* **2017**, *10*, 1238–1249. [CrossRef]
45. Iman, R.L.; Davenport, J.M. Approximations of the critical region of the Friedman statistic. *Commun. Stat. Theory Methods* **1980**, *9*, 571–595. [CrossRef]
46. Lee, W.H.; Loo, C.Y.; Ghadiri, M.; Leong, C.R.; Young, P.M.; Traini, D. The potential to treat lung cancer via inhalation of repurposed drugs. *Adv. Drug Deliv. Rev.* **2018**, *133*, 107–130. [CrossRef] [PubMed]
47. Pushpakom, S.; Iorio, F.; Eyers, P.A.; Escott, K.J.; Hopper, S.; Wells, A.; Doig, A.; Guilliams, T.; Latimer, J.; McNamee, C.; et al. Drug repurposing: Progress, challenges and recommendations. *Nat. Rev. Drug Discov.* **2019**, *18*, 41–58. [CrossRef] [PubMed]
48. Tyagi, A.; Kapoor, P.; Kumar, R.; Chaudhary, K.; Gautam, A.; Raghava, G.P.S. In silico models for designing and discovering novel anticancer peptides. *Sci. Rep.* **2013**, *3*, 2984. [CrossRef] [PubMed]

49. Gautam, A.; Chaudhary, K.; Kumar, R.; Sharma, A.; Kapoor, P.; Tyagi, A.; Raghava, G.P.S. In silico approaches for designing highly effective cell penetrating peptides. *J. Transl. Med.* **2013**, *11*, 74. [CrossRef]
50. Gupta, S.; Kapoor, P.; Chaudhary, K.; Gautam, A.; Kumar, R.; Raghava, G.P.S. In Silico Approach for Predicting Toxicity of Peptides and Proteins. *PLoS ONE* **2013**, *8*, e73957. [CrossRef]
51. Chaudhary, K.; Kumar, R.; Singh, S.; Tuknait, A.; Gautam, A.; Mathur, D.; Anand, P.; Varshney, G.C.; Raghava, G.P.S. A Web Server and Mobile App for Computing Hemolytic Potency of Peptides. *Sci. Rep.* **2016**, *6*, 22843. [CrossRef]
52. Xu, J.; Li, F.; Leier, A.; Xiang, D.; Shen, H.-H.; Marquez Lago, T.T.; Li, J.; Yu, D.-J.; Song, J. Comprehensive assessment of machine learning-based methods for predicting antimicrobial peptides. *Brief. Bioinform.* **2021**, *22*, bbab083. [CrossRef]
53. Thomsen, M.C.F.; Nielsen, M. Seq2Logo: A method for construction and visualization of amino acid binding motifs and sequence profiles including sequence weighting, pseudo counts and two-sided representation of amino acid enrichment and depletion. *Nucleic Acids Res.* **2012**, *40*, 281–287. [CrossRef]
54. Zahoránszky-Kohalmi, G.; Bologa, C.G.; Oprea, T.I. Impact of similarity threshold on the topology of molecular similarity networks and clustering outcomes. *J. Cheminform.* **2016**, *8*, 16. [CrossRef]
55. Chicco, D.; Tötsch, N.; Jurman, G. The Matthews correlation coefficient (MCC) is more reliable than balanced accuracy, bookmaker informedness, and markedness in two-class confusion matrix evaluation. *BioData Min.* **2021**, *14*, 13. [CrossRef] [PubMed]
56. Jobin, M.-L.; Blanchet, M.; Henry, S.; Chaignepain, S.; Manigand, C.; Castano, S.; Lecomte, S.; Burlina, F.; Sagan, S.; Alves, I.D. The role of tryptophans on the cellular uptake and membrane interaction of arginine-rich cell penetrating peptides. *Biochim. Biophys. Acta Biomembr.* **2015**, *1848*, 593–602. [CrossRef] [PubMed]
57. Chu, H.L.; Yip, B.S.; Chen, K.H.; Yu, H.Y.; Chih, Y.H.; Cheng, H.T.; Chou, Y.T.; Cheng, J.W. Novel antimicrobial peptides with high anticancer activity and selectivity. *PLoS ONE* **2015**, *10*, e0126390. [CrossRef] [PubMed]
58. Ellerby, H.M.; Arap, W.; Ellerby, L.M.; Kain, R.; Andrusiak, R.; Rio, G. Del; Krajewski, S.; Lombardo, C.R.; Rao, R.; Ruoslahti, E.; et al. Anti-cancer activity of targeted pro-apoptotic peptides. *Nat. Med.* **1999**, *5*, 1032–1038. [CrossRef] [PubMed]
59. Ruoslahti, E.; Pasqualini, R. Tumor Homing Molecules, Conjugates Derived Therefrom, and Methods of Using Same. Int. Pat. Appl. WO 1998/010795, 19 March 1998.
60. Bayse, C.A.; Pollard, D.B. Conformation dynamics of cyclic disulfides and selenosulfides in CXXC(U) (X = Gly, Ala) tetrapeptide redox motifs. *J. Pept. Sci.* **2019**, *25*, 16–22. [CrossRef] [PubMed]
61. Lee, S.; Kim, S.M.; Lee, R.T. Thioredoxin and thioredoxin target proteins: From molecular mechanisms to functional significance. *Antioxid. Redox Signal.* **2013**, *18*, 1165–1207. [CrossRef]
62. Ohta, T.; Hashida, Y.; Yamashita, F.; Hashida, M. Sustained Release of Mitomycin C from Its Conjugate with Single-Walled Carbon Nanotubes Associated by Pegylated Peptide. *Biol. Pharm. Bull.* **2016**, *39*, 1687–1693. [CrossRef]
63. Bailey, T.L. DREME: Motif discovery in transcription factor ChIP-seq data. *Bioinformatics* **2011**, *27*, 1653–1659. [CrossRef] [PubMed]
64. Heinz, S.; Benner, C.; Spann, N.; Bertolino, E.; Lin, Y.C.; Laslo, P.; Cheng, J.X.; Murre, C.; Singh, H.; Glass, C.K. Simple Combinations of Lineage-Determining Transcription Factors Prime cis-Regulatory Elements Required for Macrophage and B Cell Identities. *Mol. Cell* **2010**, *38*, 576–589. [CrossRef]
65. Bailey, T.L.; Boden, M.; Buske, F.A.; Frith, M.; Grant, C.E.; Clementi, L.; Ren, J.; Li, W.W.; Noble, W.S. MEME Suite: Tools for motif discovery and searching. *Nucleic Acids Res.* **2009**, *37*, 202–208. [CrossRef]
66. Asai, T.; Nagatsuka, M.; Kuromi, K.; Yamakawa, S.; Kurohane, K.; Ogino, K.; Tanaka, M.; Taki, T.; Oku, N. Suppression of tumor growth by novel peptides homing to tumor-derived new blood vessels. *FEBS Lett.* **2002**, *510*, 206–210. [CrossRef]
67. Oku, N.; Asai, T.; Watanabe, K.; Kuromi, K.; Nagatsuka, M.; Kurohane, K.; Kikkawa, H.; Ogino, K.; Tanaka, M.; Ishikawa, D.; et al. Anti-neovascular therapy using novel peptides homing to angiogenic vessels. *Oncogene* **2002**, *21*, 2662–2669. [CrossRef] [PubMed]
68. Jennings, B.H.; Pickles, L.M.; Wainwright, S.M.; Roe, S.M.; Pearl, L.H.; Ish-Horowicz, D. Molecular Recognition of Transcriptional Repressor Motifs by the WD Domain of the Groucho/TLE Corepressor. *Mol. Cell* **2006**, *22*, 645–655. [CrossRef] [PubMed]
69. Castelletto, V.; Edwards-Gayle, C.J.C.; Hamley, I.W.; Pelin, J.N.B.D.; Alves, W.A.; Aguilar, A.M.; Seitsonen, J.; Ruokolainen, J. Self-assembly of a catalytically active lipopeptide and its incorporation into cubosomes. *ACS Appl. Bio Mater.* **2019**, *2*, 3639–3647. [CrossRef] [PubMed]
70. Benjdia, A.; Berteau, O. Radical SAM Enzymes and Ribosomally-Synthesized and Post-translationally Modified Peptides: A Growing Importance in the Microbiomes. *Front. Chem.* **2021**, *9*, 678068. [CrossRef] [PubMed]
71. Yu, F.-H.; Huang, K.-J.; Wang, C.-T. C-Terminal HIV-1 Transframe p6* Tetrapeptide Blocks Enhanced Gag Cleavage Incurred by Leucine Zipper Replacement of a Deleted p6* Domain. *J. Virol.* **2017**, *91*, e00103-17. [CrossRef] [PubMed]
72. Kanehisa, M.; Goto, S.; Kawashima, S.; Nakaya, A. Thed KEGG databases at GenomeNet. *Nucleic Acids Res.* **2002**, *30*, 42–46. [CrossRef]
73. Ohlsson, B. Gonadotropin-releasing hormone and its role in the enteric nervous system. *Front. Endocrinol.* **2017**, *8*, 110. [CrossRef] [PubMed]
74. Spindel, E.R. Chapter 46—Bombesin Peptides. In *Handbook of Biologically Active Peptides*; Kastin, A.J., Ed.; Academic Press: Cambridge, MA, USA, 2013; pp. 326–330.
75. Guo, M.; Qu, X.; Qin, X.Q. Bombesin-like peptides and their receptors: Recent findings in pharmacology and physiology. *Curr. Opin. Endocrinol. Diabetes Obes.* **2015**, *22*, 3–8. [CrossRef]

antibiotics

MDPI

Article

Mining Amphibian and Insect Transcriptomes for Antimicrobial Peptide Sequences with rAMPage

Diana Lin [1], Darcy Sutherland [1,2,3], Sambina Islam Aninta [1], Nathan Louie [1], Ka Ming Nip [1,4], Chenkai Li [1,4], Anat Yanai [1], Lauren Coombe [1], René L. Warren [1], Caren C. Helbing [5], Linda M. N. Hoang [2,3] and Inanc Birol [1,2,3,*]

[1] Canada's Michael Smith Genome Sciences Centre at BC Cancer, Vancouver, BC V5Z 4S6, Canada; dlin@bcgsc.ca (D.L.); dsutherland@bcgsc.ca (D.S.); saninta@bcgsc.ca (S.I.A.); nlouie@bcgsc.ca (N.L.); kmnip@bcgsc.ca (K.M.N.); cli@bcgsc.ca (C.L.); ayanai@bcgsc.ca (A.Y.); lcoombe@bcgsc.ca (L.C.); rwarren@bcgsc.ca (R.L.W.)

[2] British Columbia Centre for Disease Control, Public Health Laboratory, Vancouver, BC V6Z R4R, Canada; linda.hoang@bccdc.ca

[3] Department of Pathology and Laboratory Medicine, University of British Columbia, Vancouver, BC V6T 1Z4, Canada

[4] Bioinformatics Graduate Program, University of British Columbia, Vancouver, BC V6T 1Z4, Canada

[5] Department of Biochemistry and Microbiology, University of Victoria, Victoria, BC V8P 5C2, Canada; chelbing@uvic.ca

* Correspondence: ibirol@bcgsc.ca

Abstract: Antibiotic resistance is a global health crisis increasing in prevalence every day. To combat this crisis, alternative antimicrobial therapeutics are urgently needed. Antimicrobial peptides (AMPs), a family of short defense proteins, are produced naturally by all organisms and hold great potential as effective alternatives to small molecule antibiotics. Here, we present rAMPage, a scalable bioinformatics discovery platform for identifying AMP sequences from RNA sequencing (RNA-seq) datasets. In our study, we demonstrate the utility and scalability of rAMPage, running it on 84 publicly available RNA-seq datasets from 75 amphibian and insect species—species known to have rich AMP repertoires. Across these datasets, we identified 1137 putative AMPs, 1024 of which were deemed novel by a homology search in cataloged AMPs in public databases. We selected 21 peptide sequences from this set for antimicrobial susceptibility testing against *Escherichia coli* and *Staphylococcus aureus* and observed that seven of them have high antimicrobial activity. Our study illustrates how in silico methods such as rAMPage can enable the fast and efficient discovery of novel antimicrobial peptides as an effective first step in the strenuous process of antimicrobial drug development.

Keywords: antimicrobial peptide, AMP discovery; genome mining; antimicrobial resistance

Citation: Lin, D.; Sutherland, D.; Aninta, S.I.; Louie, N.; Nip, K.M.; Li, C.; Yanai, A.; Coombe, L.; Warren, R.L.; Helbing, C.C.; et al. Mining Amphibian and Insect Transcriptomes for Antimicrobial Peptide Sequences with rAMPage. *Antibiotics* **2022**, *11*, 952. https://doi.org/10.3390/antibiotics11070952

Academic Editors: Guillermin Agüero-Chapin, Agostinho Antunes and Yovani Marrero-Ponce

Received: 9 June 2022
Accepted: 13 July 2022
Published: 15 July 2022

Publisher's Note: MDPI stays neutral with regard to jurisdictional claims in published maps and institutional affiliations.

Copyright: © 2022 by the authors. Licensee MDPI, Basel, Switzerland. This article is an open access article distributed under the terms and conditions of the Creative Commons Attribution (CC BY) license (https://creativecommons.org/licenses/by/4.0/).

1. Introduction

Due in large part to the overuse and misuse of antibiotics, the prevalence of multidrug-resistant bacteria is rapidly growing at a rate that cannot be matched by antibiotic discovery efforts [1]. As a consequence, the world is currently in an arms race and is at the cusp of a post-antibiotic era [1]. The slow pace of new antibiotic drug discovery, development, and regulation, combined with the accelerated emergence of resistance to existing antibiotics creates what is referred to as the "discovery void" [2]. This gap between discovery and emergence of resistance highlights an urgency to develop new antimicrobial therapeutics. One such alternative is formulations based on the antimicrobial peptides (AMPs) [3].

AMPs are short amphipathic host defense peptides that are produced in all multicellular organisms as part of the innate immune system [3]. Many AMPs operate through nonspecific mechanisms [4], such as direct electrostatic interactions with the cell membrane and immunomodulation [3], allowing for a broad spectrum of efficacy against bacteria [5], viruses [6], and fungi [7]. Furthermore, pathogens develop a slower rate of resistance to

AMPs compared to conventional antibiotics [8]. It is these qualities that position AMPs as attractive alternatives to conventional antibiotics [9].

AMPs are often produced as precursor peptides within cells that consist of an N-terminal signal peptide, followed by an acidic pro-sequence, and a C-terminal basic bioactive mature peptide sequence [3]. The acidic pro-sequence neutralizes the basic mature peptide to keep the AMP in its inactive form and the signal peptide and acidic pro-sequence together are referred to as the prepro domain [3]. AMPs are then activated by proteolytic cleavage of the prepro sequence and the release of the mature peptide [3]. While the signal peptide is often highly conserved, the acidic pro-sequence and mature AMP can be quite variable [10]. However, there is evidence that the prepro sequence can vary across different organisms [3] and even within organisms [11].

Past research has shown that amphibians, such as the American bullfrog *Rana [Lithobates] catesbeiana*, possess a rich diversity of AMPs due to their aquatic and terrestrial life cycle, where the species encounter a wide spectrum of pathogens in these two environments [11]. In amphibians, AMPs such as ranatuerin are secreted at the skin surface upon pathogen exposure and can also stimulate an adaptive immune response [12]. In contrast, insects lack a sophisticated adaptive immune system and yet are highly tolerant to bacterial infection [13,14]. This may be due to the production of AMPs by the innate immune system [14]. In insects, AMPs are found in venom or salivary gland secretions. For example, melittin, a 26 amino acid (AA) peptide is the main component of honeybee venom [13]. While there are many known amphibian AMPs, there are far fewer known insect AMPs. Amphibian AMPs have their own designated database of 1923 peptides in the Database of Anuran Defense Peptides (DADP) [15]. Additionally, they also comprise 34% (1128 sequences) of the curated Antimicrobial Peptide Database 3 (APD3) [16]. Insect AMPs, however, only contribute 10% (325 sequences) in APD3, despite being the next largest non-mammalian classification. Better characterization of these AMP arsenals holds great potential in aiding the discovery of novel AMPs.

Because most AMPs under therapeutic investigation are derived from naturally occurring AMPs in various organisms [2], effective methods to discover natural AMPs would expand the number of potential candidates. Current wet lab screening protocols consist of extraction, isolation, and purification of AMPs through laborious methods such as the collection of skin secretions followed by liquid chromatography and sequence identification using mass spectrometry [17–21]. However, these protocols are costly, time-consuming, and expertise intensive. To resolve this, a scalable, rapid, high throughput in silico methodology built on genomics technologies and able to mine RNA sequencing (RNA-seq) datasets, would greatly aid in the discovery of AMPs funneling into drug development and enhancement processes. There are in silico AMP discovery methodologies presented in earlier studies [22–26], most of which start with processed data such as assembled genomic or protein sequences. Additionally, there are several state-of-the-art tools that perform AMP prediction [27]. Because AMP precursor genes have conserved sequence characteristics, these properties can be leveraged for filtering, and their inferred mature products can be classified as an AMP or not using machine learning methods. With the current unprecedented expansion of data generation and large amounts of sequencing data available in public repositories [28], there exists a rich untapped resource for AMP discovery.

To help fill the antibiotic discovery void, we offer rAMPage: Rapid Antimicrobial Peptide Annotation and Gene Estimation, a homology-based AMP discovery pipeline to mine for putative AMP sequences in publicly available genomic resources. To classify AMP sequences, rAMPage employs AMPlify [27], an attentive deep learning model. Currently, existing AMP databases, (e.g., APD3, DADP) contain less than 4000 validated nonredundant AMP sequences in total. In comparison, we have found over 1000 putative mature AMPs in the present study, with the potential to discover thousands more. Realizing the full potential of such pipelines would require the synthesis and validation of AMP candidates. Herein, we report our results on a select list of 21 peptides we detected using rAMPage.

2. Results

2.1. Identification of Putative AMPs

Using rAMPage, we assembled ~53 million transcripts from 84 RNA-seq datasets derived from the transcriptomes of 38 amphibian (33 frogs, five toads; anurans) and 37 hymenopteran insect (eight ants, five bees, 24 wasps) species and flagged 203,758 candidate peptide sequences to be classified (Figure 1). To select a list of high-confidence putative AMPs, we collapsed duplicates from multiple samples and applied three filters: AMPlify prediction score, peptide charge, and peptide length to obtain 1137 peptide sequences. Of these, 795 originate from amphibians, and 342 from insects. Running rAMPage on all 84 datasets took one week, with all datasets (comprising < 1 billion reads) taking less than 24 h (see Supplementary Materials Figure S1 for details on the computational platform and resource usage statistics).

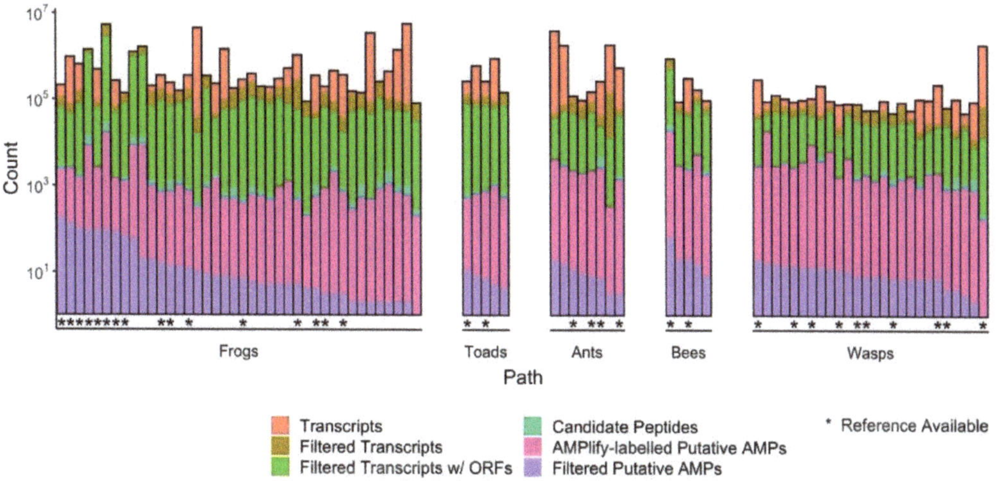

Figure 1. Statistics and attrition as the sequencing data are processed by the rAMPage AMP discovery pipeline. rAMPage processes RNA-seq datasets from raw reads to transcripts to putative AMPs. In this case, a putative AMP is defined as a sequence with an AMPlify score $\geq$10 for amphibians or $\geq$ 7 for insects, a length $\leq$ 30 AA, and a charge $\geq$ 2. Datasets with a reference transcriptome used during assembly are indicated with an asterisk. The total number of putative AMPs (n = 1478, including 341 duplicates) are shown in purple, discovered from a total of ~53 million assembled transcripts.

For each sequence, AMPlify [27] reports a prediction score s from 0 to 80, where s is a log-transformation of the AMPlify probability score p

$$s = -10 \log_{10}(1 - p), \quad (1)$$

and 80 represents the highest confidence.

We note that the training data set for the AMPlify model had an over-representation of AMPs from amphibian species [27]; hence, it is biased towards assigning higher scores for amphibian AMPs. To compensate, we have applied separate score cut-offs for the two groups: 10 for amphibians and 7 for insects. Since the majority of AMPs are positively charged, a net charge threshold of $\geq$+ 2 was applied. As for length, we filtered for sequences that are $\leq$30 AA, because shorter peptides are more cost-effective to synthesize for downstream validation studies. Figure S2 shows that the length filter used is the most restrictive filter of the three, with only 4.28% and 1.45% of the sequences for amphibians and insects, respectively, meeting this criterion.

Score, charge, length distributions, and AA compositions of the 1137 putative AMPs are characterized in Figures S1 and S4. From this set, 21 AMPs were selected for synthesis and validation, using three prioritization strategies: "Species Count", "Insect Peptide", and "AMPlify Score" (see Section 4). The peptides have been named after the species they were discovered from (Table S1), then numbered in order using their AMPlify scores.

2.2. Antimicrobial Susceptibility Testing (AST) Results

A total of 21 of the 1137 putative AMPs (Table S2) were synthesized (Genscript Biotech, Piscataway, NJ, USA) and tested for their antimicrobial activity against *Escherichia coli* ATCC 25922 and *Staphylococcus aureus* ATCC 29213 in a minimum of three independent experiments (see Figure S5 for a full set of experimental results). In these antimicrobial susceptibility tests, AMP activity was assessed using two metrics: minimum inhibitory and bactericidal concentrations (MIC and MBC, respectively). Lower MIC and MBC values are desirable as they indicate that lower AMP concentrations are sufficient for inhibitory or bactericidal activity, respectively. AMP toxicity was measured by HC_{50} hemolytic concentration values—the concentration required to lyse $\geq 50\%$ of porcine red blood cells. In contrast to MIC/MBC assays, it is desirable to have higher HC_{50} values. All 21 putative AMPs exhibited minimal to no hemolytic activity with HC_{50} values of 64 µg/mL or higher.

Of these 21 putative AMPs, three displayed moderate activity (MIC and MBC in the range 8–16 µg/mL) and four displayed high activity (≤4 µg/mL) against *E. coli* and/or *S. aureus*, all with minimal hemolytic activity, as shown in Figure 2. The characteristics of these seven sequences are described in Table 1. All seven AMPs with moderate to high antimicrobial activity have AMPlify scores greater than 25.

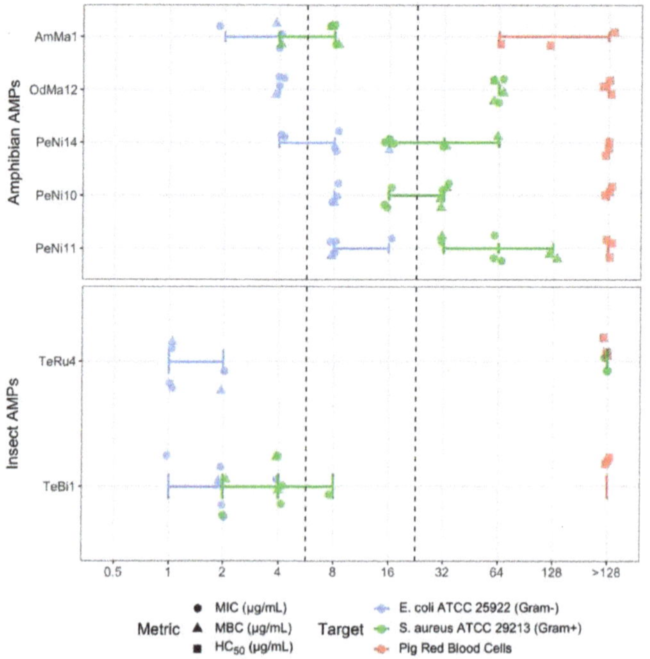

Figure 2. Antimicrobial susceptibility and hemolysis test results of seven moderately and highly active putative AMPs. AMPs were tested for their bioactivity against *E. coli* and *S. aureus* to determine minimum inhibitory and bactericidal concentrations (MIC and MBC, respectively). AMPs were also tested for their hemolytic activity using pig red blood cells to determine hemolytic concentration (HC_{50}) values. Moderate activity (MIC and MBC in the range of 8–16 µg/mL) and high activity (≤4 µg/mL) thresholds indicated by the dashed lines. AMPs are ordered by increasing MIC values against *E. coli* ATCC 25922.

Table 1. Characteristics of putative AMP sequences with moderate to high in vitro bioactivity against *E. coli* or *S. aureus*. Each sequence is separated into the prepro sequence and the predicted mature peptide sequence. Conserved proteolytic cleavage sites are underlined in the prepro sequences.

Prepro-Sequence	Putative Mature Peptide						
	Sequence	Length	Charge	AMPlify Score	MIC (μg/mL) * E. coli †	S. aureus †	Peptide ID
MFTMKKSLLVLFFLGI-VSLSLCEEERNADED-DGEMTEEVKR	GILDTLKQLGKAAVQG-LLSKAACKLAKTC	29	4	80.0	2–4	4–8	AmMa1
LGIVSLSLCQEERSA-DDEEGEVIEEEVKR	GFMDTAKNVAKNV-AVTLLYNLKCKITKAC	29	4	69.2	4	64	OdMa12
MFTMKKSLLFFFLG-TIALSLCEEERGAD-EEENGGEITDEEVKR	GLLLDTVKGAAKNVA-GILLNKLKCKVTGDC	30	3	61.8	8	16–32	PeNi10
MFTMKKSLLLVFFLG-TIALSLCEEERGAD-DDNGGEITDEEIKR	GILTDTLKGAAKNVAGVL-LDKLKCKITGGC	30	3	61.8	8–16	32–128	PeNi11
MFTLRKSLLLLFFLGM-VSLSLCEQERDAD-EDEGEVTEEVKR	GLWTTIKEGVKNFS-VGVLDKIRCKITGGC	29	3	67.5	4–8	16–64	PeNi14
MKLLALVLVLSCVV-AYTTARKRGQYWPT-NTKIFTTPYRFRREAD-QGSIVANLKNTPQLPFD-DNENLRLVLFDNDPTVDLG-EDDKEIPGPQSQPNALSNN-LHLIDENDYFSSYTSQPGT-YRSFPRNFGTSGRYRWRR-EAGGHVEPRLRFDAETQRG-NSFFTDFADLQRRANGRGI-EPTVSATAGIRFR-QEADQINPLAVRRERR	SWLSKSVKKLVNKKNY-TRLEKLAKKKLFNE	30	8	25.5	1–2	>128	TeRu4
IFLVGCKLFGNFIL-QRMQLLLALADAVA	KIKIPWGKVKDF-LVGGMKAVGKK	23	6	45.0	1–4	2–8	TeBi1

* MIC: Minimum inhibitory concentration. † *Escherichia coli* ATCC 25922; *Staphylococcus aureus* ATCC 29213.

2.3. Novelty of Discovered AMPs

To assess if the putative AMPs discovered using rAMPage are novel, a BLASTp [29] (basic local alignment search tool) protein search was performed using the 1137 sequences that met our selection criteria. Of these, 1024 sequences are reported as novel, providing no antimicrobial characterization or exact match (sequence identity = 100%; query coverage = 100%) within the NCBI non-redundant protein database [29]. The novelty analysis results for the seven moderately to highly active AMPs are presented in Table 2. Four of the queried putative AMPs (AmMa1, OdMa12, PeNi10, and PeNi14) are novel in sequence, aligning with high sequence identity (≥90%) to existing NCBI annotations [29]. Two putative AMPs (PeNi11 and TeBi1) are known and published AMPs, aligning with 100% sequence identity of the precursor protein and across the prepro and mature regions. One putative AMP (TeRu4) aligns with high sequence identity to an uncharacterized protein in the NCBI non-redundant protein database.

Table 2. Comparison of sequence identities (%) of the discovered AMPs with their best-known AMP blastp matches to the NCBI non-redundant (nr) protein database over the entire sequence (precursor), prepro or mature sequences.

Peptide ID	Source Organism	Highest Scoring Blastp Match	Sequence Identity (%)		
			Precursor	Prepro	Mature
AmMa1	*Amolops mantzorum*	Palustrin-2GN3 (ADM34231.1) [*Amolops granulosus*]	97	100	93
OdMa12	*Odorrana margaretae*	Odorranain-F2 (ABG76517.1) [*Odorrana grahami*]	98	100	97
PeNi10	*Leptobrachium boringii* *Polypedates megacephalus* *Pelophylax nigromaculatus* *Rhacophorus dennysi* *Rhacophorus omeimontis*	Pelophylaxin-1 (Q2WCN8.1) [*Pelophylax fukienensis*]	82	86	77
		Ranatuerin-2N (AEM68233.1) * [*Pelophylax nigromaculatus*]	98	97	100
PeNi11	*Leptobrachium boringii* *Polypedates megacephalus* *Pelophylax nigromaculatus* *Rhacophorus dennysi* *Rhacophorus omeimontis*	Pelophylaxin-1 (Q2WCN8.1) [*Pelophylax fukienensis*]	100	100	100
PeNi14	*Bufo gargarizans* *Polypedates megacephalus* *Pelophylax nigromaculatus* *Rhacophorus omeimontis*	Palustrin-2HB1 (AIU998997.1) [*Pelophylax hubeiensis*]	90	93	86
TeRu4	*Temnothorax rugatulus*	Uncharacterized protein (XP_024884948.1) [*Temnothorax curvispinosus*]	94	93	97
		Uncharacterized protein (TGZ47385.1) * [*Temnothorax longispinosus*]	91	90	97
TeBi1	*Tetramorium bicarinatum*	M-myrmicitoxin(01)-Tb1a (W8GNV3.1) [*Tetramorium bicarinatum*]	100	-	100

* Highest scoring blastp match when query sequence consists of only the mature sequence instead of the whole precursor. -: no significant alignment.

AmMa1, derived from the Mouping sucker frog, *A. mantzorum*, aligned with 97% sequence identity to Palustrin-2GN3 [30] from a species of the same genus, *A. granulosus*, differing only by two AA in the mature region (Figure S3a). Similarly, OdMa12, found in the green odorous frog, *O. margaretae*, aligned with 98% sequence identity to odorranain-F2 [31] from a species of the same genus, *O. grahami*, differing only by one AA in the mature region (Figure S3b). While these two sequences (AmMa1 and OdMa2) are very similar to known sequences, we have additionally discovered each of them in a different species of the same genus.

PeNi10 was detected in the dark-spotted frog *P. nigromaculatus*, and aligned with 82% identity to pelophylaxin-1 [32] from a species of the same genus, *P. fukienensis* (Figure S3c). We also identified PeNi10 in four other species of frogs: *L. boringii*, *P. megacephalus*, *R. dennysi*, *R. omeimontis* (Figure S4a). Although the PeNi10 precursor aligns best to pelophylaxin-1, the mature region aligns with complete sequence identity to ranatuerin-2N (unpublished).

PeNi14, also derived from the dark-spotted frog, *P. nigromaculatus*, aligned with 90% sequence identity to palustrin-2HB1 [33] from a species of the same genus, *P. hubeiensis* (Figure S6d). PeNi14 was also detected in three other species of frogs: *B. gargarizans*, *P. megacephalus*, *R. omeimontis* (Figure S7b).

Originating from the dark-spotted frog, *P. nigromaculatus*, PeNi11 aligned with 100% sequence identity to pelophylaxin-1 [32] from a species of the same genus, *P. fukienensis*, meaning it is identical to a known AMP precursor (Figure S6e). However, in addition to *P. nigromaculatus*, we also detected PeNi11 in four other species of frogs: *L. boringii*, *P. megacephalus*, *R. dennysi*, *R. omeimontis* (Figure S7c).

Found in the venom of tramp ant, *T. bicarinatum*, TeBi1 aligned with 100% sequence identity with bicarinalin [34,35] of the same species (Figure S6f). In the case of TeBi1, its precursor was partial on the 5′ end, accounting for no alignments in the prepro sequence.

TeRu4, discovered in the brain of the small myrmicine ant, *T. rugatulus*, aligned with 100% sequence identity to an uncharacterized protein [36] from a species of the same genus, *T. longispinosus* (Figure S6g). While TeRu4 is not a novel protein, it is a novel mature AMP as it has not been previously characterized to have antimicrobial properties.

Additional annotation of the seven bioactive peptides (five amphibians, two insects) can be found in Table S3. The underrepresentation of insect AMPs in the literature, compared to amphibians, is further demonstrated here; while the amphibian peptides have been annotated with "frog antimicrobial peptide" domains in both InterProScan [37] and Pfam [38], the insect sequences have no protein family annotations. Figure S8 illustrates the sequence identity between AMPs identified by rAMPage and known AMPs for amphibian and insect AMPs. Although the majority of putative AMPs from rAMPage were novel sequences, previously reported AMP sequences were also identified and are a good demonstration and internal validation of the robustness of this methodology.

3. Discussion

Using rAMPage, we analyzed 84 RNA-seq datasets of 38 amphibian and 37 insect species to discover 1137 putative AMPs, 1024 of which are novel. In the present study we report our validation results on 21 putative AMPs, with over 1000 additional peptide sequences left to investigate. This list is by no means exhaustive; adjusting the described filtering parameters may yield thousands more discoveries (Table S4). Further, the rAMPage pipeline can be readily used on other transcriptome sequencing datasets, though this might call for modifications in experimental designs. For instance, in the case of bacterial RNA-seq datasets with reduced post-transcriptional polyadenylation, RNA-seq data from rRNA depleted libraries would be recommended as input for the pipeline, as opposed to data from poly(A) enriched libraries [39,40].

While the sensitivity (proportion of reference AMPs captured by the three putative AMP filters) of rAMPage is <50% (Table S5 and Figure S9) with the default filtering thresholds, the filters are implemented to select for high confidence predictions that are also easier and more cost-effective to synthesize for validation. However, as more putative AMPs are discovered and the number of reference AMPs increase in public databases, the rAMPage filters can be adjusted accordingly to report more novel AMPs.

Although rAMPage captures most putative AMPs in their complete mature form, their associated precursor sequences may be incomplete, as shown using multiple sequence alignments with Clustal Omega v1.2.4 [41] (Figure S7). However, most partial transcripts are missing sequence on the 5′ end. Therefore, while the AMP precursors may be partial, the mature AMPs at the C-termini are more likely to be complete, thereby still detectable by rAMPage.

Because progress is rapid in bioinformatics, rAMPage is designed to be flexible as new technologies are developed. The pipeline is implemented as a Makefile with each step as a separate target, making the pipeline modular and providing analysis checkpoints. The tools for each step can be substituted with newer/improved tools if needed. Similarly, the pipeline is versatile and can be adapted for other sequencing technologies, for instance by assembling RNA/cDNA long reads from Pacific Biosciences of California (Menlo Park, CA, USA) or Oxford Nanopore Technologies Ltd. (Oxford, UK) instruments.

Recently, our group released AMPlify and compared its performance to other state-of-the-art tools for AMP prediction [27]. Other machine learning methods included iAMPpred [42], iAMP-2L [43], AMP Scanner Vr. 2 [44], with AMPlify outperforming all previously described AMP prediction tools in metrics of accuracy, sensitivity, and specificity [27]. For this reason, rAMPage employs AMPlify as its AMP prediction step, and will continue to until it is surpassed in performance. Machine learning in AMP discovery is a dynamic study, ranging from AMP sequence prediction and structure classification to de novo AMP sequence generation and design [45–47]. While there are existing methods to mine protein databases [48,49], rAMPage is an all-in-one tool to mine next-generation sequencing data directly from reads to AMP prediction.

While rAMPage can find a substantial number of putative AMPs, its main limitation lies in the fact that it uses homology-based sequence selection and machine learning-based sequence classification steps. These two steps are limited by the quantity and quality of data currently available for training the tools. The homology-based step of rAMPage would be less sensitive when there are more divergent signal sequences in the precursor genes. Similarly, the sequence classification engine in the pipeline, AMPlify, may be biased by known (and limited) classes of AMPs in the databases. However, this limitation is not restricted to only AMPlify, but all approaches dependent on AMP databases for training data sets [48–50].

Despite these limitations, which are expected to resolve over time as curated AMP sequence databases grow, a sizeable number (>1000 from 84 RNA-seq datasets) of AMPs were reported by the pipeline with the filters described herein. In the tested set of 21 peptides, seven demonstrated antimicrobial activity against a defined set of bacteria in vitro and 15 did not. We note that AST experiments can assess activity against the tested pathogens but cannot rule in or out an activity against other targets. Further, AMPs have multiple modes of action, and the AST protocol used in our study only validates direct action and does not test the putative immunomodulatory effects of these peptides, for instance. Of the seven active putative AMPs, three were moderately active, and all three are expressed in multiple amphibian species, potentially signaling the evolutionary significance of these AMPs.

An AMP of particular interest in the present study is TeRu4, due to its novelty and specificity in bioactivity. The precursor sequence of TeRu4 is 234 AA long, indicating that TeRu4 may be a multi-functional protein, such as a histone whose subsequence includes antimicrobial properties [51]. Additionally, TeRu4 showed a 36.84% sequence similarity to the spaetzle protein from the fruit fly *Drosophila melanogaster*, a protein in the insect Toll pathway, which triggers AMP production [52]. TeRu4 is also the most specific of the active putative AMPs we tested. While all the other active peptides tested are active against both *E. coli* and *S. aureus*, TeRu4 is active only against *E. coli*, a Gram-negative bacterium. This specificity may indicate a unique mechanism of action.

Despite the great promise of discovering putative AMPs with rAMPage, AMP-based drug development still faces some biological challenges, such as peptide stability and bacterial resistance. AMPs in their mature form are considered more unstable and more easily degraded by proteases. While synthesizing precursors for testing would increase stability, doing so would drive up the cost of synthesis using conventional synthetic chemistry methods. Although resistance to AMPs emerges at a slower rate compared to resistance to antibiotics, bacteria may develop resistance to AMPs through surface remodeling, modulation of AMP gene expression, proteolytic degradation, trapping, efflux pumps, and biofilms [4,53–55]. To combat specific mechanisms of resistance, targeted AMP discovery methods are being developed. A method to discover AMPs with anti-biofilm activity is described in a preprint [26], and a curated 3D structural and functional repository of AMPs relevant to biofilm studies called B-AMP was recently published [26]. Finding solutions to these and other challenges in developing AMPs as replacements for conventional small molecule antibiotics is an active field of research [56–58].

4. Materials and Methods

rAMPage is an AMP discovery pipeline that takes short RNA-seq reads as input, and outputs candidate putative AMPs for wet lab validation. Since it is a homology-based method to select a list of candidates for classification, a set of reference AMPs is required. Here, we describe how input datasets and reference AMPs are collated, as well as each step of rAMPage.

4.1. Collating Input RNA-Seq Datasets

The RNA-seq reads from 38 amphibian and 37 insect species were downloaded from the Sequence Read Archive (SRA) [59] using fasterq-dump v2.10.5 (http://ncbi.github.io/sra-tools/, accessed on 4 November 2019) from the NCBI SRA Tool Kit. Analyzing RNA-seq (transcriptomic) reads enables the discovery of expressed putative AMPs. Because some RNA-seq experiments were conducted with multiple tissues or treatments, there are 75 species in total, but 84 datasets are shown in Tables S6 and S7.

4.2. Collating Reference AMP Datasets

A set of 3306 AMP sequences were collated from two high-quality AMP databases: the Database of Anuran Defense Peptides (DADP; http://split4.pmfst.hr/dadp/, accessed on 6 December 2018) [15] and the Antimicrobial Peptide Database 3 (APD3; https://aps.unmc.edu, accessed on 14 September 2020) [16]. These databases are highly curated, where sequences have been validated for efficacy. To complement this list, 3835 precursor and mature AMP sequences of amphibian and insect origin were downloaded from the NCBI non-redundant (nr) protein database [29]. These sequences are less curated, including partial sequences and sequences with only in silico prediction, etc., accounting for the difference between numbers from DADP/APD3 and NCBI in Table S8.

4.3. rAMPage Pipeline

rAMPage is implemented as a Makefile and written in bash, Python3, and R. It is publicly available on GitHub (https://github.com/bcgsc/rAMPage, v1.0 accessed on 14 February 2021). The pipeline was tested for the dependencies listed in Tables S9 and S10, and is highly customizable, with its major parameter options listed in Table S4. Command and parameters for each step can be found in Table S11. A flowchart of the rAMPage pipeline is shown in Figure 3.

Because the datasets used for rAMPage originate from publicly available genomic resources and we have no control over the experimental design or protocols used, we performed rigorous quality control. The RNA-seq reads were trimmed to remove adapter sequences using fastp v0.20.0 [60], which does not require the adapter sequences to be known, and instead infers adapter sequences from sequence overlaps between reads. This is particularly convenient when dealing with multiple datasets that possibly have different sequencing protocols.

To assemble the RNA-seq reads into transcripts we used RNA-Bloom v1.3.1 [61], a de novo transcriptome assembler that works with single and paired-end reads. RNA-Bloom is able to assemble transcriptomes without a reference but also allows for reference-guided assembly if a reference is available. It also allows for multi-sample pooling, where, for instance, reads describing multiple tissues from the same individual or different treatments for the same species are assembled together while retaining the tissues or treatment specificity of assembled transcripts.

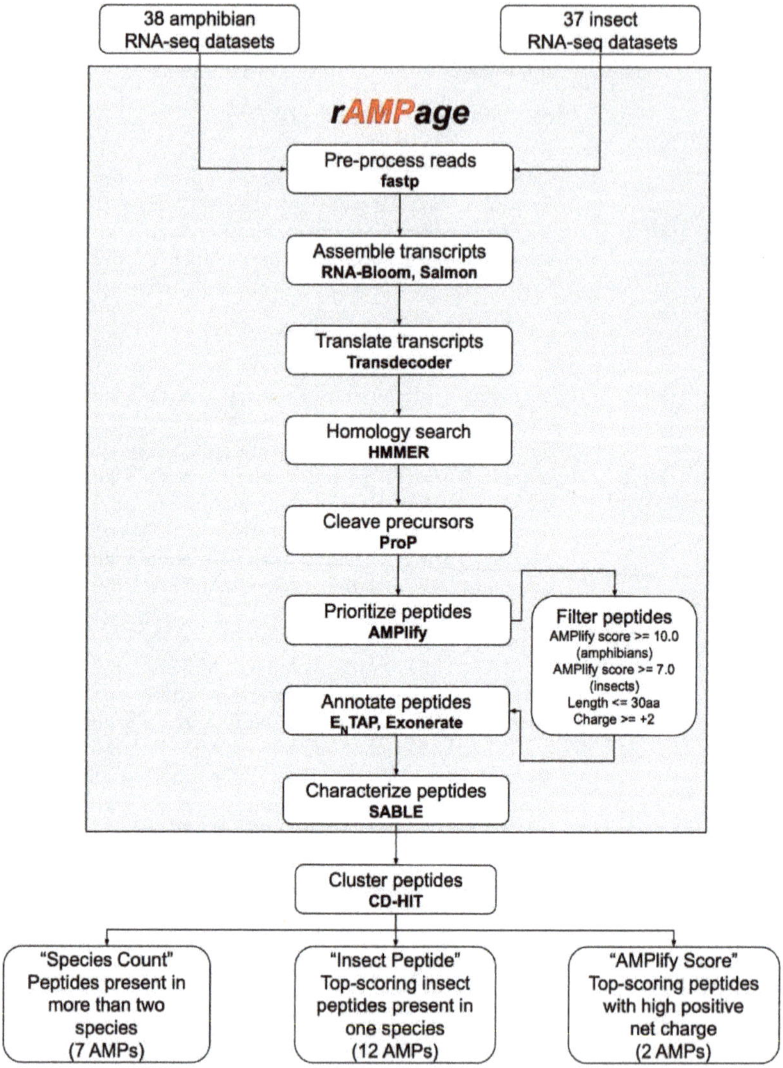

Figure 3. rAMPage workflow. The rAMPage pipeline and downstream selection of putative AMPs for validation.

We note that the transcripts with a smaller number of reads have less reconstruction evidence; thus, assembled sequences with lower measured expression levels may be enriched for misassemblies. To exclude such sequences from downstream analysis, we used Salmon v1.3.0 [62] to quantify assembled transcript expression levels, and filtered out transcripts with less than 1 TPM (transcripts per million) expression.

To obtain translated peptide sequences from the transcripts, TransDecoder v5.5.0 [63] was used to conduct an in silico six-frame open reading frame (ORF) translation, and ORFs that are at least 50 AA were selected for downstream analysis. In the case of nesting ORFs, the longest ORF was chosen.

To select putative AMP precursors from this vast pool of assembled and translated sequences, we conducted a homology search against our curated reference AMP dataset (Table S8) using HMMER v3.3.1 [64] and assigned an Expect (E) value to every sequence.

The E-value describes the number of hits expected by chance when searching a database of a particular size [65]. Sequences that share a certain degree of identity, with E-values of less than 10^{-5}, were selected as putative AMP precursors.

These putative precursor (or partial precursor) sequences were then cleaved in silico using ProP v1.0c [66] to obtain putative mature AMP sequences, to be further classified. However, cleavage prediction tools only predict where the cleavage occurs, not what each resulting cleaved peptide represents, and the AMP precursor organization shows inter- and intra-species variability [13,67,68]. While amphibian AMPs are typically cleaved at a lysine–arginine (KR) motif and their precursor structure follows a conserved structure (prepro sequence containing acidic AA residues and a mature bioactive AMP) [67], insect AMPs are typically cleaved at an RXXR motif (two arginine residues surrounding two optional AA) and the precursor structure is not always conserved [68]. Insect AMPs are more variable in structure [13], increasing the difficulty in identifying the putative mature peptide. This difficulty is especially present in precursor structures with multiple acidic regions (UniProtKB P54684.1) or multiple bioactive regions (UniProtKB P35581.1). In such multi-peptide precursors, it is unclear whether each bioactive region is its own isoform or part of a larger mature peptide. To account for this and to possibly discover novel but perhaps not naturally occurring putative AMPs, cleaved peptides were also recombined in a manner similar to alternative splicing (Figure S10). In this procedure, the order and orientation of the cleaved peptides were maintained, and cleaved peptides that originally share cleavage sites were not recombined, with a maximum of three cleaved peptides within recombination. This recombination feature can be turned off in rAMPage's options.

The collected candidate peptide sequences were classified with AMPlify v1.0.3 [27] as AMP or non-AMP sequences. When given a sequence, AMPlify calculates a score between 0 to 80, with the score ≈ 3.0103 corresponding to the classification probability cutoff of 50% through Equation (1).

To facilitate AMP synthesis for the validation experiments, we filtered the putative AMPs by length and charge, in addition to the AMPlify score. A maximum length of 30 AA was imposed to control the cost of peptide synthesis and to reduce the number of spurious hits from recombined sequences. A minimum charge of +2 was imposed as a proxy to assess the effectiveness of an AMP, as past evidence indicates that more positively charged AMPs show higher activity, especially when their mechanism of action is membrane disruption [69]. Because AMPlify was trained on mostly amphibian AMPs, different score thresholds were imposed for amphibian (≥ 10) and insect (≥ 7) datasets to compensate for the dearth of insect training AMPs.

To annotate the final set of filtered putative AMPs, E_NTAP v0.10.7, Eukaryotic Non-Model Transcriptome Annotation Pipeline [70], were used, along with UniProtKB (release 2020_06, accessed on 15 December 2020) [71], RefSeq (release 203, accessed on 15 December 2020) [72], and NCBI non-redundant (nr) (v5, accessed on 12 December 2020) [29] protein databases. For AMPs that E_NTAP failed to annotate, InterProScan 5 v5.30-69.0 [37] was run separately to annotate protein families, functions, and domains. Exonerate v2.4.0 [73] was used to align the filtered putative AMPs against the reference AMPs to assess how many of the labeled AMPs were already known AMPs. Finally, SABLE v4.0 [74] was optionally used to predict secondary structures of the filtered putative AMPs, for visualization.

4.4. Selecting Filtered Putative AMPs for Validation

To select peptides to validate from the filtered putative AMPs, we ranked their sequences using AMPlify and chose peptides based upon three selection criteria (Figure 3): "Species Count" ($n = 7$), "Insect Peptide" ($n = 12$), or "AMPlify Score" ($n = 2$), for a final total of 21 AMPs (Table S2). The sequences were first clustered using CD-HIT [75] v4.8.1 with a sequence similarity cutoff of 100%. We chose the longest sequence for each of these clusters, removing duplicate and subsumed sequences to obtain a non-redundant sequence set.

In the first selection strategy of "Species Count", sequences that were present in more than two species were chosen. In the "Insect Peptide" strategy, to balance the training bias of AMPlify towards AMPs of amphibian origin, we specifically selected insect-originating sequences using a reduced AMPlify score cutoff of >20. In the "AMPlify Score" strategy, the two highest-scoring peptides (AMPlify score = 80.0, 69.9) with the highest charge (+4) were chosen for validation.

4.5. Antimicrobial Susceptibility Testing (AST)

Twenty-one putative AMP sequences identified using the rAMPage pipeline were validated through a minimum of three AST experiments performed independently on separate days. In these tests, the AMP activity was assessed using two metrics: minimum inhibitory concentration and minimum bactericidal concentration (MIC and MBC, respectively). MIC and MBC values were determined using procedures outlined by the Clinical and Laboratory Standards Institute (CLSI), with the recommended adaptations for the testing of cationic AMPs described previously [76]. "Wild-type" strains of *Escherichia coli* (*E. coli* 25922) and *Staphylococcus aureus* (*S. aureus* 29213) were purchased from the American Type Culture Collection (ATCC; Manassas, VA, USA) and were used for screening of antimicrobial activity. Briefly, putative AMPs were synthesized by Genscript (Piscataway, NJ, USA) and received in lyophilized format. These peptides were suspended using ultrapure water (Life Technologies, Grand Island, NY, USA; Invitrogen cat# 10977-015), and an 11 µL two-fold serial dilution of 1280 to 2.5 µg/mL was prepared in duplicate rows in a 96-well microtiter plate, before being combined with 100 µL standardized bacterial inoculum yielding a final duplicate testing range of 128 to 0.25 µg/mL. The bacterial inoculum was prepared using colonies isolated on non-selective agar and combined with Mueller Hinton Broth. This suspension was measured and adjusted to achieve an optical density of 0.08–0.1, equivalent to a 0.5 McFarland standard (1–2 $\times$ 10^8 cfu/mL). The inoculum was then diluted to a target concentration of $5 \pm 3 \times 10^5$ cfu/mL; total viable counts from the final inoculum were routinely performed to confirm the target bacterial density was achieved. MIC values were reported at the concentrations in which no visible growth was detected following 20–24-h incubation at 37 °C. The MIC and adjacent wells were plated onto non-selective agar; the concentration in which killed 99.9% of the inoculum following additional overnight incubation was determined to be the MBC.

4.6. Hemolysis Experiments

The twenty-one putative AMPs were evaluated for toxicity using three independent hemolysis experiments performed on separate days. Whole blood from healthy donor pigs was purchased from Lampire Biological Laboratories (Pipersville, PA, USA). Red blood cells (RBCs) were washed and isolated by centrifugation, using Roswell Park Memorial Institute medium (RPMI) (Life Technologies, Grand Island, NY, USA; Gibco cat# 11835-030). Lyophilized AMPs were suspended and serially diluted from 128–1 µg/mL using RPMI in a 96-well plate, before being combined with 100 µL of a 1% RBC solution. Following a minimum 30 min incubation at 37 °C, plates were centrifuged and $\frac{1}{2}$ volume from each supernatant was transferred to a new 96-well plate. The absorbance of these wells was measured at 415 nm. To quantify hemolytic activity and determine the AMP concentration that kills 50% of the RBCs (HC_{50}), absorbance readings from wells containing RBCs treated with 11 µL of a 2% Triton-X100 solution or RPMI (AMP solvent-only) were used to define 100% and 0% hemolysis, respectively. All centrifugation steps were performed at 500$\times$ g for five minutes in an Allegra-6R centrifuge (Beckman Coulter, CA, USA).

5. Conclusions

rAMPage is a bioinformatics pipeline for high throughput identification of putative AMPs in RNA-seq datasets. It fills a current void in the AMP discovery process, bridging the gap between in silico and in vitro methods. The pipeline has the potential to accelerate the discovery of novel antibiotics, with the possibility to enrich existing AMP sequence repositories. The easy-to-run pipeline design with various checkpoints and the low computational resources required to run rAMPage increase its accessibility to users. By executing rAMPage on publicly available amphibian and insect transcriptome sequencing data, we have identified over 1000 putative AMPs. Of those, we performed functional tests on twenty-one putative AMPs and demonstrated that seven have moderate to high activity against *E. coli* ATCC 25922 and/or *S. aureus* ATCC 29213. As the number of tested peptides increases, the wet lab validation results can feed back into rAMPage by augmenting the reference AMP datasets, helping refine the underlying homology and machine learning approaches. We expect rAMPage to have broad utility in the discovery of novel antimicrobials from a wide variety of transcriptome sequencing datasets.

6. Patents

Patent applications pending on the reported novel peptides.

Supplementary Materials: The following supporting information can be downloaded at: https://www.mdpi.com/article/10.3390/antibiotics11070952/s1, Figure S1: Putative AMP filters used for amphibians and insects; Figure S2: Runtime and memory of each dataset through rAMPage; Figure S3: Score, length, and charge distribution of filtered putative AMPs; Figure S4: Amino acid composition of filtered putative AMPs; Figure S5: Antimicrobial susceptibility and hemolysis testing of 21 putative AMPs; Figure S6: Multiple sequence alignments of moderately to highly active AMPs; Figure S7: Multiple sequence alignments of moderately to highly active AMP precursors; Figure S8: Distribution of alignment of filtered putative AMPs to mature reference AMPs; Figure S9: Distribution of reference mature AMPs; Figure S10: Approach for peptides with multiple cleavage sites; Table S1: Peptide naming convention; Table S2: Subset of 21 putative AMPs synthesized and validated against *E. coli* and *S. aureus*; Table S3: Annotation of moderately to highly active putative mature AMPs; Table S4: Major options for rAMPage; Table S5: Sensitivity of all putative AMP filter combinations; Table S6: Amphibian RNA-seq datasets; Table S7: Insect RNA-seq datasets; Table S8: Breakdown of AMP sequences in AMP databases; Table S9: Shell scripting dependencies of rAMPage; Table S10: Bioinformatic tool dependencies of rAMPage; Table S11: Command and parameters for each step of rAMPage. References [11,27,29,30,41,59–64,73–75,77–117] are cited in the supplementary materials.

Author Contributions: Conceptualization, I.B., C.C.H. and L.M.N.H.; methodology, I.B., R.L.W., L.C., D.L. and D.S.; software, D.L., S.I.A., K.M.N. and C.L.; validation, D.S., A.Y. and N.L.; data curation, D.L. and C.L.; writing—original draft preparation, D.L.; writing—review and editing, I.B., R.L.W., L.C., D.S., A.Y., C.L., D.L. and C.C.H., funding acquisition, I.B., C.C.H. and L.M.N.H. All authors have read and agreed to the published version of the manuscript.

Funding: This work was supported by funds from Genome Canada, and Genome BC as part of the PeptAid (291PEP) and AnnoVis (281ANV) projects. Additional support was provided by the Canadian Agricultural Partnership, a federal–provincial–territorial initiative. The program is delivered by the Investment Agriculture Foundation of BC (INV106). Further funds were received from the Office of the Vice President, Research and Innovation of the University of British Columbia. Opinions expressed in this document are those of the author and not necessarily those of the Governments of Canada and British Columbia or the Investment Agriculture Foundation of BC. The Governments of Canada and British Columbia, and the Investment Agriculture Foundation of BC, and their directors, agents, employees, or contractors will not be liable for any claims, damages, or losses of any kind whatsoever arising out of the use of, or reliance upon, this information.

Institutional Review Board Statement: Not applicable.

Informed Consent Statement: Not applicable.

Data Availability Statement: Accessions for input RNA-seq datasets can be found in Tables S6 and S7. rAMPage code is publicly available at https://github.com/bcgsc/rAMPage (v1.0, accessed on 14 February 2021).

Acknowledgments: This work was based on a prototype pipeline created by S. Austin Hammond.

Conflicts of Interest: I.B. is the founder of, and a shareholder in, Amphoraxe Life Sciences Inc.

References

1. Hede, K. Antibiotic Resistance: An Infectious Arms Race. *Nature* **2014**, *509*, S2–S3. [CrossRef] [PubMed]
2. Koo, H.B.; Seo, J. Antimicrobial Peptides under Clinical Investigation. *Pept. Sci.* **2019**, *111*, e24122. [CrossRef]
3. Zhang, L.; Gallo, R.L. Antimicrobial Peptides. *Curr. Biol.* **2016**, *26*, R14–R19. [CrossRef] [PubMed]
4. Andersson, D.I.; Hughes, D.; Kubicek-Sutherland, J.Z. Mechanisms and Consequences of Bacterial Resistance to Antimicrobial Peptides. *Drug Resist. Updat.* **2016**, *26*, 43–57. [CrossRef] [PubMed]
5. Brandenburg, K.; Heinbockel, L.; Correa, W.; Lohner, K. Peptides with Dual Mode of Action: Killing Bacteria and Preventing Endotoxin-Induced Sepsis. *Biochim. Biophys. Acta BBA-Biomembr.* **2016**, *1858*, 971–979. [CrossRef]
6. Klotman, M.E.; Chang, T.L. Defensins in Innate Antiviral Immunity. *Nat. Rev. Immunol.* **2006**, *6*, 447–456. [CrossRef] [PubMed]
7. De Lucca, A.J.; Walsh, T.J. Antifungal Peptides: Novel Therapeutic Compounds against Emerging Pathogens. *Antimicrob. Agents Chemother.* **1999**, *43*, 1–11. [CrossRef]
8. Hancock, R.E.W.; Sahl, H.-G. Antimicrobial and Host-Defense Peptides as New Anti-Infective Therapeutic Strategies. *Nat. Biotechnol.* **2006**, *24*, 1551–1557. [CrossRef]
9. Moravej, H.; Moravej, Z.; Yazdanparast, M.; Heiat, M.; Mirhosseini, A.; Moosazadeh Moghaddam, M.; Mirnejad, R. Antimicrobial Peptides: Features, Action, and Their Resistance Mechanisms in Bacteria. *Microb. Drug Resist.* **2018**, *24*, 747–767. [CrossRef]
10. Vanhoye, D.; Bruston, F.; Nicolas, P.; Amiche, M. Antimicrobial Peptides from Hylid and Ranin Frogs Originated from a 150-Million-Year-Old Ancestral Precursor with a Conserved Signal Peptide but a Hypermutable Antimicrobial Domain. *Eur. J. Biochem.* **2003**, *270*, 2068–2081. [CrossRef]
11. Helbing, C.C.; Hammond, S.A.; Jackman, S.H.; Houston, S.; Warren, R.L.; Cameron, C.E.; Birol, I. Antimicrobial Peptides from Rana [Lithobates] Catesbeiana: Gene Structure and Bioinformatic Identification of Novel Forms from Tadpoles. *Sci. Rep.* **2019**, *9*, 1529. [CrossRef] [PubMed]
12. Conlon, J.M.; Mechkarska, M. Host-Defense Peptides with Therapeutic Potential from Skin Secretions of Frogs from the Family Pipidae. *Pharmaceuticals* **2014**, *7*, 58–77. [CrossRef]
13. Wu, Q.; Patočka, J.; Kuča, K. Insect Antimicrobial Peptides, a Mini Review. *Toxins* **2018**, *10*, 461. [CrossRef]
14. Sheehan, G.; Farrell, G.; Kavanagh, K. Immune Priming: The Secret Weapon of the Insect World. *Virulence* **2020**, *11*, 238–246. [CrossRef] [PubMed]
15. Novković, M.; Simunić, J.; Bojović, V.; Tossi, A.; Juretić, D. DADP: The Database of Anuran Defense Peptides. *Bioinformatics* **2012**, *28*, 1406–1407. [CrossRef] [PubMed]
16. Wang, G.; Li, X.; Wang, Z. APD3: The Antimicrobial Peptide Database as a Tool for Research and Education. *Nucleic Acids Res.* **2016**, *44*, D1087–D1093. [CrossRef] [PubMed]
17. Zhang, R.-W.; Liu, W.-T.; Geng, L.-L.; Chen, X.-H.; Bi, K.-S. Quantitative Analysis of a Novel Antimicrobial Peptide in Rat Plasma by Ultra Performance Liquid Chromatography–Tandem Mass Spectrometry. *J. Pharm. Anal.* **2011**, *1*, 191–196. [CrossRef] [PubMed]
18. Shen, W.; Chen, Y.; Yao, H.; Du, C.; Luan, N.; Yan, X. A Novel Defensin-like Antimicrobial Peptide from the Skin Secretions of the Tree Frog, Theloderma Kwangsiensis. *Gene* **2016**, *576*, 136–140. [CrossRef]
19. Pei, J.; Feng, Z.; Ren, T.; Sun, H.; Han, H.; Jin, W.; Dang, J.; Tao, Y. Purification, Characterization and Application of a Novel Antimicrobial Peptide from Andrias Davidianus Blood. *Lett. Appl. Microbiol.* **2018**, *66*, 38–43. [CrossRef]
20. Chen, W.; Hwang, Y.Y.; Gleaton, J.W.; Titus, J.K.; Hamlin, N.J. Optimization of a Peptide Extraction and LC–MS Protocol for Quantitative Analysis of Antimicrobial Peptides. *Future Sci. OA* **2019**, *5*, FSO348. [CrossRef]
21. Chowdhury, T.; Mandal, S.M.; Kumari, R.; Ghosh, A.K. Purification and Characterization of a Novel Antimicrobial Peptide (QAK) from the Hemolymph of Antheraea Mylitta. *Biochem. Biophys. Res. Commun.* **2020**, *527*, 411–417. [CrossRef] [PubMed]
22. Amaral, A.C.; Silva, O.N.; Mundim, N.C.C.R.; de Carvalho, M.J.A.; Migliolo, L.; Leite, J.R.S.A.; Prates, M.V.; Bocca, A.L.; Franco, O.L.; Felipe, M.S.S. Predicting Antimicrobial Peptides from Eukaryotic Genomes: In Silico Strategies to Develop Antibiotics. *Peptides* **2012**, *37*, 301–308. [CrossRef]
23. Prichula, J.; Primon-Barros, M.; Luz, R.C.Z.; Castro, Í.M.S.; Paim, T.G.S.; Tavares, M.; Ligabue-Braun, R.; d'Azevedo, P.A.; Frazzon, J.; Frazzon, A.P.G.; et al. Genome Mining for Antimicrobial Compounds in Wild Marine Animals-Associated Enterococci. *Mar. Drugs* **2021**, *19*, 328. [CrossRef]
24. De la Lastra, J.M.P.; Garrido-Orduña, C.; Borges, A.A.; Jiménez-Arias, D.; García-Machado, F.J.; Hernández, M.; González, C.; Boto, A. Bioinformatics discovery of vertebrate cathelicidins from the mining of available genomes. In *Drug Discovery—Concepts to Market*; Bobbarala, V., Ed.; InTech: London, UK, 2018; ISBN 978-1-78923-696-5.
25. Tomazou, M.; Oulas, A.; Anagnostopoulos, A.K.; Tsangaris, G.T.; Spyrou, G.M. In Silico Identification of Antimicrobial Peptides in the Proteomes of Goat and Sheep Milk and Feta Cheese. *Proteomes* **2019**, *7*, 32. [CrossRef]

26. Mhade, S.; Panse, S.; Tendulkar, G.; Awate, R.; Kadam, S.; Kaushik, K.S. AMPing Up the Search: A Structural and Functional Repository of Antimicrobial Peptides for Biofilm Studies, and a Case Study of Its Application to Corynebacterium striatum, an Emerging Pathogen. *Front. Cell. Infect. Microbiol.* **2021**, *11*, 803774. [CrossRef]
27. Li, C.; Sutherland, D.; Hammond, S.A.; Yang, C.; Taho, F.; Bergman, L.; Houston, S.; Warren, R.L.; Wong, T.; Hoang, L.M.N.; et al. AMPlify: Attentive Deep Learning Model for Discovery of Novel Antimicrobial Peptides Effective against WHO Priority Pathogens. *BMC Genom.* **2022**, *23*, 77. [CrossRef]
28. Muir, P.; Li, S.; Lou, S.; Wang, D.; Spakowicz, D.J.; Salichos, L.; Zhang, J.; Weinstock, G.M.; Isaacs, F.; Rozowsky, J.; et al. The Real Cost of Sequencing: Scaling Computation to Keep Pace with Data Generation. *Genome Biol.* **2016**, *17*, 53. [CrossRef]
29. NCBI Resource Coordinators. Database Resources of the National Center for Biotechnology Information. *Nucleic Acids Res.* **2016**, *44*, D7–D19. [CrossRef]
30. Guo, R.; Chen, D.; Diao, Q.; Xiong, C.; Zheng, Y.; Hou, C. Transcriptomic Investigation of Immune Responses of the Apis Cerana Cerana Larval Gut Infected by Ascosphaera Apis. *J. Invertebr. Pathol.* **2019**, *166*, 107210. [CrossRef]
31. Li, J.; Xu, X.; Xu, C.; Zhou, W.; Zhang, K.; Yu, H.; Zhang, Y.; Zheng, Y.; Rees, H.H.; Lai, R.; et al. Anti-Infection Peptidomics of Amphibian Skin. *Mol. Cell. Proteom.* **2007**, *6*, 882–894. [CrossRef]
32. Song, Y.; Ji, S.; Liu, W.; Yu, X.; Meng, Q.; Lai, R. Different Expression Profiles of Bioactive Peptides in Pelophylax Nigromaculatus from Distinct Regions. *Biosci. Biotechnol. Biochem.* **2013**, *77*, 1075–1079. [CrossRef] [PubMed]
33. Wang, X.; Ren, S.; Guo, C.; Zhang, W.; Zhang, X.; Zhang, B.; Li, S.; Ren, J.; Hu, Y.; Wang, H. Identification and Functional Analyses of Novel Antioxidant Peptides and Antimicrobial Peptides from Skin Secretions of Four East Asian Frog Species. *Acta Biochim. Biophys. Sin.* **2017**, *49*, 550–559. [CrossRef] [PubMed]
34. Rifflet, A.; Gavalda, S.; Téné, N.; Orivel, J.; Leprince, J.; Guilhaudis, L.; Génin, E.; Vétillard, A.; Treilhou, M. Identification and Characterization of a Novel Antimicrobial Peptide from the Venom of the Ant Tetramorium Bicarinatum. *Peptides* **2012**, *38*, 363–370. [CrossRef] [PubMed]
35. Téné, N.; Bonnafé, E.; Berger, F.; Rifflet, A.; Guilhaudis, L.; Ségalas-Milazzo, I.; Pipy, B.; Coste, A.; Leprince, J.; Treilhou, M. Biochemical and Biophysical Combined Study of Bicarinalin, an Ant Venom Antimicrobial Peptide. *Peptides* **2016**, *79*, 103–113. [CrossRef] [PubMed]
36. Kaur, R.; Stoldt, M.; Jongepier, E.; Feldmeyer, B.; Menzel, F.; Bornberg-Bauer, E.; Foitzik, S. Ant Behaviour and Brain Gene Expression of Defending Hosts Depend on the Ecological Success of the Intruding Social Parasite. *Philos. Trans. R. Soc. Lond. B Biol. Sci.* **2019**, *374*, 20180192. [CrossRef] [PubMed]
37. Jones, P.; Binns, D.; Chang, H.-Y.; Fraser, M.; Li, W.; McAnulla, C.; McWilliam, H.; Maslen, J.; Mitchell, A.; Nuka, G.; et al. InterProScan 5: Genome-Scale Protein Function Classification. *Bioinformatics* **2014**, *30*, 1236–1240. [CrossRef]
38. Finn, R.D.; Bateman, A.; Clements, J.; Coggill, P.; Eberhardt, R.Y.; Eddy, S.R.; Heger, A.; Hetherington, K.; Holm, L.; Mistry, J.; et al. Pfam: The Protein Families Database. *Nucleic Acids Res.* **2014**, *42*, D222–D230. [CrossRef]
39. Sarkar, N. Polyadenylation of MRNA in Prokaryotes. *Annu. Rev. Biochem.* **1997**, *66*, 173–197. [CrossRef]
40. Wangsanuwat, C.; Heom, K.A.; Liu, E.; O'Malley, M.A.; Dey, S.S. Efficient and Cost-Effective Bacterial MRNA Sequencing from Low Input Samples through Ribosomal RNA Depletion. *BMC Genom.* **2020**, *21*, 717. [CrossRef]
41. Sievers, F.; Wilm, A.; Dineen, D.; Gibson, T.J.; Karplus, K.; Li, W.; Lopez, R.; McWilliam, H.; Remmert, M.; Söding, J.; et al. Fast, Scalable Generation of High-Quality Protein Multiple Sequence Alignments Using Clustal Omega. *Mol. Syst. Biol.* **2011**, *7*, 539. [CrossRef]
42. Meher, P.K.; Sahu, T.K.; Saini, V.; Rao, A.R. Predicting Antimicrobial Peptides with Improved Accuracy by Incorporating the Compositional, Physico-Chemical and Structural Features into Chou's General PseAAC. *Sci. Rep.* **2017**, *7*, 42362. [CrossRef] [PubMed]
43. Xiao, X.; Wang, P.; Lin, W.-Z.; Jia, J.-H.; Chou, K.-C. IAMP-2L: A Two-Level Multi-Label Classifier for Identifying Antimicrobial Peptides and Their Functional Types. *Anal. Biochem.* **2013**, *436*, 168–177. [CrossRef] [PubMed]
44. Veltri, D.; Kamath, U.; Shehu, A. Deep Learning Improves Antimicrobial Peptide Recognition. *Bioinformatics* **2018**, *34*, 2740–2747. [CrossRef]
45. Das, P.; Wadhawan, K.; Chang, O.; Sercu, T.; Santos, C.D.; Riemer, M.; Chenthamarakshan, V.; Padhi, I.; Mojsilovic, A. PepCVAE: Semi-Supervised Targeted Design of Antimicrobial Peptide Sequences. *arXiv* **2018**, arXiv:1810.07743. [CrossRef]
46. Dean, S.N.; Alvarez, J.A.E.; Zabetakis, D.; Walper, S.A.; Malanoski, A.P. PepVAE: Variational Autoencoder Framework for Antimicrobial Peptide Generation and Activity Prediction. *Front. Microbiol.* **2021**, *12*, 725727. [CrossRef] [PubMed]
47. Szymczak, P.; Możejko, M.; Grzegorzek, T.; Bauer, M.; Neubauer, D.; Michalski, M.; Sroka, J.; Setny, P.; Kamysz, W.; Szczurek, E. HydrAMP: A Deep Generative Model for Antimicrobial Peptide Discovery. *bioRxiv* **2022**. [CrossRef]
48. Porto, W.F.; Pires, A.S.; Franco, O.L. Computational Tools for Exploring Sequence Databases as a Resource for Antimicrobial Peptides. *Biotechnol. Adv.* **2017**, *35*, 337–349. [CrossRef]
49. Ramazi, S.; Mohammadi, N.; Allahverdi, A.; Khalili, E.; Abdolmaleki, P. A Review on Antimicrobial Peptides Databases and the Computational Tools. *Database* **2022**, *2022*, baac011. [CrossRef]
50. Aronica, P.G.A.; Reid, L.M.; Desai, N.; Li, J.; Fox, S.J.; Yadahalli, S.; Essex, J.W.; Verma, C.S. Computational Methods and Tools in Antimicrobial Peptide Research. *J. Chem. Inf. Model.* **2021**, *61*, 3172–3196. [CrossRef]
51. Cho, J.H.; Sung, B.H.; Kim, S.C. Buforins: Histone H2A-Derived Antimicrobial Peptides from Toad Stomach. *Biochim. Biophys. Acta BBA-Biomembr.* **2009**, *1788*, 1564–1569. [CrossRef]

52. De Gregorio, E.; Spellman, P.T.; Tzou, P.; Rubin, G.M.; Lemaitre, B. The Toll and Imd Pathways Are the Major Regulators of the Immune Response in Drosophila. *EMBO J.* **2002**, *21*, 2568–2579. [CrossRef] [PubMed]
53. Guilhelmelli, F.; Vilela, N.; Albuquerque, P.; Derengowski, L.D.S.; Silva-Pereira, I.; Kyaw, C.M. Antibiotic Development Challenges: The Various Mechanisms of Action of Antimicrobial Peptides and of Bacterial Resistance. *Front. Microbiol.* **2013**, *4*, 353. [CrossRef] [PubMed]
54. Rodríguez-Rojas, A.; Baeder, D.Y.; Johnston, P.; Regoes, R.R.; Rolff, J. Bacteria Primed by Antimicrobial Peptides Develop Tolerance and Persist. *PLoS Pathog.* **2021**, *17*, e1009443. [CrossRef]
55. da Cunha, N.B.; Cobacho, N.B.; Viana, J.F.C.; Lima, L.A.; Sampaio, K.B.O.; Dohms, S.S.M.; Ferreira, A.C.R.; de la Fuente-Núñez, C.; Costa, F.F.; Franco, O.L.; et al. The next Generation of Antimicrobial Peptides (AMPs) as Molecular Therapeutic Tools for the Treatment of Diseases with Social and Economic Impacts. *Drug Discov. Today* **2017**, *22*, 234–248. [CrossRef]
56. Cao, J.; de la Fuente-Nunez, C.; Ou, R.W.; Torres, M.D.T.; Pande, S.G.; Sinskey, A.J.; Lu, T.K. Yeast-Based Synthetic Biology Platform for Antimicrobial Peptide Production. *ACS Synth. Biol.* **2018**, *7*, 896–902. [CrossRef] [PubMed]
57. Hazam, P.K.; Goyal, R.; Ramakrishnan, V. Peptide Based Antimicrobials: Design Strategies and Therapeutic Potential. *Prog. Biophys. Mol. Biol.* **2019**, *142*, 10–22. [CrossRef] [PubMed]
58. Hirano, M.; Saito, C.; Goto, C.; Yokoo, H.; Kawano, R.; Misawa, T.; Demizu, Y. Rational Design of Helix-Stabilized Antimicrobial Peptide Foldamers Containing α,α-Disubstituted AAs or Side-Chain Stapling. *ChemPlusChem* **2020**, *85*, 2731–2736. [CrossRef]
59. Leinonen, R.; Sugawara, H.; Shumway, M.; On behalf of the International Nucleotide Sequence Database Collaboration. Sequence Read Archive. *Nucleic Acids Res.* **2011**, *39*, D19–D21. [CrossRef]
60. Chen, S.; Zhou, Y.; Chen, Y.; Gu, J. Fastp: An Ultra-Fast All-in-One FASTQ Preprocessor. *Bioinformatics* **2018**, *34*, i884–i890. [CrossRef]
61. Nip, K.M.; Chiu, R.; Yang, C.; Chu, J.; Mohamadi, H.; Warren, R.L.; Birol, I. RNA-Bloom Enables Reference-Free and Reference-Guided Sequence Assembly for Single-Cell Transcriptomes. *Genome Res.* **2020**, *30*, 1191–1200. [CrossRef]
62. Patro, R.; Duggal, G.; Love, M.I.; Irizarry, R.A.; Kingsford, C. Salmon Provides Fast and Bias-Aware Quantification of Transcript Expression. *Nat. Methods* **2017**, *14*, 417–419. [CrossRef] [PubMed]
63. Haas, B.J.; Papanicolaou, A.; Yassour, M.; Grabherr, M.; Blood, P.D.; Bowden, J.; Couger, M.B.; Eccles, D.; Li, B.; Lieber, M.; et al. De Novo Transcript Sequence Reconstruction from RNA-Seq Using the Trinity Platform for Reference Generation and Analysis. *Nat. Protoc.* **2013**, *8*, 1494–1512. [CrossRef] [PubMed]
64. Johnson, L.S.; Eddy, S.R.; Portugaly, E. Hidden Markov Model Speed Heuristic and Iterative HMM Search Procedure. *BMC Bioinform.* **2010**, *11*, 431. [CrossRef] [PubMed]
65. Finn, R.D.; Clements, J.; Eddy, S.R. HMMER Web Server: Interactive Sequence Similarity Searching. *Nucleic Acids Res.* **2011**, *39*, W29–W37. [CrossRef]
66. Duckert, P.; Brunak, S.; Blom, N. Prediction of Proprotein Convertase Cleavage Sites. *Protein Eng. Des. Sel.* **2004**, *17*, 107–112. [CrossRef]
67. Wang, X.; Song, Y.; Li, J.; Liu, H.; Xu, X.; Lai, R.; Zhang, K. A New Family of Antimicrobial Peptides from Skin Secretions of Rana Pleuraden. *Peptides* **2007**, *28*, 2069–2074. [CrossRef]
68. Yi, H.-Y.; Chowdhury, M.; Huang, Y.-D.; Yu, X.-Q. Insect Antimicrobial Peptides and Their Applications. *Appl. Microbiol. Biotechnol.* **2014**, *98*, 5807–5822. [CrossRef]
69. Jiang, Z.; Vasil, A.I.; Hale, J.D.; Hancock, R.E.W.; Vasil, M.L.; Hodges, R.S. Effects of Net Charge and the Number of Positively Charged Residues on the Biological Activity of Amphipathic Alpha-Helical Cationic Antimicrobial Peptides. *Biopolymers* **2008**, *90*, 369–383. [CrossRef]
70. Hart, A.J.; Ginzburg, S.; Xu, M.; Fisher, C.R.; Rahmatpour, N.; Mitton, J.B.; Paul, R.; Wegrzyn, J.L. EnTAP: Bringing Faster and Smarter Functional Annotation to Non-model Eukaryotic Transcriptomes. *Mol. Ecol. Resour.* **2020**, *20*, 591–604. [CrossRef]
71. The UniProt Consortium; Bateman, A.; Martin, M.-J.; Orchard, S.; Magrane, M.; Agivetova, R.; Ahmad, S.; Alpi, E.; Bowler-Barnett, E.H.; Britto, R.; et al. UniProt: The Universal Protein Knowledgebase in 2021. *Nucleic Acids Res.* **2021**, *49*, D480–D489. [CrossRef]
72. O'Leary, N.A.; Wright, M.W.; Brister, J.R.; Ciufo, S.; Haddad, D.; McVeigh, R.; Rajput, B.; Robbertse, B.; Smith-White, B.; Ako-Adjei, D.; et al. Reference Sequence (RefSeq) Database at NCBI: Current Status, Taxonomic Expansion, and Functional Annotation. *Nucleic Acids Res.* **2016**, *44*, D733–D745. [CrossRef] [PubMed]
73. Slater, G.; Birney, E. Automated Generation of Heuristics for Biological Sequence Comparison. *BMC Bioinform.* **2005**, *6*, 31. [CrossRef]
74. Adamczak, R.; Porollo, A.; Meller, J. Combining Prediction of Secondary Structure and Solvent Accessibility in Proteins. *Proteins* **2005**, *59*, 467–475. [CrossRef] [PubMed]
75. Fu, L.; Niu, B.; Zhu, Z.; Wu, S.; Li, W. CD-HIT: Accelerated for Clustering the next-Generation Sequencing Data. *Bioinformatics* **2012**, *28*, 3150–3152. [CrossRef]
76. Wiegand, I.; Hilpert, K.; Hancock, R.E.W. Agar and Broth Dilution Methods to Determine the Minimal Inhibitory Concentration (MIC) of Antimicrobial Substances. *Nat. Protoc.* **2008**, *3*, 163–175. [CrossRef] [PubMed]
77. Sanchez, E.; Rodríguez, A.; Grau, J.H.; Lötters, S.; Künzel, S.; Saporito, R.A.; Ringler, E.; Schulz, S.; Wollenberg Valero, K.C.; Vences, M. Transcriptomic Signatures of Experimental Alkaloid Consumption in a Poison Frog. *Genes* **2019**, *10*, 733. [CrossRef]

78. Siu-Ting, K.; Torres-Sánchez, M.; San Mauro, D.; Wilcockson, D.; Wilkinson, M.; Pisani, D.; O'Connell, M.J.; Creevey, C.J. Inadvertent Paralog Inclusion Drives Artifactual Topologies and Timetree Estimates in Phylogenomics. *Mol. Biol. Evol.* **2019**, *36*, 1344–1356. [CrossRef]
79. Xia, Y.; Luo, W.; Yuan, S.; Zheng, Y.; Zeng, X. Microsatellite Development from Genome Skimming and Transcriptome Sequencing: Comparison of Strategies and Lessons from Frog Species. *BMC Genom.* **2018**, *19*, 886. [CrossRef]
80. Fan, W.; Jiang, Y.; Zhang, M.; Yang, D.; Chen, Z.; Sun, H.; Lan, X.; Yan, F.; Xu, J.; Yuan, W. Comparative Transcriptome Analyses Reveal the Genetic Basis Underlying the Immune Function of Three Amphibians' Skin. *PLoS ONE* **2017**, *12*, e0190023. [CrossRef]
81. Reilly, B.D.; Schlipalius, D.I.; Cramp, R.L.; Ebert, P.R.; Franklin, C.E. Frogs and Estivation: Transcriptional Insights into Metabolism and Cell Survival in a Natural Model of Extended Muscle Disuse. *Physiol. Genom.* **2013**, *45*, 377–388. [CrossRef]
82. Liscano Martinez, Y.; Arenas Gómez, C.M.; Smith, J.; Delgado, J.P. A Tree Frog (Boana Pugnax) Dataset of Skin Transcriptome for the Identification of Biomolecules with Potential Antimicrobial Activities. *Data Brief* **2020**, *32*, 106084. [CrossRef] [PubMed]
83. Grogan, L.F.; Mulvenna, J.; Gummer, J.P.A.; Scheele, B.C.; Berger, L.; Cashins, S.D.; McFadden, M.S.; Harlow, P.; Hunter, D.A.; Trengove, R.D.; et al. Survival, Gene and Metabolite Responses of Litoria Verreauxii Alpina Frogs to Fungal Disease Chytridiomycosis. *Sci. Data* **2018**, *5*, 180033. [CrossRef] [PubMed]
84. Qiao, L.; Yang, W.; Fu, J.; Song, Z. Transcriptome Profile of the Green Odorous Frog (Odorrana Margaretae). *PLoS ONE* **2013**, *8*, e75211. [CrossRef] [PubMed]
85. Chang, L.; Zhu, W.; Shi, S.; Zhang, M.; Jiang, J.; Li, C.; Xie, F.; Wang, B. Plateau Grass and Greenhouse Flower? Distinct Genetic Basis of Closely Related Toad Tadpoles Respectively Adapted to High Altitude and Karst Caves. *Genes* **2020**, *11*, 123. [CrossRef]
86. Caty, S.N.; Alvarez-Buylla, A.; Byrd, G.D.; Vidoudez, C.; Roland, A.B.; Tapia, E.E.; Budnik, B.; Trauger, S.A.; Coloma, L.A.; O'Connell, L.A. Molecular Physiology of Chemical Defenses in a Poison Frog. *J. Exp. Biol.* **2019**, *222*, jeb.204149. [CrossRef]
87. Shu, Y.; Xia, J.; Yu, Q.; Wang, G.; Zhang, J.; He, J.; Wang, H.; Zhang, L.; Wu, H. Integrated Analysis of MRNA and MiRNA Expression Profiles Reveals Muscle Growth Differences between Adult Female and Male Chinese Concave-Eared Frogs (Odorrana Tormota). *Gene* **2018**, *678*, 241–251. [CrossRef]
88. Yoshida, N.; Kaito, C. Dataset for de Novo Transcriptome Assembly of the African Bullfrog Pyxicephalus Adspersus. *Data Brief* **2020**, *30*, 105388. [CrossRef]
89. Bossuyt, F.; Schulte, L.M.; Maex, M.; Janssenswillen, S.; Novikova, P.Y.; Biju, S.D.; Van de Peer, Y.; Matthijs, S.; Roelants, K.; Martel, A.; et al. Multiple Independent Recruitment of Sodefrin Precursor-Like Factors in Anuran Sexually Dimorphic Glands. *Mol. Biol. Evol.* **2019**, *36*, 1921–1930. [CrossRef]
90. Zhang, Y.; Li, Y.; Qin, Z.; Wang, H.; Li, J. A Screening Assay for Thyroid Hormone Signaling Disruption Based on Thyroid Hormone-Response Gene Expression Analysis in the Frog Pelophylax Nigromaculatus. *J. Environ. Sci.* **2015**, *34*, 143–154. [CrossRef]
91. Eskew, E.A.; Shock, B.C.; LaDouceur, E.E.B.; Keel, K.; Miller, M.R.; Foley, J.E.; Todd, B.D. Gene Expression Differs in Susceptible and Resistant Amphibians Exposed to Batrachochytrium Dendrobatidis. *R. Soc. Open sci.* **2018**, *5*, 170910. [CrossRef]
92. Stuckert, A.M.M.; Chouteau, M.; McClure, M.; LaPolice, T.M.; Linderoth, T.; Nielsen, R.; Summers, K.; MacManes, M.D. The Genomics of Mimicry: Gene Expression throughout Development Provides Insights into Convergent and Divergent Phenotypes in a Müllerian Mimicry System. *Mol. Ecol.* **2021**, *30*, 4039–4061. [CrossRef] [PubMed]
93. Christenson, M.K.; Trease, A.J.; Potluri, L.-P.; Jezewski, A.J.; Davis, V.M.; Knight, L.A.; Kolok, A.S.; Davis, P.H. De Novo Assembly and Analysis of the Northern Leopard Frog Rana Pipiens Transcriptome. *J. Genom.* **2014**, *2*, 141–149. [CrossRef] [PubMed]
94. Price, S.J.; Garner, T.W.J.; Balloux, F.; Ruis, C.; Paszkiewicz, K.H.; Moore, K.; Griffiths, A.G.F. A de Novo Assembly of the Common Frog (Rana Temporaria) Transcriptome and Comparison of Transcription Following Exposure to Ranavirus and Batrachochytrium Dendrobatidis. *PLoS ONE* **2015**, *10*, e0130500. [CrossRef]
95. Furman, B.L.S.; Evans, B.J. Sequential Turnovers of Sex Chromosomes in African Clawed Frogs (Xenopus) Suggest Some Genomic Regions Are Good at Sex Determination. *G3 (Bethesda)* **2016**, *6*, 3625–3633. [CrossRef] [PubMed]
96. Birol, I.; Behsaz, B.; Hammond, S.A.; Kucuk, E.; Veldhoen, N.; Helbing, C.C. De Novo Transcriptome Assemblies of Rana (Lithobates) Catesbeiana and Xenopus Laevis Tadpole Livers for Comparative Genomics without Reference Genomes. *PLoS ONE* **2015**, *10*, e0130720. [CrossRef]
97. Barbosa-Morais, N.L.; Irimia, M.; Pan, Q.; Xiong, H.Y.; Gueroussov, S.; Lee, L.J.; Slobodeniuc, V.; Kutter, C.; Watt, S.; Colak, R.; et al. The Evolutionary Landscape of Alternative Splicing in Vertebrate Species. *Science* **2012**, *338*, 1587–1593. [CrossRef]
98. Arvidson, R.; Kaiser, M.; Lee, S.S.; Urenda, J.-P.; Dail, C.; Mohammed, H.; Nolan, C.; Pan, S.; Stajich, J.E.; Libersat, F.; et al. Parasitoid Jewel Wasp Mounts Multipronged Neurochemical Attack to Hijack a Host Brain. *Mol. Cell. Proteom.* **2019**, *18*, 99–114. [CrossRef]
99. Yek, S.H.; Boomsma, J.J.; Schiøtt, M. Differential Gene Expression in Acromyrmex Leaf-Cutting Ants after Challenges with Two Fungal Pathogens. *Mol. Ecol.* **2013**, *22*, 2173–2187. [CrossRef]
100. Yoon, K.A.; Kim, K.; Kim, W.-J.; Bang, W.Y.; Ahn, N.-H.; Bae, C.-H.; Yeo, J.-H.; Lee, S.H. Characterization of Venom Components and Their Phylogenetic Properties in Some Aculeate Bumblebees and Wasps. *Toxins* **2020**, *12*, 47. [CrossRef]
101. McNamara-Bordewick, N.K.; McKinstry, M.; Snow, J.W. Robust Transcriptional Response to Heat Shock Impacting Diverse Cellular Processes despite Lack of Heat Shock Factor in Microsporidia. *mSphere* **2019**, *4*, e00219-19. [CrossRef]
102. Becchimanzi, A.; Avolio, M.; Bostan, H.; Colantuono, C.; Cozzolino, F.; Mancini, D.; Chiusano, M.L.; Pucci, P.; Caccia, S.; Pennacchio, F. Venomics of the Ectoparasitoid Wasp Bracon Nigricans. *BMC Genom.* **2020**, *21*, 34. [CrossRef]

103. de Bekker, C.; Ohm, R.A.; Loreto, R.G.; Sebastian, A.; Albert, I.; Merrow, M.; Brachmann, A.; Hughes, D.P. Gene Expression during Zombie Ant Biting Behavior Reflects the Complexity Underlying Fungal Parasitic Behavioral Manipulation. *BMC Genom.* **2015**, *16*, 620. [CrossRef] [PubMed]
104. von Wyschetzki, K.; Lowack, H.; Heinze, J. Transcriptomic Response to Injury Sheds Light on the Physiological Costs of Reproduction in Ant Queens. *Mol. Ecol.* **2016**, *25*, 1972–1985. [CrossRef]
105. Zhao, W.; Shi, M.; Ye, X.; Li, F.; Wang, X.; Chen, X. Comparative Transcriptome Analysis of Venom Glands from Cotesia Vestalis and Diadromus Collaris, Two Endoparasitoids of the Host Plutella Xylostella. *Sci. Rep.* **2017**, *7*, 1298. [CrossRef]
106. Coffman, K.A.; Harrell, T.C.; Burke, G.R. A Mutualistic Poxvirus Exhibits Convergent Evolution with Other Heritable Viruses in Parasitoid Wasps. *J. Virol.* **2020**, *94*, e02059-19. [CrossRef] [PubMed]
107. Burke, G.R.; Strand, M.R. Systematic Analysis of a Wasp Parasitism Arsenal. *Mol. Ecol.* **2014**, *23*, 890–901. [CrossRef] [PubMed]
108. Robinson, S.D.; Mueller, A.; Clayton, D.; Starobova, H.; Hamilton, B.R.; Payne, R.J.; Vetter, I.; King, G.F.; Undheim, E.A.B. A Comprehensive Portrait of the Venom of the Giant Red Bull Ant, Myrmecia Gulosa, Reveals a Hyperdiverse Hymenopteran Toxin Gene Family. *Sci. Adv.* **2018**, *4*, eaau4640. [CrossRef]
109. Martinson, E.O.; Mrinalini; Kelkar, Y.D.; Chang, C.-H.; Werren, J.H. The Evolution of Venom by Co-Option of Single-Copy Genes. *Curr. Biol.* **2017**, *27*, 2007–2013. [CrossRef]
110. Cook, N.; Boulton, R.A.; Green, J.; Trivedi, U.; Tauber, E.; Pannebakker, B.A.; Ritchie, M.G.; Shuker, D.M. Differential Gene Expression Is Not Required for Facultative Sex Allocation: A Transcriptome Analysis of Brain Tissue in the Parasitoid Wasp *Nasonia vitripennis*. *R. Soc. Open sci.* **2018**, *5*, 171718. [CrossRef]
111. Sim, A.D.; Wheeler, D. The Venom Gland Transcriptome of the Parasitoid Wasp Nasonia Vitripennis Highlights the Importance of Novel Genes in Venom Function. *BMC Genom.* **2016**, *17*, 571. [CrossRef]
112. Kazuma, K.; Masuko, K.; Konno, K.; Inagaki, H. Combined Venom Gland Transcriptomic and Venom Peptidomic Analysis of the Predatory Ant Odontomachus Monticola. *Toxins* **2017**, *9*, 323. [CrossRef] [PubMed]
113. Smith, C.R.; Helms Cahan, S.; Kemena, C.; Brady, S.G.; Yang, W.; Bornberg-Bauer, E.; Eriksson, T.; Gadau, J.; Helmkampf, M.; Gotzek, D.; et al. How Do Genomes Create Novel Phenotypes? Insights from the Loss of the Worker Caste in Ant Social Parasites. *Mol. Biol. Evol.* **2015**, *32*, 2919–2931. [CrossRef] [PubMed]
114. Özbek, R.; Wielsch, N.; Vogel, H.; Lochnit, G.; Foerster, F.; Vilcinskas, A.; von Reumont, B.M. Proteo-Transcriptomic Characterization of the Venom from the Endoparasitoid Wasp Pimpla Turionellae with Aspects on Its Biology and Evolution. *Toxins* **2019**, *11*, 721. [CrossRef] [PubMed]
115. Yang, L.; Yang, Y.; Liu, M.-M.; Yan, Z.-C.; Qiu, L.-M.; Fang, Q.; Wang, F.; Werren, J.H.; Ye, G.-Y. Identification and Comparative Analysis of Venom Proteins in a Pupal Ectoparasitoid, Pachycrepoideus Vindemmiae. *Front. Physiol.* **2020**, *11*, 9. [CrossRef]
116. Bouzid, W.; Verdenaud, M.; Klopp, C.; Ducancel, F.; Noirot, C.; Vétillard, A. De Novo Sequencing and Transcriptome Analysis for Tetramorium Bicarinatum: A Comprehensive Venom Gland Transcriptome Analysis from an Ant Species. *BMC Genom.* **2014**, *15*, 987. [CrossRef]
117. Negroni, M.A.; Foitzik, S.; Feldmeyer, B. Long-Lived Temnothorax Ant Queens Switch from Investment in Immunity to Antioxidant Production with Age. *Sci. Rep.* **2019**, *9*, 7270. [CrossRef]

antibiotics

MDPI

Article

Novel Alligator Cathelicidin As-CATH8 Demonstrates Anti-Infective Activity against Clinically Relevant and Crocodylian Bacterial Pathogens

Felix L. Santana [1,2], Karel Estrada [3], Morgan A. Alford [2], Bing C. Wu [2], Melanie Dostert [2], Lucas Pedraz [2], Noushin Akhoundsadegh [2], Pavneet Kalsi [2], Evan F. Haney [2], Suzana K. Straus [4], Gerardo Corzo [1,*] and Robert E. W. Hancock [2,*]

[1] Departamento de Medicina Molecular y Bioprocesos, Instituto de Biotecnología, Universidad Nacional Autónoma de México, Cuernavaca 62210, Mexico
[2] Centre for Microbial Diseases and Immunity Research, University of British Columbia, Vancouver, BC V6T 1Z4, Canada
[3] Unidad de Secuenciación Masiva y Bioinformática, Instituto de Biotecnología, Universidad Nacional Autónoma de México, Cuernavaca 62210, Mexico
[4] Department of Chemistry, University of British Columbia, Vancouver, BC V6T 1Z1, Canada
* Correspondence: gerardo.corzo@ibt.unam.mx (G.C.); bob@hancocklab.com (R.E.W.H.)

Abstract: Host defense peptides (HDPs) represent an alternative way to address the emergence of antibiotic resistance. Crocodylians are interesting species for the study of these molecules because of their potent immune system, which confers high resistance to infection. Profile hidden Markov models were used to screen the genomes of four crocodylian species for encoded cathelicidins and eighteen novel sequences were identified. Synthetic cathelicidins showed broad spectrum antimicrobial and antibiofilm activity against several clinically important antibiotic-resistant bacteria. In particular, the As-CATH8 cathelicidin showed potent in vitro activity profiles similar to the last-resort antibiotics vancomycin and polymyxin B. In addition, As-CATH8 demonstrated rapid killing of planktonic and biofilm cells, which correlated with its ability to cause cytoplasmic membrane depolarization and permeabilization as well as binding to DNA. As-CATH8 displayed greater antibiofilm activity than the human cathelicidin LL-37 against methicillin-resistant *Staphylococcus aureus* in a human organoid model of biofilm skin infection. Furthermore, As-CATH8 demonstrated strong antibacterial effects in a murine abscess model of high-density bacterial infections against clinical isolates of *S. aureus* and *Acinetobacter baumannii*, two of the most common bacterial species causing skin infections globally. Overall, this work expands the repertoire of cathelicidin peptides known in crocodylians, including one with considerable therapeutic promise for treating common skin infections.

Keywords: cathelicidins; antimicrobial peptides; LL-37; biofilms; abscess model; skin model; reptiles

Citation: Santana, F.L.; Estrada, K.; Alford, M.A.; Wu, B.C.; Dostert, M.; Pedraz, L.; Akhoundsadegh, N.; Kalsi, P.; Haney, E.F.; Straus, S.K.; et al. Novel Alligator Cathelicidin As-CATH8 Demonstrates Anti-Infective Activity against Clinically Relevant and Crocodylian Bacterial Pathogens. *Antibiotics* **2022**, *11*, 1603. https://doi.org/10.3390/antibiotics11111603

Academic Editors: Agostinho Antunes, Guillermin Agüero-Chapin and Yovani Marrero-Ponce

Received: 28 September 2022
Accepted: 6 November 2022
Published: 11 November 2022

Publisher's Note: MDPI stays neutral with regard to jurisdictional claims in published maps and institutional affiliations.

Copyright: © 2022 by the authors. Licensee MDPI, Basel, Switzerland. This article is an open access article distributed under the terms and conditions of the Creative Commons Attribution (CC BY) license (https://creativecommons.org/licenses/by/4.0/).

1. Introduction

The rise of antibiotic resistance in bacterial pathogens across all drug classes poses a serious global public health issue. Recent data showed that, in 2019, antimicrobial resistance directly caused 1.27 million deaths and was associated with 4.9 million deaths worldwide [1]. Furthermore, human health issues, such as the severe acute respiratory syndrome coronavirus 2 (SARS-CoV-2) global pandemic, have recently aggravated this problem [2].

Especially concerning are bacteria of the ESKAPE group (*Enterococcus faecium*, *Staphylococcus aureus*, *Klebsiella pneumoniae*, *Acinetobacter baumannii*, *Pseudomonas aeruginosa*, *Enterobacter* sp.) [3]. These recalcitrant pathogens have been classified by the World Health Organization (WHO) as priorities for the development of new treatments, given their high levels of resistance to almost all common antibiotics and their substantial impact on human health worldwide [3,4]. Perhaps underappreciated is the fact that many of these ESKAPE bacteria can form biofilms, bacterial communities that are responsible for over 65% of bacterial infections in the clinics and are more resistant to conventional antibiotic treatments and many host immune responses [5,6]. Consequently, biofilm infections often become persistent and must be dealt with by surgical debridement [6]. Therefore, to adequately address infections due to ESKAPE pathogens, it is essential to identify antimicrobial compounds with activity against both the planktonic and biofilm growth state.

Host defense peptides (HDPs) have been described as an alternative to conventional antibiotics [7,8]. HDPs have broad-spectrum activity against free-swimming (planktonic) bacteria and in some instances biofilms, multitarget mechanisms of action that ensure a lower propensity to induce resistance, and additional assets such as anti-inflammatory properties [9,10]. Cathelicidins are one of the largest families of HDPs in vertebrates and can be recognized by their conserved pre-pro domains despite a broad diversity of mature sequences and structures [7]. They are multifunctional peptides with great potential for the development of new therapeutic agents, and several cathelicidins, or their derivatives, have been evaluated in clinical trials, including the human cathelicidin LL-37 [11].

Crocodylians (crocodiles, alligators, caimans, gavials and false gavials) possess a robust immune system [12,13] that allows them to deal with environmental microorganisms, as well as potential pathogens that are found in their natural microbiota [14,15]. These include several bacterial species that are pathogenic to humans and belong to the ESKAPE group [14–17]. Thus, crocodylian cathelicidins (crocCATHs) constitute a potential source of natural HDPs that might prove useful as novel anti-infectives.

Six crocCATHs have been previously identified in the Chinese alligator (*Alligator sinensis*) [18] and one was predicted from the American alligator (*Alligator mississippiensis*) [19]. Most of these peptides displayed moderate broad spectrum antimicrobial activity, as well as immunomodulatory properties [18,20,21]. However, the peptide sequences were identified based on either putative functional genome annotation or by BLAST search in combination with expression analysis at transcriptional level. Although these methodologies made it possible to identify novel sequences in these two species, a comprehensive analysis of cathelicidin sequences encoded in several different crocodylian species is lacking. Furthermore, the antibiofilm activities of crocodylian cathelicidins have been poorly characterized, despite the clinical relevance of biofilm infections in humans.

Profile hidden Markov models (HMMs) of multiple sequence alignments are complex statistical models that capture position-specific information about the likelihood of particular residues and the frequency of insertions/deletions in each position of the alignment [22]. They have shown higher accuracy for the detection of remote homologs compared to other methods, such as BLAST [23]. Using a strategy based on profile HMMs, we identified novel crocCATHs in *A. mississippiensis*, *A. sinensis*, *Crocodylus porosus* and *Gavialis gangeticus* and subsequently synthesized four of these. Synthetic crocCATHs demonstrated broad-spectrum in vitro antimicrobial and antibiofilm activities against several bacterial strains, including clinical isolates of ESKAPE pathogens. In addition, we characterized the antibiofilm properties of these crocCATHs in a human skin organoid model and investigated the in vivo anti-infective activity of As-CATH8, the most potent peptide here identified.

2. Results

2.1. Bioinformatic Screen of Crocodylian Genomes Identified 18 Novel crocCATHs

Analysis of crocodylian genomes using profile hidden Markov models (HMMs) from an alignment of 140 vertebrate (reptiles, birds and mammals) cathelicidins led to the identification of 18 novel cathelicidin sequences (Supplementary Table S1 and Figure S1). Overall, six sequences were identified in *A. mississippiensis*, two in *A. sinensis*, four in *C. porosus* and another six in *G. gangeticus*. Due to the somewhat low quality of the current genome assemblies, particular identified sequences were missing parts of their N-terminal domain (especially the signal peptide region) and were reported as partial (Supplementary

Table S2). Nevertheless, they did contain most of the cathelin domain—including the four well-conserved cysteines (Supplementary Figure S1)—as well as a mature peptide region, and were therefore considered new cathelicidins. Furthermore, according to the NCBI BLASTp tool, most of the new peptide sequences (including the signal peptide and cathelin domain regions) shared high identity with complete cathelicidin sequences from crocodylians (>78%) and other reptiles (>46%). Our work also identified five *A. mississippiensis* sequences with 100% identity with crocCATHs labeled as predicted in the NCBI nucleotide and protein databases.

Novel cathelicidins were named according to their orthology with the previously described As-CATH1–6 sequences from *A. sinensis* [18]. Phylogenetic analysis, including sequences from reptiles, birds and mammals, indicated that the crocCATHs grouped into seven well-defined clusters (Figure 1). Interestingly, cluster 4 appeared more distant from most crocCATHs and was grouped together with some snake and turtle sequences, which might indicate that this is the most ancient cluster in the family. Our analysis successfully identified orthologous sequences in most crocodylian clusters. Nevertheless, some cathelicidin sequences were identified with less well-defined orthology relationships (e.g., Am-CATH11 and Cp-CATH10). Moreover, our analysis identified a completely new cluster (cluster 7 in Figure 1) composed of sequences from three crocodylian species, with more distant relationships with Am-CATH8 and As-CATH8. Interestingly, As-CATH7 and As-CATH8 partially overlapped in the same region of the *A. sinensis* genome (Supplementary Table S2).

2.2. *Mature crocCATHs Displayed Characteristic Properties of α-Helical Cathelicidins*

To further study some of the identified crocCATHs, four sequences were selected for chemical synthesis. The sequences As-CATH7 and Gg-CATH7 were selected from the novel cluster 7, whereas the sequence As-CATH8 was selected due to its partial overlap with As-CATH7. The fourth peptide was chosen based on previous studies demonstrating that *A. sinensis* cathelicidin (As-CATH5) has broad-spectrum in vitro antimicrobial activity and is effective against bacterial infections in several in vivo models [18,20,24]. Consequently, the orthologous sequence Gg-CATH5 from *G. gangeticus* was chosen.

The region corresponding to the mature peptide of the selected crocCATHs was manually predicted, as previously described for the As-CATH1–6 sequences [18]. Most of the predicted mature sequences started after a valine residue (Supplementary Table S1), likely part of an elastase cleavage site, located at a residue within positions 138–140 in the multiple sequence alignment (Supplementary Figure S1). The exceptions were the sequences Cp-CATH3 from *C. porosus* and Gg-CATH4 from *G. gangeticus*, which contained an isoleucine and an aspartic acid, respectively. In this case, mature peptides were predicted based on inferred cleavage sites in orthologous cathelicidins from other crocodylian species.

The physicochemical properties of the chosen mature peptides are shown in Table 1. In general, the synthetic crocCATHs were short peptides (20–24 amino acids), with net positive charge (from 3.76 to 4.76) and variable hydrophobicity (from −0.39 to 0.06). Gg-CATH7 displayed the lowest net positive charge, whereas As-CATH8 showed the highest total hydrophobicity index. Notably, all crocodylian peptides displayed somewhat lower net charge and higher hydrophobicity when compared to the human cathelicidin LL-37.

The crocCATHs were structurally characterized using computational tools and circular dichroism spectroscopy. Since the human cathelicidin LL-37 has been extensively characterized as being α-helical [25], it was not included in this analysis. Structural modeling suggested that all four crocCATHs adopted an α-helix conformation (Figure 2A) with an asymmetric distribution of charged and hydrophobic residues on both sides of the helix (Figure 2B), suggesting amphipathicity. Calculation of the mean hydrophobic moments, a numerical estimate of the amphipathicity of a peptide structure [26], indicated differences among the peptides in terms of the magnitude and direction of this vector (Table 1 and Figure 2B). Overall, Gg-CATH5 was the most amphipathic sequence of all crocCATHs, although it showed lower values than those estimated for LL-37 (Table 1).

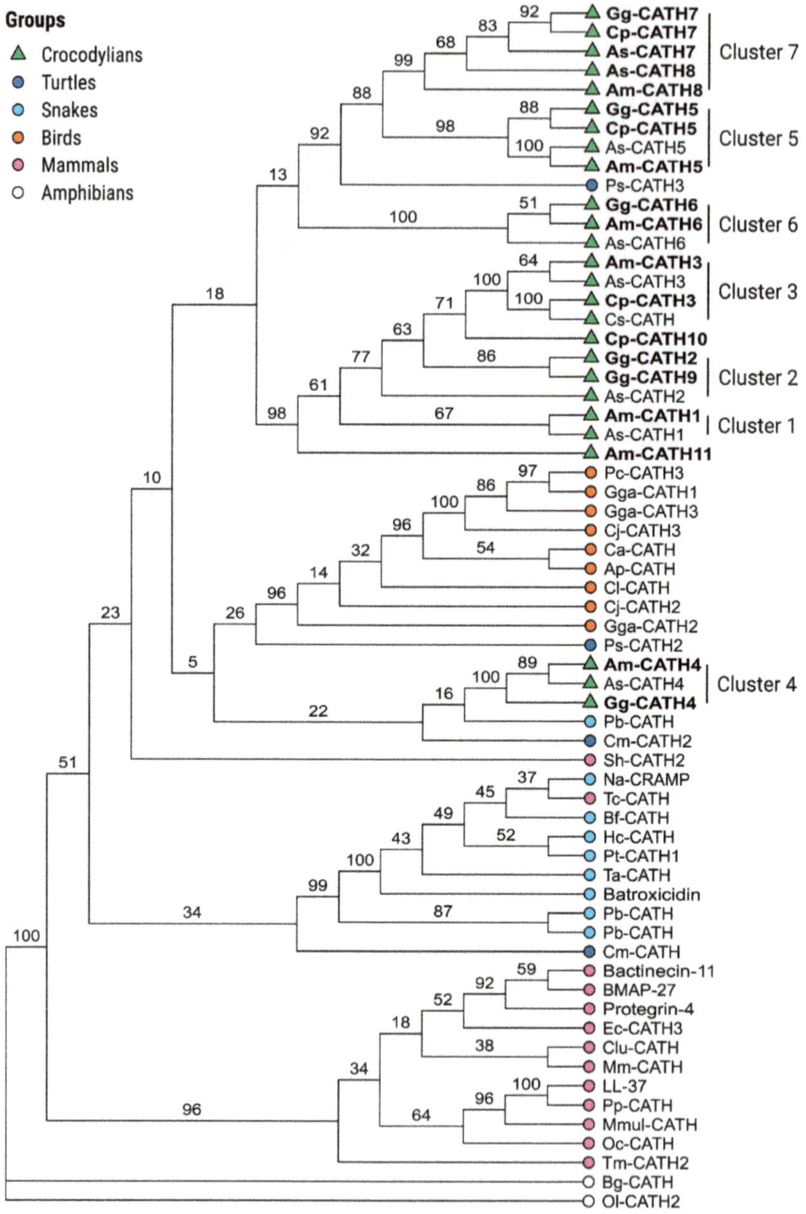

Figure 1. Phylogenetic analysis of crocCATH sequences. The tree was generated using the maximum likelihood criterion implemented in the RaxML program. The analysis included the full-length crocodylian amino acid sequences, as well as sequences from other reptilian, avian and mammalian species. Newly identified crocCATH sequences are displayed in bold. The amphibian cathelicidins Bg-CATH and Ol-CATH2 were used as outgroups to root the tree. Branch numbers indicate statistical support as percent after 1000 bootstrap replicates. The seven identified crocodylian clusters are indicated in the figure, which were named according to the previously described *A. sinensis* cathelicidins [18]. The alligator cathelicidin AM-36 [19] was renamed here as Am-CATH4. NCBI accession numbers of all cathelicidin sequences can be found in Supplementary Tables S1 and S3.

Table 1. Physicochemical properties of synthetic croCATHs and human LL-37. Properties were calculated using the Peptides and modlAMP packages in R and Python, respectively.

Name	Sequence	Length	MW	Charge	HI	HM
As-CATH7	KRVNWRKVGRNTALGASYVLSFLG	24	2693	4.76	−0.15	0.25
As-CATH8	KRVNWAKVGRTALKLLPYIFG	21	2431	4.76	0.06	0.29
Gg-CATH5	TRRKWWKKVLNGAIKIAPYILD	22	2670	4.76	−0.39	0.40
Gg-CATH7	KRVNWRKVGLGASYVMSWLG	20	2308	3.76	−0.11	0.23
LL-37	LLGDFFRKSKEKIGKEFKRIVQRIKDFLRNLVPRTES	37	4493	5.76	−0.72	0.56

As: A. sinensis, Gg: G. gangeticus. Length: number of amino acid residues; MW: theoretical molecular weight in daltons, rounded values; charge: net charge according to the Bjellqvist; HI: hydrophobicity index according to the Kyte–Doolittle scale scale; HM: mean hydrophobic moment (amphipathicity), numerical values of the vectors shown in the wheel representations in Figure 2.

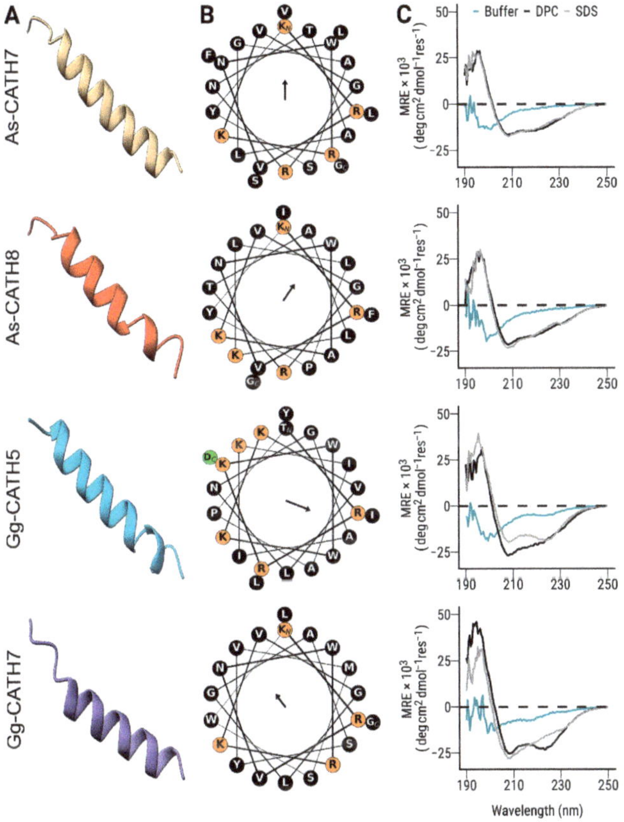

Figure 2. Structural analysis of the synthetic crocCATHs. (**A**) Three-dimensional structures were modeled using the AlphaFold algorithm and visualized in Chimera X. (**B**) Helical wheel representations were generated using the Python package modlAMP. Residues with positive and negative charges are highlighted in orange and green, respectively, whereas the remaining amino acids in the sequence (largely hydrophobic) are shown in black. The orientation of the vector mean hydrophobic moment (amphipathicity) for each sequence is displayed in the center of the wheel. The length of the arrow is proportional to the numerical values shown in Table 1. (**C**) Circular dichroism spectra of crocCATHs were obtained in sodium phosphate buffer (aqua), as well as in the presence of SDS (grey) and DPC (black) micelles. The results are shown as mean residual ellipticity (MRE).

Circular dichroism spectroscopy studies showed that the synthetic crocCATHs exhibited a largely disordered structure in sodium phosphate buffer (Figure 2C), characterized by low ellipticity above 210 nm and the presence of negative bands near 195 nm in the spectrum [27]. In the presence of dodecyl phosphocholine (DPC, a neutral membrane mimic), all the crocCATHs acquired a helical conformation, as revealed by minima in the ellipticity profile at around 208–210 nm and 222–225 nm (Figure 2C) [27], with some variance from ideal spectra indicating the potential contributions from other structural configurations. Similar spectra were observed in sodium dodecyl sulfate (SDS, an anionic membrane mimic). While cathelicidins can be very diverse in structure [7], crocCATHs displayed similar structural properties to other α-helical members of the cathelicidin family in reptiles, birds and mammals [28–30].

2.3. As-CATH8 and Gg-CATH5 Exhibited Broad In Vitro Activities against Planktonic and Biofilm Bacteria

The antibacterial activity of the synthetic crocCATHs was evaluated against several medically important pathogens, including those from the ESKAPE group. These peptides showed broad antimicrobial activity against Gram-positive and Gram-negative pathogenic bacteria (Table 2), with the exception of *E. faecium*. In general, minimum inhibitory concentrations (MICs) ranged from 0.25 to 4 μM (~0.6–10 μg/mL). Overall, As-CATH8 and Gg-CATH5 were the most active peptides and showed potency similar to the last-resort antibiotics polymyxin B and vancomycin against Gram-negative and Gram-positive bacteria, respectively, but with activity profiles that overlapped for both types of bacteria. Interestingly, *Proteus vulgaris* was considerably (>8-fold) more susceptible to the cathelicidin peptides As-CATH8 and Gg-CATH5 than to polymyxin B. In addition, these peptides showed better activity than the human cathelicidin LL-37 against *Escherichia coli* and *Salmonella* Typhimurium, with for example, MIC values (in μg/mL) that were 8–16-fold higher than As-CATH8 against both strains (Supplementary Table S4).

Table 2. Antimicrobial activity of the crocCATHs. The MIC values of the synthetic peptides were determined in a microdilution assay in MHB. The antibiotic vancomycin was used against Gram-positive *S. aureus* and *E. faecium* whereas polymyxin B was employed against the remaining Gram-negative strains. Values in μg/mL can be found in Supplementary Table S4.

Bacteria	MIC in μM					
	As-CATH7	**As-CATH8**	**Gg-CATH5**	**Gg-CATH7**	**Polymyxin B**	**Vancomycin**
E. cloacae	0.5	0.5	0.5	2	0.5	n.d.
S. aureus	4	0.5	1	16	n.d.	0.5
K. pneumoniae	1	0.5	0.5	4	0.5	n.d.
A. baumannii	0.25	0.25	0.5	1	0.5	n.d.
P. aeruginosa	4	1	1	8	0.5	n.d.
E. faecium	>64	>64	>64	64	n.d.	>64
E. coli	2	1	4	4	0.5	n.d.
S. Typhimurium	2	1	0.5	4	1	n.d.
P. vulgaris	>64	4	8	>64	>64	n.d.

n.d.: not determined.

The inhibitory activity of the crocCATHs against bacterial biofilms was determined using a microtiter assay against six of these species. The antibiofilm activities showed similar trends to those observed in the MIC assays, although, generally speaking, higher concentrations were required to observe an effect. As-CATH8 was the most active peptide with minimal biofilm inhibitory concentrations ($MBIC_{95}$ in the range of 1–4 μM) against five of six species (except *P. aeruginosa*), while Gg-CATH5 had good activity against four of the six species (Table 3 and Supplementary Figure S2).

Table 3. Biofilm inhibitory activity of the crocCATHs. The $MBIC_{95}$ values of the synthetic peptides were determined by a microdilution assay using crystal violet to stain the adhered bacterial biomass. $MBIC_{95}$ was defined as the minimal peptide concentration capable of inhibiting mean biofilm growth by at least 95% compared to the untreated control. Values in μg/mL can be found in Supplementary Table S5.

Bacteria	$MBIC_{95}$ in μM			
	As-CATH7	As-CATH8	Gg-CATH5	Gg-CATH7
E. cloacae	32	4	4	16
S. aureus	4	1	1	4
A. baumannii	1	0.5	0.5	1
P. aeruginosa	>64	64	32	>64
E. coli	32	1	32	32
S. Typhimurium	1	1	1	4

The cytotoxicity towards human cells was also investigated and compare to the human cathelicidin LL-37. Lactate dehydrogenase (LDH) release assays showed that As-CATH8 and Gg-CATH5 were moderately cytotoxic against human bronchial epithelial (HBE) cells and peripheral blood mononuclear cells (PBMCs) (Supplementary Figure S3), at the highest concentrations tested (5 and 10 μM). This effect was similar to that observed for the natural human cathelicidin LL-37, which has been used in a phase 1 human clinical trial [31]. In contrast, the crocodylian peptides As-CATH7 and Gg-CATH7 showed low cytotoxicity against both cell types, comparable to the immunomodulatory peptide IDR-1018 used as control.

2.4. *As-CATH8 and Gg-CATH5 Completely Eradicated S. aureus Biofilms in a Human Organoid Skin Model*

Synthetic crocCATHs were tested in a more complex system; namely, a human skin organoid model where bacteria grow as biofilms. In this model, no peptide-induced cytotoxic effects were observed according to LDH release assays and histology studies. In contrast to mono-layer cell models, the skin organoid model demonstrates fully stratified epidermal skin layers, which strongly resemble the morphology and permeability of human skin [32]. Therefore, it is arguably a more relevant model to assess the biological activities of antimicrobial molecules under in vivo-like conditions. Since most crocCATHs had good in vitro activity against *S. aureus*, we tested this organism in the skin model.

The results obtained in the skin-biofilm infection model highlighted the antibiofilm activity of As-CATH8 and Gg-CATH5 cathelicidins (Figure 3A). Treatment with 200 μg of these peptides completely eradicated *S. aureus* biofilms after 24 h. This effect was significant for both peptides when compared to the negative control and was superior to the human cathelicidin LL-37, which showed low and insignificant biofilm eradication activity (3-fold; $p > 0.05$) in this assay. As-CATH7 and Gg-CATH7 had greater antibiofilm activity than LL-37 (4877-fold and 425-fold reductions, respectively) but failed to eliminate bacterial biofilms in most replicates. These results supported As-CATH8 and Gg-CATH5 as the peptides with the highest direct antibiofilm activity of the crocCATHs in this in vivo-like model.

2.5. *As-CATH8 Showed a Strong Anti-Infective Effect in a Murine Abscess Model*

The antibacterial capacities of As-CATH8 and Gg-CATH5 were further evaluated in the murine skin infection/abscess model. Mice were inoculated with clinical isolates of *S. aureus* and *A. baumannii*, two frequent causes of human skin infections [8]. Subcutaneous administration of the crocCATHs or LL-37 alone (15 mg/kg) into uninfected animals showed no evidence of tissue damage or peptide precipitation at the site of injection. Therefore, the peptides were considered non-toxic at the doses used.

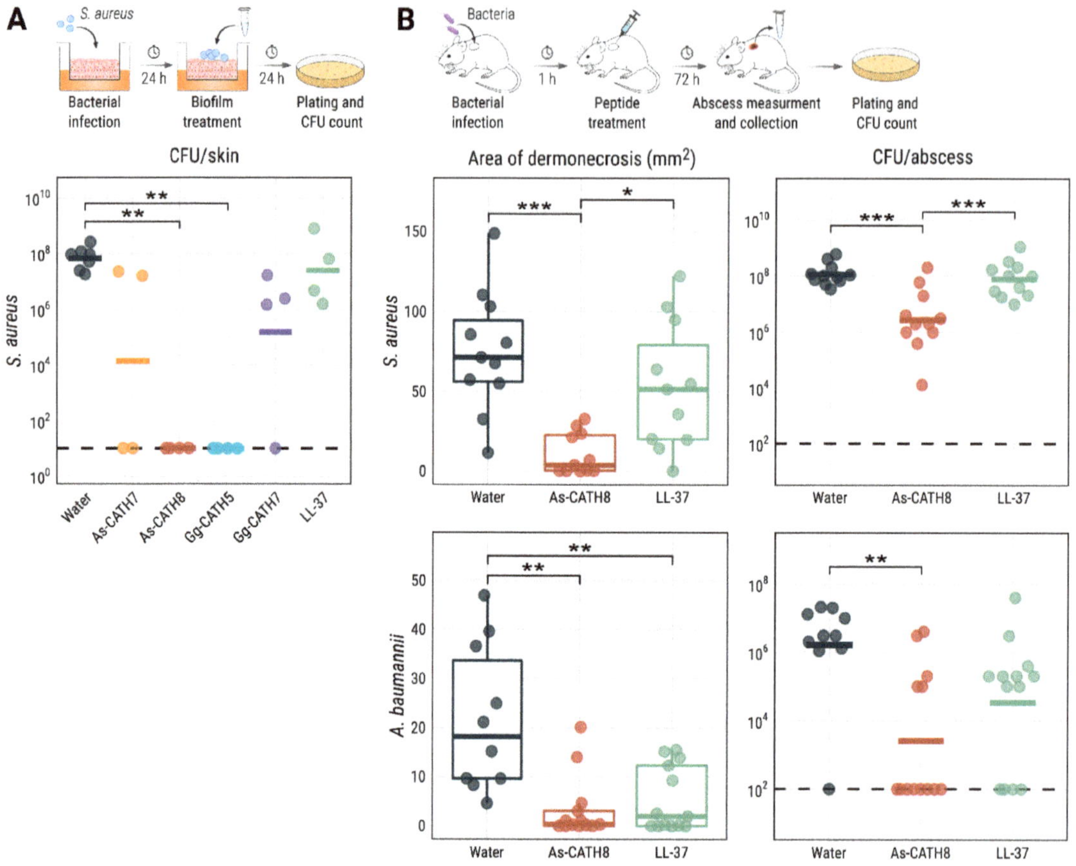

Figure 3. Anti-infective capacity of As-CATH8 and LL-37 in a human skin organoid (**A**) and a murine abscess (**B**) model. (**A**) The ability of crocCATHs to eradicate pre-formed *S. aureus* biofilms was evaluated in a human skin air–liquid interface organoid model. Biofilms were treated with 200 µg of each peptide or with distilled water as a negative control and bacteria were recovered after 24 h. Results are presented as geometric mean per treatment (horizontal bars) of at least four independent biological replicates (dots). Data were statistically analyzed using the Kruskal–Wallis test followed by Dunn's post hoc test with the Benjamini–Hochberg correction. (**B**) The anti-infective activity of cathelicidin peptides was assessed in a murine abscess model against *S. aureus* and *A. baumannii*. Mice were inoculated with each bacterium for 1 h and then treated intra abscess with 15 mg/kg of peptides or distilled water as a negative control. The area of dermonecrosis and bacterial load in the abscesses was quantified after three days. Results corresponding to the abscess area are shown as box plots and were statistically analyzed using the Kruskal–Wallis test followed by Dunn's post hoc test with the Benjamini–Hochberg correction. CFU results are shown as geometric mean per treatment (horizontal bars) and were statistically analyzed using ANOVA followed by the Tukey's post hoc test. Each mouse is represented by individual data points in the abscess experiments. In all the plots, asterisks represent statistically significant differences (* = $p < 0.05$, ** = $p < 0.01$, *** = $p < 0.001$). Detection limits of the bacterial enumeration assays are shown as dashed lines.

In this high-density infection model, Gg-CATH5 showed only weak activity against *S. aureus*. In contrast, As-CATH8 showed a stronger antibacterial effect and was able to substantially decrease the area of dermonecrosis formed above the abscess with both pathogens (Figure 3B). Dermonecrosis is a skin pathology where the skin cells are killed, leaving a visible lesion (the abscess) [33]. The reductions in the *S. aureus* area of dermonecrosis (19-fold) and bacterial burden (42-fold) observed for As-CATH8 were significant when compared to the negative control (distilled water) and LL-37. For the *A. baumannii* infections, treatment with As-CATH8 also reduced both the area of dermonecrosis (61-fold) and the bacterial load (632-fold) when compared to untreated mice (Figure 3B). More importantly, complete eradication of *A. baumannii* was observed in the majority (62%) of mice treated with As-CATH8. Treatment with LL-37 significantly decreased the area of dermonecrosis (ninefold) formed by *A. baumannii* but relatively moderately impacted bacterial recovery in most animals (48-fold).

2.6. As-CATH8 Was More Bactericidal and Killed Faster Than Antibiotics

To further study the antimicrobial activity of As-CATH8, time–kill curves were plotted for planktonic *S. aureus* and *A. baumannii* cells and biofilms (Figure 4A). When compared to vancomycin or polymyxin B, As-CATH8 at its MIC was faster in killing planktonic cells from both bacterial species. Specifically, the crocodylian peptide showed a time-dependent effect on *S. aureus* CFU counts and significantly reduced bacterial survival within 0.5 h of treatment. Furthermore, As-CATH8 was more effective than vancomycin against this bacterium at all time points. While complete killing of planktonic *A. baumannii* by As-CATH8 was seen as soon as 0.5 h after treatment, it took polymyxin B up to 20 h to achieve the same effect.

Biofilm eradication experiments showed similar trends (Figure 4A). In this case, As-CATH8 at 64-fold the MIC nearly eradicated *S. aureus* biofilms within 2 h, while vancomycin showed only a modest effect at that time point. However, vancomycin did show potent activity against *S. aureus* biofilms after 20 h of treatment. As-CATH8 acted rapidly against *A. baumannii* and was able to completely eradicate bacterial biofilms within 1 h of treatment. Notably, polymyxin B showed strong overall activity against this bacterium, although complete eradication was observed only at the 20 h time point.

2.7. Potential Role of Interaction with Bacterial Membranes and DNA in the Antibacterial Activity of As-CATH8

To elucidate possible bacterial targets important for the antimicrobial activity of As-CATH8, its effect on bacterial membranes was investigated. Membrane depolarization was assessed using the membrane potential-sensitive dye $DiSC_3(5)$ (3,3′-dipropylthiadicarbocyanine iodide) [34,35]. This hydrophobic dye with a caged cationic interior can concentrate in bacterial cytoplasmic membranes according to the magnitude of the membrane potential (which is oriented toward the negatively charged interior). A high concentration in the membrane leads to self-quenching of $DiSC_3(5)$ fluorescence, while depolarization of the bacterial membrane promotes the collapse of the membrane potential, the release of this dye and the subsequent increase of its fluorescence emission [35,36]. In addition, cytoplasmic membrane permeability was investigated using propidium iodide (PI). PI is a commonly used dye that becomes fluorescent when it binds to the DNA. However, it is membrane-impermeant and can only enter cells if cytoplasmic membranes are damaged [36].

The effect of several concentrations of As-CATH8 on *S. aureus* and *A. baumannii* membranes was compared to that of vancomycin and polymyxin B after 1 h treatment (Figure 4B). The membrane-permeabilizing wasp peptide mastoparan [37,38] served as a positive control. While almost no effect was observed for vancomycin and polymyxin B, consistent with a mechanism of action independent of the disruption of the cytoplasmic bacterial membrane [39,40], As-CATH8 showed a concentration-dependent effect on membrane depolarization ($DiSC_3(5)$ fluorescence) and permeabilization (PI fluorescence) against both bacteria (Figure 4B). This effect was particularly noticeable at concentrations above the MIC of As-CATH8 for *S. aureus* (0.5 μM) and *A. baumannii* (0.25 μM), and it was similar to that observed for mastoparan at high peptide concentrations. As-CATH8 was also able to permeabilize *S. aureus* membranes at concentrations below its MIC (even 16-fold lower). In this case, the PI signal reached the maximal intensity at lower concentrations when compared to *A. baumannii*, for which $DiSC_3(5)$ and PI signals reached their highest fluorescence values at 2–8 μM As-CATH8 (8- to 32-fold the MIC). Interestingly, maximum values of depolarization or permeabilization did not always lead to notable bacterial killing by As-CATH8, since a 1000-fold reduction in CFU counts was only observed at concentrations higher than 1 μM against *S. aureus* and 8 μM against *A. baumannii* (Figure 4B and Supplementary Figure S4). This suggested that other targets beside the cytoplasmic membrane might be relevant for the mode of action of As-CATH8.

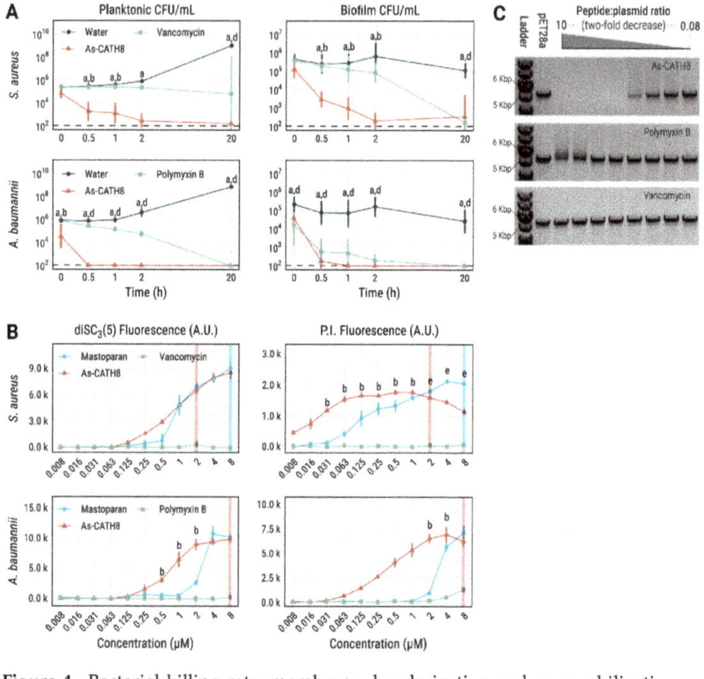

Figure 4. Bacterial killing rate, membrane depolarization and permeabilization and DNA binding capacity of As-CATH8. (**A**) Killing of planktonic *S. aureus* and *A. baumannii* cells at the MIC in MHB media. Antibiofilm activity was assessed in 10% TSB supplemented with 0.1% glucose at 64-fold MIC. CFU data are displayed as geometric mean ×/geometric standard deviation. (**B**) Cytoplasmic membrane depolarization and permeabilization were assessed after 1 h treatment of planktonic cells using $DiSC_3(5)$ and PI, respectively. Membrane-permeabilizing wasp peptide mastoparan was used as a positive control. Shown are fluorescence readings (mean ± standard error in arbitrary units). Perpendicular lines represent the minimal peptide concentration leading to at least 1000-fold CFU reduction compared to the untreated control (see also Supplementary Figure S4). (**C**) Gel electrophoretic mobility shift assay demonstrating the DNA binding capacity of As-CATH8, employing the linearized plasmid pET28a at 2-fold decreasing peptide:plasmid weight ratios (see Supplementary Figure S5 for an uncropped image). Peptidic antibiotics vancomycin (active against *S. aureus*) and polymyxin B (active against *A. baumannii*) were used as comparisons. Letters denote statistically significant differences ($p < 0.05$) between As-CATH8 and water (a), As-CATH8 and antibiotics (b), As-CATH8 and mastoparan (c), antibiotics and water (d) or antibiotics and Mastoparan (e) according to the Kruskal–Wallis test followed by Dunn's post hoc test with the Benjamini-Hochberg p-value correction. All experiments were performed at least three times independently.

Therefore, the DNA binding capacity of As-CATH8 was evaluated in a gel electrophoretic mobility shift assay [41] using the linearized plasmid pET28a (Figure 4C). The peptidic antibiotics vancomycin and polymyxin B showed no and weak capacities for binding to DNA, respectively. In contrast, As-CATH8 was able to affect DNA migration at peptide:plasmid ratios exceeding 0.63:1. This suggested that, when As-CATH8 enters the cells, it could interact with nucleic acids to affect cellular processes, such as replication, transcription, and translation.

3. Discussion

Skin and soft tissue infections (SSTIs) are among the most prevalent bacterial diseases in humans and constitute one of the main precursors of severe sepsis [8]. Furthermore, they pose a significant financial burden on the healthcare system [6]. *S. aureus* has been identified among the most frequent bacteria isolated from SSTIs worldwide, whereas Gram-negative ESKAPE bacteria, such as *A. baumnannii*, are more frequently associated with chronic or postoperative wounds [8]. Treatment of biofilm-associated SSTIs, which usually exhibit higher antibiotic resistance, is particularly difficult [5]. More efficacious treatments are therefore desperately needed. In this context, HDPs have shown promising results for the treatment of this type of infections [8].

Bioinformatic strategies have enabled new possibilities for the identification of HDPs in lesser-studied species, such as crocodylians [42]. Previously, HMMs have been successfully used to explore cathelicidin peptides in several vertebrate species [43,44]. Using a similar strategy, 18 cathelicidins were identified in four crocodylian species (i.e., *A. mississippiensis*, *A. sinensis*, *C. porosus* and *G. gangeticus*), which showed broad and potent antimicrobial activity against most ESKAPE pathogens and *P. vulgaris*. In particular, As-CATH8, the most active crocodylian peptide, showed similar MIC values to the last-resort antibiotic vancomycin and polymyxin B (Table 2). It also impaired biofilm formation in all bacterial strains tested (Table 3). Additionally, As-CATH8 was generally faster than both antibiotics at killing *S. aureus* and *A. baumannii* planktonic cells and pre-formed biofilms (Figure 4A), highlighting the advantages of As-CATH8 compared to vancomycin and polymyxin B in treating infections and limiting the development of bacterial resistance.

It is well-known that HDPs can interact with multiple extracellular and intracellular targets to exert their antimicrobial and antibiofilm effects [9,11]. Experiments using fluorescent probes showed that As-CATH8 was able to depolarize and permeabilize *S. aureus* and *A. baumannii* membranes (Figure 4B). Although it seems likely that compromising the integrity of the membrane is a key component of the killing mechanism of As-CATH8, this may not always be a fatal event and additional or alternative activities might also play a significant role. Two main elements support this idea: first, maximum values of depolarization ($DiSC_3(5)$ fluorescence) and permeabilization (PI fluorescence) did not always lead to a notable reduction in CFU counts (Supplementary Figure S4), suggesting that bacteria can recover to some extent from this perturbation, as discussed previously for cationic peptides [45]. Second, at concentrations near the MIC, As-CATH8 showed only modest effects on the membranes, while peptide internalization and intracellular signaling may still have occurred at these concentrations. Interaction with bacterial DNA has been shown to be important for the antimicrobial mechanism of several vertebrate cathelicidins, including LL-37 [46–48]. This interaction can potentially interfere with several bacterial processes, such as replication and transcription, and usually leads to bacterial death [47,49]. In this study, As-CATH8 displayed stronger DNA binding capacity than vancomycin or polymyxin B, even at peptide ratios equivalent to the MIC against most pathogens (0.8–6.3 μg/mL). Differences in DNA binding affinity between As-CATH8 and antibiotics cannot only be attributed to differences in net charge, since polymyxin B (+5) [50] and As-CATH8 (+4.76) have similar positive charges. In contrast, vancomycin was the least charged of all the molecules (net charge +1) [51] and this could explain the lack of affinity observed for vancomycin to the negatively charged pET28a plasmid (Figure 4C). Taken together, we propose that As-CATH8 kills pathogens through both membrane disruption and alternative mechanisms of action, possibly through interaction with DNA, as suggested for other reptilian cathelicidins [47].

In line with observations for LL-37, cytotoxicity experiments showed that As-CATH8 and Gg-CATH5 were moderately toxic towards HBE cells and PBMCs, whereas As-CATH7 and Gg-CATH7 showed negligible effects. In this regard, other crocodylian cathelicidins have also demonstrated relatively high in vitro cytotoxicity against some cell lines, albeit at higher concentrations than those used here [18]. Although further investigation of their cytotoxic properties is warranted before crocCATHs can be used systemically to treat bacterial infections, it is important to note that in more complex systems, such as the human skin organoid and murine abscess models, no appreciable cytotoxicity was observed upon treatment with As-CATH8 or Gg-CATH5. These results therefore reaffirmed the known limitations of cell lines for assessing peptide cytotoxicity [52] and emphasize the importance of physiologically relevant environments for examining the biological activity of HDPs.

The in vivo anti-infective capacity of As-CATH8 was evaluated in a high-density murine bacterial abscess model. This high-density infection model is difficult to treat with conventional antibiotics but peptides have shown some success. Under these conditions, As-CATH8 decreased the area of dermonecrosis and bacterial load (Figure 3B) in abscesses formed by both *S. aureus* and *A. baumannii* and overall was more effective than the human cathelicidin LL-37. In particular, *A. baumannii* was quite sensitive to treatment with As-CATH8, which caused a reduction of at least 4-fold in bacterial load in most mice (Figure 3B). These results aligned with previous studies that have shown the therapeutic potential of crocCATHs against bacterial infections. For example, the cathelicidin peptides As-CATH2, As-CATH3 and As-CATH5 from *A. sinensis* demonstrated anti-infective properties against *E. coli* and *S. aureus* in a murine peritonitis model [18], while the protective capacity of As-CATH4 and As-CATH5 against bacterial infections was also revealed using invertebrate models [21]. Interestingly, Gg-CATH5, the *G. gangeticus* novel ortholog of the As-CATH5 peptide from *A. sinensis* [18], did not show significant anti-infective capacity as As-CATH8 in the abscess model against *S. aureus*, despite showing similar activity in other assays, including the skin organoid model. Studies involving reptile cathelicidins have suggested that the immunomodulatory activity of these molecules plays an important role in their activity in vivo [18,53,54]. Therefore, the evaluation of As-CATH8 in other animal models that allow the characterization of its immunomodulatory effects at non-toxic concentrations could provide more information about its optimal biological targets.

Overall, this work expands the repertoire of cathelicidins known in crocodylians and highlights the potential of bioinformatic tools to screen reptilian species that are attractive for the identification of natural HDPs. Moreover, we identified the As-CATH8 peptide, which has substantial therapeutic promise for treatment of *S. aureus* and *A. baumannii* skin infections, two of the most prevalent bacterial species causing SSTIs worldwide.

4. Material and Methods

4.1. Identification of Cathelicidin Sequences Using HMMs

To identify novel crocCATHs, the versions ASM28112v4 (assembly accession number: GCA_000281125.4) for *A. mississippiensis*, ASM45574v1 (assembly accession number: GCA_000455745.1) for *A. sinensis* [55], CroPor_comp1 (assembly accession number: GCA_001723895.1) for *C. porosus* and GavGan_comp1 (assembly accession number: GCA_001723915.1) for *G. gangeticus* were downloaded from NCBI. The initial versions of the genome assemblies generated by St John et al. [56] were also employed.

An automated workflow was established using Snakemake version 5.3.0 [57]. First, profile HMMs were generated using HMMER3 version 3.21 (http://hmmer.org/, accessed on 20 July 2018) from a multiple sequence alignment comprising 140 cathelicidin amino acid sequences of different vertebrate species (reptiles, birds and mammals), retrieved from publicly available sequence databases.

Multiple sequence alignment was performed using MAFFT version 7.310 [58] employing the iterative method with refinement (L-INS-i) and manually curated using the program

AliView version 1.26 [59]. Six open reading frames for each version of the genomes were searched for the generated profile HMMs. Matched regions were extracted and expanded 5 kbp upstream and downstream. Expanded regions were then aligned to the initial amino acid sequences using the Exonerate software version 2.4 [60] to obtain the best exon/intron prediction for each crocodylian sequence. These steps were repeated until no new sequences were found, each time starting from a new alignment comprising all crocodylian sequences identified in the previous iterations.

The signal peptide domains in the identified crocCATH sequences were predicted by the SignalP 5.0 server [61]. The prediction of the mature peptide regions was based on information from previously published reptilian cathelicidins [18,62]. Neutrophil elastase was assumed to be the enzyme responsible for processing the mature crocodylian peptides, as suggested for other vertebrate cathelicidins [63–65].

4.2. Phylogenetic Analysis of the Cathelicidin Sequences

Phylogenetic analysis of the identified crocCATH sequences was performed with RaxML (Randomized Axelerated Maximum Likelihood) software version 8.2.12 [66] using the maximum likelihood criterion. Full-length cathelicidin sequences from various reptilian, avian and mammalian species were also included. The amphibian Ol-CATH2 sequences from *Odorrana livida* (NCBI accession number: AXR75914) and Bg-CATH from *Bufo gargarizans* (NCBI accession number: ANV28414) were used as outgroups to root the tree. The VT + G4 model was adopted as the best amino acid substitution model in accordance with the Aikaike's and Bayesian information criteria implemented in ModelTest-NG software version 0.1.6 [67]. Rapid analysis with 1000 bootstrap replicates and determination of the highest-scoring maximum likelihood tree was performed in the same run in RaxML. The resulting phylogenetic tree was edited using treeio version 1.18.1 [68] and visualized with ggtree version 3.2.1 [69] in R version 4.2.1 [70] and RStudio version 2022.2.0.443 [71].

4.3. Prediction of Physicochemical and Structural Characteristics of Mature crocCATHs

Physicochemical properties of mature cathelicidins including length, net charge and hydrophobicity index were predicted with the Peptides package version 2.4.4 [72] in RStudio. Net charge was estimated using the Bjellqvist scale [73], assuming an environmental pH = 7.0. This pKa scale is based on the polypeptide migration in an immobilized pH gradient. In addition, the hydrophobicity index was calculated using the Kyte–Doolittle scale, which is based on an amalgam of experimental observations derived from the literature [74]. Both the Bjellqvist and the Kyte–Doolittle scales are implemented in extensively used bioinformatic software, such as the ProtParam tool from the ExPASy server [75]. The mean hydrophobic moment was estimated with the modlAMP package version 4.3.0 [76] in Python version 3.9.6, employing an angle of 100°, which is recommended for α-helical structures [26]. Wheel representations of the distribution of hydrophobic and charged residues of the crocCATHs were also generated using the same package.

Three-dimensional models of the crocCATH mature peptides were obtained using a freely available and slightly simplified version of the AlphaFold algorithm version 2.0 [77], which was implemented in Google colab [78]. The structures were visualized in Chimera X version 1.2.5 [79].

4.4. Peptides, Reagents and Culture Media

The amino acid sequences of the synthetic crocCATH peptides and the human cathelicidin LL-37 are shown in Table 1. Crocodylian peptides were chemically synthesized by Genscript (Piscataway, NJ, USA), whereas the LL-37 and the innate defense regulator peptide 1018 (VRLIVAVRIWRR-NH_2) [80] were purchased from CPC Scientific Inc. (Sunnyvale, CA, USA). The wasp venom-derived peptide mastoparan (INLKALAALAKKIL-NH_2, also named mastoparan-L) [37,81] was acquired from Peptide 2.0 Inc. (Chantilly, VA, USA) All synthetic peptides were obtained with purity higher than 95%.

Peptide stocks were prepared in sterile endotoxin-free water (Baxter, Classic Health, Edmonton, AB, Canada) and adjusted to the desired concentration (usually 2 or 2.5 mM), which was estimated by absorbance at 280 nm in a Nanodrop ND-1000 (ThermoFisher Scientific, Waltham, MA, USA). Concentration values were corrected using the theoretical extinction coefficients of each peptide estimated with the ProtParam tool (https://web.expasy.org/protparam/, accessed on 30 July 2019) from the ExPASy server. Since LL-37 and mastoparan do not contain aromatic residues that absorb at 280 nm, their concentrations were estimated by weight, assuming the lyophilizates contained 70% peptide mass.

The antibiotics polymyxin B and vancomycin were obtained from MilliporeSigma (Burlington, MA, USA) and were resuspended in water to the desired stock concentrations. The DiSC$_3$(5) dye was obtained from MilliporeSigma (Burlington, MA, USA) and the PI dye was from ThermoFisher Scientific (Waltham, MA, USA). Working aliquots of DiSC$_3$(5) were prepared in 100% DMSO, kept at −20 °C and freeze-thawed no more than three times.

The bacterial culture media Luria-Bertani (LB) broth, brain heart infusion (BHI), tryptic soy broth (TSB), Todd Hewitt broth (THB) and Mueller Hinton broth (MHB) were obtained from ThermoFisher Scientific (Waltham, MA, USA).

All other culture media and supplements used in the human skin organoid model were purchased from MilliporeSigma (Burlington, MA, USA).

4.5. Determination of the Secondary Structure of Synthetic Cathelicidins

Circular dichroism experiments were carried out using a JASCO J-815 spectropolarimeter (Jasco, Easton, MD, USA) at room temperature as previously described [82]. All samples were prepared in 25 mM sodium phosphate buffer (pH 7.4) at a final peptide concentration of 100 µM. Spectra were obtained in buffer solution and in the presence of 10 mM sodium dodecyl sulfate (SDS) and 7.5 mM dodecyl phosphocholine (DPC) micelles.

Spectra were corrected by subtracting the buffer background and data were analyzed as mean residual ellipticity values and plotted in RStudio. Final spectra represent an average of three scans.

4.6. Bacterial Strains and Culture Conditions

The following bacterial pathogens were used in this study: *S. enterica* subsp. *enterica* serovar Typhimurium ATCC 14028, *E. coli* O157:H7 [83], the clinical isolates *S. aureus* SAP0017 [84] and USA300 LAC [85], *E. faecium* #1-1 [85], *A. baumannii* Ab5075 [85] and *E. cloacae* 218R1 [85], as well as *P. aeruginosa* PAO1 [34], *P. vulgaris* HSC7200-T2 (Hancock Lab strain collection) and *K. pneumoniae* KPLN49 [85].

Overnight cultures were grown in LB at 37 °C with shaking at 250 rpm, except for *E. faecium*, which was grown in BHI medium.

4.7. Antimicrobial Activity and Biofilm Inhibition Assays

The antimicrobial activity of the crocCATHs was evaluated with the broth microdilution method as described previously [86]. MIC was defined as the first peptide or antibiotic concentration without visible bacterial growth. Reported values are the statistical mode of at least three independent experiments.

Bacterial biofilm inhibition assays were performed using a microtiter assay as described by Haney et al. [87]. For *E. cloacae*, *E. coli*, *P. aeruginosa* and *S.* Typhimurium, assays were performed using BM2 minimal medium (62 mM potassium phosphate, 7 mM ammonium sulfate, 0.5 mM magnesium sulfate, pH 7.0) supplemented with 0.4% glucose (*w*/*v*). Antibiofilm activity against *A. baumannii* and *S. aureus* SAP0017 was evaluated in 10% TSB (*v*/*v*) media supplemented with 0.1% glucose (*w*/*v*), whereas 10% THB (*v*/*v*) medium was employed for *P. vulgaris*.

Data from at least three independent experiments were analyzed as the percentage of biofilm mass compared to the untreated control. After crystal violet staining, MBIC$_{95}$ was then calculated for each peptide, defined as the minimal peptide concentration capable of inhibiting mean biofilm growth by at least 95% compared to the untreated control [87].

4.8. Cell Lines and Peripheral Blood Mononuclear Cells (PBMCs)

Immortalized human bronchial epithelial (HBE) cells (16HBE14o-) were used for in vitro cytotoxicity experiments as described elsewhere [52,88].

The human N/TERT keratinocyte cells used in the skin model experiments were provided by Dr. Peter Nibbering (Leiden University Medical Center, The Netherlands) and cultured as detailed by Wu et al. [32].

Human PBMCs were isolated from human blood following the ethics protocols of the University of British Columbia, Canada. Consent was obtained from healthy volunteers before blood donation. Isolation and treatment of unstimulated PBMC was performed as previously described [80].

4.9. Lactate Dehydrogenase (LDH) Release Assays

Peptide-induced cytotoxicity was assessed by measuring the extracellular activity of the LDH enzyme using the Cytotoxicity Detection Kit (MilliporeSigma, Burlington, MA, USA) as previously described [80,88]. The percentage of LDH release relative to the untreated (negative) and Triton X-100 (positive, 100% cytotoxicity) control was assessed for at least three biological replicates and recorded as percent cytotoxicity.

4.10. Skin Model Experiments

The human N/TERT epidermal skin models were established as previously published [32]. Briefly, models were cultured in 12-well plates seeded with N/TERT keratinocyte cells at a density of 3×10^5 cells/insert in DermaLife K Keratinocyte complete medium supplemented with LifeFactors (Lifeline Cell Technology, Oceanside, CA, USA). Skin models were cultured at the air–liquid interface for 10 days at 37 °C with 7.3% CO_2 before being used in experiments.

To investigate the antibiofilm capacity of the cathelicidin peptides, 5 μL (~10^6 CFU) of *S. aureus* SAP0017 grown to mid-log phase was applied to the center of the N/TERT skin and plates were incubated for 24 h. Skin biofilms were then treated with 30 μL (200 μg) of each crocodylian peptide or the human LL-37 as a comparison. Sterile distilled water was used as a negative control. After 24 h of treatment, skin samples were excised from the culture inserts, sonicated for 5 min in sterile PBS and vortexed for 30 s. Bacterial counts were determined by serial dilution and plating on LB agar. The detection limit of the assay was 10 CFU/skin.

4.11. Bacterial Abscess Formation and Peptide Treatment

The animals used in this study were female CD-1 mice purchased from Charles River Laboratories Inc. (Wilmington, MA, USA), 5–7 weeks old and weighing 25 ± 5 g at the time of the experiment. Mice were housed in cohorts of 4–5 littermates exposed to the same pathogen. Standard animal husbandry protocols were employed.

The in vivo activity of As-CATH8 was examined in a subcutaneous abscess infection model as previously described [33] using *S. aureus* USA300 LAC and *A. baumannii*. Fifty microliters of the bacterial culture were injected subcutaneously into the shaved left dorsum of mice at an inoculum density of 5–15 × 10^7 CFU. One hour later, abscesses were treated with either 15 mg/kg As-CATH8 or LL-37 or sterile endotoxin-free water (Baxter, Classic Health, Edmonton, AB, Canada) as a negative control. Daily clinical grading of the animals was recorded post-treatment for 72 h; mice were then euthanized by exposure to CO_2 followed by cervical dislocation. Visible dermonecrosis was measured using a caliper and abscesses were harvested in PBS and homogenized using a Mini-Beadbeater (BioSpec Products, Bartlesville, OK, USA). Bacterial counts were determined by serial dilution and plating on LB agar. Two or three independent experiments were performed, each containing 2–4 biological replicates. The detection limit of this model was 100 CFU/abscess.

4.12. *Planktonic and Biofilm-Killing Assays*

The bactericidal activity of As-CATH8 and antibiotics was evaluated against planktonic *S. aureus* SAP0017 and *A. baumannii* cells under similar conditions to those used in the antimicrobial assays. Bacteria were grown overnight in LB media and diluted to ~5 × 10^5 CFU/mL in MHB. Bacterial cultures (1 mL) were treated with As-CATH8 or antibiotics (vancomycin for *S. aureus* or polymyxin B for *A. baumannii*) at the MIC and tubes were incubated at 37 °C with gentle shaking. Samples were taken at 0, 0.5, 1, 2 and 20 h after treatment and CFU counts determined by serial dilution and plating on LB agar.

Biofilm-killing assays were set up like the biofilm inhibition assays previously described. After forming the biofilms for 24 h in 10% TSB (*v*/*v*) supplemented with 0.1% glucose (*w/v*), *S. aureus* SAP0017 and *A. baumannii* biofilms were treated with As-CATH8 or antibiotics (vancomycin or polymyxin B) at 64 × MIC. Plates were incubated at 37 °C and bacterial biomass was scraped out of the wells with cotton swabs at 0, 0.5, 1, 2 and 20 h after treatment. Cotton tips were placed in 1 mL of LB and sonicated for 5 min, and bacterial numbers were determined by serial dilution and plating on LB agar.

4.13. *Membrane Depolarization and Permeabilization Assays*

The cytoplasmic membrane depolarization and permeabilization activities of As-CATH8 compared to those of antibiotics (vancomycin or polymyxin B) were assessed against *S. aureus* SAP0017 and *A. baumannii* using the membrane-potential sensitive dye $DiSC_3(5)$ and the cell viability dye PI [36]. The membrane-permeabilizing peptide mastoparan [37] was included as a positive control and water served as a negative (untreated) control.

An end-point assay was performed as suggested by Boix-Lemonche et al. [89] with several modifications. Briefly, after growth in LB, mid-log phase bacteria were centrifuged and washed twice with 5 mM HEPES buffer supplemented with 20 mM glucose (HEPES-Gluc). Cell density was adjusted to ~10^7 CFU/mL in (HEPES-Gluc) supplemented with 0.1 M KCl. A fraction (10 mL) of the culture was treated with 0.8 μM $DiSC_3(5)$ and incubated for 1 h at 23 °C protected from the light. Another 10 mL were then treated with 3.5 μM PI and incubated under the same conditions for 15 min. After incubation, 190 μL/well of the cultures were added to black opaque 96-well plates (Corning Inc.) and pre-treatment fluorescence was monitored every 2 min for a total of 10 min using a Synergy H1 Hybrid Multi-Mode Reader (BioTek, Winooski, VT, USA). The excitation and emission wavelengths were the following: for $DiSC_3(5)$, 305 nm excitation and 617 nm emission; for PI, 622 nm excitation and 700 nm emission. The digital gain was adjusted to 150/255 for DiSC3(5) and 110/255 for PI. After assessing that fluorescence values remained stable, bacteria were treated with 10 μL/well of peptide, antibiotic or water. Fluorescence was quantified 1 h after treatment under the same conditions and represented as a function of peptide concentration, subtracting the background of untreated cells.

To assess bacterial survival after treatment, supernatants from the fluorescence assays were serial diluted and plated for CFU enumeration. Since neither $DiSC_3(5)$ nor PI affected bacterial growth or treatment susceptibility under our experimental conditions, supernatants from wells with the same treatment but different dyes were pooled together. Recovered bacterial counts (CFU/mL) were represented as a function of peptide concentration.

4.14. *Agarose Gel Electrophoretic Mobility Shift Assay*

To investigate the DNA binding capacity of As-CATH8, vancomycin and polymyxin B, an agarose gel electrophoretic mobility shift assay was performed as previously described [41]. Briefly, overnight cultures of *E. coli* BL21 Star cells harboring the pET28a plasmid were grown in LB supplemented with kanamycin (30 μg/mL). The pET28a plasmid was purified using the QIAprep Spin Miniprep Kit (QIAGEN Inc., Hilden, Germany) and linearized with the *Sma*I endonuclease (Thermofisher Scientific, Waltham, MA, USA).

Linear pET28a was purified from an agarose gel using the QIAquick Gel Extraction Kit (QIAGEN Inc., Hilden, Germany).

Twofold decreasing amounts of As-CATH8 or antibiotics were incubated for 1 h at room temperature with 100 ng of linear pET28a in 10 μL of binding buffer (5% glycerol, 10 mM Tris-HCl pH 8.0, 1 mM EDTA, 1 mM DTT, 20 mM KCl and 50 μg/mL BSA). After this, 2 μL of 6× DNA Loading Dye (Thermofisher Scientific, Waltham, MA, USA) was added and the mixture was loaded onto a 1% agarose gel in TAE buffer containing SYBR Safe (Thermofisher Scientific, Waltham, MA, USA). The gel was run at 100 V for 1 h and the GeneRuler 1 kb DNA ladder (Thermofisher Scientific, Waltham, MA, USA) was used as a molecular weight marker. Finally, the gel was imaged on a ChemiDoc Touch Imaging System (BioRad Laboratories, Montreal, QC, Canada).

4.15. Statistical Analysis

Statistical processing was performed in RStudio using the R packages DescTools version 0.99.44 and rstatix version 0.7.0 [90]. Data normality was assessed using visual methods (Q-Q and density plots), as well as with the Shapiro–Wilk statistical test. Homogeneity of variance was analyzed using residual plots and Levene's statistical test. The parametric ANOVA test was used for comparison between groups, followed by Tukey's post hoc test. The Kruskal–Wallis test was used as a non-parametric method, followed by Dunn's multiple comparison test with the Benjamini–Hochberg *p*-value correction. In all cases, p-values < 0.05 were considered statistically significant.

Supplementary Materials: The following supporting information can be downloaded at: https://www.mdpi.com/article/10.3390/antibiotics11111603/s1. Table S1: Cathelicidin sequences identified in *Alligator mississippiensis, Alligator sinensis, Crocodylus porosus, and Gavialis gangeticus*; Table S2: Summary of prediction of identified cathelicidin sequences from *A. mississippiensis, A. sinensis, C. porosus*, and *G. gangeticus*; Table S3: Vertebrate cathelicidins peptides included in the phylogenetic analysis; Table S4: Antimicrobial activity of the crocodylian cathelicidins; Table S5: Biofilm inhibitory activity of the crocodylian cathelicidins; Figure S1: Multiple sequence alignment of novel and previously identified crocodylian cathelicidins; Figure S2: Biofilm inhibitory activity of crocodylian cathelicidin peptides against different bacterial pathogens; Figure S3: Cytotoxic activity of crocodylian cathelicidins against human cells; Figure S4: Bacterial membrane depolarization and permeabilization capacity of As-CATH8; Figure S5: DNA binding activity of As-CATH8 [18,19,91].

Author Contributions: Conceptualization: F.L.S., G.C. and R.E.W.H.; methodology: F.L.S., K.E., M.A.A., B.C.W., E.F.H. and L.P.; software: F.L.S. and K.E.; validation: F.L.S., M.A.A., B.C.W., M.D., L.P., N.A., E.F.H. and S.K.S.; formal analysis: F.L.S. and K.E.; investigation: F.L.S., K.E., M.A.A., B.C.W., M.D., L.P., N.A., E.F.H. and S.K.S.; resources: S.K.S., G.C. and R.E.W.H.; data curation: F.L.S., K.E., P.K. and E.F.H.; writing—original draft preparation: F.L.S.; writing—review and editing: all authors; visualization: F.L.S.; supervision: G.C. and R.E.W.H.; project administration: F.L.S.; funding acquisition: G.C. and R.E.W.H. All authors have read and agreed to the published version of the manuscript.

Funding: Research work was funded by the Canadian Institutes of Health Research (CIHR, grant number FDN-154287) awarded to REWH, as well as by Dirección General de Asuntos del Personal Académico—Universidad Nacional Autónoma de México (DGAPA-UNAM, grant number IT200321) and by Consejo Nacional de Ciencia y Tecnología (CONACyT)—Fondo Institucional de Fomento Regional para el Desarrollo Científico, Tecnológico y de Innovación (grant number 303045) awarded to GC as part of the Alagon-Becerril-Corzo-Possani research group consortium. Additionally, GC obtained economic support from Programa Iberoamericano de Ciencia y Tecnología para el Desarrollo (CYTED, project 219RT0573). SKS gratefully acknowledges funding from the Natural Sciences and Engineering Research Council (NSERC, grant number RGPIN-2017-03831). The content presented here is solely the responsibility of the authors and does not necessarily represent the official views of the CIHR. F.L.S. was a Ph.D. fellow on the Programa de Doctorado en Ciencias Biomédicas (PDCB) from UNAM and was supported by a Ph.D. scholarship (number 595253) from CONACyT. M.A.A. held a CIHR Vanier Doctoral Scholarship, a University of British Columbia (UBC) Killam Doctoral Scholarship and a UBC Four-Year Fellowship. M.D. was funded through the Graduate Award

Program from the Center for Blood Research. L.P. received a postdoctoral fellowship from the Ramón Areces Foundation (Life and Matter Sciences). R.E.W.H. held a Canada Research Chair in Health and Genomics and holds a UBC Killam Professorship.

Institutional Review Board Statement: The study was conducted in accordance with the Declaration of Helsinki and in accordance with the UBC ethics guidelines (certificate number H04-70232). Animal experiments were conducted in accordance with the Canadian Council on Animal Care guidelines, following approval by the University of British Columbia Animal Care Committee (protocol code A14-0253).

Informed Consent Statement: Informed consent was obtained from all healthy volunteers involved in the study.

Data Availability Statement: Sequences generated as part of this study with their NCBI accession numbers can be found in Supplementary Table S1. Accession numbers of the vertebrate sequences included in the phylogenetic analysis are included in Supplementary Table S3.

Acknowledgments: The authors would like to thank the Instituto de Biotecnología—UNAM for giving access to its computer cluster to perform the bioinformatic analysis presented in this work. We also acknowledge the Shared Instrument Facility (SIF) in the Department of Chemistry of UBC for use of the circular dichroism instrument, funded through the Canada Foundation for Innovation (CFI).

Conflicts of Interest: The authors declare no conflict of interest. EFH and REWH have invented and filed for patent protection on unrelated antibiofilm peptide sequences. Their patents have been assigned to their employer, the UBC, and have been licensed to ABT Innovations Inc., in which both have an ownership position. ABT Innovations Inc. is a subsidiary of ASEP Medical Holdings. EFH is employed by ASEP and receives a salary, while REWH holds an executive position and is on the Board of ASEP.

References

1. Antimicrobial Resistance Collaborators. Global Burden of Bacterial Antimicrobial Resistance in 2019: A Systematic Analysis. *Lancet* **2022**, *399*, 629–655. [CrossRef]
2. Mahoney, A.R.; Safaee, M.M.; Wuest, W.M.; Furst, A.L. The Silent Pandemic: Emergent Antibiotic Resistances Following the Global Response to SARS-CoV-2. *iScience* **2021**, *24*, 102304. [CrossRef] [PubMed]
3. De Oliveira, D.M.P.; Forde, B.M.; Kidd, T.J.; Harris, P.N.A.; Schembri, M.A.; Beatson, S.A.; Paterson, D.L.; Walker, M.J. Antimicrobial Resistance in ESKAPE Pathogens. *Clin. Microbiol. Rev.* **2020**, *33*, e00181-19. [CrossRef]
4. Tacconelli, E.; Carrara, E.; Savoldi, A.; Harbarth, S.; Mendelson, M.; Monnet, D.L.; Pulcini, C.; Kahlmeter, G.; Kluytmans, J.; Carmeli, Y.; et al. Discovery, Research, and Development of New Antibiotics: The WHO Priority List of Antibiotic-Resistant Bacteria and Tuberculosis. *Lancet Infect. Dis.* **2018**, *18*, 318–327. [CrossRef]
5. Dostert, M.; Trimble, M.J.; Hancock, R.E.W. Antibiofilm Peptides: Overcoming Biofilm-Related Treatment Failure. *RSC Adv.* **2021**, *11*, 2718–2728. [CrossRef]
6. Cámara, M.; Green, W.; MacPhee, C.E.; Rakowska, P.D.; Raval, R.; Richardson, M.C.; Slater-Jefferies, J.; Steventon, K.; Webb, J.S. Economic Significance of Biofilms: A Multidisciplinary and Cross-Sectoral Challenge. *NPJ Biofilms Microbiomes* **2022**, *8*, 42. [CrossRef]
7. Alford, M.A.; Baquir, B.; Santana, F.L.; Haney, E.F.; Hancock, R.E.W. Cathelicidin Host Defense Peptides and Inflammatory Signaling: Striking a Balance. *Front. Microbiol.* **2020**, *11*, 1902. [CrossRef]
8. Pfalzgraff, A.; Brandenburg, K.; Weindl, G. Antimicrobial Peptides and Their Therapeutic Potential for Bacterial Skin Infections and Wounds. *Front. Pharmacol.* **2018**, *9*, 281. [CrossRef]
9. Hancock, R.E.W.; Alford, M.A.; Haney, E.F. Antibiofilm Activity of Host Defence Peptides: Complexity Provides Opportunities. *Nat. Rev. Microbiol.* **2021**, *19*, 786–797. [CrossRef]
10. Drayton, M.; Deisinger, J.P.; Ludwig, K.C.; Raheem, N.; Müller, A.; Schneider, T.; Straus, S.K. Host Defense Peptides: Dual Antimicrobial and Immunomodulatory Action. *Int. J. Mol. Sci.* **2021**, *22*, 11172. [CrossRef]
11. Mookherjee, N.; Anderson, M.A.; Haagsman, H.P.; Davidson, D.J. Antimicrobial Host Defence Peptides: Functions and Clinical Potential. *Nat. Rev. Drug Discov.* **2020**, *19*, 311–332. [CrossRef] [PubMed]
12. Webb, G.J.W.; Messel, H. Abnormalities and Injuries in the Estuarine Crocodile Crocodylus Porosus. *Wildl. Res.* **1977**, *4*, 311–319. [CrossRef]
13. Merchant, M.E.; Mills, K.; Leger, N.; Jerkins, E.; Vliet, K.A.; McDaniel, N. Comparisons of Innate Immune Activity of All Known Living Crocodylian Species. *Comp. Biochem. Physiol. B Biochem. Mol. Biol.* **2006**, *143*, 133–137. [CrossRef] [PubMed]
14. Charruau, P.; Pérez-Flores, J.; Pérez-Juárez, J.G.; Cedeño-Vázquez, J.R.; Rosas-Carmona, R. Oral and Cloacal Microflora of Wild Crocodiles Crocodylus Acutus and C. Moreletii in the Mexican Caribbean. *Dis. Aquat. Org.* **2012**, *98*, 27–39. [CrossRef] [PubMed]

15. Silva, J.S.A.; Mota, R.A.; Pinheiro Júnior, J.W.; Almeida, M.C.S.; Silva, D.R.; Ferreira, D.R.A.; Azevedo, J.C.N. Aerobic Bacterial Microflora of Broad-Snouted Caiman (*Caiman latirostris*) Oral Cavity and Cloaca, Originating from Parque Zoológico Arruda Câmara, Paraíba, Brazil. *Braz. J. Microbiol.* **2009**, *40*, 194–198. [CrossRef]
16. Lovely, C.J.; Leslie, A.J. Normal Intestinal Flora of Wild Nile Crocodiles (*Crocodylus niloticus*) in the Okavango Delta, Botswana. *J. S. Afr. Vet. Assoc.* **2008**, *79*, 67–70. [CrossRef] [PubMed]
17. Flandry, F.; Lisecki, E.J.; Domingue, G.J.; Nichols, R.L.; Greer, D.L.; Haddad, R.J. Initial Antibiotic Therapy for Alligator Bites: Characterization of the Oral Flora of Alligator Mississippiensis. *South. Med. J.* **1989**, *82*, 262–266. [CrossRef] [PubMed]
18. Chen, Y.; Cai, S.; Qiao, X.; Wu, M.; Guo, Z.; Wang, R.; Kuang, Y.-Q.; Yu, H.; Wang, Y. As-Cath1-6, Novel Cathelicidins with Potent Antimicrobial and Immunomodulatory Properties from Alligator Sinensis, Play Pivotal Roles in Host Antimicrobial Immune Responses. *Biochem. J.* **2017**, *474*, 2861–2885. [CrossRef] [PubMed]
19. Barksdale, S.M.; Hrifko, E.J.; van Hoek, M.L. Cathelicidin Antimicrobial Peptide from Alligator Mississippiensis Has Antibacterial Activity Against Multi-Drug Resistant Acinetobacter Baumanii and Klebsiella Pneumoniae. *Dev. Comp. Immunol.* **2017**, *70*, 135–144. [CrossRef]
20. Guo, Z.; Qiao, X.; Cheng, R.; Shi, N.; Wang, A.; Feng, T.; Chen, Y.; Zhang, F.; Yu, H.; Wang, Y. As-Cath4 and 5, Two Vertebrate-Derived Natural Host Defense Peptides, Enhance the Immuno-Resistance Efficiency Against Bacterial Infections in Chinese Mitten Crab, Eriocheir Sinensis. *Fish Shellfish Immunol.* **2017**, *71*, 202–209. [CrossRef]
21. Chen, Z.; Zhang, J.; Ming, Z.; Tong, H.; Wu, J.; Chen, Q.; Wang, Y.; Luo, F.; Wang, Y.; Feng, T. As-Cathelicidin4 Enhances the Immune Response and Resistance Against Aeromonas Hydrophila in Caridean Shrimp. *J. Fish Dis.* **2022**, *45*, 743–754. [CrossRef] [PubMed]
22. Eddy, S.R. Hidden Markov Models. *Curr. Opin. Struct. Biol.* **1996**, *6*, 361–365. [CrossRef]
23. Eddy, S.R. Accelerated Profile HMM Searches. *PLoS Comput. Biol.* **2011**, *7*, e1002195. [CrossRef] [PubMed]
24. Xie, Q.; Liu, Y.; Luo, F.; Yi, Q.; Wang, Y.; Deng, L.; Dai, J.; Feng, T. Antiviral Activity of Cathelicidin 5, a Peptide from Alligator Sinensis, Against WSSV in Caridean Shrimp Exopalaemon Modestus. *Fish Shellfish Immunol.* **2019**, *93*, 82–89. [CrossRef]
25. Xhindoli, D.; Pacor, S.; Benincasa, M.; Scocchi, M.; Gennaro, R.; Tossi, A. The Human Cathelicidin LL-37 Pore-Forming Antibacterial Peptide and Host-Cell Modulator. *Biochim. Biophys. Acta* **2016**, *1858*, 546–566. [CrossRef]
26. Phoenix, D.A.; Harris, F. The Hydrophobic Moment and Its Use in the Classification of Amphiphilic Structures (Review). *Mol. Membr. Biol.* **2002**, *19*, 1–10. [CrossRef]
27. Greenfield, N.J. Using Circular Dichroism Spectra to Estimate Protein Secondary Structure. *Nat. Protoc.* **2006**, *1*, 2876–2890. [CrossRef]
28. Wei, L.; Gao, J.; Zhang, S.; Wu, S.; Xie, Z.; Ling, G.; Kuang, Y.-Q.; Yang, Y.; Yu, H.; Wang, Y. Identification and Characterization of the First Cathelicidin from Sea Snakes with Potent Antimicrobial and Anti-Inflammatory Activity and Special Mechanism. *J. Biol. Chem.* **2015**, *290*, 16633–16652. [CrossRef]
29. Yu, K.; Park, K.; Kang, S.-W.; Shin, S.Y.; Hahm, K.-S.; Kim, Y. Solution Structure of a Cathelicidin-Derived Antimicrobial Peptide, CRAMP as Determined by NMR Spectroscopy. *J. Pept. Res.* **2002**, *60*, 1–9. [CrossRef]
30. Gao, W.; Xing, L.; Qu, P.; Tan, T.; Yang, N.; Li, D.; Chen, H.; Feng, X. Identification of a Novel Cathelicidin Antimicrobial Peptide from Ducks and Determination of Its Functional Activity and Antibacterial Mechanism. *Sci. Rep.* **2015**, *5*, 17260. [CrossRef]
31. Mahlapuu, M.; Sidorowicz, A.; Mikosinski, J.; Krzyżanowski, M.; Orleanski, J.; Twardowska-Saucha, K.; Nykaza, A.; Dyaczynski, M.; Belz-Lagoda, B.; Dziwiszek, G.; et al. Evaluation of LL-37 in Healing of Hard-to-Heal Venous Leg Ulcers: A Multicentric Prospective Randomized Placebo-Controlled Clinical Trial. *Wound Repair Regen.* **2021**, *29*, 938–950. [CrossRef] [PubMed]
32. Wu, B.C.; Haney, E.F.; Akhoundsadegh, N.; Pletzer, D.; Trimble, M.J.; Adriaans, A.E.; Nibbering, P.H.; Hancock, R.E.W. Human Organoid Biofilm Model for Assessing Antibiofilm Activity of Novel Agents. *NPJ Biofilms Microbiomes* **2021**, *7*, 8. [CrossRef] [PubMed]
33. Pletzer, D.; Mansour, S.C.; Wuerth, K.; Rahanjam, N.; Hancock, R.E.W. New Mouse Model for Chronic Infections by Gram-negative Bacteria Enabling the Study of Anti-Infective Efficacy and Host-Microbe Interactions. *mBio* **2017**, *8*, e00140-17. [CrossRef] [PubMed]
34. Zhang, L.; Dhillon, P.; Yan, H.; Farmer, S.; Hancock, R.E. Interactions of Bacterial Cationic Peptide Antibiotics with Outer and Cytoplasmic Membranes of Pseudomonas Aeruginosa. *Antimicrob. Agents Chemother.* **2000**, *44*, 3317–3321. [CrossRef]
35. Sims, P.J.; Waggoner, A.S.; Wang, C.H.; Hoffman, J.F. Studies on the Mechanism by Which Cyanine Dyes Measure Membrane Potential in Red Blood Cells and Phosphatidylcholine Vesicles. *Biochemistry* **1974**, *13*, 3315–3330. [CrossRef]
36. Benfield, A.H.; Henriques, S.T. Mode-of-Action of Antimicrobial Peptides: Membrane Disruption Vs. Intracellular Mechanisms. *Front. Med. Technol.* **2020**, *2*, 610997. [CrossRef]
37. dos Santos Cabrera, M.P.; Alvares, D.S.; Leite, N.B.; de Souza, B.M.; Palma, M.S.; Riske, K.A.; Neto, J.R. New Insight into the Mechanism of Action of Wasp Mastoparan Peptides: Lytic Activity and Clustering Observed with Giant Vesicles. *Langmuir* **2011**, *27*, 10805–10813. [CrossRef]
38. Kristensen, K.; Ehrlich, N.; Henriksen, J.R.; Andresen, T.L. Single-Vesicle Detection and Analysis of Peptide-Induced Membrane Permeabilization. *Langmuir* **2015**, *31*, 2472–2483. [CrossRef]
39. Mühlberg, E.; Umstätter, F.; Kleist, C.; Domhan, C.; Mier, W.; Uhl, P. Renaissance of Vancomycin: Approaches for Breaking Antibiotic Resistance in Multidrug-Resistant Bacteria. *Can. J. Microbiol.* **2020**, *66*, 11–16. [CrossRef]

40. Trimble, M.J.; Mlynárčik, P.; Kolář, M.; Hancock, R.E.W. Polymyxin: Alternative Mechanisms of Action and Resistance. *Cold Spring Harb. Perspect. Med.* **2016**, *6*, a025288. [CrossRef]
41. Haney, E.F.; Petersen, A.P.; Lau, C.K.; Jing, W.; Storey, D.G.; Vogel, H.J. Mechanism of Action of Puroindoline Derived Tryptophan-Rich Antimicrobial Peptides. *Biochim. Biophys. Acta* **2013**, *1828*, 1802–1813. [CrossRef] [PubMed]
42. Santana, F.L.; Estrada, K.; Ortiz, E.; Corzo, G. Reptilian β-Defensins: Expanding the Repertoire of Known Crocodylian Peptides. *Peptides* **2021**, *136*, 170473. [CrossRef] [PubMed]
43. Cheng, Y.; Prickett, M.D.; Gutowska, W.; Kuo, R.; Belov, K.; Burt, D.W. Evolution of the Avian β-Defensin and Cathelicidin Genes. *BMC Evol. Biol.* **2015**, *15*, 188. [CrossRef] [PubMed]
44. Whelehan, C.J.; Barry-Reidy, A.; Meade, K.G.; Eckersall, P.D.; Chapwanya, A.; Narciandi, F.; Lloyd, A.T.; O'Farrelly, C. Characterisation and Expression Profile of the Bovine Cathelicidin Gene Repertoire in Mammary Tissue. *BMC Genom.* **2014**, *15*, 128. [CrossRef]
45. Wu, M.; Maier, E.; Benz, R.; Hancock, R.E. Mechanism of Interaction of Different Classes of Cationic Antimicrobial Peptides with Planar Bilayers and with the Cytoplasmic Membrane of *Escherichia coli*. *Biochemistry* **1999**, *38*, 7235–7242. [CrossRef]
46. Hsu, C.-H.; Chen, C.; Jou, M.-L.; Lee, A.Y.-L.; Lin, Y.-C.; Yu, Y.-P.; Huang, W.-T.; Wu, S.-H. Structural and DNA-binding Studies on the Bovine Antimicrobial Peptide, Indolicidin: Evidence for Multiple Conformations Involved in Binding to Membranes and DNA. *Nucleic Acids Res.* **2005**, *33*, 4053–4064. [CrossRef]
47. Liu, C.; Shan, B.; Qi, J.; Ma, Y. Systemic Responses of Multidrug-Resistant Pseudomonas Aeruginosa and Acinetobacter Baumannii Following Exposure to the Antimicrobial Peptide Cathelicidin-BF Imply Multiple Intracellular Targets. *Front. Cell. Infect. Microbiol.* **2017**, *7*, 466. [CrossRef]
48. Limoli, D.H.; Rockel, A.B.; Host, K.M.; Jha, A.; Kopp, B.T.; Hollis, T.; Wozniak, D.J. Cationic Antimicrobial Peptides Promote Microbial Mutagenesis and Pathoadaptation in Chronic Infections. *PLoS Pathog.* **2014**, *10*, e1004083. [CrossRef]
49. Scheenstra, M.R.; van den Belt, M.; Tjeerdsma-van Bokhoven, J.L.M.; Schneider, V.A.F.; Ordonez, S.R.; van Dijk, A.; Veldhuizen, E.J.A.; Haagsman, H.P. Cathelicidins PMAP-36, LL-37 and CATH-2 Are Similar Peptides with Different Modes of Action. *Sci. Rep.* **2019**, *9*, 4780. [CrossRef]
50. Velkov, T.; Thompson, P.E.; Nation, R.L.; Li, J. Structure-Activity Relationships of Polymyxin Antibiotics. *J. Med. Chem.* **2010**, *53*, 1898–1916. [CrossRef]
51. Jia, Z.; O'Mara, M.L.; Zuegg, J.; Cooper, M.A.; Mark, A.E. The Effect of Environment on the Recognition and Binding of Vancomycin to Native and Resistant Forms of Lipid II. *Biophys. J.* **2011**, *101*, 2684–2692. [CrossRef] [PubMed]
52. Arenas, I.; Ibarra, M.A.; Santana, F.L.; Villegas, E.; Hancock, R.E.W.; Corzo, G. In Vitro and in Vivo Antibiotic Capacity of Two Host Defense Peptides. *Antimicrob. Agents Chemother.* **2020**, *64*, e00145-20. [CrossRef] [PubMed]
53. Shi, N.; Cai, S.; Gao, J.; Qiao, X.; Yang, H.; Wang, Y.; Yu, H. Roles of Polymorphic Cathelicidins in Innate Immunity of Soft-Shell Turtle, Pelodiscus Sinensis. *Dev. Comp. Immunol.* **2019**, *92*, 179–192. [CrossRef] [PubMed]
54. Cai, S.; Qiao, X.; Feng, L.; Shi, N.; Wang, H.; Yang, H.; Guo, Z.; Wang, M.; Chen, Y.; Wang, Y.; et al. Python Cathelicidin CATHPb1 Protects Against Multidrug-Resistant Staphylococcal Infections by Antimicrobial-Immunomodulatory Duality. *J. Med. Chem.* **2018**, *61*, 2075–2086. [CrossRef] [PubMed]
55. Wan, Q.-H.; Pan, S.-K.; Hu, L.; Zhu, Y.; Xu, P.-W.; Xia, J.-Q.; Chen, H.; He, G.-Y.; He, J.; Ni, X.-W.; et al. Genome Analysis and Signature Discovery for Diving and Sensory Properties of the Endangered Chinese Alligator. *Cell Res.* **2013**, *23*, 1091–1105. [CrossRef]
56. St John, J.A.; Braun, E.L.; Isberg, S.R.; Miles, L.G.; Chong, A.Y.; Gongora, J.; Dalzell, P.; Moran, C.; Bed'hom, B.; Abzhanov, A.; et al. Sequencing Three Crocodilian Genomes to Illuminate the Evolution of Archosaurs and Amniotes. *Genome Biol.* **2012**, *13*, 415. [CrossRef]
57. Köster, J.; Rahmann, S. Snakemake—A Scalable Bioinformatics Workflow Engine. *Bioinformatics* **2012**, *28*, 2520–2522. [CrossRef]
58. Katoh, K.; Standley, D.M. MAFFT Multiple Sequence Alignment Software Version 7: Improvements in Performance and Usability. *Mol. Biol. Evol.* **2013**, *30*, 772–780. [CrossRef]
59. Larsson, A. AliView: A Fast and Lightweight Alignment Viewer and Editor for Large Datasets. *Bioinformatics* **2014**, *30*, 3276–3278. [CrossRef]
60. Slater, G.S.C.; Birney, E. Automated Generation of Heuristics for Biological Sequence Comparison. *BMC Bioinform.* **2005**, *6*, 31. [CrossRef]
61. Almagro Armenteros, J.J.; Tsirigos, K.D.; Sønderby, C.K.; Petersen, T.N.; Winther, O.; Brunak, S.; von Heijne, G.; Nielsen, H. SignalP 5.0 Improves Signal Peptide Predictions Using Deep Neural Networks. *Nat. Biotechnol.* **2019**, *37*, 420–423. [CrossRef] [PubMed]
62. Zhao, H.; Gan, T.-X.; Liu, X.-D.; Jin, Y.; Lee, W.-H.; Shen, J.-H.; Zhang, Y. Identification and Characterization of Novel Reptile Cathelicidins from Elapid Snakes. *Peptides* **2008**, *29*, 1685–1691. [CrossRef] [PubMed]
63. Xiao, Y.; Cai, Y.; Bommineni, Y.R.; Fernando, S.C.; Prakash, O.; Gilliland, S.E.; Zhang, G. Identification and Functional Characterization of Three Chicken Cathelicidins with Potent Antimicrobial Activity. *J. Biol. Chem.* **2006**, *281*, 2858–2867. [CrossRef] [PubMed]
64. Lu, X.J.; Chen, J.; Huang, Z.A.; Shi, Y.H.; Lv, J.N. Identification and Characterization of a Novel Cathelicidin from Ayu, Plecoglossus Altivelis. *Fish Shellfish Immunol.* **2011**, *31*, 52–57. [CrossRef]

65. Hao, X.; Yang, H.; Wei, L.; Yang, S.; Zhu, W.; Ma, D.; Yu, H.; Lai, R. Amphibian Cathelicidin Fills the Evolutionary Gap of Cathelicidin in Vertebrate. *Amino Acids* **2012**, *43*, 677–685. [CrossRef]
66. Stamatakis, A. RAxML Version 8: A Tool for Phylogenetic Analysis and Post-Analysis of Large Phylogenies. *Bioinformatics* **2014**, *30*, 1312–1313. [CrossRef]
67. Darriba, D.; Posada, D.; Kozlov, A.M.; Stamatakis, A.; Morel, B.; Flouri, T. ModelTest-NG: A New and Scalable Tool for the Selection of Dna and Protein Evolutionary Models. *Mol. Biol. Evol.* **2020**, *37*, 291–294. [CrossRef]
68. Wang, L.-G.; Lam, T.T.-Y.; Xu, S.; Dai, Z.; Zhou, L.; Feng, T.; Guo, P.; Dunn, C.W.; Jones, B.R.; Bradley, T.; et al. Treeio: An R Package for Phylogenetic Tree Input and Output with Richly Annotated and Associated Data. *Mol. Biol. Evol.* **2020**, *37*, 599–603. [CrossRef]
69. Yu, G. Using Ggtree to Visualize Data on Tree-Like Structures. *Curr. Protoc. Bioinform.* **2020**, *69*, e96. [CrossRef]
70. R Core Team. *R: A Language and Environment for Statistical Computing*; R Foundation for Statistical Computing: Vienna, Austria, 2022.
71. RStudio Team. *Rstudio: Integrated Development Environment for R*; RStudio, PBC.: Boston, MA, USA, 2022.
72. Osorio, D.; Rondon-Villarreal, P.; Torres, R. Peptides: A Package for Data Mining of Antimicrobial Peptides. *R J.* **2015**, *7*, 4–14. [CrossRef]
73. Bjellqvist, B.; Hughes, G.J.; Pasquali, C.; Paquet, N.; Ravier, F.; Sanchez, J.C.; Frutiger, S.; Hochstrasser, D. The Focusing Positions of Polypeptides in Immobilized pH Gradients Can Be Predicted from Their Amino Acid Sequences. *Electrophoresis* **1993**, *14*, 1023–1031. [CrossRef] [PubMed]
74. Kyte, J.; Doolittle, R.F. A Simple Method for Displaying the Hydropathic Character of a Protein. *J. Mol. Biol.* **1982**, *157*, 105–132. [CrossRef]
75. Walker, J.M. (Ed.) *The Proteomics Protocols Handbook*, 3rd ed.; Humana Press: Totowa, NJ, USA, 2005; ISBN 978-1-58829-343-5.
76. Müller, A.T.; Gabernet, G.; Hiss, J.A.; Schneider, G. modlAMP: Python for Antimicrobial Peptides. *Bioinformatics* **2017**, *33*, 2753–2755. [CrossRef] [PubMed]
77. Jumper, J.; Evans, R.; Pritzel, A.; Green, T.; Figurnov, M.; Ronneberger, O.; Tunyasuvunakool, K.; Bates, R.; Žídek, A.; Potapenko, A.; et al. Highly Accurate Protein Structure Prediction with AlphaFold. *Nature* **2021**, *596*, 583–589. [CrossRef] [PubMed]
78. Mirdita, M.; Ovchinnikov, S.; Steinegger, M. ColabFold—Making Protein Folding Accessible to All. *bioRxv* **2021**. [CrossRef]
79. Pettersen, E.F.; Goddard, T.D.; Huang, C.C.; Meng, E.C.; Couch, G.S.; Croll, T.I.; Morris, J.H.; Ferrin, T.E. UCSF ChimeraX: Structure Visualization for Researchers, Educators, and Developers. *Protein Sci.* **2021**, *30*, 70–82. [CrossRef]
80. Haney, E.F.; Wu, B.C.; Lee, K.; Hilchie, A.L.; Hancock, R.E.W. Aggregation and Its Influence on the Immunomodulatory Activity of Synthetic Innate Defense Regulator Peptides. *Cell Chem. Biol.* **2017**, *24*, 969–980.e4. [CrossRef]
81. Hilchie, A.L.; Sharon, A.J.; Haney, E.F.; Hoskin, D.W.; Bally, M.B.; Franco, O.L.; Corcoran, J.A.; Hancock, R.E.W. Mastoparan Is a Membranolytic Anti-Cancer Peptide That Works Synergistically with Gemcitabine in a Mouse Model of Mammary Carcinoma. *Biochim. Biophys. Acta* **2016**, *1858*, 3195–3204. [CrossRef]
82. Raheem, N.; Kumar, P.; Lee, E.; Cheng, J.T.J.; Hancock, R.E.W.; Straus, S.K. Insights into the Mechanism of Action of Two Analogues of Aurein 2.2. *Biochim. Biophys. Acta Biomembr.* **2020**, *1862*, 183262. [CrossRef]
83. Chase-Topping, M.; Gally, D.; Low, C.; Matthews, L.; Woolhouse, M. Super-Shedding and the Link Between Human Infection and Livestock Carriage of *Escherichia coli* O157. *Nat. Rev. Microbiol.* **2008**, *6*, 904–912. [CrossRef]
84. Mansour, S.C.; Pletzer, D.; de la Fuente-Núñez, C.; Kim, P.; Cheung, G.Y.C.; Joo, H.-S.; Otto, M.; Hancock, R.E.W. Bacterial Abscess Formation Is Controlled by the Stringent Stress Response and Can Be Targeted Therapeutically. *EBioMedicine* **2016**, *12*, 219–226. [CrossRef] [PubMed]
85. Pletzer, D.; Mansour, S.C.; Hancock, R.E.W. Synergy Between Conventional Antibiotics and Anti-Biofilm Peptides in a Murine, Sub-Cutaneous Abscess Model Caused by Recalcitrant ESKAPE Pathogens. *PLoS Pathog.* **2018**, *14*, e1007084. [CrossRef] [PubMed]
86. Wiegand, I.; Hilpert, K.; Hancock, R.E.W. Agar and Broth Dilution Methods to Determine the Minimal Inhibitory Concentration (MIC) of Antimicrobial Substances. *Nat. Protoc.* **2008**, *3*, 163–175. [CrossRef] [PubMed]
87. Haney, E.F.; Trimble, M.J.; Hancock, R.E.W. Microtiter Plate Assays to Assess Antibiofilm Activity Against Bacteria. *Nat. Protoc.* **2021**, *16*, 2615–2632. [CrossRef]
88. Santana, F.L.; Arenas, I.; Haney, E.F.; Estrada, K.; Hancock, R.E.W.; Corzo, G. Identification of a Crocodylian -Defensin Variant from Alligator Mississippiensis with Antimicrobial and Antibiofilm Activity. *Peptides* **2021**, *141*, 170549. [CrossRef]
89. Boix-Lemonche, G.; Lekka, M.; Skerlavaj, B. A Rapid Fluorescence-Based Microplate Assay to Investigate the Interaction of Membrane Active Antimicrobial Peptides with Whole Gram-Positive Bacteria. *Antibiotics* **2020**, *9*, 92. [CrossRef]
90. Kassambara, A. *Practical Statistics in R for Comparing Groups: Numerical Variables*; Practical statistics in R series; Independently Published, 2019; ISBN 978-1-71233-088-3.
91. Tankrathok, A.; Punpad, A.; Kongchaiyapoom, M.; Sosiangdi, S.; Jangpromma, N.; Daduang, S.; Klaynongsruang, S. Identification of the First Crocodylus Siamensis Cathelicidin Gene and Rn15 Peptide Derived from Cathelin Domain Exhibiting Antibacterial Activity. *Biotechnol. Appl. Biochem.* **2019**, *66*, 142–152. [CrossRef]

antibiotics MDPI

Article

Revealing Genome-Based Biosynthetic Potential of *Streptomyces* sp. BR123 Isolated from Sunflower Rhizosphere with Broad Spectrum Antimicrobial Activity

Neelma Ashraf [1,2,*], Sana Zafar [1], Roman Makitrynskyy [3], Andreas Bechthold [3], Dieter Spiteller [2], Lijiang Song [4], Munir Ahmad Anwar [1], Andriy Luzhetskyy [5], Ali Nisar Khan [1], Kalsoom Akhtar [1] and Shazia Khaliq [1,*]

1 Industrial Biotechnology Division, National Institute for Biotechnology and Genetic Engineering (NIBGE), Constituent College of Pakistan Institute of Engineering and Applied Sciences (PIEAS), Jhang Road, P.O. Box 577, Faisalabad 38000, Pakistan
2 Department of Chemical Ecology/Biological Chemistry, University of Konstanz, 78457 Konstanz, Germany
3 Department of Pharmaceutical Biology and Biotechnology, Institute of Pharmaceutical Sciences, University of Freiburg, 79104 Freiburg im Breisgau, Germany
4 Department of Chemistry, University of Warwick Coventry, Coventry CV4 7AL, UK
5 Pharmaceutical Biotechnology Campus, Saarland University, Building C2.3, 66123 Saarbrucken, Germany
* Correspondence: neelma.ashraf@uni-konstanz.de (N.A.); skhaliq1976@gmail.com (S.K.); Tel.: +92-41-9201316 (S.K.); Fax: +92-41-92014722 (S.K.)

Citation: Ashraf, N.; Zafar, S.; Makitrynskyy, R.; Bechthold, A.; Spiteller, D.; Song, L.; Anwar, M.A.; Luzhetskyy, A.; Khan, A.N.; Akhtar, K.; et al. Revealing Genome-Based Biosynthetic Potential of *Streptomyces* sp. BR123 Isolated from Sunflower Rhizosphere with Broad Spectrum Antimicrobial Activity. *Antibiotics* **2022**, *11*, 1057. https://doi.org/10.3390/antibiotics11081057

Academic Editors: Agostinho Antunes, Guillermin Agüero-Chapin and Yovani Marrero-Ponce

Received: 2 July 2022
Accepted: 1 August 2022
Published: 4 August 2022

Publisher's Note: MDPI stays neutral with regard to jurisdictional claims in published maps and institutional affiliations.

Copyright: © 2022 by the authors. Licensee MDPI, Basel, Switzerland. This article is an open access article distributed under the terms and conditions of the Creative Commons Attribution (CC BY) license (https://creativecommons.org/licenses/by/4.0/).

Abstract: Actinomycetes, most notably the genus *Streptomyces*, have great importance due to their role in the discovery of new natural products, especially for finding antimicrobial secondary metabolites that are useful in the medicinal science and biotechnology industries. In the current study, a genome-based evaluation of *Streptomyces* sp. isolate BR123 was analyzed to determine its biosynthetic potential, based on its in vitro antimicrobial activity against a broad range of microbial pathogens, including gram-positive and gram-negative bacteria and fungi. A draft genome sequence of 8.15 Mb of *Streptomyces* sp. isolate BR123 was attained, containing a GC content of 72.63% and 8103 protein coding genes. Many antimicrobial, antiparasitic, and anticancerous compounds were detected by the presence of multiple biosynthetic gene clusters, which was predicted by in silico analysis. A novel metabolite with a molecular mass of 1271.7773 in positive ion mode was detected through a high-performance liquid chromatography linked with mass spectrometry (HPLC-MS) analysis. In addition, another compound, meridamycin, was also identified through a HPLC-MS analysis. The current study reveals the biosynthetic potential of *Streptomyces* sp. isolate BR123, with respect to the synthesis of bioactive secondary metabolites through genomic and spectrometric analysis. Moreover, the comparative genome study compared the isolate BR123 with other *Streptomyces* strains, which may expand the knowledge concerning the mechanism involved in novel antimicrobial metabolite synthesis.

Keywords: *Streptomyces*; secondary metabolites; genome; biosynthetic gene clusters; high-performance liquid chromatography (HPLC); mass spectrometry

1. Introduction

The growing resistance of pathogenic microorganisms to antimicrobial agents has become a global problem [1]. There is a dire need to discover newer antibiotics and techniques that can overcome this problem [2,3]. In the development of new therapeutical agents, natural products play a vital role. More than 2200 biologically active compounds have been isolated from naturally abundant microorganisms [4,5]. Many novel antibiotics were discovered from soil bacteria as well as from marine habitats.

Actinomycetes are a group of aerobic, gram-positive, sporulating, and filamentous bacteria that have aerial and substrate mycelium, with the ability to produce many bioactive secondary metabolites [6]. Among the class Actinobacteria, the genus *Streptomyces*, primarily found in the soil and aquatic habitats, has gained much attention because of its role in the production of novel antimicrobial metabolites. More than 7630 bioactive compounds have been reported to be only produced by this genus [7]. These bioactive compounds are the result of an unprecedented genetic potential through biosynthetic gene clusters (BGCs), which are harbored in their genomes and contain genes arranged in close vicinity. The BGCs are under the control of a sophisticated regulatory network and the laboratory conditions used [8]. Hence, the same species isolated from different habitats can have different sets of biosynthetic gene clusters, which may be lost or gained when a particular strain is transferred to a new environment [9]. Biosynthetic gene clusters (BGCs) have been classified into two main pathways based on their products, i.e., nonribosomal peptide synthetases (NRPSs) and polyketide synthases (PKSs), for the biosynthesis of potent secondary metabolites. Polyketide synthases (PKSs) are further divided into PKS-I and PKS-II gene clusters, where the diversity evolution of PKSs can be achieved by using fragments of genes PKS-I ketosynthase and PKS-II KSα domains. Conversely, NRPSs are produced by nonribosomal peptide synthase (NRPS) gene clusters and to achieve their diversity evolution, their adenylation (AD) domains are used. Both the NRPS and PKS products are comprised of remarkably long genes (>5 kb) that encode multi-modular enzymes with repetitive domain structures. In addition, other well-known classes of BGCs are terpenoids, saccharides and lanthipeptides [10,11].

The conventional approach to discovering antibiotics from *Streptomyces* is through the bioactivity-based identification of a compound, using mass spectrometry and nuclear magnetic resonance (NMR) analyses [12]. However, the genome-based approaches have divulged that most of the BGCs are not expressed under certain laboratory conditions, proposing that the capability of *Streptomyces* to produce secondary compounds has been underestimated [13,14]. On average, each *Streptomyces* has the potential to produce more than 30 secondary metabolites, meaning that they are a valuable source of natural product discovery [15]. The genomic data of over 1141 strains of *Streptomyces* are deposited and available in the GenBank database. In this study, we conducted a detailed analysis of *Streptomyces* sp. BR123, which was isolated from the rhizosphere of a sunflower plant. The analysis was based on its in vitro antimicrobial activities in relation to the whole genome sequencing data and a general comparison with other reported strains of the genus *Streptomyces*.

2. Materials and Methods

2.1. Isolation and Cultivation Conditions of Streptomyces sp. BR123

Soil samples were collected from the rhizosphere of sunflower plants located in various agricultural fields of Faisalabad, Pakistan for the purpose of isolating *Streptomyces* colonies. From each sample, 1 g of dried soil was added into 9 mL of double distilled autoclaved water and mixed well. The diluted aliquots (0.1 mL), 10^{-1}, 10^{-2}, 10^{-3}, 10^{-4}, and 10^{-5} were spread into petri plates containing a starch casein agar (SCA) medium, composed of: soluble starch 10.0 g, KNO_3 2.0 g, casein 0.3 g, K_2HPO_4 2.0 g, NaCl 2.0 g, $MgSO_4{\cdot}7H_2O$ 0.05 g, $FeSO_4{\cdot}7H_2O$ 0.01 g, $CaCO_3$ 0.02, agar 20 g, and distilled water 1 L [16]. The pH of the medium was adjusted to be 7.0–7.2. The medium was supplemented with an antifungal solution of cycloheximide (100 µg/mL) to inhibit fungus growth, and plates were incubated at 30 °C for 5–7 days. Colonies that showed hard texture and filamentous mycelium when observed under a phase contrast microscope were picked and purified by using an agar streak method [17]. The purified stock cultures were preserved in glycerol (40% *v*/*v*) at −80 °C. Moreover, *Streptomyces* sp. BR123 was cultivated in a starch casein broth at 30 °C, rotated at 180 rpm for 7 days for later analysis.

2.2. Sequencing and Assembly of the Genome

To perform the genome-based comparative analysis, the biosynthetic potential of *Streptomyces* isolate BR123 was investigated at the level of draft genome sequence. The biomass of the isolate BR123 was separated from the liquid culture and grown for 72 h at 30 °C in casein-starch-peptone-yeast extract-malt extract (CSPY-ME) broth with the composition (in g/L): K_2HPO_4 0.5, starch 10, casein 3, yeast extract 1, malt extract 10, and peptone 1. The broth's final pH was 7.2. Genomic DNA of high quality was obtained through the bead method and quantification was performed by a high-sensitivity (HS) assay of Quant-iT double-stranded DNA (dsDNA) (ThermoFisher Scientific, Waltham, MA, USA). The genomic DNA was sequenced at MicrobesNG using the Nextera XT Library Preparation Kit (Illumina, San Diego, CA, USA). For the generation and quantification of the Illumina library, the KAPA Biosystems Library Quantification Kit was used. The genomic data were deposited at the National Centre for Biotechnology Information (NCBI) under the accession number PRJNA643667. Trimmomatic 0.30 was used to compile raw reads, with a quality cutoff of Q15 [18].

2.3. *Annotation of Genome and Bioinformatics Analysis*

For the annotation of the genome, Rapid Annotation using Subsystem Technology (RAST) version 2.0 was used [19]. For the assembly of matrices, PGAP (Prokaryotic Genome Annotation Pipeline) v4.2 from the NCBI was used. The predictions of gene clusters with the potential to produce secondary metabolites were analyzed by using the online antiSMASH (antibiotics & Secondary Metabolite Analysis Shell) bacterial version, accessed on 22 April 2022.

2.4. *Amplification of NRPS and PKS Genes by PCR*

The PKS-I, PKS-II, and NRPS genes were amplified using the following primer sets, K1F (5′-TSAAGTCSAACATCCGBCA-3′)/M6R (5′-CGCAGGTTSCSGTACCAG TA-3′) [20], KSα (5′-TSGCSTGCTTGGAYGCSATC-3′)/KSβ (5′-TGGAANCCGCCGAABCCGCT-3′), and A3F (5′-GCSTACSYSATSTACACSTCSGG-3′)/A7R (5′-SASGTCVCCSGTSGCGTA S-3′). The reaction for NRPS and PKS genes was made with the final volume of 50 μL containing 1.5 μL of extracted genomic DNA, 1 μL of each primer (10 pmol), 21.5 μL of nuclease-free water, and 25 μL of dream taq (PCR master mix). The amplification process was performed in Analytik Jena Flex Thermal cycler block assembly 96 G, according to the following specified conditions for each primer: 5 minutes at 95 °C for denaturation and 35 cycles of 30 seconds at 95 °C; 2 minutes at 57 °C, 63 °C, and 59.7 °C for K1F/M6R, KSα/KSβ, and A3F/A7R, respectively; 4 minutes at 72 °C; and 10 minutes at 72 °C. Gel electrophoresis was used to analyze the PCR products using 1% agarose gel final stained with ethidium bromide and the end product was purified with the help of GeneJET PCR Purification Kit K0721 (Thermo scientific/Vilnius, Lithuania).

2.5. *Assessment of Antimicrobial Potential*

The isolate BR123 was checked for antimicrobial potential through the agar-well diffusion method [21] against 2 gram-positive bacteria (*Staphylococcus aureus* and *Bacillus subitilis*), 4 gram-negative bacteria (*Salmonella typhi, Xanthomonas oryzae, Escherichia coli* and *Pseudomonas aeruginosa*), and 4 fungi (*Aspergillus flavus, Aspergillus niger, Fusarium solani* and *Fusarium oxysporum*) by using 7 different media (Supplementary Table S1). Plates were overlaid with the test culture and wells were filled with the supernatant of BR123. These plates were incubated for 24 h at 30 °C in case of bacteria and for 5–7 days in the case of fungal for the examination of clear zones formation.

2.6. *Analysis of Metabolites through HPLC-MS from Streptomyces sp. BR123*

2.6.1. Sample Preparation

Streptomyces sp. BR123 was pre-cultivated in a starch casein (SC) broth (pH 7.2). After cultivating for 4 days in a rotary shaker at 180 rpm and 28 °C, 5 mL of the culture was used to inoculate 1 L of casein-starch-peptone-yeast extract-malt extract (CSPY-ME) broth in a 2.8 L flask [17]. Twice extraction of the entire culture was performed with an equal volume of ethyl acetate (EtOAc) by adjusting the pH of the broth to 3.5. To obtain solid material, the ethyl acetate extract was concentrated in a rotary evaporator.

2.6.2. Analysis of Metabolites

Low resolution electrospray ionization source mass spectra were recorded using a UHPLC focused Thermo Scientific Dionex UltiMate 3000 auto-sampler (Dionex, Thermo Fisher Scientific, Freiburg, Germany), coupled with a TSQ Quantum Access MAX diode array detector (DAD, Thermo Fisher Scientific, Germany). The diode array detector allows for the relative qualification of non-volatile components. Using a mobile phase of water (A) and acetonitrile (B) both containing 0.5% acetic acid, the separation of compounds was performed on a C18 HPLC column (Waters, 3.5 m, 4.6 100 mm). The gradient started by washing for the following durations and concentrations: 0.5 min in 95% A; 19.5 min in 5% A; 23.5 min in 5% A; 24 min in 95% A; 27 min in 95% A; followed by a final washing in 95% A and 5% B solution for 5 min. The column was re-equilibrated. The method lasted a total of 27 min. The flow rate was 0.5 mL/min, column temperature was 30 ± 10 °C, and pressure was adjusted from 5×10^2 to 4×10^4 kPa. Further analysis of the compounds was determined using high resolution Bruker MaXis II Q-TOF (Bruker, Warwick, UK) mass spectrometer coupled with a Dionex 3000RS UHPLC (Bruker, Warwick, UK). The analysis was performed by keeping a mass range of 50–3000 m/z and using a mobile phase of water (A) and acetonitrile (B), both containing 0.1% formic acid. Separation was again performed by C18 HPLC column. The gradient for the high resolution started from 5% to 100% in 25 min, keeping a flow rate of 0.2 mL/min. The column was washed and re-equilibrated. Mass spectra were recorded in both negative and positive modes and Xcalibur version 4.3 was used for the data analysis.

2.7. Comparative Genome Analysis

The complete 16S rRNA sequence data from the genome of all strains were retrieved from TrueBacTMIDBeta [19]. Alignment of the extracted 16S rRNA sequences was achieved through the ClustalW tool available in MEGA Software version 7 [22] and the phylogenetic tree was constructed using the neighbor-joining method with a bootstrap value of 1000. Additionally, the whole genome phylogeny was determined by using the online available version of KBase software. The average nucleotide identity scores were calculated using the FastANI algorithm [23].

2.8. Accession Number of Genome Sequence

The genome sequence of *Streptomyces* sp. BR123 has been submitted to GenBank under the bio project number PRJNA643667, genome sequencing project number JACBGN000000000, and SRA number SRR12527047. Moreover, the 16S rRNA gene sequence has been submitted to GenBank under the accession number MT799988.

3. Results and Discussion

3.1. General Genomic Characteristics and Phylogenetic Analysis of Streptomyces sp. BR123

A genomic sequence with a total stretch of 8,158,025 bp was obtained, and the length of the shortest contig at value N50 was observed to be 22,797 (Figure 1).

An average GC content of 72.63% was observed in the isolate BR123, which is close to that of previously reported *Streptomyces* strains [24–26]. A total of 8103 protein coding sequences (CDS), 281 pseudo genes, 8 rRNA genes, and 68 tRNA genes were predicted through Rapid Annotation using Subsystem Technology (RAST) [27,28]. Table 1 provides the genomic characteristics of *Streptomyces* sp. BR123 in comparison to certain other available genomes of *Streptomyces* strains.

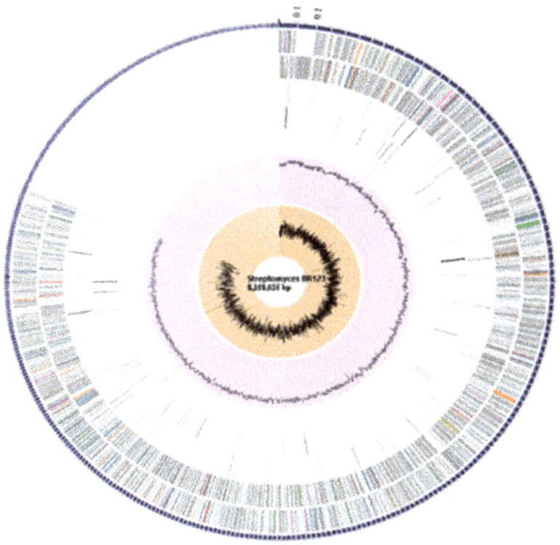

Figure 1. Circular map of the *Streptomyces* isolate BR123 genome, retrieved from PATRIC version 3.6.9. Description of each circle is given from outside in: CDS on the forward strand, CDS on the reverse strand, RNA genes, CDS with homology to known antimicrobial resistance genes, CDS with homology to known virulence factors, GC content, and GC skew.

Table 1. General genomic features of *Streptomyces* sp. isolate BR123 and other species used in this study.

Strain	Bio-Project Accession	Size (Mbps)	No. of Contigs	% G + C	CDS	tRNA	rRNA
Streptomyces sp. isolate BR123	PRJNA643667	8.16	723	72.63	8103	68	8
Streptomyces globosus LZH-48	PRJNA428275	7.54	-	73.62	6524	71	3
Streptomyces katrae NRRL ISP-5550	PRJNA238534	8.05	1874	72.69	7305	56	2
Streptomyces virginiae NRRL ISP-5094	PRJNA238534	8.32	133	72.4	7245	74	13
Streptomyces clavuligerus F1D7	PRJNA679926	7.59	-	72.5	6122	65	18
Streptomyces diastaticus NBRC 15402	PRJDB6184	7.85	32	72.7	-	75	8
Streptomyces bacillaris ATCC 15855	PRJNA471017	7.89	-	72.0	6746	65	18
Streptomyces cyaneofuscatus SID 10855	PRJNA603111	7.88	52	71.6	6755	66	12
Streptomyces griseus NBRC 13350	PRJDA20085	8.55	-	72.2	7087	67	18
Streptomyces lavendulae YAKB-15	PRJNA526603	7.77	100	72.2	7009	70	21

The taxonomic position of the *Streptomyces* sp. BR123 was determined within the genus *Streptomyces* (Supplementary Figure S2). Additional confirmation of this was performed by a genome-based phylogenetic analysis of the isolate BR123 in comparison with other *Streptomyces* strains [29,30]. *Streptomyces* sp. BR123 was closely branched with three other *Streptomyces* species and most closely branched with *Streptomyces globosus* (Figure 2).

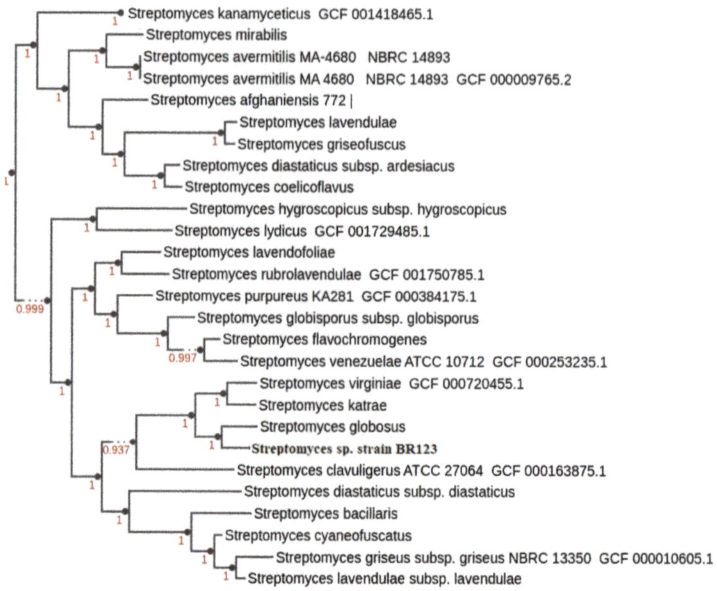

Figure 2. Whole genome-based tree of *Streptomyces* isolate BR123 with other *Streptomyces* strains, inferred using Kbase.

The relationship with other species was verified by average nucleotide identity (ANI) scores, based on a previously used strategy [31,32]. The ANI value between *Streptomyces* sp. BR123 and *Streptomyces globosus* was found to be the maximum (87.3066) compared to the other *Streptomyces* species (Table 2) and the alignment between the two strains was strong (Figure 3).

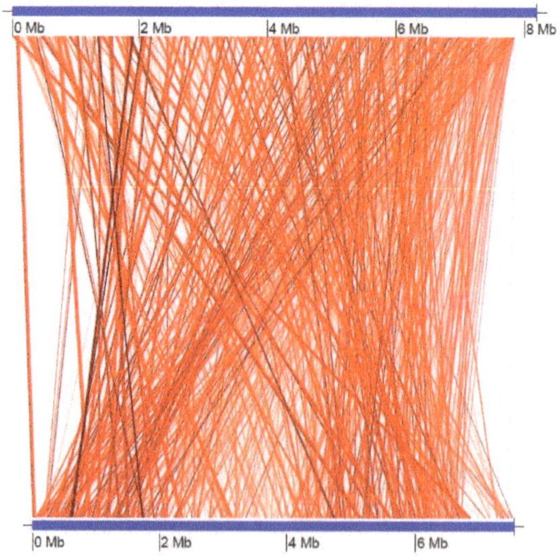

Figure 3. Genome alignment between *Streptomyces* isolate BR123 and *Streptomyces globosus*. Alignment was performed using the online KBase tool with default parameters. Synteny regions are represented by red lines, whereas breaks in synteny are the blank regions. Genome sizes are marked in the horizontal panels and conserved regions are linked.

Table 2. Average nucleotide identity (ANI) between all *Streptomyces* species used in this study.

Query	Reference	ANI Estimate	Matches	Total
Streptomyces lavendulae subsp. *lavendulae*	*Streptomyces* sp. isolate BR123	81.6134	1070	2300
Streptomyces sp. isolate BR123	*Streptomyces lavendulae* subsp. *lavendulae*	81.673	1050	2391
Streptomyces sp. isolate BR123	*Streptomyces virginiae*	86.0723	1576	2391
Streptomyces virginiae	*Streptomyces* sp. isolate BR123	86.0802	1554	2721
Streptomyces globosus	*Streptomyces* sp. isolate BR123	87.1686	1630	2510
Streptomyces sp. isolate BR123	*Streptomyces globosus*	87.3066	1626	2391
Streptomyces sp. isolate BR123	*Streptomyces katrae*	87.1854	1671	2391
Streptomyces katrae	*Streptomyces* sp. isolate BR123	87.2335	1635	2813

3.2. Annotation and Assembly of Genome Sequence

Automatic annotation performed by using the RAST server yielded 8038 features related to the protein coding genes. A total of 333 subsystems were identified using RAST genome analysis, which represented: the amino acid and derivative metabolism (448 ORFs); cofactors, vitamins, prosthetic groups, pigments (194 ORFs); and protein metabolism (236 ORFs). Ninety four open reading frames (ORFs) were involved in DNA metabolism, whereas 15 ORFs were found to code for secondary metabolites (Figure 4).

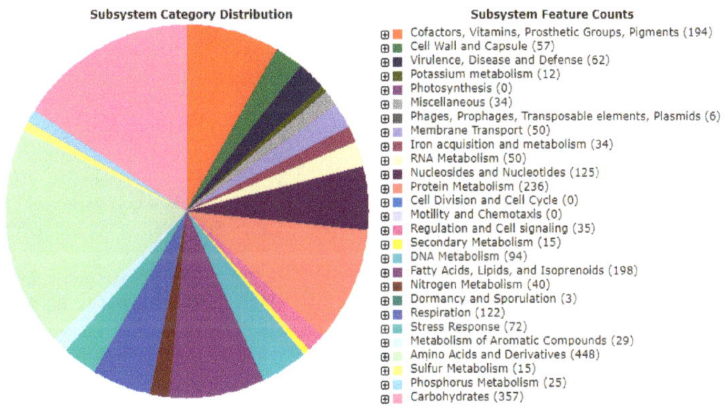

Figure 4. An overview of the subsystems for the genome of *Streptomyces* isolate BR123.

3.3. Biosynthetic Secondary Metabolite Gene Clusters of Streptomyces sp. BR123

About 70–80% of the total bioactive metabolites discovered so far relate to the genus *Streptomyces* [33]. Consequently, similar types of antimicrobial metabolites were found to be produced by *Streptomyces* strains, isolated from different environments [34]. Due to this de-duplication, rare actinobacteria have been targeted for the search of novel antimicrobial compounds [35]. The exploration of a genome-based biosynthetic potential of new isolates may be useful for finding novel compounds. In this study, a total of 44 clusters were identified in this strain, responsible for the production of secondary metabolites. This included 4 types of NRPS (nonribosomal peptide synthetase), 9 types of PKS (polyketide synthase), and 7 types of hybrid biosynthetic gene clusters. The hybrids featured melanin-terpene, lanthipeptide-3-NRPS, NRPS-transAT-PKS, T1 PKS-NRPS-like, T3 PKS-guanidinotides-RiPP-like, T1 PKS-NAPAA, and RRE-containing-thiopeptide. Most of the gene clusters detected in the isolate BR123 were related to polyketide biosynthesis. Out of the 44 biosynthetic gene clusters, 33 clusters represented differing percentages of resemblance with known BGCs, whereas 11 exhibited no similarity with known homologous gene clusters. The latter clusters were considered as orphan biosynthetic gene clusters [36] (Table 3). Particularly, the NRPS, NRPS-like, hybrid gene clusters, and majority of the peptide butyrolactone shared resemblance with antibacterial compounds, while most polyketides and other gene clusters shared similarity with anticancer and pigmented compounds. However, low degree of similarity was observed in most cases, suggesting the occurrence of possibly novel biosynthetic gene clusters [37,38].

Table 3. List of putative secondary metabolites producing biosynthetic gene clusters as predicted by antiSMASH.

Cluster	Size (bp)	Most Similar Known Biosynthetic Gene Cluster	MIBG BGC-ID
Siderophores:			
3	11,590	-	-
56	6349	-	-
226	8264	Desferrioxamin B (100%)	BGC0000941
261	8036	Ficellomycin (7%)	BGC0001593
279	6963	Ficellomycin (7%)	BGC0001593
Terpenes:			
9	16,885	-	-
11	21,676	Hopene (61%)	BGC0000663
16	21,086	-	-
19	13,165	-	-
24	25,408	Isorenieratene (63%)	BGC0001227
69	13,506	Ebelactone (5%)	BGC0001580
PKS:			
2 (Type I)	103,249	Concanamycin A (21%)	BGC0000040
4 (Type I)	46,281	Clifednamide A (30%)	BGC0001553
94 (Type I)	23,404	Tetrocarcin A (8%)	BGC0000162
129 (Type I)	19,401	-	-
320(Type I)	7593	-	-
350(Type I)	6899	-	-
58 (Type II)	34,290	Granaticin (16%)	BGC0000227
89 (Type III)	24,296	Alkylresorcinol (100%)	BGC0000282
338 (Type III)	7187	Flaviolin (75%)	BGC0000902
NRPS:			
104	23,007	Lactonamycin (5%)	BGC0000238
271	9618	Griseoviridin/Fijimycin A (8%)	BGC0000459
239	11,133	-	-
401	5437	Virginiamycin S1 (11%)	BGC0001116
Peptides:			
59 (Lanthipeptide class II)	13,149	-	-
76 (Lanthipeptide class I)	23,247	Chejuenolide A/Chejuenolide B (7%)	BGC0001543
Butyrolactones:			
100	6302	Griseoviridin/Fijimycin A (8%)	BGC0000459
NRPS/PKS-like:			
221 (NRPS-like)	12,004	Lipstatin (14%)	BGC0000382
429 (NRPS-like)	4493	Glycinocin A (4%)	BGC0000379
243 (PKS-like)	10,893	Virginiamycin S1 (33%)	BGC0001116
Hybrids:			
3 (Melanin, terpene)	33,435	Melanin (40%)	BGC0000909
29 (Lanthipeptide-3, NRPS)	43,146	Azicemicin (8%)	BGC0000202
46 (NRPS, transAT-PKS)	36,866	Virgimiamycin S1 (55%)	BGC0001116
62 (Type I PKS, NRPS-like)	29,119	Monensin (26%)	BGC0000100
98 (Type III PKS, guanidinotides, RiPP-like)	23,202	Pheganomycin (52%)	BGC0001148
149 (Type I PKS, NAPAA)			
433 (RRE-containing, thiopeptide)	17,747	Mediomycin A (34%)	BGC0001661
	4312	Lactazol (33%)	BGC0000606

The core structure of 15 clusters was predicted, which include 4 NRPS, 1 NRPS-like, 5 type I PKS, 1 PKS-like and 4 hybrid gene clusters. Moreover, a putative class II of lanthipeptide with a core peptide was also predicted (Supplementary File S1). Out of these clusters, 1 NRPS, 2 type-1 PKS, and the lanthipeptides were the orphan BGCs in *Streptomyces* sp. BR123 predicted by antiSMASH. The class II lanthipeptides are produced by the lanthionine synthase C (LanC) family protein that is present in cluster 59. Moreover, in the LanC enzyme of lanthipeptide class II, di-dehydroalanine (Dha) and di-dehydrobutyrine (Dhb) were well conserved.

Besides the core biosynthetic genes in *Streptomyces* isolate BR123, there were 10 clusters (clusters 9, 19, 24, 29, 40, 62, 89, 149, 183, 221) with transcription regulation and 8 clusters (clusters 11, 53, 76, 98, 157, 239, 279, 338) with transport genes, and there 7 clusters observed (clusters 3, 4, 16, 46, 59, 100, 104) with both transcription regulation and transport genes.

3.4. Detection of NRPS and PKS Genes in Streptomyces sp. BR123

The amplification and detection of NRPS and PKS genes via PCR further confirmed their presence in this *Streptomyces* strain (Supplementary Figure S3). *Streptomyces* sp. BR123 was also found to be active against a broad range of pathogenic microorganisms, including gram-positive and gram-negative bacteria and fungi. However, the activity was based on the media supplements used, and the maximum activity observed in the enrichment medium CSPY-ME resulted in the formation of the largest zone of inhibitions against some of the fungal and all of the tested bacterial strains. The maximum inhibitory effect was observed against *Bacillus* subtilis, showing a zone of inhibition with a diameter of 24.1 ± 0.12, followed by *E. coli* (23.5 ± 0.10) and *Aspergillus niger* (20.2 ± 0.08). No significant activities were observed in the ISP1 and ISP4 media (Supplementary Table S1), and the zone of inhibition in the ISP3 medium was only observed in Aspergillus niger (13.4 ± 0.05). Such a variation in activity could be due to different growth proportion in a minimal medium. Inhibition causes a greater effect in a minimal medium compared to a complex medium, where the medium's ingredients may compensate for the inhibitory effect of the product formation [39].

3.5. Production of Secondary Metabolites by Streptomyces sp. BR123

The production of various metabolites were verified through HPLC-MS [40–42]. A compound detected in the UV spectrum, with absorption maxima at 219 nm, 288 nm, and 369 nm, and a mass spectrum at positive ion mode with m/z ratio of 822.22 was identified as meridamycin, with a molecular mass of 821.5 (Figure 5).

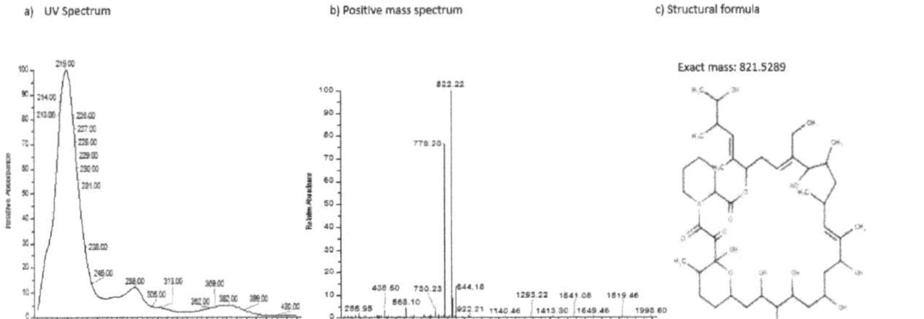

Figure 5. Characteristics of meridamycin, a metabolite observed from isolate BR123, calculated using HPLC-MS analysis. (**a**) The UV-visible spectrum; (**b**) the positive ion mass spectrum; and (**c**) the structural formula.

Meridamycin is a macrocyclic polyketide which possesses non-immunosuppressive, neuroprotective activity by acting on dopaminergic receptors and has been found to be suitable for the treatment of neurological diseases [43]. A small number of studies have reported the production of this compound from the genus *Streptomyces* during the last few years [43,44], and evidence on the presence of the biosynthetic pathway of this compound in *Streptomyces* sp. DSM 4137 has been published [44]. Moreover, various therapeutically important metabolites analogous to meridamycin have also been previously identified [45]. Another compound with absorbance maxima at 221 nm, 333 nm, and 351 nm and a molecular mass of 1271 at positive ion mode (Figure 6) was also observed. Upon library screening, it was observed to not correspond with any known compound, thus further characterization is required. The compound analysis of *Streptomyces* sp. BR123 indicated the potential of this strain as a candidate for the production of novel secondary metabolites.

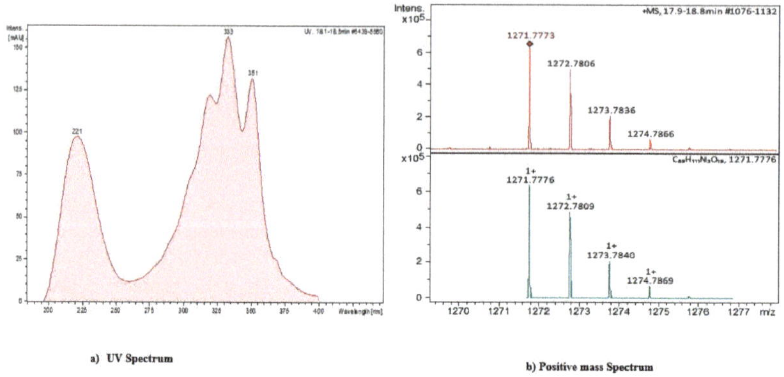

Figure 6. Characteristics of unidentified metabolite from the *Streptomyces* isolate BR123 based on (**a**) UV spectrum; (**b**) HPLC-MS analysis.

4. Conclusions

Due to the development of multi-drug resistance (MDR) by emerging pathogens against the available antibiotics, there is a dire need to find new sources of antibiotics. The genus *Streptomyces* has massively contributed to the field of medicine through the synthesis of antibacterial, antifungal, antiparasitic, and anticancerous compounds. In the current study, we explored an indigenously isolated potent bioactive *Streptomyces* strain, and added another draft genome sequence to the rising number of *Streptomyces* sequences in the repository. Moreover, a few already known compounds in addition to some new and uncharacterized compounds were also detected using the HPLC-MS technique. This genome insight study of *Streptomyces* sp. BR123 and the information about the biosynthetic clusters of some uncharacterized natural compounds may prove to be a valuable addition to prior knowledge, assisting in the search for novel compounds as well as providing the much-needed structural diversity required for a new generation of antibiotics designed for pathogens with MDR.

Supplementary Materials: The following supporting information can be downloaded at https://www.mdpi.com/article/10.3390/antibiotics11081057/s1, Figure S1: A plot representing the number of contigs of the *Streptomyces* sp. BR123 genome with the GC percentage in a certain range; Figure S2: The phylogenetic tree of *Streptomyces* isolate BR123 and other *Streptomyces* species based on 16S rRNA sequences; Figure S3: PCR-based identification of NRPS and PKS genes in isolate BR123. (a) NRPS (b) PKS-I (c) PKS-II; File S1: Biosynthetic gene clusters predicted by antiSMASH and their core structures; Table S1: Antimicrobial activity of *Streptomyces* strain BR123 in different growth media.

Author Contributions: N.A. conducted research, composed the first draft, and edited it; S.Z. partially contributed in experimental procedures and writing of manuscript; R.M. contributed in experiment design and conducting LCMS; A.B. assisted in methodology, data quality and editing; D.S. analyzed the data and helped in sequencing; L.S. helped in interpretation of LCMS data; M.A.A. worked on the manuscript's investigation and editing; A.L. assisted in the formal analysis, revision, and editing of the manuscript; A.N.K. was involved in the development and analysis of the approach; final reviewing and editing was all done by K.A.; S.K. supervised the entailed conception, project administration, resource provision, writing, reviewing, and editing. All authors have read and agreed to the published version of the manuscript.

Funding: This research received no external funding.

Institutional Review Board Statement: Not applicable.

Informed Consent Statement: Informed consent was obtained from all subjects involved in the study.

Data Availability Statement: https://www.ncbi.nlm.nih.gov/assembly/GCF_013401435.1/ (10 July 2020).

Acknowledgments: We acknowledge "Zukunftskolleg" for funding and supporting the current research by providing "ZUKOnnect Fellowship". We also acknowledge the University of Konstanz for providing the scientific environment and facilities needed for the research. We thank Mi-crobesNG for their genome sequencing services.

Conflicts of Interest: Authors have no conflict of interest to declare.

References

1. Jakubiec-Krzesniak, K.; Rajnisz-Mateusiak, A.; Guspiel, A.; Ziemska, J.; Solecka, J. Secondary metabolites of actinomycetes and their antibacterial, antifungal and antiviral properties. *Pol. J. Microbiol.* **2018**, *67*, 259–272. [CrossRef] [PubMed]
2. Falzone, M.; Crespo, E.; Jones, K.; Khan, G.; Korn, V.L.; Patel, A.; Patel, M.; Patel, K.; Perkins, C.; Siddiqui, S.; et al. Nutritional control of antibiotic production by *Streptomyces platensis* MA7327: Importance of L-aspartic acid. *J. Antibiot.* **2017**, *70*, 828–831. [CrossRef] [PubMed]
3. Quinn, G.A.; Banat, A.M.; Abdelhameed, A.M.; Banat, I.M. *Streptomyces* from traditional medicine: Sources of new innovations in antibiotic discovery. *J. Med. Microbiol.* **2020**, *69*, 1040–1048. [CrossRef] [PubMed]
4. Metsämuuronen, S.; Sirén, H. Bioactive phenolic compounds, metabolism and properties: A review on valuable chemical compounds in Scots pine and Norway spruce. *Phytochem. Rev.* **2019**, *18*, 623–664. [CrossRef]
5. Park, S.R.; Yoon, Y.J.; Pham, J.V.; Yilma, M.A.; Feliz, A.; Majid, M.T.; Maffetone, N.; Walker, J.R.; Kim, E.; Reynolds, J.M. A review of the microbial production of bioactive natural products and biologics. *Front. Microbiol.* **2019**, *10*, 1404.
6. Dholakiya, R.N.; Kumar, R.; Mishra, A.; Mody, K.H.; Jha, B. Antibacterial and antioxidant activities of novel actinobacteria strain isolated from Gulf of Khambhat, Gujarat. *Front. Microbiol.* **2017**, *8*, 2420. [CrossRef]
7. Das, R.; Romi, W.; Das, R.; Sharma, H.K.; Thakur, D. Antimicrobial potentiality of actinobacteria isolated from two microbiologically unexplored forest ecosystems of Northeast India. *BMC Microbiol.* **2018**, *18*, 71. [CrossRef]
8. Guerrero-Garzón, J.F.; Zehl, M.; Schneider, O.; Rückert, C.; Busche, T.; Kalinowski, J.; Bredholt, H.; Zotchev, S.B. *Streptomyces* spp. from the marine sponge Antho dichotoma: Analyses of secondary metabolite biosynthesis gene clusters and some of their products. *Front. Microbiol.* **2020**, *11*, 437. [CrossRef]
9. Ziemert, N.; Lechner, A.; Wietz, M.; Millán-Aguiñaga, N.; Chavarria, K.L.; Jensen, P.R. Diversity and evolution of secondary metabolism in the marine actinomycete genus Salinispora. *Proc. Natl. Acad. Sci. USA* **2014**, *111*, E1130–E1139. [CrossRef]
10. Komaki, H.; Sakurai, K.; Hosoyama, A.; Kimura, A.; Igarashi, Y.; Tamura, T. Diversity of nonribosomal peptide synthetase and polyketide synthase gene clusters among taxonomically close *Streptomyces* strains. *Sci. Rep.* **2018**, *8*, 6888. [CrossRef]
11. Xu, L.; Ye, K.-X.; Dai, W.-H.; Sun, C.; Xu, L.-H.; Han, B.-N. Comparative Genomic Insights into Secondary Metabolism Biosynthetic Gene Cluster Distributions of Marine *Streptomyces*. *Mar. Drugs* **2019**, *17*, 498. [CrossRef]
12. Betancur, L.A.; Forero, A.M.; Vinchira-Villarraga, D.M.; Cardenas, J.D.; Romero-Otero, A.; Chagas, F.O.; Pupo, M.T.; Castellanos, L.; Ramos, F.A. NMR-based metabolic profiling to follow the production of anti-phytopathogenic compounds in the culture of the marine strain *Streptomyces* sp. PNM-9. *Microbiol. Res.* **2020**, *239*, 126507. [CrossRef]
13. Rebets, Y.; Brötz, E.; Tokovenko, B.; Luzhetskyy, A. Actinomycetes biosynthetic potential: How to bridge in silico and in vivo? *J. Ind. Microbiol. Biotechnol.* **2014**, *41*, 387–402. [CrossRef]
14. Ziemert, N.; Alanjary, M.; Weber, T. The evolution of genome mining in microbes—A review. *Nat. Prod. Rep.* **2016**, *33*, 988–1005. [CrossRef]
15. Lacey, H.J.; Rutledge, P.J. Recently discovered secondary metabolites from *Streptomyces* species. *Molecules* **2022**, *27*, 887. [CrossRef]
16. Mohseni, M.; Norouzi, H.; Hamedi, J.; Roohi, A. Screening of antibacterial producing actinomycetes from sediments of the Caspian Sea. *Int. J. Mol. Cell. Med.* **2013**, *2*, 64–71.
17. Ashraf, N.; Bechthold, A.; Anwar, M.A.; Ghauri, M.A.; Anjum, M.S.; Khan, A.N.; Akhtar, K.; Khaliq, S. Production of a broad spectrum streptothricin like antibiotic from halotolerant *Streptomyces fimbriatus* isolate G1 associated with marine sediments. *Folia Microbiol.* **2021**, *66*, 639–649. [CrossRef]
18. Ashraf, N.; Bechthold, A.; Anwar, M.A.; Khaliq, S. Draft Genome Sequence of *Streptomyces* sp. Strain BR123, Endowed with Broad-Spectrum Antimicrobial Potential. *Microbiol. Resour. Announc.* **2020**, *9*, e00972-20. [CrossRef]
19. Akhtar, N.; Ghauri, M.A.; Akhtar, K.; Parveen, S.; Farooq, M.; Ali, A.; Schierack, P. Comparative analysis of draft genome sequence of *Rhodococcus* sp. Eu-32 with other *Rhodococcus* species for its taxonomic status and sulfur metabolism potential. *Curr. Microbiol.* **2019**, *76*, 1207–1214. [CrossRef]
20. Escalante-Réndiz, D.; de-la-Rosa-García, S.; Tapia-Tussell, R.; Martín, J.; Reyes, F.; Vicente, F.; Gamboa-Angulo, M. Molecular identification of selected *Streptomyces* strains isolated from Mexican tropical soils and their anti-Candida activity. *Int. J. Environ. Res. Public Health* **2019**, *16*, 1913. [CrossRef]

21. Asma Azmani, A.; Lemriss, S.; Barakate, M.; Souiri, A.; Dhiba, D.; Hassani, L.; Hamdali, H. Screening and characterization of *Streptomyces* spp. isolated from three moroccan ecosystems producing a potential. *BioTech* **2022**, *11*, 22. [CrossRef] [PubMed]
22. Chaves, J.V.; Ojeda, C.P.O.; da Silva, I.; de Lima Procopio, R. Identification and Phylogeny of *Streptomyces* Based on Gene Sequences. *Res. J. Microbiol.* **2017**, *13*, 13–20.
23. Jain, C.; Rodriguez-R, L.M.; Phillippy, A.M.; Konstantinidis, K.T.; Aluru, S. High throughput ANI analysis of 90 K prokaryotic genomes reveals clear species boundaries. *Nat. Commun.* **2018**, *9*, 5114. [CrossRef] [PubMed]
24. Gomez-Escribano, J.P.; Castro, J.F.; Razmilic, V.; Chandra, G.; Andrews, B.; Asenjo, J.A.; Bibb, M.J. The *Streptomyces leeuwenhoekii* genome: De novo sequencing and assembly in single contigs of the chromosome, circular plasmid pSLE1 and linear plasmid pSLE2. *BMC Genom.* **2015**, *16*, 485. [CrossRef]
25. Subramaniam, G.; Thakur, V.; Saxena, R.K.; Vadlamudi, S.; Purohit, S.; Kumar, V.; Rathore, A.; Chitikineni, A.; Varshney, R.K. Complete genome sequence of sixteen plant growth promoting *Streptomyces* strains. *Sci. Rep.* **2020**, *10*, 10294. [CrossRef]
26. Wang, C.; Wang, Y.; Ma, J.; Hou, Q.; Liu, K.; Ding, Y.; Du, B. Screening and whole-genome sequencing of two *Streptomyces* species from the rhizosphere soil of peony reveal their characteristics as plant growth-promoting rhizobacteria. *BioMed Res. Int.* **2018**, *2018*, 2419686. [CrossRef]
27. Ser, H.-L.; Tan, W.-S.; Ab Mutalib, N.-S.; Yin, W.-F.; Chan, K.-G.; Goh, B.-H.; Lee, L.-H. Genome sequence of *Streptomyces mangrovisoli* MUSC 149T isolated from intertidal sediments. *Braz. J. Microbiol.* **2018**, *49*, 13–15. [CrossRef]
28. Franco, C.M.; Adetutu, E.M.; Le, H.X.; Ballard, R.A.; Araujo, R.; Tobe, S.S.; Paul, B.; Mallya, S.; Satyamoorthy, K. Complete genome sequences of the endophytic *Streptomyces* sp. strains LUP30 and LUP47B, isolated from lucerne plants. *Genome Announc.* **2017**, *5*, e00556-17. [CrossRef]
29. Alam, M.T.; Merlo, M.E.; Takano, E.; Breitling, R. Genome-based phylogenetic analysis of *Streptomyces* and its relatives. *Mol. Phylogenet. Evol.* **2010**, *54*, 763–772. [CrossRef]
30. Heinsch, S.C.; Hsu, S.-Y.; Otto-Hanson, L.; Kinkel, L.; Smanski, M.J. Complete genome sequences of *Streptomyces* spp. isolated from disease-suppressive soils. *BMC Genom.* **2019**, *20*, 994. [CrossRef]
31. Majer, H.M.; Ehrlich, R.L.; Ahmed, A.; Earl, J.P.; Ehrlich, G.D.; Beld, J. Whole genome sequencing of *Streptomyces actuosus* ISP-5337, *Streptomyces sioyaensis* B-5408, and Actinospica acidiphila B-2296 reveals secondary metabolomes with antibiotic potential. *Biotechnol. Rep.* **2021**, *29*, e00596. [CrossRef]
32. Vicente, C.M.; Thibessard, A.; Lorenzi, J.-N.; Benhadj, M.; Hôtel, L.; Gacemi-Kirane, D.; Lespinet, O.; Leblond, P.; Aigle, B. Comparative genomics among closely related *Streptomyces* strains revealed specialized metabolite biosynthetic gene cluster diversity. *Antibiotics* **2018**, *7*, 86. [CrossRef]
33. Qian, P.-Y.; Li, Z.; Xu, Y.; Li, Y.; Fusetani, N. Mini-review: Marine natural products and their synthetic analogs as antifouling compounds: 2009–2014. *Biofouling* **2015**, *31*, 101–122. [CrossRef]
34. Matsumoto, A.; Takahashi, Y. Endophytic actinomycetes: Promising source of novel bioactive compounds. *J. Antibiot.* **2017**, *70*, 514–519. [CrossRef]
35. Demain, A.L. Importance of microbial natural products and the need to revitalize their discovery. *J. Ind. Microbiol. Biotechnol.* **2014**, *41*, 185–201. [CrossRef]
36. Malik, A.; Kim, Y.R.; Jang, I.H.; Hwang, S.; Oh, D.-C.; Kim, S.B. Genome-based analysis for the bioactive potential of *Streptomyces yeochonensis* CN732, an acidophilic filamentous soil actinobacterium. *BMC Genom.* **2020**, *21*, 118. [CrossRef]
37. Siupka, P.; Hansen, F.T.; Schier, A.; Rocco, S.; Sørensen, T.; Seget, Z.P. Antifungal activity and biosynthetic potential of new *Streptomyces* sp. MW-W600-10 strain isolated from coal mine water. *Int. J. Mol. Sci.* **2021**, *22*, 7441. [CrossRef]
38. Peña, A.; Del Carratore, F.; Cummings, M.; Takano, E.; Breitling, R. Output ordering and prioritisation system (OOPS): Ranking biosynthetic gene clusters to enhance bioactive metabolite discovery. *J. Ind. Microbiol. Biotechnol.* **2018**, *45*, 615–619. [CrossRef]
39. Davis, K.E.R.; Joseph, S.J.; Janssen, P.H. Effects of Growth Medium, Inoculum Size, and Incubation Time on Culturability and Isolation of Soil Bacteria. *Appl. Environ. Microbiol.* **2005**, *71*, 826–834. [CrossRef]
40. Čihák, M.; Kameník, Z.; Šmídová, K.; Bergman, N.; Benada, O.; Kofroňová, O.; Petříčková, K.; Bobek, J. Secondary metabolites produced during the germination of *Streptomyces coelicolor*. *Front. Microbiol.* **2017**, *8*, 2495. [CrossRef]
41. Lu, L.; Wang, J.; Xu, Y.; Wang, K.; Hu, Y.; Tian, R.; Yang, B.; Lai, Q.; Li, Y.; Zhang, W. A high-resolution LC-MS-based secondary metabolite fingerprint database of marine bacteria. *Sci. Rep.* **2014**, *4*, 6537. [CrossRef] [PubMed]
42. Tangerina, M.M.; Furtado, L.C.; Leite, V.M.; Bauermeister, A.; Velasco-Alzate, K.; Jimenez, P.C.; Garrido, L.M.; Padilla, G.; Lopes, N.P.; Costa-Lotufo, L.V.; et al. Metabolomic study of marine *Streptomyces* sp.: Secondary metabolites and the production of potential anticancer compounds. *PLoS ONE* **2020**, *15*, e0244385. [CrossRef] [PubMed]
43. He, M.; Haltli, B.; Summers, M.; Feng, X.; Hucul, J. Isolation and characterization of meridamycin biosynthetic gene cluster from *Streptomyces* sp. NRRL 30748. *Gene* **2006**, *377*, 109–118. [CrossRef] [PubMed]
44. Sun, Y.; Hong, H.; Samborskyy, M.; Mironenko, T.; Leadlay, P.F.; Haydock, S.F. Organization of the biosynthetic gene cluster in *Streptomyces* sp. DSM 4137 for the novel neuroprotectant polyketide meridamycin. *Microbiology* **2006**, *152*, 3507–3515.
45. Liu, M.; Lu, C.; Shen, Y. Four New Meridamycin Congeners *Streptomyces* sp. SR107. *RSC Adv.* **2016**, *6*, 49792–49796. [CrossRef]

antibiotics

MDPI

Review

Bioactive Peptides against Human Apicomplexan Parasites

Norma Rivera-Fernández [1,*], Jhony Anacleto-Santos [1], Brenda Casarrubias-Tabarez [2,3], Teresa de Jesús López-Pérez [1], Marcela Rojas-Lemus [2], Nelly López-Valdez [2] and Teresa I. Fortoul [2]

1 Departamento de Microbiología y Parasitología, Facultad de Medicina, Universidad Nacional Autónoma de México (UNAM), Ciudad Universitaria, Mexico City 04510, Mexico
2 Departamento de Biología Celular y Tisular, Facultad de Medicina, Universidad Nacional Autónoma de México (UNAM), Ciudad Universitaria, Mexico City 04510, Mexico
3 Posgrado en Ciencias Biológicas, Universidad Nacional Autónoma de México (UNAM), Ciudad Universitaria, Mexico City 04510, Mexico
* Correspondence: normariv@unam.mx

Abstract: Apicomplexan parasites are the causal agents of different medically important diseases, such as toxoplasmosis, cryptosporidiosis, and malaria. Toxoplasmosis is considered a neglected parasitosis, even though it can cause severe cerebral complications and death in immunocompromised patients, including children and pregnant women. Drugs against *Toxoplasma gondii*, the etiological agent of toxoplasmosis, are highly toxic and lack efficacy in eradicating tissue cysts, promoting the establishment of latent infection and acute relapsing disease. Cryptosporidiosis has been recognized as the most frequent waterborne parasitosis in US outbreaks; anti-cryptosporidium drug discovery still faces a major obstacle: drugs that can act on the epicellular parasite. Severe malaria is most commonly caused by the progression of infection with *Plasmodium falciparum*. In recent years, great progress has been made in the field of antimalarial drugs and vaccines, although the resistance of *P. falciparum* to artemisinin has recently gained a foothold in Africa. As seen, the search for new drugs against these parasites remains a challenge. Peptide-based drugs seem to be attractive alternative therapeutic agents recently recognized by the pharmaceutical industry, as they can kill different infectious agents and modulate the immune response. A review of the experimental effects of bioactive peptides on these parasites follows, along with comments. In addition, some biological and metabolomic generalities of the parasites are reviewed to elucidate peptide mechanisms of action on Apicomplexan targets.

Keywords: Apicomplexan; bioactive peptides; toxoplasmosis; cryptosporidiosis; malaria

Citation: Rivera-Fernández, N.; Anacleto-Santos, J.; Casarrubias-Tabarez, B.; López-Pérez, T.d.J.; Rojas-Lemus, M.; López-Valdez, N.; Fortoul, T.I. Bioactive Peptides against Human Apicomplexan Parasites. *Antibiotics* **2022**, *11*, 1658. https://doi.org/10.3390/antibiotics11111658

Academic Editors: Agostinho Antunes, Guillermin Agüero-Chapin and Yovani Marrero-Ponce

Received: 10 October 2022
Accepted: 16 November 2022
Published: 19 November 2022

Publisher's Note: MDPI stays neutral with regard to jurisdictional claims in published maps and institutional affiliations.

Copyright: © 2022 by the authors. Licensee MDPI, Basel, Switzerland. This article is an open access article distributed under the terms and conditions of the Creative Commons Attribution (CC BY) license (https://creativecommons.org/licenses/by/4.0/).

1. Introduction

Parasitism is a biological interaction present in nature. Some parasites can cause a severe clinical picture, and others can even cause host death. Millions of people are infected by parasites worldwide, mainly in lower- and middle-income countries. Among the most important human parasites are single-cell protozoan organisms, which are divided into different phyla [1,2]. The protozoan phylum Apicomplexa is a large group of intracellular alveolates; its name is derived from the complex of organelles located at the apical end that allow them to survive in the host cell. Apicomplexan parasites cause important infectious diseases in humans, including malaria, toxoplasmosis, and cryptosporidiosis [3]. Some intestinal coccidian infections and toxoplasmosis are considered by the World Health Organization (WHO), neglecting parasitosis; therefore, they are not a priority for pharmaceuticals to invest in the research of new compounds for their control, and malaria is one of the most dangerous infections that caused approximately 627,000 human deaths in 2020 [4]. Anti-*Toxoplasma* drugs are highly toxic and ineffective in destroying tissue cysts, and cryptosporidiosis treatments are partially effective mostly in immunocompromised patients. Despite antimalarial drug research on the development of novel treatments, the emergence of strains resistant to first-line drugs is increasing; therefore, new alternatives are necessary [5,6]. Based on this background, a search for active molecules is needed. Drug development against these parasites has been approached from different perspectives, including in silico models, hybrid compound design, bio-guided studies in natural products, and even the use of combined therapies with known antibiotic drugs [7].

An interesting emerging category of active molecules is antimicrobial peptides (AMPs), which are attractive alternative therapeutic agents. Peptides are a diverse group of proteins of 10–100 amino acid residues. They have amphipathic structures, contain up to 50% hydrophobic residues, and possess a net positive charge of +2 to +9 [8]. AMPs are found naturally in tissues and cells from multicellular organisms and play a crucial role in the innate immune response to protect themselves since these organisms do not develop an adaptive immune system such as vertebrates. The interest in these compounds is due to their biochemical features that can interfere with ion channels and structural components of the cell membrane [9,10]. The first AMP was identified in mid-1990 from *Drosophila melanogaster;* at the time of this writing, at least 5000 AMPs have been reported [11,12].

The applications of AMPs are still under constant investigation, and in the last decade, their interesting antibacterial drug resistance, anticancer, anti-inflammatory, immunomodulatory, and antiparasitic activities have been reported [13–15]. However, the clinical application of AMPs has been limited due to the toxicity and stability of these molecules and other drawbacks, such as high production costs compared to conventional antibiotics. Although there are no commercial AMP products to date, we cannot ignore the great potential of AMPs. These molecules offer great alternatives due to their results in in vitro models [16,17].

In this review, we provide an in-depth overview of the main Apicomplexan human parasites and AMPs with antiparasitic activity, as well as their mechanisms of action.

1.1. Toxoplasmosis

This parasitic infection is caused by *Toxoplasma gondii,* an obligate intracellular distributed worldwide that infects a wide range of homothermic animals, including humans [18,19]. It is recognized as the main public health problem in human and veterinary medicine and is one of the five neglected parasitic infections cited by the WHO. *T. gondii* sexual reproduction involves species from the Felidae family, including domestic cats [20]. *T. gondii* affect approximately one-third of the human population, and climate change is increasing its prevalence of infection [21,22]. Epidemiological studies worldwide revealed that the prevalence in pregnant women is approximately 1.1% and could be related to cultural habits, such as eating undercooked meat (one of the main risk factors for *T. gondii* infection), especially of pork, lamb, or venison [23–25]. Humans can also be infected by eating raw shellfish (like oysters, clams, and mussels), by accidental ingestion of oocysts in contaminated soil, or by congenital transmission [25].

The toxoplasmosis incubation period is 10 to 14 days, and 90% of cases are asymptomatic. In symptomatic individuals, lymphadenitis, lymphadenopathy, fever, sore throat, headache, and myalgia have been reported [26]. The presence of hepatosplenomegaly, pulmonary or cardiac symptoms, conjunctivitis, and skin rash were recorded. Clinical manifestations are generally self-limited within 3–4 weeks. In immunocompetent individuals, neurological symptoms rarely occur; in some exceptional cases, moderate cognitive impairment has been reported [26]. In immunocompromised people with toxoplasmosis, parasites have a predilection for immune privilege sites, and extensive cell lesions are present, which can lead to encephalitis, retinochoroiditis, pericarditis, interstitial pneumonia, and Guillain-Barre syndrome. Encephalitis is an important clinical manifestation, especially in patients with AIDS, and congenital infections can lead to death [27].

In the biological life cycle of *T. gondii,* four parasitic forms are involved: tachyzoites, bradyzoites, tissue cysts, and oocysts. Definitive hosts ingest prey infected with tissue cysts, mainly in the skeletal muscle or brain. Due to digestive action, the bradyzoites contained in the tissue cysts invade the enterocytes and, through schizogony replication, differentiate into macro- and microgametes. Subsequently, fertilization takes place, which gives rise to a zygote. This zygote transforms into an immature, noninfectious oocyst that is released into the environment along with the host's feces. The noninfecting oocyst sporulates and becomes infective, and contaminates water, soil, and food in favorable environmental conditions. Intermediate hosts (i.e., warm-blooded animals, including humans) become infected through the consumption of water and food contaminated with sporulated oocysts or raw or undercooked meat with tissue cysts. Oocysts and tissue cysts release sporozoites and bradyzoites, respectively, and differentiate into tachyzoites within the intestinal epithelium. After replication, the tachyzoites exit the cell, destroying it, and the infection spreads to neighboring cells. The immune response will eliminate most parasites; those that are not removed will become bradyzoites and will form tissue cysts that can remain in the host's organs and tissues throughout life (chronic infection). In immunocompromised individuals, bradyzoites differentiate back to tachyzoites, causing severe or fatal acute disseminated infection [18,28,29] (Figure 1).

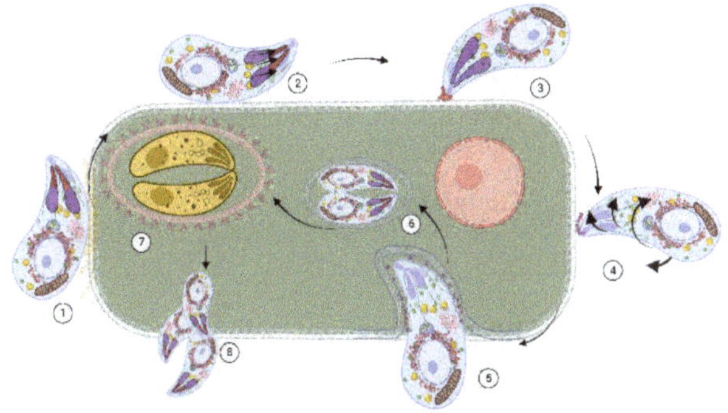

Figure 1. Active invasion of *T. gondii*. In Apicomplexan, three types of secretory organelles are observed: micronemes, rhoptries, and dense granules, carrying characteristic proteins. Attachment to host cell membrane via micronemes (MIC) proteins (**1**). Invasion and moving junction development by secretion of proteins from rhoptries neck (RON) and rhoptires (ROP) (**2**,**3**). Internalization via secretion of RON/AMA proteins (**4**). Parasitophorous vacuole development via granule dense proteins (GRA) (**5**). Proliferation and tachyzoite asexual replication (**6**). Increases immune response, interconversion to bradyzoite, and tissue cyst formation (**7**). Decreases immune response, interconversion to bradyzoites-tachyzoites, and dissemination of the parasite (**8**). Tachyzoites cause acute infection, leading to severe toxoplasmosis. While several drugs are available against tachyzoites, there is no treatment against tissue cysts, which are responsible for chronic infection. An ideal anti-*Toxoplasma* drug should be effective against both stages and prevent interconversion. Protein targeting secretory organelles is a matter of interest. Created with BioRender.com under license to publish by Anacleto SJ.

A combination of dihydrofolate reductase inhibitors such as pyrimethamine and trimethoprim, and dihydropteroate synthetase inhibitors (sulfonamides) are currently used as the first-choice treatment for toxoplasmosis; nevertheless, drug-resistant strains have been reported. It is worth mentioning that in the last decade, more than 50 resistant strains were identified and have developed resistance mainly to sulfonamides [30,31]. In addition to this, the presence of adverse effects and the fact that treatments are only effective in the acute phase of infection, turn out necessary to have new alternatives to treatment that are safe, effective, affordable, and active against the tissue cysts. For this reason, the recent emergence of AMPs offers wide potential for the discovery of new anti-*Toxoplasma* drugs. In Figure 2, drugs that have been tested against *Toxoplasma* are described.

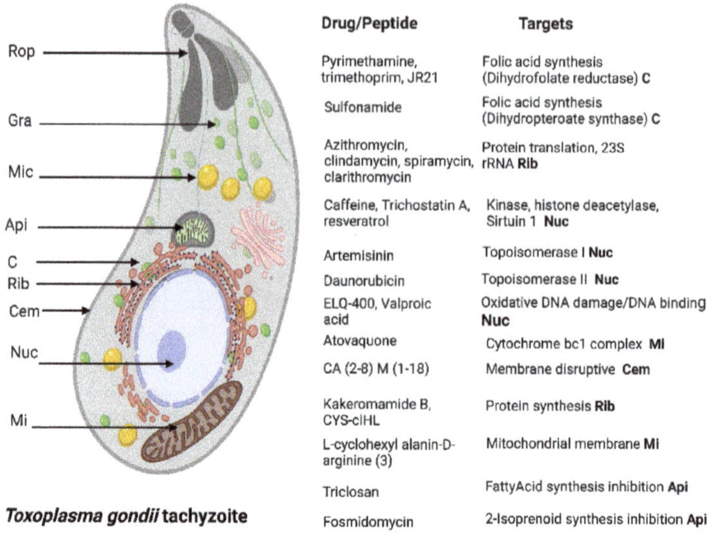

Figure 2. *T. gondii* tachyzoite drug targets. Rop, rohptry. Gra, dense granule. Mic micronemes. Api, apicoplast. C, cytoplasm. Cem, cell membrane. Rib, ribosome. Nuc, nucleus. Mi, mitochondrion. Created with BioRender.com under license to publish by Anacleto SJ.

1.2. Cryptosporidiosis

Cryptosporidium spp. is an important public health problem currently recognized as the main cause of diarrhea in humans and farm animals, causing significant morbidity and mortality worldwide, mainly in children. Approximately 40 species have been described in the *Cryptosporidium* genus. Two species are the most common, *Cryptosporidium hominis* and *C. parvum*, both of which can infect humans. *C. parvum* also infects cattle [32,33]. In low-income countries, 54% of children have had diarrhea associated with cryptosporidiosis. Children and immunocompromised patients are the most vulnerable groups to *Cryptosporidium* infections. It is estimated that two million children die worldwide annually, and 7 million cases are associated with morbidity in Asian and African populations [34]. In the last seventeen years, the incidence of *Cryptosporidium* infection in HIV-positive patients has increased up to 41.3% in Russia [35].

Cryptosporidium incubation period takes a week after the ingestion of infective oocysts. The clinical manifestations include diarrhea, fever, nausea, vomiting, abdominal pain, general malaise, and malnutrition. Chronic diarrhea in HIV patients is recognized as a classical clinical manifestation, and severe dehydration, weight loss, and malnutrition that can lead to death have been observed [36,37].

There are different parasitic stages in the life cycle of *Cryptosporidium* spp.: oocysts, sporozoites, trophozoites, and merozoites. The oocyst is the infective stage and can be consumed in contaminated water or food. Four sporozoites are contained inside each oocyst and are released by digestive processes in the intestinal epithelium. A schizogonic division takes place, resulting in the production of eight merozoites (type I merozoites), which reinvade new cells, and after a period of intracellular growth (type II merozoite), merozoites differentiate into micro and macrogametocytes that lead to fertilization and zygote formation. Mature zygotes develop into infective thin or thick-walled oocysts that are released from enterocytes. Infective thin-walled oocysts are broken in the intestine and lead to reinfections, while infective thick-walled oocysts are released into the environment through feces, contaminating water, soil, and food [38–41] (Figure 3).

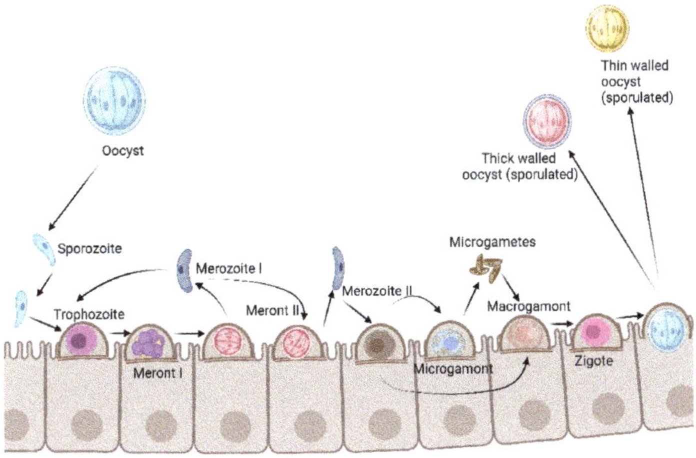

Figure 3. *Cryptosporidium* spp. development in the host cell. Anti-cryptosporidial drug development challenges a major problem: the discovery of systemic drugs that can reach epicellular parasites (preventing schizogonic reproduction); and the absorption by patients undergoing diarrhea. Created with BioRender.com under license to publish by Anacleto SJ.

Only nitazoxanide has demonstrated efficacy in human cryptosporidiosis. A number of new targets have been identified for chemotherapy, and progress has been made in developing drugs for these targets (Figure 4).

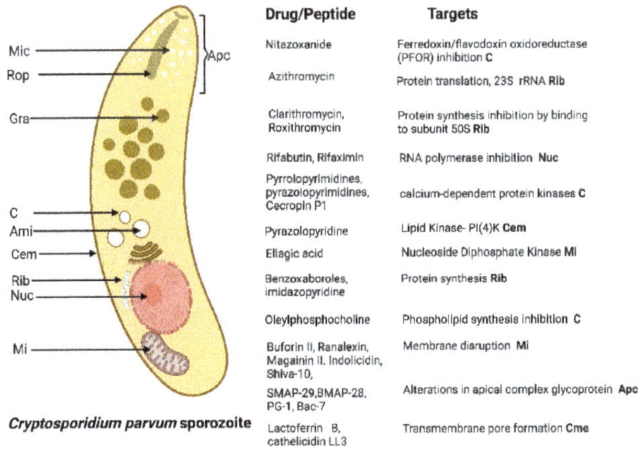

Figure 4. *Cryptosporidium* drug targets. *Cryptosporodium* lacks many drug targets present in other Apicomplexans because of a simplified metabolism and the absence of de novo nutrient synthetic pathways. Mic micronemes. Rop, rohptry. Gra, dense ganule. Apc, apical complex. C, cytoplasm. Ami, amylopectin granules. Cem, cell membrane. Rib, ribosome. Nuc, nucleus. Mi, mitochondrion. Created with BioRender.com under license to publish by Anacleto SJ.

1.3. Malaria

Malaria is a parasitic disease considered a major public health problem because it causes a great number of morbidity and mortality cases, mostly in tropical and subtropical zones worldwide. In 2020, 241 million malaria cases were reported, and 627,000 deaths occurred, which represented a substantial increase compared to what was reported in 2019 [42]. Malaria is caused by *Plasmodium* parasites, which are intracellular Parasites transmitted mainly by the bite of female mosquitoes of the genus *Anopheles*. There are more than 120 *Plasmodium* species capable of infecting mammals, birds, and reptiles; nevertheless, only five species can infect humans, *P. malariae*, *P. falciparum*, *P. knowlesi*, *P. ovale*, and *P. vivax* [43,44].

In humans, parasites replicate asexually, while sexual reproduction takes place in *Anopheles* mosquitoes. Sporozoites injected by the *Anopheles* mosquito while feeding, reach the liver through the bloodstream and invade hepatocytes forming merozoites [45]. In the liver, *P. ovale* and *P. vivax* sporozoites can convert into hypnozoites, which are dormant forms that can relapse months or years later [44]. After liver parasite replication, merozoites are released into the bloodstream, and the intraerythrocytic cycle begins, in which rings, trophozoites, schizonts, merozoites, and gametocytes are developed [43]. Gametocytes are ingested by *Anopheles* mosquitos, and the cycle begins again. In the midgut of the mosquito, gametocytes develop a zygote, then a mobile ookinete capable of traversing the intestinal wall and forming an oocyst that, when mature, will develop sporozoites that will be released to invade the salivary glands [46,47]. During the intraerythrocytic cycle (Figure 5), the clinical features observed include high fever, chills, headache, myalgias, arthralgias, nausea, vomiting, and diarrhea [48,49]. *P. falciparum* infections can cause complicated malaria as a consequence of the cytoadherence phenomenon in which infected erythrocytes adhere to the vascular endothelium of different organs, causing cerebral malaria, acute respiratory distress syndrome, acute renal failure, anemia, thrombocytopenia, and placental malaria [48]. The intensity of clinical manifestation during complicated malaria varies according to age and the intensity of transmission, and if not treated promptly, mortality is high [40].

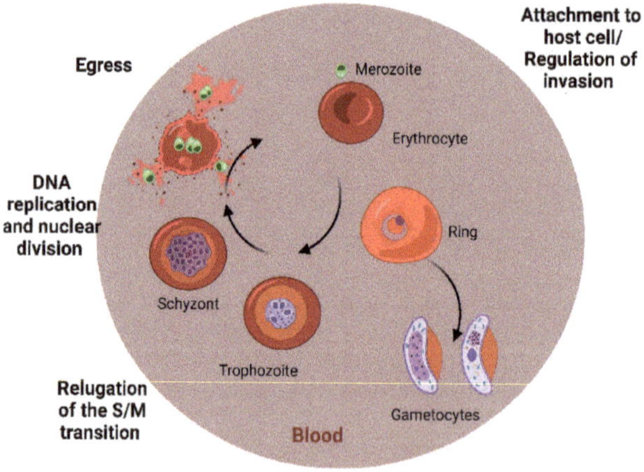

Figure 5. *Plasmodium* spp. intraerythrocytic cycle. Most antimalarial drugs target the asexual erythrocytic stages (rings, throphozoites, and schyzonts).

Multiple antimalarial drugs are used, including chloroquine, mefloquine, pyrimethamine, primaquine, and artemisinin derivatives [49] (Figure 6). Unfortunately, it is estimated that malaria morbidity and mortality have increased since 2020 due to the convergence of multiple factors, such as COVID-19 and Ebola outbreaks, natural disasters, and drug resistance, mainly to chloroquine and recently to artemisinin derivatives [44]. Malaria parasites have developed immune evasion strategies. Therefore, it is essential to find new alternatives for malaria control [42,44,50].

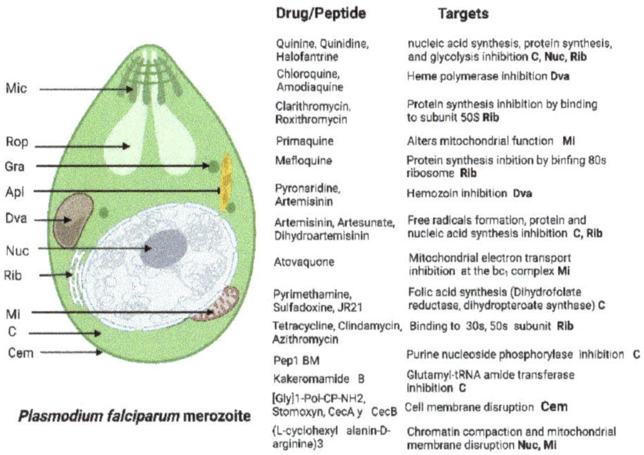

Figure 6. *Plasmodium* spp. drug targets. Antimalarial drugs such as aryl amino alcohol (chloroquine, mefloquine, primaquine), antifolate compounds (pyrimethamine), and artemisinin derivatives (artesunate, artemether) target the asexual erythrocytic stages of the parasite. Mic micronemes. Rop, rohptry. Gra, dense ganule. Api, apicoplast. Dva, digestive vacuole. Nuc, nucleus. Rib, ribosome. Mi, mitochondrion. C, cytoplasm. Cem, cell membrane. Created with BioRender.com under license to publish by Anacleto SJ.

2. Antimicrobial Peptide Classification

The need to categorize everything that is known has facilitated the management of information in different settings, and chemical structures also have their own classification according to the functional groups present in their chemical structures. However, peptides are made up of a series of amino acids that are present in different functional groups depending on their biological activities. According to various authors, AMPs can be categorized according to different features, such as their charges (cationic, anionic), biological activities (antibacterial, antifungal, antiprotozoal, etc.), mechanisms of action, and even the source from which they were isolated (either from natural sources or synthetically) (Figure 7). A general form of classification is based on their physicochemical characteristics, which can be divided into four main groups: (1) α-helices, (2) β-pleated sheets, (3) those with mixed structures, and (4) those with atypical conformations [51–53]. The α helical structure is characterized by coiling on itself through peptide bonds and creating a type of tube. This conformation, in addition to providing amphipathic characteristics, allows it to be easily inserted into the cell membrane, creating channels [54]. β-pleated sheets are structures that fold back on themselves through N-H bonds of amino acids that conform by forming hydrogen bonds with the C=O groups of the opposite amino acids. Mixed structures can be present, within the same chain of amino acids, of the two conformations, both helical and β-pleated sheets. Finally, the atypical structures present forms that do not correspond to those mentioned above [55–57].

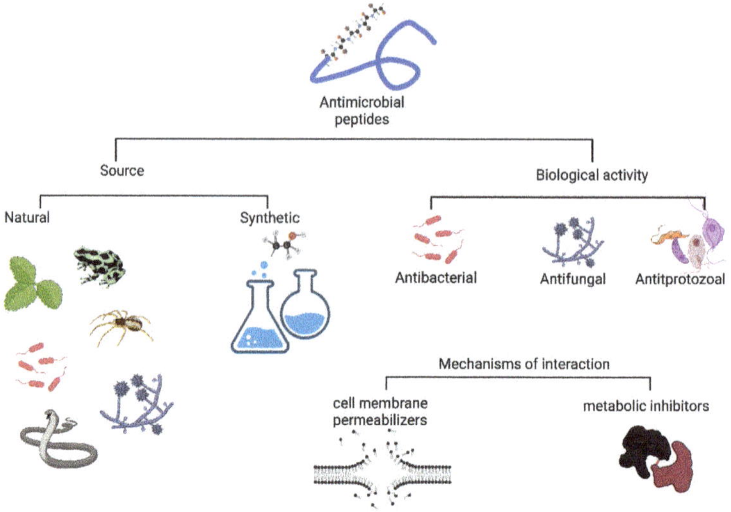

Figure 7. Antimicrobial peptides classification and interaction.

3. Mechanisms of Interaction by AMPs

Currently, research on AMPs has constantly been increasing, together with new research techniques such as bio-guided studies, in silico analysis, and synthesis, offering a broad number of peptides that have been described and evaluated in different biological models and clinical phases. To date, according to the Database of the Antimicrobial Activity and Structure of Peptides, 19,398 have been described, 82.5% of which are synthetic, and the rest have been isolated by natural sources, such as animals (75%), bacteria (12%), plants (9%) and fungi (4%) [58]. The knowledge of their mechanisms of action is continually increasing. It is noted that several peptides active against Apicomplexa parasites act directly on components of the cell membrane and extracellular components and the mechanism of surface membranes, mainly because AMPS are cationic and amphipathic molecules [59]. Most AMPs interfere with the correct functioning of the cytoplasmic membrane. With the progress in the discovery of AMPs and the elucidation of their mechanisms of action, researchers managed to understand different pathways by which they interact in both the host and host cells. Once the AMPs enter the cell, they can interact with components of the cytoplasm, altering the electrochemical balance as well as inhibiting metabolic processes essential for the survival of the parasite, altering cellular homeostasis and essential processes for cell replication [60].

AMPs' mechanisms of action have been categorized into two main groups: those that exert a direct effect on killing cells and those that modulate the immune response. The first group is subdivided into two subgroups, those that kill directly by permeabilizing the cell membrane due to hydrophobic and electrostatic interactions of the peptides, and the second group, those peptides that kill by affecting the internal components of the cell acting as metabolic inhibitors [60–63].

4. Peptides Active against Apicomplexan Parasites

4.1. *Toxoplasma gondii*

Regarding AMPs that can modulate the immune response, it has been shown in vivo that HPRP-A1/A2 (amphipathic α-helical peptide) treatment induced a Th1/Tc1 response and elicited proinflammatory cytokines in mice infected with *T. gondii*; it is the only peptide with this type of mechanism of action in the parasite. These peptides affect the viability of tachyzoites at low concentrations; in addition, their activities against gram-negative and gram-positive bacteria and some pathogenic fungi have been reported [64]. A group of peptides that weaken the cell membrane, CA (2–8) M (1–18), lycosin-I, XYP1, XYP2, XYP3, longicin and longicin P4, have been tested in in vitro models against *T. gondii*. Lycosin-I was the most active, with an IC_{50} of 10 µM. However, other effects on the integrity of the tachyzoites were reported, such as the aggregation of the parasites induced by longicin P4, which in an in vivo model has managed to prolong the survival of mice for up to 11 days compared to the control [64–70].

Venoms from invertebrates such as spiders, scorpions, amphibians, and some reptiles are composed of different peptides, which in turn act mainly as modulators of ion channels and have been widely investigated in the pharmacological field for different diseases such as cancer and AIDS [71]. Some of these toxins have been evaluated against *Toxoplasma* [71]; however, peptides responsible for this activity have not been identified, although it is worth continuing with this research to identify the active peptides and elucidate their mechanisms of action. It should be noted that of the venoms and secretions evaluated, those obtained from the spiders *Ornitoctonus huwena* and *Chilobrachys jingzhao* were active against *T. gondii* tachyzoites at 3 µg/mL and increased the survival rate in vivo. There is only one study reporting peptide efficacy against *T. gondii* tissue cysts. The venom of the scorpion *Tityus serrulatus* was evaluated, and the Pep 1 peptide decreased the number of cerebral tissue cysts in infected mice, although its mechanism of action is still unknown [72–74].

Peptides with interesting biological activities have also been detected in marine organisms, as is the case of the conotoxin isolated from *Conus californicus* that affected tachyzoites in concentrations from 10 nM; of all the peptides investigated, it showed the highest activity [75].

Synthetic peptides represent an important component of known peptides to date, many of which have been identified from natural sources. Of the five synthetic peptides evaluated, Ac2-26 identified in human cells was able to reduce the parasite load from a concentration of 5 µM. (Table 1) [76].

Table 1. AMPs with in vitro anti-*Toxoplasma* activity on tachyzoites.

AMP Name	Type	Source	Evaluated Concentrations	Cytotoxicity	Activity and Possible Mechanism of Action	IC_{50}
Frog skin secretion [71]	ND	*Phyllomedusa distincta* [Amphibia] *Corythomanti greening* [Amphibia]	25 µg/mL and 22 µg/mL respectively	None in human Fibroblasts	Inhibits invasion	ND
CA (2–8) M(1–18) [65]	Cecropin/ melittin hybrid peptide	Synthetic	5 µM	None in human fibroblasts	Reduces viability Membrane lytic activity	ND
Ac2-26 peptide mimetic of Annexin A1 [76]	Human peptide	Synthetic	5 µM	ND	Decreases proliferation rate	ND
Lycosin-I [68]	Linear peptide	*Lycosa singoriensis* [Arachnida]	20 µM	Cytotoxic at 34.69 µM in human fibroblasts	Invasion and proliferation inhibition. Cell membrane alteration	28 and 10.08 µM for intracellular and extracellular tachyzoites, respectively
Longicin [69]	Cationic	*Haemaphysalis longicornis* [Arachnida]	50 µM	ND	Reduces proliferation. Cell membrane disruption	ND
ND [72]	Venoms	*Ornitoctonus huwena* *Chilobrachys jingzhao* [Arachnida]	12.5 µg/mL	Cytotoxic to Hella cells	Proliferation and invasion reduction	ND
XYP1 [67]	Cationic	synthesized	2.5–40 µM	Low cytotoxicity at 20 µM in human fibroblasts	Inhibition of viability, invasion, and proliferation. Damage to membrane associated proteins (HSP29)	38.79 µM

Table 1. *Cont.*

AMP Name	Type	Source	Evaluated Concentrations	Cytotoxicity	Activity and Possible Mechanism of Action	IC_{50}
cal14.1a [75]	Conotoxin	*Conus californicus* [Gastropoda]	10–50 μM	Not detected up to 50 μM in Hep-2 cells	Affects viability and replication by disrupting cell membrane	ND
ND [73]	Venom	*Hemiscorpius Lepturus* [Arachnida]	50 μg/mL	CC_{50} 72.46 μg/mL (Vero cells)	Reduces viability and invasion. Probably damaging ion channels and enzymatic activity	39.06 μg/mL
Killer peptide (KP) [77]	Decapeptide	Synthetic	25–200 μg/mL	Nontoxic to Vero cells. Genotoxic effects were reported	Reduces invasion and proliferation. Maybe triggers an apoptosis like cell death	ND
Longicin P4 [70]	ND	*Haemaphysalis Longicornis* [Arachnida]	50 μM	Nontoxic up to 25 μM	Reduces proliferation. Induces aggregation and affects membrane integrity	ND
HPRP-A1/A2 [64]	Cationic peptide	Synthetic	10–40 μg/mL	Nontoxic in peritoneal macrophages.	Reduces viability, adhesion, and invasion	ND
Sub6-B, Pep1, Pep2a and Pep2b [74]	Venom fractions	*Tityus serrulatus* [Arachnida]	100 μg/mL	Nontoxic in peritoneal macrophages	Reduces invasion and replication. Disruption of cell membrane	ND

ND: Not Determined.

4.2. *Cryptosporidium spp.*

AMPs that have been active in in vivo and in vitro evaluations against specific parasitic states of *Cryptosporidium* spp. are summarized in Table 2. Although human cryptosporidiosis is mainly caused by two species, *Cryptosporidium hominis* and *Cryptosporidium parvum*, AMP investigations against this parasite have specifically used *C. parvum* in both its sporozoite and oocyst forms and through evaluations in cell cultures and in vivo. The use of the meront phase has also been reported to determine the parasite load in these investigations. Approximately 16 cationic peptides have been tested to determine their anti-*Cryptosporidium* activity; three of them have been evaluated in more than one trial with similar results, and even combined treatments have been carried out to improve activity, as in the case of indolicidin, ranalexin, and magainin II. However, these combinations cannot be effectively compared because the pharmacological parameters of IC_{50} are not reported, and even in most of these evaluations, only 1 to 3 different concentrations up to 50 mM were evaluated. Evaluating these AMPs at different concentrations to determine their IC_{50} values, as well as their average cytotoxicity is of great importance to continue their research. Those with the best activity were the Buforin II and Magainin II peptides, which affected approximately 99.8% of the parasites in vitro at a concentration of 10 μg/mL [78–85]. However, the coupling of the peptide octarginine and the antibiotic nitazoxanide showed excellent results, lowering the IC_{50} value to 2.9 nM compared to the IC_{50} of nitozoanide alone, which was 197 nM. Of all the peptides evaluated, this combination showed the best results [86].

In in vivo experiments, peptides, such as glucagon-like peptides, in a treatment of 50 µg/kg of weight in calves infected with *C. parvum*, managed to reduce the symptoms of the infection, and eliminate the release of oocysts in the feces. Other peptides that act by regulating the immune response, SA35, and SA40, were isolated from *C. parvum*. These peptides were tested in mice infected and immunized with 5 µg of each peptide. Evaluations of the parasite load generate specific IgA antibodies and reductions of up to 96% of all intestinal forms of the parasite (Table 2) [87,88]. To date, the efficacies of none of these peptides have been demonstrated in clinical trials. However, it should not be ignored the biological activities that they present in low concentrations, and the synergistic effects that some reported peptides exert in combination with commercial antibiotics. The search for new alternatives for the treatment of cryptosporidiosis should focus on not only AMPs but also their combination with other active molecules, with the goal of attacking the parasite by different mechanisms of action.

Table 2. Synthetic AMPs with in vitro anti-*Cryptosporidium* activity.

AMP Name	Type	Evaluated Concentrations	Cytotoxicity	Activity and Possible Mechanisms of Action
Buforin II [85]	α-Helical	20 µM	None in A549 cells.	Reduces sporozoites viability. Cell membrane Disruption
Ranalexin [84]	Cationic	64 µg/mL	Non in A549 cells.	Sporozoites growth suppression. Cell membrane Disruption
Ranalexin, Magainin II. Indolicidin [82]	Cationic, helix and tridecapeptide	50 mM	Non in A549 cells	Sporozoites growth suppression. Cell membrane damage by synergic effect between peptide and lipophilic antibiotics
Shiva-10 [89]	Lytic peptide	10 µM	ND	Reduces sporozoite viability. Membrane lytic effect
Cecropin P1, magainin II, ranalexin, and indolicidin [83]	Cationic peptides	50 µM	ND	Reduction in the proliferation of schizonts. Inhibition of Na/H and Na/Ca^2 exchanges in the cell membrane
KFFKFFKFF and IKFLKFLKFL [81]	Cationic peptides	100 µg/mL	ND	Reduction in the viability of sporozoites. Cell membrane disruption
SMAP-29, BMAP-28, PG-1, Bac-7 [80]	Helical peptides	100 µg/mL	ND	Strong cytotoxic effect on sporozoites. Alterations in the glycoprotein of the apical complex
Indolicidin, Magainin II, Ranalexin [79]	Cathionic peptides	50 µM	ND	Reduction in merozoites proliferation
Octaarginine-6-FAM-Nitazoanide combination [86]	Cathionic peptides	197 nM	No cytotoxic effects in human ileocecal adenocarcinoma cells	Reduction in trophozoites and meronts replication
Lactoferrin B, cathelicidin LL3, indolicidin, βdefens1in, ß defensin 2. [90]	Cathionic peptides	10 µg/mL	Low cytotoxic effect in human colorectal adenocarcinoma cells	Inhibition of sporozoites attachment and invasion. Transmembrane pore formation
Buforin II, Magainin II, Lasalocid. [78]	Cathionic peptides	10 µg/mL	ND	Reduction in oocysts infectivity. Membrane disruption

ND: Not determined. IC_{50} values were not established.

4.3. Peptides Active against Plasmodium spp.

Peptides against *Plasmodium* have multiple mechanisms of action that cause decreases in parasitemia (Table 3), and one of the predominant mechanisms is the interaction of peptides with enzymes causing their inhibition and, consequently damage to the metabolic pathways in which they participate. For example, for the maintenance and processing of genetic material, peptides can inhibit the enzyme purine nucleoside phosphorylase of *P. falciparum*, and the enzyme dihydrofolate reductase-thymidylate synthase, resulting in the death of the parasite [91,92]. Another example of enzyme inhibition occurs during the erythrocyte cycle, during the digestion of hemoglobin in the digestive vacuole for protein biosynthesis and heme crystallization, a process that is catalyzed by enzymes such as falcispainins that, if their function is inhibited, the parasite cannot obtain the amino acids necessary for protein synthesis and therefore would die; this strategy is used by certain peptides, such as CYS-IHL and CYS-cIHL, that are capable of inhibiting these enzymes [93,94].

Table 3. AMPs with in vitro anti-Malarial activity.

AMP Name	Type	Source	Evaluated Concentration	Cytotoxicity	Activity and Possible Mechanisms of Action	IC_{50}
Pep1 BM [91]	ND	Synthetic	20 µL	ND	Inhibition of purine nucleoside phosphorylase in *P. falciparum* rings	16.14 µg/mL
JR21 [92]	ND	Synthetic	10 µM	ND	Dihydrofolate reductase-thymidylate synthase inhibition in *P. falciparum* rings	3.87 µM
CYS-IHL [94]	Linear	Synthetic	69.91 µM	Noncytotoxic in human liver carcinoma cell.	Hemoglobinase activity inhibition in late *P. falciparum* Trophozoites	27.55 µM
Kakeromamide B [95]	Cyclic	*Moorea producens* [Cyanobacteria]	11 µM	Noncytotoxic in HEK293T and HepG2 cells	Reduction in proliferation of *P. falciparum* sexual blood-stages and *P. berghei* liver-stage. High affinity to actin, sortilin and subunit A of glutamyl-tRNA amide transferase	8.9 µM
[Gly]1-Pol-CP-NH2 [96]	ND	Synthetic derived from Pol-CP-NH2	6.25 µM	Cytotoxic in human mammary adenocarcinoma, Hep G2, SHSY-5Y, and SK-mel-147	Cell membrane disruption in *P. falciparum* sporozoites	ND
Crotamine [97,98]	Cationic	*Crotalusdurissusterrificus* [Lepidosauria]	20 µM	No hemolytic activity in human erythrocytes	Peptide–membrane interactions and H+ homeostasis disruption in *P. falciparum* asexual blood stages	1.87 µM
(L-cyclohexyl alanin-D-arginine) 3 [99]	ND	Synthetic	59.16 ng/mL	No cytotoxic effects in human erythrocytes and leukocytes	Chromatin compaction and mitochondrial membrane disruption in *P. falciparum* asexual blood stages	8.94 ng/mL
rR8-JR21 [92]	ND	Synthetic	13.22	ND	Dihydrofolate reductase-thymidylate synthase inhibition in *P. falciparum* ring stages	1.53 µM
LZ1 [100]	Linear peptide	Synthetic derived fromcathelicidin-BF	25 µM and 4 mg/kg	ND	Blockade of ATP production by selective inhibition of pyruvate kinase activity in *P. falciparum* blood stages.	3.045 µM
Mtk-1 y Mtk-2 [101]	Rich in proline	*Drosophila melanogaster* [Insecta]	50 µM	Hemolytic activity in pig and mouse (CD1) erythrocytes	Cell membrane disruption in *P. falciparum* asexual blood stages	ND
Stomoxyn [101]	ND	*Lucilia sericata* [Insecta]	50 µM	Hemolytic activity in highest concentrations in pig and mouse (CD1) erythrocytes	Cell membrane disruption in *P. falciparum* asexual blood stages	ND

Table 3. *Cont.*

AMP Name	Type	Source	Evaluated Concentration	Cytotoxicity	Activity and Possible Mechanisms of Action	IC_{50}
CecA y CecB [101]	Linear cations	*Galleria mellonella* [Insecta]	50 μM	Hemolytic activity in highest concentrations in pig and mouse (CD1) erythrocytes	Cell membrane disruption in *P. falciparum* asexual blood stages.	ND
[Arg]3-VmCT1-NH2, [Arg]7-VmCT1-NH2 [102]		Synthetic	5 μM/L	Lower Cytotoxic effects in MCF-7 human breast epithelial cells, CC_{50} 20 and 18 μM/L	Cell membrane disruption in *P. gallinaceum* sporozoites	0.57, 0.51 μM/L
VmCT1-NH2 [102]		*Vaejovis mexicanus* [Arachnida]	5 μM/L	CC_{50} 8.3 μM/L in MCF-7 human breast epithelial cells	Cell membrane disruption in *P. gallinaceum* sporozoites	0.49 μM/L

ND: not determined.

Peptide–membrane interactions and H+ homeostasis disruption in *P. falciparum* asexual blood stages

Other targets of peptides are proteins and membranes, which, if damaged, can modify the morphology of the parasite; however, not all peptides have parasiticidal effect, and some only stop the development of *Plasmodium* spp., which is reflected in the slowed kinetics of the life cycle [92,94–98].

In addition to reducing parasitemia, some peptides are capable of modifying the immune response in the host by reducing the overproduction of proinflammatory cytokines and, as a consequence, modulating damage to organs that are severely affected, such as the liver [99].

Nevertheless, more information is needed to elucidate the mechanisms of action of antimicrobial peptides against *Plasmodium* spp.

5. Concluding Remarks and Future Research Directions

Antimicrobial peptides have been described in many species, including fungi, plants, insects, and humans (allowing access to an endless number of possible peptides with diverse biological activities), and are currently presented as a therapeutic solution to control different pathogenic microorganisms. Microorganisms that cause diseases in humans are constantly evolving, which represents a challenge in the pursuit of effective treatments against these pathogens. Some characteristics that make peptides attractive as potential drugs are that they have been evolving for almost the same amount of time as the species that produce them, and their effects on the control of microorganisms are very remarkable. Some peptides are being used in experimental phases, and others are already marketed, e.g., peptides against fungal agents such as *Candida albicans*, *Cryptococcus neoformans*, and *Fusarium oxysporum*. Some peptides have been developed for topical application against human papilloma virus, and others have been developed against protozoa and nematodes, gram-negative bacteria, tumors, and as neuroprotectors.

Endogenous bioactive peptides can be produced in different cell types, such as neural cells, immune cells, or glands, while exogenous peptides can be obtained from nutrients, insects, nematodes, or marine organisms. Cecropin is one of the most explored insect peptides that can destroy cell membranes and inhibit proline uptake.

Unlike other parasites, Apicomplexans have complex life cycles comprised of different stages characterized by rapid replication, which enables adaptation to drug treatment. The Apicomplexa invasion process involves secretory organelles housing proteins that allow host-cell entrance and the development of an intracellular compartment in which the parasites reproduce asexually. As intracellular organisms, their nutritional needs rely on biosynthetic pathways or salvaging metabolites from their host [103]. Apicomplexa drug targets include calcium-dependent protein kinases, mitochondrial electron transport chain, proteins secretion pathways, type II fatty acid synthesis, DNA synthesis and replication, and, DNA expression, among others [104]. Most of the peptides reviewed in this text produce the disruption of parasite cell membranes, in contrast to conventional chemotherapeutic drugs, which act on precise targets such as DNA or specific enzymes. Nonetheless, plasma membrane disruption, produces fast depolarization triggering protein and DNA/RNA inhibition synthesis, which can lead to parasite death. Some peptides are rich in amino acids, such as tryptophan and lysine, that might have an effect on anionic biological membranes, producing pores, which allow peptides to distribute into internal membranes and organelles [64].

Unlike Apicomplexan, hemoflagellate protozoa, such as *Trypanosoma* and *Leishmania*, have less complex life cycles. Various research groups have been dedicated to the discovery and structural elucidation of novel peptides against these parasites since the early 90s. Extracellular forms (promastigote and trypomastigote) are the most common stages used for the screening of peptides' activity [105]. The antiprotozoal activity is supposed to occur by membrane disruption, apoptosis, or by immunomodulatory responses. In vivo assessments are considerably underexplored, due to their rapid degradation by endogenous proteases [105]. It seems that peptide-based antiprotozoal drug development, presents several challenges related to the complex life cycles. Therefore, computational models and tools for the prediction of peptide activity are urgently needed. However, peptides have some advantages over traditional drugs, such as slower emergence of resistance [106].

There are some issues to consider while scaling up peptide design. Peptides have various limitations that could hinder their anti-Apicomplexa therapeutic use. They have unfavorable plasma stability, are unable to cross the cell membrane to target intracellular targets, degrade easily, and have poor penetration of the intestinal mucosa; thus, it can be assumed that they are not good candidates to treat intracellular parasites. [107]. Nonetheless, the results obtained so far show that they can be a good alternative to control these parasites. It must be taken into consideration, that novel peptides must easily reach intracellular targets with little or no toxicity to mammalian cells. To improve these disadvantages, encapsulation into a micro- or nanoparticle, can be achieved, as well as in silico sequence-based prediction of cell-penetrating and toxicity. Penetratin-like peptides bind to glycosaminoglycans at the cell surface. Natural DNA-binding peptides can be the source for designing cell-penetrating peptides, such as those rich in lysine, or arginine [107].

Although there are currently some pharmacological alternatives for the control of Apicomplexan parasites, these are sometimes inefficient, especially due to resistance mechanisms and severe side effects, and they do not act against all parasite stages and sometimes restrict access to some intracellular locations. Based upon the abovementioned results, it seems that synthetic peptides, as well as those derived from natural sources, could be promising alternatives for the treatment of infectious diseases. It is necessary to develop new anti-Apicomplexan compounds combining drug research pathways, such as in silico rational drug design and bio-guided natural substance studies, to identify new molecules that might be able to act directly in the parasites or indirectly by activating the host immune system.

As reported in the literature, peptides show a broad antimicrobial spectrum; therefore, it would be recommended to explore their synergistic ability in combination with those drugs in which resistance is reported, their capacity to decrease or increase the adverse effects of currently used drugs, and their distribution in the parasite and in the host cell. Genetic engineering or chemical modification of these peptides to improve their functional properties would also be recommended. There is a high potential for the use of antimicrobial peptides, and more research in this field can lead to promising results that can have considerable effects on the control of human Apicomplexan parasites.

Author Contributions: Conceptualization: N.R.-F.; investigation: J.A.-S. and B.C.-T.; resources: T.d.J.L.-P. and M.R.-L.; writing—original draft preparation: all authors; writing—review and editing:

all authors; visualization: all authors; supervision: all authors; project administration: N.R.-F.; funding acquisition: N.R.-F. All authors have read and agreed to the published version of the manuscript.

Funding: This research was funded by Dirección General de Asuntos del Personal Académico (DGAPA) Programa de Apoyo a Proyectos de Investigación e Innovación Tecnológica (PAIIT)-Universidad Nacional Autónoma de México (UNAM) proyect IN200721.

Institutional Review Board Statement: Not applicable.

Informed Consent Statement: Not applicable.

Data Availability Statement: Not applicable.

Conflicts of Interest: The authors declare no conflict of interest.

References

1. Cummings, R.D.; Hokke, C.H.; Haslam, S.M. Parasitic infections. In *Essentials of Glycobiology*, 4th ed.; Spring Harbor Laboratory Press: Cold Spring Harbor, NY, USA, 2022.
2. Memariani, H.; Memariani, M. Melittin as a promising anti-protozoan peptide: Current knowledge and future prospects. *AMB Express* **2021**, *11*, 69. [CrossRef] [PubMed]
3. Harding, C.R.; Frischknecht, F. The Riveting Cellular Structures of Apicomplexan Parasites. *Trends Parasitol.* **2020**, *36*, 979–991. [CrossRef] [PubMed]
4. Chan, K.; Tusting, L.S.; Bottomley, C.; Saito, K.; Djouaka, R.; Lines, J. Malaria transmission and prevalence in rice-growing versus non-rice-growing villages in Africa: A systematic review and meta-analysis. *Lancet Planet. Health* **2022**, *6*, e257–e269. [CrossRef]
5. Shammaa, A.M.; Powell, T.G.; Benmerzouga, I. Adverse outcomes associated with the treatment of *Toxoplasma* infections. *Sci. Rep.* **2021**, *11*, 1035. [CrossRef] [PubMed]
6. Gargala, G. Drug treatment and novel drug target against *Cryptosporidium*. *Parasite* **2008**, *15*, 275–281. [CrossRef]
7. Alven, S.; Aderibigbe, B. Combination Therapy Strategies for the Treatment of Malaria. *Molecules* **2019**, *24*, 3601. [CrossRef]
8. Zhu, Y.; Hao, W.; Wang, X.; Ouyang, J.; Deng, X.; Yu, H.; Wang, Y. Antimicrobial peptides, conventional antibiotics, and their synergistic utility for the treatment of drug-resistant infections. *Med. Res. Rev.* **2022**, *42*, 1377–1422. [CrossRef]
9. Erdem Büyükkiraz, M.; Kesmen, Z. Antimicrobial peptides (AMPs): A promising class of antimicrobial compounds. *J. Appl. Microbiol.* **2022**, *132*, 1573–1596. [CrossRef]
10. Mahlapuu, M.; Håkansson, J.; Ringstad, L.; Björn, C. Antimicrobial peptides: An emerging category of therapeutic agents. *Front. Cell. Infect.* **2016**, *6*, 194. [CrossRef]
11. Cardoso, P.; Glossop, H.; Meikle, T.G.; Aburto-Medina, A.; Conn, C.E.; Sarojini, V.; Valery, C. Molecular engineering of antimicrobial peptides: Microbial targets, peptide motifs and translation opportunities. *Biophys. Rev.* **2021**, *13*, 35–69. [CrossRef]
12. Lemaitre, B.; Nicolas, E.; Michaut, L.; Reichhart, J.-M.; Hoffmann, J.A. The Dorsoventral Regulatory Gene Cassette spätzle/Toll/cactus Controls the Potent Antifungal Response in *Drosophila* Adults. *Cell* **1996**, *86*, 973–983. [CrossRef]
13. Kardani, K.; Bolhassani, A. Antimicrobial/anticancer peptides: Bioactive molecules and therapeutic agents. *Immunotherapy* **2021**, *13*, 669–684. [CrossRef]
14. Guryanova, S.V.; Ovchinnikova, T.V. Immunomodulatory and allergenic properties of antimicrobial peptides. *Int. J. Mol. Sci.* **2022**, *23*, 2499. [CrossRef]
15. Nogrado, K.; Adisakwattana, P.; Reamtong, O. Antimicrobial peptides: On future antiprotozoal and anthelminthic applications. *Acta. Trop.* **2022**, *235*, 106665. [CrossRef] [PubMed]
16. Fry, D.E. Antimicrobial peptides. *Surg. Infect.* **2018**, *19*, 804–811. [CrossRef] [PubMed]
17. Zhang, C.; Yang, M. Antimicrobial Peptides: From Design to Clinical Application. *Antibiotics* **2022**, *11*, 349. [CrossRef] [PubMed]
18. Aguirre, A.A.; Longcore, T.; Barbieri, M.; Dabritz, H.; Hill, D.; Klein, P.N.; Lepczyk, C.; Lilly, E.L.; McLeod, R.; Milcarsky, J.; et al. The One Health Approach to Toxoplasmosis: Epidemiology, Control, and Prevention Strategies. *Ecohealth* **2019**, *16*, 378–390. [CrossRef] [PubMed]
19. Cossu, G.; Preti, A.; Gyppaz, D.; Gureje, O.; Carta, M.G. Association between toxoplasmosis and bipolar disorder: A systematic review and meta-analysis. *J. Psychiatr. Res.* **2022**, *153*, 284–291. [CrossRef]
20. Hajimohammadi, B.; Ahmadian, S.; Firoozi, Z.; Askari, M.; Mohammadi, M.; Eslami, G.; Askari, V.; Loni, E.; Barzegar-Bafrouei, R.; Boozhmehrani, M.J. A Meta-Analysis of the Prevalence of Toxoplasmosis in Livestock and Poultry Worldwide. *EcoHealth* **2022**, *19*, 55–74. [CrossRef]
21. De Barros, R.A.M.; Torrecilhas, A.C.; Marciano, M.A.M.; Mazuz, M.L.; Pereira-Chioccola, V.L.; Fux, B. Toxoplasmosis in Human and Animals Around the World. Diagnosis and Perspectives in the One Health Approach. *Acta Trop.* **2022**, *231*, 106432. [CrossRef]
22. Molan, A.; Nosaka, K.; Hunter, M.; Wang, W. Global status of *Toxoplasma gondii* infection: Systematic review and prevalence snapshots. *Trop. Biomed.* **2019**, *36*, 898–925. [PubMed]
23. Robinson, E.; de Valk, H.; Villena, I.; Le Strat, Y.; Tourdjman, M. National perinatal survey demonstrates a decreasing seroprevalence of *Toxoplasma gondii* infection among pregnant women in France, 1995 to 2016: Impact for screening policy. *Eurosurveillance* **2021**, *26*, 1900710. [CrossRef] [PubMed]

24. Rostami, A.; Riahi, S.M.; Contopoulos-Ioannidis, D.G.; Gamble, H.R.; Fakhri, Y.; Shiadeh, M.N.; Foroutan, M.; Behniafar, H.; Taghipour, A.; Maldonado, Y.A.; et al. Acute Toxoplasma infection in pregnant women worldwide: A systematic review and meta-analysis. *PLoS Negl. Trop. Dis.* **2019**, *13*, e0007807. [CrossRef] [PubMed]
25. López-Fabal, F.; Gómez-Garcés, J.L. Marcadores serológicos de gestantes españolas e inmigrantes en un área del sur de Madrid durante el periodo 2007–2010. *Rev. Esp. Quimioter.* **2013**, *26*, 108–111. [PubMed]
26. Dubey, J.P. Outbreaks of clinical toxoplasmosis in humans: Five decades of personal experience, perspectives and lessons learned. *Parasites Vectors* **2021**, *14*, 263. [CrossRef]
27. McLeod, R.; Cohen, W.; Dovgin, S.; Finkelstein, L.; Boyer, K.M. Human toxoplasma infection. In *Toxoplasma Gondii*; Elsevier: Amsterdam, The Netherlands, 2020; pp. 117–227.
28. Attias, M.; Teixeira, D.E.; Benchimol, M.; Vommaro, R.C.; Crepaldi, P.H.; De Souza, W. The life-cycle of *Toxoplasma gondii* reviewed using animations. *Parasites Vectors* **2020**, *13*, 588. [CrossRef]
29. Dubey, J.P. The history and life cycle of *Toxoplasma gondii*. In *Toxoplasma Gondii*; Elsevier: Amsterdam, The Netherlands, 2020; pp. 1–19.
30. Montazeri, M.; Mehrzadi, S.; Sharif, M.; Sarvi, S.; Tanzifi, A.; Aghayan, S.A.; Daryani, A. Drug Resistance in *Toxoplasma gondii*. *Front. Microbiol.* **2018**, *9*, 2587. [CrossRef]
31. Dunay Ildiko, R.; Gajurel, K.; Dhakal, R.; Liesenfeld, O.; Montoya Jose, G. Treatment of Toxoplasmosis: Historical Perspective, Animal Models, and Current Clinical Practice. *Clin. Microbiol. Rev.* **2018**, *31*, e00057-17. [CrossRef]
32. Adkins, P.R.F. Cryptosporidiosis. *Vet. Clin. N. Am. Food Anim.* **2022**, *38*, 121–131. [CrossRef]
33. Feng, Y.; Ryan, U.M.; Xiao, L. Genetic Diversity and Population Structure of *Cryptosporidium*. *Trends Parasitol.* **2018**, *34*, 997–1011. [CrossRef]
34. Korpe, P.S.; Valencia, C.; Haque, R.; Mahfuz, M.; McGrath, M.; Houpt, E.; Kosek, M.; McCormick, B.J.J.; Penataro Yori, P.; Babji, S.; et al. Epidemiology and Risk Factors for Cryptosporidiosis in Children From 8 Low-income Sites: Results From the MAL-ED Study. *Clin. Infect. Dis.* **2018**, *67*, 1660–1669. [CrossRef] [PubMed]
35. Ahmadpour, E.; Safarpour, H.; Xiao, L.; Zarean, M.; Hatam-Nahavandi, K.; Barac, A.; Picot, S.; Rahimi, M.T.; Rubino, S.; Mahami-Oskouei, M.; et al. Cryptosporidiosis in HIV-positive patients and related risk factors: A systematic review and meta-analysis. *Parasite* **2020**, *27*, 27. [CrossRef] [PubMed]
36. Ryan, U.; Hill, K.; Deere, D. Review of generic screening level assumptions for quantitative microbial risk assessment (QMRA) for estimating public health risks from Australian drinking water sources contaminated with *Cryptosporidium* by recreational activities. *Water. Res.* **2022**, *220*, 118659. [CrossRef] [PubMed]
37. Urrea-Quezada, A.; González-Díaz, M.; Villegas-Gómez, I.; Durazo, M.; Hernández, J.; Xiao, L.; Valenzuela, O. Clinical manifestations of cryptosporidiosis and identification of a new *Cryptosporidium* subtype in patients from Sonora, Mexico. *J. Pediatr. Infect. Dis.* **2018**, *37*, e136–e138. [CrossRef] [PubMed]
38. Guérin, A.; Striepen, B. The Biology of the Intestinal Intracellular Parasite *Cryptosporidium*. *Cell Host Microbe* **2020**, *28*, 509–515. [CrossRef]
39. English, E.D.; Guérin, A.; Tandel, J.; Striepen, B. Live imaging of the *Cryptosporidium parvum* life cycle reveals direct development of male and female gametes from type I meronts. *PLoS Biol.* **2022**, *20*, e3001604. [CrossRef]
40. Tandel, J.; English, E.D.; Sateriale, A.; Gullicksrud, J.A.; Beiting, D.P.; Sullivan, M.C.; Pinkston, B.; Striepen, B. Life cycle progression and sexual development of the Apicomplexan parasite *Cryptosporidium parvum*. *Nat. Microbiol.* **2019**, *4*, 2226–2236. [CrossRef]
41. Borowski, H.; Thompson, R.C.A.; Armstrong, T.; Clode, P.L. Morphological characterization of *Cryptosporidium parvum* life-cycle stages in an in vitro model system. *Parasitology* **2010**, *137*, 13–26. [CrossRef]
42. WHO. World Malaria Report 2021. Available online: https://www.who.int/publications/i/item/9789240040496 (accessed on 26 September 2022).
43. Su, X.-z.; Lane, K.D.; Xia, L.; Sá, J.M.; Wellems, T.E. Plasmodium Genomics and Genetics: New Insights into Malaria Pathogenesis, Drug Resistance, Epidemiology, and Evolution. *Clin. Microbiol. Rev.* **2019**, *32*, e00019-19. [CrossRef]
44. Ashley, E.A.; Pyae Phyo, A.; Woodrow, C.J. Malaria. *Lancet* **2018**, *391*, 1608–1621. [CrossRef]
45. Sinnis, P.; Zavala, F. The skin: Where malaria infection and the host immune response begin. *Semin. Immunopathol.* **2012**, *34*, 787–792. [CrossRef] [PubMed]
46. Drahansky, M. Liveness Detection in Biometrics. Available online: https://www.intechopen.com/chapters/17746 (accessed on 26 September 2022).
47. Abugri, J.; Ayariga, J.; Sunwiale, S.S.; Wezena, C.A.; Gyamfi, J.A.; Adu-Frimpong, M.; Agongo, G.; Dongdem, J.T.; Abugri, D.; Dinko, B. Targeting the *Plasmodium falciparum* proteome and organelles for potential antimalarial drug candidates. *Heliyon* **2022**, *8*, e10390. [CrossRef] [PubMed]
48. Trampuz, A.; Jereb, M.; Muzlovic, I.; Prabhu, R.M. Clinical review: Severe malaria. *Crit. Care Med.* **2003**, *7*, 315. [CrossRef]
49. Schofield, L.; Grau, G.E. Immunological processes in malaria pathogenesis. *Nat. Rev. Immunol.* **2005**, *5*, 722–735. [CrossRef]
50. Siddiqui, F.A.; Liang, X.; Cui, L. *Plasmodium falciparum* resistance to ACTs: Emergence, mechanisms, and outlook. *Int. J. Parasitol. Drugs Drug Resist.* **2021**, *16*, 102–118. [CrossRef]
51. Hernández-Aristizábal, Antimicrobial Peptides with Antibacterial Activity against Vancomycin-Resistant *Staphylococcus aureus* Strains: Classification, Structures, and Mechanisms of Action. *Int. J. Mol. Sci.* **2021**, *22*, 7927. [CrossRef] [PubMed]

52. Luong, H.X.; Thanh, T.T.; Tran, T.H. Antimicrobial peptides—Advances in development of therapeutic applications. *Life Sci.* **2020**, *260*, 118407. [CrossRef]
53. Lima, A.M.; Azevedo, M.I.G.; Sousa, L.M.; Oliveira, N.S.; Andrade, C.R.; Freitas, C.D.T.; Souza, P.F.N. Plant antimicrobial peptides: An overview about classification, toxicity and clinical applications. *Int. J. Biol. Macromol.* **2022**, *214*, 10–21. [CrossRef]
54. Böhmová, E.; Machová, D.; Pechar, M.; Pola, R.; Venclíková, K.; Janoušková, O.; Etrych, T. Cell-Penetrating peptides: A useful tool for the delivery of various cargoes into cells. *Physiol. Res.* **2018**, *67*, S267–S279. [CrossRef]
55. Huan, Y.; Kong, Q.; Mou, H.; Yi, H. Antimicrobial peptides: Classification, design, application and research progress in multiple fields. *Front. Microbiol.* **2020**, *11*, 2559. [CrossRef]
56. Lee, H.-T.; Lee, C.-C.; Yang, J.-R.; Lai, J.Z.C.; Chang, K.Y. A large-scale structural classification of antimicrobial peptides. *Biomed. Res. Int.* **2015**, *2015*, 475062. [CrossRef] [PubMed]
57. Hafeez, A.; Jiant, X.; Bergen, P.; Zhu, Y. Antimicrobial Peptides: An Update on Classifications and Databases. *Int. J. Mol. Sci.* **2021**, *22*, 11691. [CrossRef] [PubMed]
58. Pirtskhalava, M.; Amstrong, A.A.; Grigolava, M.; Chubinidze, M.; Alimbarashvili, E.; Vishnepolsky, B.; Gabrielian, A.; Rosenthal, A.; Hurt, D.E.; Tartakovsky, M. DBAASP v3: Database of antimicrobial/cytotoxic activity and structure of peptides as a resource for development of new therapeutics. *Nucleic Acids Res.* **2021**, *49*, D288–D297. [CrossRef] [PubMed]
59. Straub, K.W.; Cheng, S.J.; Sohn, C.S.; Bradley, P.J. Novel components of the Apicomplexan moving junction reveal conserved and coccidia-restricted elements. *Cell. Microbiol.* **2009**, *11*, 590–603. [CrossRef]
60. Sabiá Júnior, E.F.; Menezes, L.F.S.; de Araújo, I.F.S.; Schwartz, E.F. Natural occurrence in venomous arthropods of antimicrobial peptides active against protozoan parasites. *Toxins* **2019**, *11*, 563. [CrossRef]
61. Brogden, K.A. Antimicrobial peptides: Pore formers or metabolic inhibitors in bacteria? *Nat. Rev. Microbiol.* **2005**, *3*, 238–250. [CrossRef]
62. Kumar, P.; Kizhakkedathu, J.; Straus, S. Antimicrobial Peptides: Diversity, Mechanism of Action and Strategies to Improve the Activity and Biocompatibility In Vivo. *Biomolecules* **2018**, *8*, 4. [CrossRef]
63. Raheem, N.; Straus, S.K. Mechanisms of action for antimicrobial peptides with antibacterial and antibiofilm functions. *Front. Microbiol.* **2019**, *10*, 2866. [CrossRef]
64. Liu, R.; Ni, Y.; Song, J.; Xu, Z.; Qiu, J.; Wang, L.; Zhu, Y.; Huang, Y.; Ji, M.; Chen, Y. Research on the effect and mechanism of antimicrobial peptides HPRP-A1/A2 work against *Toxoplasma gondii* infection. *Parasite Immunol.* **2019**, *41*, e12619. [CrossRef]
65. Seeber, F. An enzyme-release assay for the assessment of the lytic activities of complement or antimicrobial peptides on extracellular *Toxoplasma gondii*. *J. Microbiol. Methods* **2000**, *39*, 189–196. [CrossRef]
66. Shin, I.S.; Seo, C.S.; Lee, M.Y.; Ha, H.K.; Huh, J.I.; Shin, H.K. In vitro and in vivo evaluation of the genotoxicity of Gumiganghwal-tang, a traditional herbal prescription. *J. Ethnopharmacol.* **2012**, *141*, 350–356. [CrossRef] [PubMed]
67. Liu, Y.; Tang, Y.; Tang, X.; Wu, M.; Hou, S.; Liu, X.; Li, J.; Deng, M.; Huang, S.; Jiang, L. Anti-*Toxoplasma gondii* Effects of a Novel Spider Peptide XYP1 In Vitro and In Vivo. *Biomedicines* **2021**, *9*, 934. [CrossRef] [PubMed]
68. Tang, Y.; Hou, S.; Li, X.; Wu, M.; Ma, B.; Wang, Z.; Jiang, J.; Deng, M.; Duan, Z.; Tang, X.; et al. Anti-Parasitic effect on *Toxoplasma gondii* induced by a spider peptide lycosin-I. *Exp. Parasitol.* **2019**, *198*, 17–25. [CrossRef] [PubMed]
69. Tanaka, T.; Maeda, H.; Galay, R.L.; Boldbattar, D.; Umemiya-Shirafuji, R.; Suzuki, H.; Xuan, X.; Tsuji, N.; Fujisaki, K. Tick longicin implicated in the arthropod transmission of *Toxoplasma gondii*. *J. Vet. Sci. Technol.* **2012**, *3*, 3633–3640. [CrossRef]
70. Tanaka, T.; Maeda, H.; Matsuo, T.; Boldbattar, D.; Umemiya-Shirafuji, R.; Kume, A.; Suzuki, H.; Xuan, X.; Tsuji, N.; Fujisaki, K. Parasiticidal activity of *Haemaphysalis longicornis* longicin P4 peptide against *Toxoplasma gondii*. *Peptides* **2012**, *34*, 242–250. [CrossRef]
71. Gustavo Tempone, A.; de Souza Carvalho Melhem, M.; Oliveira Prado, F.; Motoie, G.; Mitsuyoshi Hiramoto, R.; Maria Antoniazzi, M.; Fernando Baptista Haddad, C.; Jared, C. Amphibian secretions for drug discovery studies: A search for new antiparasitic and antifungal compounds. *Lett. Drug Des. Discov.* **2007**, *4*, 67–73. [CrossRef]
72. Hou, S.; Liu, Y.; Tang, Y.; Wu, M.; Guan, J.; Li, X.; Wang, Z.; Jiang, J.; Deng, M.; Duan, Z. Anti-*Toxoplasma gondii* effect of two spider venoms in vitro and in vivo. *Toxicon* **2019**, *166*, 9–14. [CrossRef]
73. Khaleghi Rostamkolaie, L.; Hamidinejat, H.; Razi Jalali, M.H.; Jafari, H.; Najafzadeh Varzi, H.; Seifi Abadshapouri, M.R. In vitro therapeutic effect of *Hemiscorpius lepturus* venom on tachyzoites of *Toxoplasma gondii*. *J. Parasit. Dis.* **2019**, *43*, 472–478. [CrossRef]
74. De Assis, D.R.R.; Pimentel, P.M.d.O.; Dos Reis, P.V.M.; Rabelo, R.A.N.; Vitor, R.W.A.; Cordeiro, M.d.N.; Felicori, L.F.; Olórtegui, C.D.C.; Resende, J.M.; Teixeira, M.M. *Tityus Serrulatus* (Scorpion): From the Crude Venom to the Construction of Synthetic Peptides and Their Possible Therapeutic Application Against *Toxoplasma gondii* Infection. *Front. Cell. Infect. Microbiol.* **2021**, *11*, 706618. [CrossRef]
75. De León-Nava, M.A.; Romero-Núñez, E.; Luna-Nophal, A.; Bernáldez-Sarabia, J.; Sánchez-Campos, L.N.; Licea-Navarro, A.F.; Morales-Montor, J.; Muñiz-Hernández, S. In vitro effect of the synthetic cal14.1a conotoxin, derived from *Conus californicus*, on the human parasite *Toxoplasma gondii*. *Mar. Drugs* **2016**, *14*, 66. [CrossRef]
76. De Oliveira Cardoso, M.F.; Moreli, J.B.; Gomes, A.O.; de Freitas Zanon, C.; Silva, A.E.; Paulesu, L.R.; Ietta, F.; Mineo, J.R.; Ferro, E.A.; Oliani, S.M. Annexin A1 peptide is able to induce an anti-parasitic effect in human placental explants infected by *Toxoplasma gondii*. *Microb. Pathog.* **2018**, *123*, 153–161. [CrossRef] [PubMed]
77. Giovati, L.; Santinoli, C.; Mangia, C.; Vismarra, A.; Belletti, S.; 'Adda, T.; Fumarola, C.; Ciociola, T.; Bacci, C.; Magliani, W. Novel activity of a synthetic decapeptide against *Toxoplasma gondii* tachyzoites. *Front. Microbiol.* **2018**, *9*, 753. [CrossRef] [PubMed]

78. Giacometti, A.; Cirioni, O.; Del Prete, M.S.; Barchiesi, F.; Scalise, G. Short-term exposure to membrane-active antibiotics inhibits *Cryptosporidium parvum* infection in cell culture. *Antimicrob. Agents Chemother.* **2000**, *44*, 3473–3475. [CrossRef]
79. Giacometti, A.; Cirioni, O.; Barchiesi, F.; Caselli, F.; Scalise, G. In vitro activity of polycationic peptides against *Cryptosporidium parvum, Pneumocystis carinii* and yeast clinical isolates. *J. Antimicrob. Chemother.* **1999**, *44*, 403–406. [CrossRef] [PubMed]
80. Giacometti, A.; Cirioni, O.; Del Prete, M.S.; Skerlavaj, B.; Circo, R.; Zanetti, M.; Scalise, G. In vitro effect on *Cryptosporidium parvum* of short-term exposure to cathelicidin peptides. *J. Antimicrob. Chemother.* **2003**, *51*, 843–847. [CrossRef]
81. Giacometti, A.; Cirioni, O.; Kamysz, W.; Kasprzykowski, F.; Barchiesi, F.; Del Prete, M.S.; Maćkiewicz, Z.; Scalise, G. In vitro effect of short-term exposure to two synthetic peptides, alone or in combination with clarithromycin or rifabutin, on *Cryptosporidium parvum* infectivity. *Peptides* **2002**, *23*, 1015–1018. [CrossRef]
82. Giacometti, A.; Cirioni, O.; Barchiesi, F.; Fortuna, M.; Scalise, G. In vitro anticryptosporidial activity of ranalexin alone and in combination with other peptides and with hydrophobic antibiotics. *Eur. J. Clin. Microbiol.* **1999**, *18*, 827–829. [CrossRef]
83. Giacometti, A.; Cirioni, O.; Barchiesi, F.; Ancarani, F.; Scalise, G. In vitro anti-cryptosporidial activity of cationic peptides alone and in combination with inhibitors of ion transport systems. *J. Antimicrob. Chemother.* **2000**, *45*, 651–654. [CrossRef]
84. Giacometti, A.; Cirioni, O.; Barchiesi, F.; Scalise, G. Anticryptosporidial activity of ranalexin, lasalocid and azithromycin alone and in combination in cell lines. *J. Antimicrob. Chemother.* **2000**, *45*, 375–377. [CrossRef]
85. Giacometti, A.; Cirioni, O.; Del Prete, M.S.; Barchiesi, F.; Fineo, A.; Scalise, G. Activity of buforin II alone and in combination with azithromycin and minocycline against *Cryptosporidium parvum* in cell culture. *J. Antimicrob. Chemother.* **2001**, *47*, 97–99. [CrossRef]
86. Nguyen-Ho-Bao, T.; Ambe, L.A.; Berberich, M.; Hermosilla, C.; Taubert, A.; Daugschies, A.; Kamena, F. Octaarginine Improves the Efficacy of Nitazoxanide against *Cryptosporidium parvum*. *Pathogens* **2022**, *11*, 653. [CrossRef] [PubMed]
87. Tosini, F.; Ludovisi, A.; Tonanzi, D.; Amati, M.; Cherchi, S.; Pozio, E.; Gómez-Morales, M.A. Delivery of SA35 and SA40 peptides in mice enhances humoral and cellular immune responses and confers protection against *Cryptosporidium parvum* infection. *Parasites Vectors* **2019**, *12*, 233. [CrossRef] [PubMed]
88. Kessler, M.; Connor, E.; Lehnert, M. Volatile organic compounds in the strongly fragrant fern genus Melpomene (Polypodiaceae). *Plant. Biol.* **2015**, *17*, 430–436. [CrossRef] [PubMed]
89. Arrowood, M.J.; Jaynes, J.M.; Healey, M.C. In vitro activities of lytic peptides against the sporozoites of *Cryptosporidium parvum*. *Antimicrob. Agents Chemother.* **1991**, *35*, 224–227. [CrossRef] [PubMed]
90. Carryn, S.; Schaefer, D.A.; Imboden, M.; Homan, E.J.; Bremel, R.D.; Riggs, M.W. Phospholipases and cationic peptides inhibit *Cryptosporidium parvum* sporozoite infectivity by parasiticidal and non-parasiticidal mechanisms. *J. Parasitol.* **2012**, *98*, 199–204. [CrossRef]
91. Martins, G.G.; de Jesus Holanda, R.; Alfonso, J.; Gómez Garay, A.F.; dos Santos, A.P.d.A.; de Lima, A.M.; Francisco, A.F.; Garcia Teles, C.B.; Zanchi, F.B.; Soares, A.M. Identification of a peptide derived from a *Bothrops moojeni* metalloprotease with in vitro inhibitory action on the *Plasmodium falciparum* purine nucleoside phosphorylase enzyme (PfPNP). *Biochimie* **2019**, *162*, 97–106. [CrossRef]
92. Chaianantakul, N.; Sungkapong, T.; Supatip, J.; Kingsang, P.; Kamlaithong, S.; Suwanakitti, N. Antimalarial effect of cell penetrating peptides derived from the junctional region of *Plasmodium falciparum* dihydrofolate reductase-thymidylate synthase. *Peptides* **2020**, *131*, 170372. [CrossRef]
93. Teixeira, C.; Gomes, J.R.; Gomes, P. Falcipains, *Plasmodium falciparum* cysteine proteases as key drug targets against malaria. *Curr. Med. Chem.* **2011**, *18*, 1555–1572. [CrossRef]
94. Mishra, M.; Singh, V.; Tellis, M.B.; Joshi, R.S.; Pandey, K.C.; Singh, S. Cyclic peptide engineered from phytocystatin inhibitory hairpin loop as an effective modulator of falcipains and potent antimalarial. *J. Biomol. Struct. Dyn.* **2022**, *40*, 3642–3654. [CrossRef]
95. Sweeney-Jones, A.M.; Gagaring, K.; Antonova-Koch, J.; Zhou, H.; Mojib, N.; Soapi, K.; Skolnick, J.; McNamara, C.W.; Kubanek, J. Antimalarial Peptide and Polyketide Natural Products from the Fijian Marine *Cyanobacterium Moorea* producens. *Mar. Drugs* **2020**, *18*, 167. [CrossRef]
96. Torres, M.D.T.; Silva, A.F.; Andrade, G.P.; Pedron, C.N.; Cerchiaro, G.; Ribeiro, A.O.; Oliveira, V.X., Jr.; de la Fuente-Nunez, C. The wasp venom antimicrobial peptide polybia-CP and its synthetic derivatives display antiplasmodial and anticancer properties. *Bioeng. Transl. Med.* **2020**, *5*, e10167. [CrossRef] [PubMed]
97. El Chamy Maluf, S.; Hayashi, M.A.F.; Campeiro, J.D.; Oliveira, E.B.; Gazarini, M.L.; Carmona, A.K. South American rattlesnake cationic polypeptide crotamine trafficking dynamic in *Plasmodium falciparum*-infected erythrocytes: Pharmacological inhibitors, parasite cycle and incubation time influences in uptake. *Toxicon* **2022**, *208*, 47–52. [CrossRef] [PubMed]
98. El Chamy Maluf, S.; Dal Mas, C.; Oliveira, E.B.; Melo, P.M.; Carmona, A.K.; Gazarini, M.L.; Hayashi, M.A.F. Inhibition of malaria parasite *Plasmodium falciparum* development by crotamine, a cell penetrating peptide from the snake venom. *Peptides* **2016**, *78*, 11–16. [CrossRef] [PubMed]
99. Somsri, S.; Mungthin, M.; Klubthawee, N.; Adisakwattana, P.; Hanpithakpong, W.; Aunpad, R. A Mitochondria-Penetrating Peptide Exerts Potent Anti-Plasmodium Activity and Localizes at Parasites' Mitochondria. *Antibiotics* **2021**, *10*, 1560. [CrossRef] [PubMed]
100. Fang, Y.; He, X.; Zhang, P.; Shen, C.; Mwangi, J.; Xu, C.; Mo, G.; Lai, R.; Zhang, Z. In Vitro and In Vivo Antimalarial Activity of LZ1, a Peptide Derived from Snake Cathelicidin. *Toxins* **2019**, *11*, 379. [CrossRef]

101. Tonk, M.; Pierrot, C.; Cabezas-Cruz, A.; Rahnamaeian, M.; Khalife, J.; Vilcinskas, A. The *Drosophila melanogaster* antimicrobial peptides Mtk-1 and Mtk-2 are active against the malarial parasite *Plasmodium falciparum*. *Parasitol. Res.* **2019**, *118*, 1993–1998. [CrossRef]
102. Pedron, C.N.; Silva, A.F.; Torres, M.D.T.; de Oliveira, C.S.; Andrade, G.P.; Cerchiaro, G.; Pinhal, M.A.S.; de la Fuente-Nunez, C.; Oliveira, V.X., Jr. Net charge tuning modulates the antiplasmodial and anticancer properties of peptides derived from scorpion venom. *J. Pept. Sci.* **2021**, *27*, e3296. [CrossRef]
103. Rangel, G.W.; Llinás, M. Re-Envisioning Anti-Apicomplexan Parasite Drug Discovery Approaches. *Front. Cell. Infect. Microbiol.* **2021**, *11*, 691121. [CrossRef]
104. Kloehn, J.; Harding, C.R.; Soldati-Favre, D. Supply and demand—Heme synthesis, salvage and utilization by Apicomplexa. *FEBS Lett.* **2021**, *288*, 382–404. [CrossRef]
105. Robles-Loaiza, A.A.; Pinos-Tamayo, E.A.; Mendes, B.; Teixeira, C.; Alves, C.; Gomes, P.; Almeida, J.R. Peptides to Tackle Leishmaniasis: Current Status and Future Directions. *Int. J. Mol. Sci.* **2021**, *22*, 4400. [CrossRef]
106. Apostolopoulos, V.; Bojarska, J.; Chai, T.-T.; Elnagdy, S.; Kaczmarek, K.; Matsoukas, J.; New, R.; Parang, K.; Lopez, O.P.; Parhiz, H.; et al. A Global Review on Short Peptides: Frontiers and Perspectives. *Molecules* **2021**, *26*, 430. [CrossRef] [PubMed]
107. Juretić, D. Designed Multifunctional Peptides for Intracellular Targets. *Antibiotics* **2022**, *11*, 1196. [CrossRef] [PubMed]

antibiotics

MDPI

Review

Designed Multifunctional Peptides for Intracellular Targets

Davor Juretić [1,2]

1 Mediterranean Institute for Life Sciences, 21000 Split, Croatia; djuretic@medils.org
2 Faculty of Science, University of Split, 21000 Split, Croatia; juretic@pmfst.hr

Abstract: Nature's way for bioactive peptides is to provide them with several related functions and the ability to cooperate in performing their job. Natural cell-penetrating peptides (CPP), such as penetratins, inspired the design of multifunctional constructs with CPP ability. This review focuses on known and novel peptides that can easily reach intracellular targets with little or no toxicity to mammalian cells. All peptide candidates were evaluated and ranked according to the predictions of low toxicity to mammalian cells and broad-spectrum activity. The final set of the 20 best peptide candidates contains the peptides optimized for cell-penetrating, antimicrobial, anticancer, antiviral, antifungal, and anti-inflammatory activity. Their predicted features are intrinsic disorder and the ability to acquire an amphipathic structure upon contact with membranes or nucleic acids. In conclusion, the review argues for exploring wide-spectrum multifunctionality for novel nontoxic hybrids with cell-penetrating peptides.

Keywords: amphipathic peptides; multifunctional; design; penetratins; antimicrobial; antiviral; anticancer; anti-inflammatory; cell-penetrating; non-toxic

Citation: Juretić, D. Designed Multifunctional Peptides for Intracellular Targets. *Antibiotics* **2022**, *11*, 1196. https://doi.org/10.3390/antibiotics11091196

Academic Editors: Agostinho Antunes, Guillermin Agüero-Chapin and Yovani Marrero-Ponce

Received: 8 August 2022
Accepted: 29 August 2022
Published: 3 September 2022

Publisher's Note: MDPI stays neutral with regard to jurisdictional claims in published maps and institutional affiliations.

Copyright: © 2022 by the author. Licensee MDPI, Basel, Switzerland. This article is an open access article distributed under the terms and conditions of the Creative Commons Attribution (CC BY) license (https://creativecommons.org/licenses/by/4.0/).

1. Introduction

Bioactive peptides are all around us, including host defense peptides (HFD) in our bodies. We can regard them as templates developed by natural evolution that are lead compounds for creating commercial products or drugs. Various chemical modifications are employed to increase their stability for different applications. Bioactive peptides are often multifunctional. Some are hidden within proteins and liberated to perform their functions only when needed. Others can be designed in silico by combining several shorter peptides. In any case, there is a fast-growing field of design and applications for peptides that may have multifaceted performance. Such candidate therapeutics may help treat complex diseases often associated with opportunistic infections. Dual antibacterial and anticancer activity has been frequently observed [1–6]. For instance, wide-range antibacterial peptide aurein 1.2 exhibits high activity against 52 cancer cell lines [7]. Another nontoxic antimicrobial peptide, buforin IIb, is active against 60 human tumor cell lines [8]. The bimodal function can encompass antimicrobial and anti-inflammatory activity [9–11]. Hilchie et al. [9] mention 18 biological activities of cationic host defense peptides and their synthetic derivatives. In their 2019 review [12], Hilchie et al. stressed that "cationic amphipathic peptides may exhibit any combination of antimicrobial, anticancer, or immune-modulatory properties".

Regarding antimicrobial performance, antifungal and antiviral activity are of particular interest due to difficulties in the development of safe, low molecular weight antibiotics against such targets [13–17]. The penetration inside cells also belongs to the coveted multifunctional property, firstly for the ability of cell-penetrating peptides (CPP) to interact with the cellular membrane in a non-invasive manner [18,19], and secondly for acting on hard-to-reach intracellular targets [20,21].

Current algorithms for predicting the activity of multifunctional peptides have limited accuracy. However, they are still helpful indicators of which natural peptides or in silico constructs are promising for much more expensive verifications in vitro and in vivo. A plethora of user-friendly servers has appeared during recent years for sequence-based prediction of cell-penetrating (CPP), antimicrobial (AMP), anticancer (ACP), antiviral (AVP), antifungal (AFP), and anti-inflammatory (AIP) peptides [22–35]. An older server by Hwang et al. [36] can be used to predict DNA binding. A valuable feature is when servers allow for designing novel peptides with improved function [35] or decreased toxicity [37]. The goal of combining all six activities (CPP, AMP, ACP, AVP, AFP, and AIP) in a single peptide construct is possible, but two caveats should be considered. We do not want to invest time and money into examining strongly toxic peptides. Fortunately, in silico prediction by dedicated servers for toxicity [37–39] and hemolytic activity [40] can be used to prune designed candidates with high predicted hemolytic activity or toxicity to healthy human cells. Secondly, all predictions are questionable in the absence of experimental validation. Hence, whenever possible, we must compare predictions with observations to obtain insight into the reliability of employed "in silico" expectations.

We shall describe in this review several classes of peptides that have confirmed or predicted high multifunctional potential. Our approach is to start with some natural or artificial peptides with proven cell-transduction efficiency. It is the parent peptide for in silico exploration on how it can be modified or fused to other bioactive peptides for acquiring multifunctional activity without losing its cell-penetrating ability. Such peptides have a better chance of reaching intracellular pathogens that are difficult to eradicate with conventional antibiotics.

Regarding predictions, there are several additional caveats to using publicly accessible web servers for predicting sequence-based functionality for a peptide. The most important one is reproducibility. Free assistance to the scientific community via such web servers is never cost-free for those who maintain them. Suppose larger organizations up to the state or international level are not involved in maintaining long-term reproducibility. In that case, the half-life of servers for scientific calculations is measured in years, not decades. The most severe reproducibility problem is when the server's output (score) is different for each submission of an identical peptide. That may happen when recent algorithms are still riddled with bugs; although, their link is in the public domain and the description is published in a high-impact journal. The case example is the ToxIBTL server for predicting peptide toxicity [41].

Different artificial intelligence algorithms are becoming ever more popular in constructing predictive algorithms. However, most suffer from well-known weaknesses. They are essentially black boxes containing some rules learned during the training procedure. There is no easy way to discover and formulate these rules, however useful they may be in raising the prediction accuracy. Overly intensive training does not help either because it can decrease the performance when the AI algorithm is presented with the testing dataset, which differs in some properties from the training dataset.

When large enough datasets of non-redundant and non-homologous peptides are collected, one can separate the training and testing datasets by choosing some compromise for the cut-off in similarity among these datasets. It is an excellent practice when several benchmarking datasets are used for testing. However, the proper training procedure should be such that testing datasets are never examined during the training procedure. Tests with the benchmark datasets should be done only once. Frequent jackknife tests of the training dataset amount to additional training procedures and should be avoided if possible. It may not be possible when different descriptors are tested as well.

The fourth caveat is connected to the choice of features or descriptors. It is subjective and usually limited to overly simple ideas about what is essential for peptides' activity. Atomic composition, amino acid composition, dipeptides composition, charges, and other amino acid features (hydrophobicity) completely neglect the sequence order of amino acid residues in a peptide, sequence profile of hydrophobicity and hydrophobic moments, dipole moments, and many other structure-associated physicochemical features. These are features and descriptors we described in our publications when we were constructing descriptors for predicting selectivity and a membrane-induced increase in helical conformation [42–46].

Recently developed AI algorithms, which we mentioned in Methods, incorporate interpretable features and in-depth analysis of peptides' biophysical and biochemical properties. We have used them on many occasions during the past several years. There were only occasional short service disruptions for some of them, probably due to maintenance. Our last accession was on 7 August 2022.

We shall firstly examine in this work the multitude of natural penetratin analogs with special attention to those of ancient origin. Secondly, we shall use the hybrid constructs with penetratin analogs and optimized penetratin to find promising lead compounds for strong multifunctional activity. Thirdly, novel peptide conjugates for intracellular targets will be proposed too. Next, shorter CPPs unrelated to penetratin, either known or novel, will be examined regarding predicted multifunctional activities when conjugated to peptides with verified activity for promising broad-spectrum applications.

Conclusions will gather the best compromise for all peptide constructs among strongly predicted six multifunctional activities (CPP, AMP, ACP, AVP, AFP, and AIP) and low toxicity estimates in the hope of future experimental verifications and appropriate chemical modifications for various applications. The class of highly charged temporin analogs fused to short CPP ended up as 50% of the 20 best peptides that have promising therapeutic potential. They are not overly expensive for synthesis, with a length ranging from 22 to 31 amino acid residues.

2. Sequence-Based Servers for Predicting Peptide Activity and Proposed Ranking Methods

The choice of online available predictive algorithms is according to (a) their online persistence, (b) the usage simplicity when peptide sequence is submitted, and (c) claimed accuracy. The last requirement (accuracy) is challenging to estimate independently from the authors' claims. Prediction results are commented on in the paper when they indicate some algorithm shortcomings.

The **MLCPP** server, www.thegleelab.org/MLCPP/ (accessed on 7 August 2022) by Manavalan et al. [22], is used to predict peptide cell-penetrating probability and uptake efficiency. We also consulted the **C2Pred** server by Tang et al. [23] (http://lin-group.cn/server/C2Pred, (accessed on 7 August 2022)) for the CPP probability.

The **DP-Bind** server http://lcg.rit.albany.edu/dp-bind/ (accessed on 7 August 2022) by Hwang et al. [36] is used for sequence-based prediction of DNA-binding residues in DNA-binding proteins and peptides. In some cases, the **dSPRINT** server http://protdomain.princeton.edu/dsprint, (accessed on 7 August 2022)) by Etzion-Fuchs et al. [47] provided the confirmation of the DNA-binding preference for sequence domains.

The antimicrobial peptide probability for a query peptide is found by applying the Support Vector Machine (SVM) algorithm from the **CAMP$_{R3}$** web server http://www.camp.bicnirrh.res.in/predict (accessed on 7 August 2022) [24]. We also used the **AmpGram** server (http://biongram.biotech.uni.wroc.pl/AmpGram/ (accessed on 7 August 2022) [25]) to identify antimicrobial peptides.

Two web servers are used to predict the peptide's anticancer activity. These are the **ACPred** server http://codes.bio/acpred/ (accessed on 7 August 2022) [26] and the **mACPred** server http://thegleelab.org/mACPpred/ (accessed on 7 August 2022) by Boopathi et al. [27].

Three web servers are used to predict the peptide's antiviral activity. These are the **ENNAVIA** server https://research.timmons.eu/ennavia (accessed on 7 August 2022) by Timmons and Hewage [28], the **FIRM-AVP** server https://msc-viz.emsl.pnnl.gov/AVPR/ (accessed on 7 August 2022) by Chowdhury et al. [29], and the **Meta-iAVP** server http://codes.bio/meta-iavp/ (accessed on 7 August 2022) by Schaduangrat et al. [30].

The **iAMPpred** web server http://cabgrid.res.in:8080/amppred/server.php (accessed on 7 August 2022) of Meher et al. [31] gives predictions for antibacterial, antiviral, and antifungal activity, but we reported only the last one. We also used the **AntiFungal** server of Zhang et al. [32] (https://www.chemoinfolab.com/antifungal/, (accessed on 7 August 2022)) to predict the antifungal activity.

For the prediction of anti-inflammatory activity, we used the **AIPpred** server (http://www.thegleelab.org/AIPpred/ (accessed on 7 August 2022) [33]), the **PreAIP** server (http://kurata14.bio.kyutech.ac.jp/PreAIP/ (accessed on 7 August 2022) [34]), and the scoring output of the **AntiInflam** server (http://metagenomics.iiserb.ac.in/antiinflam/ (accessed on 7 August 2022) [35]) when it predicts the anti-inflammatory activity. We used the AntiInfam server to design peptides with a better anti-inflammatory score.

Two different methods estimated peptide toxicity. Firstly, the probability that the peptide has hemolytic activity was assessed using the **HAPPENN** server https://research.timmons.eu/happenn (accessed on 7 August 2022) by Timmons et al. [40]. Secondly, the peptide toxicity was predicted by the **ToxinPred** server https://webs.iiitd.edu.in/raghava/toxinpred/ (accessed on 7 August 2022) [37–39]. We used the server modules for batch submission and designing peptides with decreased toxicity. To verify peptide toxicity class (toxic or nontoxic), a more recent **ToxIBTL** server http://server.wei-group.net/ToxIBTL (accessed on 7 August 2022) [41] was also employed. Besides toxicity class, that server's output contains an irreproducible and meaningless score because the user is given a different score for an identical peptide in each submission.

We employed older reliable servers, **SPLIT 3.5** [42] and **SPLIT 4.0** [43], for predicting the sequence profile of hydrophobicities, optimal hydrophobic moments, and membrane preference for amphipathic and membrane-associated segments: http://split.djpept.com/split/ (accessed on 7 August 2022) and http://split.djpept.com/split/4/ (accessed on 7 August 2022). Our **Mutator** tool [46] served to design anuran-like peptide antibiotics with a predicted high selectivity index: http://mutator.djpept.com/ (accessed on 7 August 2022) or http://splitbioinf.pmfst.hr/mutator/ (accessed on 7 August 2022).

For each of the considered peptides, we presented predicted results in Tables 1–5. The summary Table 6 for ranking the best peptide constructs presents only mean scores for each of the predicted activities. The mean score for anti-inflammatory activity can be higher than 1.0 because the AntiInflam server reports the score for the AIP activity that can be higher than 1.0. The arithmetic average of mean CPP, AMP, ACP, AVP, AFP, and AIP scores served to rank all peptides regardless of their toxicity to healthy human cells. We then introduced the reward for predicted low toxicity and hemolytic activity to obtain the overall ranking for all nontoxic multifunctional constructs. The reward score is calculated as a negative mean of toxicity score (negative) by the ToxinPred server and the HAPPENN server output (positive). Mean scores for six activities and the reward score are then averaged to obtain the overall score. It ranges from 0.873 to 0.927 for the 20 best peptides, while the reward score ranges from 0.346 to 0.867.

Table 1. Penetratin-like peptides within homeodomains.

Organism/ Common Name	Parent Protein or Gene/ GenBank or Uniprot Link	* Penetratin or Penetratin Analog Sequence	#Arg /#Lys/CPP Probability $
Drosophilamelanogaster/fruit fly	pAntp/P02833	RQIKIWFQNRRMKWKK	3/4/1.00
Homo sapiens/human	Hox-A5/P20719 PDX-1/P52945 HXD8/P13378 Hox-C12/ P31275	**RQIKIWFQNRRMKWKK** **RHIKIWFQNRRMKWKK** **RQVKIWFQNRRMKWKK** **QQVKIWFQNRRMKKKR**	3/4/1.00 3/4/0.997 3/4/0.97 3/4/0.97
Homo sapiens/human	Pax-6/P26367 Pax-7/P23759 and Pax-3/P23760	ARIQV**WFSNRRAKW**RR ARVQV**WFSNRRARW**RK	5/1/0.94 5/1/0.94
Homo sapiens/human	PITX2/D6RFI4	ARVRV**WFKNRRAKW**RKR	5/3/0.97
Ciona intestinalis/sea squirt tunicate	Pax3/7-like/NP_001071798.1	ARVQV**WFSNRRAKW**RR	5/1/0.94
Acropora millepora/stony coral	Pax-6/XP_029212196.2	ARIQV**WFSNRRAKW**RK	4/2/0.94
Capitella teleta/annelid worm	Ct-Pax3/7 (Pax6)/A1XC54, ABC68267.1	ARVQV**WFSNRRARW**RK	5/1/0.94
Nematostella vectensis/sea anemone	PaxC homeodomain transcription factor/Q5IGV4	ARVQV**WFSNRRAKW**RR	5/1/0.94
Mnemiopsis leidyi/comb jelly	PRD10a homeobox trancription factor/ ADO22618.1	ARIQV**WFQNRRAKW**RK	4/2/0.93
Amphimedon queenslandica/sponge	Pax-6/XP_003387530.1	SRVQV**WFQNRRAKW**RK	4/2/0.93
Trichoplax adhaerens	PaxB/ACH57172.1	ARVQV**WFSNRRAKW**RK	4/2/0.92
Ceratocystis platani/fungi	Pax-6/KKF93291.1	AKINN**WFQNRRAK**AKL	2/3/0.86
Galerina marginata/Dykaria higher fungi	Homeobox containing protein fragment/ A0A067SZU8	ARIQV**WFSNRRAKW**RR	5/1/0.94
Planoprotostelium fungivorum/amoeba	Arf-GAP with homeobox domain/ A0A2P6NXG8	ARIQV**WFSNRRAKW**RR	5/1/0.94
Monosiga brevicollis (Choanoflagellate)	Mb_hbx2 homeobox-domain protein/ A9UP33	**QQI**NN**WFINAR**RRLLNR	4/0/0.76
Capsaspora owczarzaki amoebae(*Filasterea clade)*	CAOG_004648 Homeobox domain-containing protein/ A0A0D2VSA1	**RVIRIWFQNRRAK**QRR RRQKARRNQFWIRIVRR§	6/1/0.96 7/1/0.96

Table 1. *Cont.*

Organism/ Common Name	Parent Protein or Gene/ GenBank or Uniprot Link	* Penetratin or Penetratin Analog Sequence	#Arg /#Lys/CPP Probability $
Candida glabrata/budding yeast	Homeobox containing protein PHO2/ Q6FKZ3	KNVRIWFQNRRAKVRK KNVRIWFQNRRAKVRKKGKL	4/3/0.95 4/5/0.95
Hanseniaspora osmophila/ wine-making yeast	Regulatory protein PHO2 with homobox domain 1/ A0A1E5RMZ3	TQVKIWFQNRRMKWKR	3/3/0.94
Acinetobacter baumannii/Gram- bacteria	Homeobox domain-containing protein (partial)/ WP_139162288.1	RQVAVWFQNRRARWKT	4/1/0.87
Klebsiella pneumoniae/Gram- bacteria	Homeobox domain-containing protein WP_185963280.1	TQIKIWFQNRRAK*D*HR	3/2/0.76
Euryarchaeota archaeon	RYE98021.1	RQVSVWFTNARKRIWL	3/1/0.77
Acanthamoeba polyphaga mimivirus/ giant virus	Putative homeobox protein/ AKI80488.1	RQIQIWFQNRRCK*D*RK	4/2/0.87
Moumouvirus maliensis/giant virus	Homeodomain containing protein/ QGR53678.1	KQISIWFANRRAY*D*ARK RKNGVKMTKVKKIRRSR[&]	3/2/0.63 4/5/0.94
Megavirus chiliensis/giant virus	Putative homeobox protein/ YP_004894234.1	RQIQIWFQNRRAR*D*SKKNR	5/2/0.85
Bandra megavirus/	Homeobox/ AUV58136.1	RQIQIWFQNRRAR*D*SKKIR	5/2/0.85
Unclassified Mimivirus/ giant virus	Homeobox protein/ QZX43434.1	RQIQIWFQNRRAR*D*SRKNR	6/1/0.86

* Bold font is for amino acid residues that are identical in type and sequence location to *Drosophila* pAntp penetratin; underlined residues are for extended penetratin analog at its C-terminal; All examined viruses and some Gram-negative bacteria have aspartate (D) highlighted with italic font instead of tryptophan (W) at the 14th sequence location. $ #Arg/#Lys are the numbers of arginines and lysines in the sequence. The third number after the slash symbol is the cell-penetrating probability (CPP), according to www.thegleelab.org/MLCPP/ (accessed on 7 August 2022) server. § Reversed amoebae penetratin (Filasterea clade) with added arginine. & Homeodomain motif upstream from penetratin analog is also predicted as the CPP.

The overall score ranking is highly dependent on estimated toxicity. Peptide toxicity is usually firstly examined as hemolytic potency. Minimizing hemolytic activity can improve the therapeutic potential of peptides. The HAPPENN server [40] employs the threshold value of 0.5 to distinguish hemolytic from non-hemolytic peptides. Its valuable feature is distinguishing C-terminal amidated from non-amidated peptides. Amidated peptides are more active antimicrobials but can be associated with increased hemolytic activity. Magainin-2 in its C-terminal amidated form is the best-known antimicrobial peptide. More than 500 μM concentration of MG2 is needed to cause 50% hemolysis. Its hemolytic probability is 0.83 (see Table 5, peptide 6 for the HAPPENN output). Therefore, a peptide with a probability for hemolytic activity between 0.50 and 0.83 or less can still be a good candidate for synthesis, purification, and testing.

3. Under-Appreciated Versatility of Penetratins

3.1. The Evolutionary Depth of Homeobox Domains and Penetratin-like Cryptides in the Animalia Kingdom

Natural DNA-binding peptides can be the inspiration for designing cell-penetrating peptides (CPP) with DNA-binding and other multifunctional activities. We shall first explore this idea for the penetratin-like peptides. Le Roux et al. published in 1993 [48], the primary structure of 35 amino acid long cryptide L(322)TRRRRIEIAHALCLTE **RQIKIWFQNRRMKWKK**EN(356) rich in arginines from the homeodomain of the Drosophila melanogaster (fruit fly) protein Antennapedia (pAntp). The highlighted sequence (with bold font residues) was named the penetratin peptide. Remarkably, that 16-residues long cryptide (hidden peptide) from homeodomain proteins connected fruit flies to humans (Table 1). One can speculate that DNA-binding and cell-penetrating functions are related and equally ancient for penetratin analogs found in homeobox-like proteins (Tables 1 and 2). More to the point, membrane activity, cell-penetrating ability, antimicrobial potency, and anticancer activity are also related to the highly cationic and moderately amphipathic structure of the penetratin and its natural or synthetic analogs [49–58].

Identical hexadecapeptide penetratin analog is present in Drosophila O18381, mouse P63015, and human P26367 Pax-6 parent proteins. It is the arginine-rich ARIQV**WFSNRR**A **KW**RR sequence (residues identical to *Drosophila* pAntp penetratin are in a bold font). We can estimate its evolutionary depth by performing the peptide search for that arginine-rich sequence in the UniProt database. There are about two thousand hits for invertebrate and vertebrate animals, most associated with the Pax-6 annotation. The *Pax-6* gene is a master control gene responsible for developing photodetection and eye morphogenesis in flies, mice, and humans. Walter Gehring and his co-authors postulated that the strikingly diverse eyes found in the most primitive to the most advanced animals derived from an ancestral eye and ancestral organ selector genes [59–63]. Pax and Pax-like genes coding for penetratin analogs were found not only in flatworms, insects, and mammals but also in sponges lacking a nervous system [64–66].

Corresponding proteins are transcription factors containing two to three domains with three α-helices. The first two domains belong to the defining Pax signature of the 128-amino acid DNA-binding paired domain [67]. The third DNA-binding domain with three helices is the 60-amino acid homeobox domain. Binding to DNA as homodimers or heterodimers is often essential for the transcriptional activity of homeobox-containing proteins [68]. An unresolved question is the functional importance of penetratin analogs found in a homeobox-like sequence of the simplest and most ancient animals devoid of organs. Another underexplored question regards the possible toxicity of natural or designed penetratin analogs. When substituted amino acids change peptide–DNA or parent protein–DNA interaction, the results can be either beneficial or harmful in vivo. Disease-causing mutations in the human Pax3 gene belong to the latter examples.

From the UniProt entry P23760 the homeobox sequence is Q(219)RRSRTTFT AEQLEEL(234)ERAF(238)ERTHYPDIYTREELAQRAKLTEARVQV(265)W(266)FSNR(270) R(271)AR(273)WRKQA(278) for human Pax3 (we underlined helices α1, α2, and α3). The substitution of residues V(265), W(266), R(270), R(271), and R(273) from recognition helix α3 with, respectively, F, C, C, C, and K, may result in the Waardenburg syndrome (WS1) with impaired hearing and other disorders. Presumably, Phe (F) and Cys (C) cannot maintain crucial DNA–homeodomain interactions provided by V(265), W(266), and R(271). Substitutions P for L(234) and S for F(238) are also causing WS1 syndrome probably by destabilizing the hydrophobic interactions for the homeodomain fold (see Birrane et al., 2009 paper [69], where L(16) and F(20) correspond to L(234) and F(238)). Birrane et al. [69] concluded that Pax3 has no DNA-interacting residue in its first homeodomain helix (α1). It has one DNA-interacting residue in its second helix (α2) and eight such residues in its third DNA-recognition helix (α3). Other authors also concluded that the penetratin-like helix α3 has the strongest contact with the major DNA groove [70,71].

We restricted Table 1 examples of metazoan penetratins to phylums Chordata (Mammalia class), Tunicata (subphylum, Ascidiacea class, which includes sea squirts), Antrophod (Insecta class), Annelida (Polychaeta class worm), Cnidaria (Anthozoa class, including stony corals), Ctenophora (Tentaculata class, which includes comb jellies), Porifera (Despongiae class), and Placozoa (*T. adhaerens*). In all subkingdoms of Animalia, we can easily find those penetratin analogs that are essential motifs in transcription factors regulating the development.

Given examples from Table 1, let us elaborate on the evolutionary depth of the conserved role for Pax, Pax-like genes, homeotic genes, and associated penetratin-like DNA-binding motifs. It is not only penetratin-like peptides from animals without eyes, eye spots, and neurons (Table 1 examples for Porifera and Placozoa). Surprisingly, such peptides are also present in fungi, yeasts, bacteria, Archaea, and viruses. In his 2013 review, Peter Holland observed that homeotic genes were not found in Archaea or bacteria [72]. However, additional Archaea and bacterial genomes have been decoded during the past decade. The last nine rows from Table 1 illustrate that homeobox domains and penetratin analogs can be found as cryptides among proteins from prokaryotic cells and viruses. The bacterial origin is more likely than the Archaea origin for a recognizable homeodomain with the helix-loop-helix-turn-helix motif. Only marginal similarity to pAntp or human Pax-6 penetratin is found for natural penetratin analogs from Archaea because at least 50% of the residues from these hexadecapeptides are different. Recent whole-genome decoding of giant viruses also revealed putative homeodomains and penetratin analogs [73,74]. The conserved motif WFXNRR is shared among all kingdoms of life, but it is too short to find significant similarities. In any case, prokaryotes and viruses also use regulatory transcription factors, and some of them may have been the progenitors of homeotic proteins in eukaryotes.

Ed Lewis, the first expert on homeotic genes, quipped in a letter to Walter Gehring: "Dear Walter, you made the homeobox our flying carpet." The penetratin analog segments are our time-machine part of the "flying carpet" for reaching the distant past of Life development. Let us show several examples to support that claim. We used our PROSITE motifs, BLASTP, and UniProt searches to investigate the evolutionary roots. That is the origin of some of the cited penetratin analogs (see Tables 1 and 2).

Example 1: Human penetratin-like sequences

There are more than 500 human homeotic proteins. Some human proteins contain two homeobox domains and two different penetratin-like peptides (see some examples at UniProt links O43812, Q96PT3, A6NLW8, and P0CJ85). Human Zink finger homeobox protein 3 has four homeobox domains in its long sequence of 3703 residues (see Q15911) with four associated penetratins, which are, however, of low similarity to pAntp penetratin.

Example 2: Nematodes, cnidarians, and tunicates

Previously mentioned arginine-rich analog ARIQVWFSNRRAKWRR is present in the Vab-3 transcription factor G5EDS1 from the worm *Caenorhabditis elegans*. The worm does not have eyespots, much less fully developed eyes. Since it lives underground or inside rotting fruits, it does not require image-forming eyes, however primitive. Still, the worm has consistently expressed the Pax6 gene [66], which must be somehow involved in developing its miniature brain. *C. elegans* uses rhodopsin-like sensory receptor protein Q10042 annotated with a G protein-coupled receptor activity, but molecular details of its function are unknown. Color-perceiving systems without eyes and without "seeing" color may exist. The *C. elegans* animal model is probably the best for discovering neural circuits and previously unrecognized proteins that have evolved to capture light and react to rich information within the light spectrum. Its nervous system consists of only 302 neurons and performs miracles of sensing mechanical forces, chemicals, temperature, humidity, and electromagnetic fields. The Vab-3 involvement (if any) in *C. elegans* neural circuits for eyeless light detection is still the subject of active research.

The same arginine-rich sequence is present in the *Nematostella vectensis* (sea anemone) PaxC homeodomain from the transcription factor Q5IGV4. That cnidarian has a variable number of neurons (several hundred at most [75]) in decentralized nerve nets and poorly understood eyeless photodetection [76]). Another cnidarian, the *Acropora millepora* stony coral, can tune spawning behavior with the phases of the moonlight [77]. It is unknown whether the penetratin analog ARIQVWFSNRRAKWRK from Q5IGV4 protein, with a conservative Arg to Lys substitution, plays a role in light sensing by coral larva or not. It would not be surprising that more ancient eyeless vision needed penetratin analogs for its development. The arginine-rich hexadecapeptide connects worms, corals, and starlet sea anemones to insects and mammals. Its sequence can be as good a, if not a better, vehicle than pAntp penetratin for trans-membrane transport.

Tunicates are the sister group to vertebrates. The *Ciona intestinalis* larva (sea squirt tunicate) has the smallest brain of any chordate, with only 231 neurons [78]. Still, it needs the transcription factor protein NP_001071798.1 containing the penetratin-like ARVQVWFSNRRAKWRR sequence. Larva's simple eye-spot ocellus has a pigment cell and vertebrate type ciliary opsin Ci-opsin1 [79], showing significant homology to vertebrate rhodopsins [80]. The retinal chromophore, Ci-opsin1, ocellus, and homeobox-containing transcription factors are the connection to the evolution of complex vertebrate eyes.

Example 3: Placozoans

Placozoans are the simplest animals in the evolutionary tree of Metazoa. The expression of homeobox-containing proteins has been confirmed in *Trichoplax adhaerens* and other placozoans [81–83]. *T. adhaerens* express genes encoding for proteins implicated in morphogenesis [84], innate immunity [85–90], and motility [91]. Moving and sensing are possible without brain cells but not without specialized proteins. The ARVQVWFSNRRAKWRR penetratin analog from the *T. adhaerens* ACH57174.1 Pax-3-like protein is different from corresponding human analogs only in one or two conservative amino acid substitutions (only V↔I or R↔K)! The TriPaxB penetratin RVVQVWFQNQRAKLKK from the *Trichoplax adhaerens* protein Lim1 (UniProt entry B5LDT8) served as a query (named TriPaxB) for extended penetratins in other simple organisms (see Table 2).

T. adhaerens has a high regeneration and rejuvenation potential, partially due to the regulated expression of homeotic genes Not and Trox-2 [92]). The best-conserved regions of corresponding proteins contain penetratin-like peptides A**QVKVWFQNRRIKWRK** and K**QVKIWFQNRR**V**KWKK**. We used the bold font for residues from the *T. adhaerens* peptides are identical to Drosophila pAntp penetratin residues.

Example 4: Poriferans

The Pax-6 protein XP_003387530.1 (or Uniprot entry A0A1X7UM72) from the embryo of the sponge *Amphimedon queenslandica* is annotated as the homeobox domain-containing protein (by UniProt) and as paired box protein Pax-6-like (by NCBI genome annotation data). In both databases, the DNA binding is predicted as the transcription factor activity. The PaxB penetratin from *T. adhaerens* with the sequence ARVQVWFSNRRAKWRK is similar to the SRVQVWFQNRRAKWRK peptide in the sponge's Pax-6. Substituted residues are in bold font and underlined.

Example 5: Amoeboid protist

The amoeboid holozoan *Capsaspora owczarzaki* is one close unicellular relative of animals [84]. Authors labeled as Co_5 the homeobox domain from the protein A0A0D2VSA1.

It contains six arginines within the penetratin sequence RVIRIWFQNRRAKQRR. Other natural penetratins have a high number of Arg and Lys residues (Table 1). These sequences are still underexplored candidates for transporting bioactive cargo into the cell.

3.2. *The Penetratin-like Cryptides from Other Kingdoms*

The search among ascomycetes (fungi) also resulted in diverse penetratins. One hit with the Pax-6 annotation is for the *Ceratocystis platani* fungus causing disease on sycamore trees. It is the Paired box protein Pax-6 (KKF93291.1) with 639 residues. The penetratin analog from its homeobox region has a 56% identity to pAntp penetratin (see Table 1).

Another regulatory protein PHO2 (A0A1E5RMZ3) with the homeobox domain from Hanseniaspora osmophila (wine-making yeast) has an associated penetratin analog, which is similar in its sequence TQVKIWFQNRRMKWKR to the pAntp. The budding yeast penetratin analog KNVRIWFQNRRAKVRKKGKL extended at its C-terminal (underlined) from the PHO2 (Q6FKZ3) protein has a high positive charge and unknown abilities. Its CPP probability prediction by the MLCPP server is similar (0.93) to pAntp (0.98). Hemolytic activity prediction by the HAPPENN server is a strikingly low probability of 0.018 compared to pAntp's 0.936. Thus, exploring natural penetratin analogs from all available sources can be the first stepping stone toward discovering nontoxic CPP candidates with a peptide backbone.

Two representative bacterial and one archeon species are included in Table 1 because at least one homeobox domain-containing motif with penetratin analog is found among their expressed proteins. The similarity is modest or low to pAntp. Archeon penetratin analog **RQ**VSV**WFTNAR**KRIWL is only 38% identical to pAntp penetratin (residues with bold font are 6 out of 16 residues), raising doubts about similar functions.

Some viral proteins contain remarkably efficient CPP, such as the TAT peptide from HIV [93,94], which has as promising drug-delivery therapeutic potential as penetratin [95]. The TAT peptide sequence GRKKRRQRRRPPQ is, however, easily cleaved by furin. Thus, CPP is not stable enough in vivo for efficient cargo delivery [96]. Hemmati et al. [97] identified 310 decapeptides with predicted CPP activity in the proteome of severe acute respiratory syndrome coronavirus 2 (SARS-CoV-2). In the surface glycoprotein S (spike protein) alone, there are 24 CPP candidates, some rich in Arg residues. Nucleocapsid protein N is even richer in CPP candidates (54). Arginines are required firstly for binding to negatively charged groups of viral nucleic acid [98] and secondly for penetrating the eukaryotic cell membrane.

The superkingdom of viruses includes the class of giant viruses. The genomes with accession numbers: NC_014649, NC_020104, and NC_016072 contain homeobox proteins. The dSPRINT server [47] examines whether the protein domain query binds DNA, RNA, small molecules, ions, or peptides and assigns corresponding interaction probabilities to each interaction type for each residue. Figure 1 illustrates these probabilities for predicted CPP peptide and penetratin analog present within the homeodomain-containing protein QGR53678.1 of a giant *Moumouvirus maliensis* virus. The corresponding residues Arg-44 to Arg-112 with underlined Table 1 peptides for that virus are: RKNGVKMTKV(10)KKIR**RSRLFT**(20)**T**TQ**L**QILEET(30) YKTNK**YISLN**(40)EKINLSKNFG(50)VTVK**QISIWF**(60)**ANRRA**YDAR, where we highlighted with a bold font those residues for which DNA-binding probability is higher than 0.95. The probability of binding ligands other than DNA is less than 0.05 for all residues within both predicted homeodomain motifs. Thus, three C-terminal residues from the predicted CPP peptide (underlined N-terminal 17 residues) and ten residues from the predicted penetratin analog (underlined C-terminal 16 residues) are strongly predicted DNA-binding residues (Figure 1).

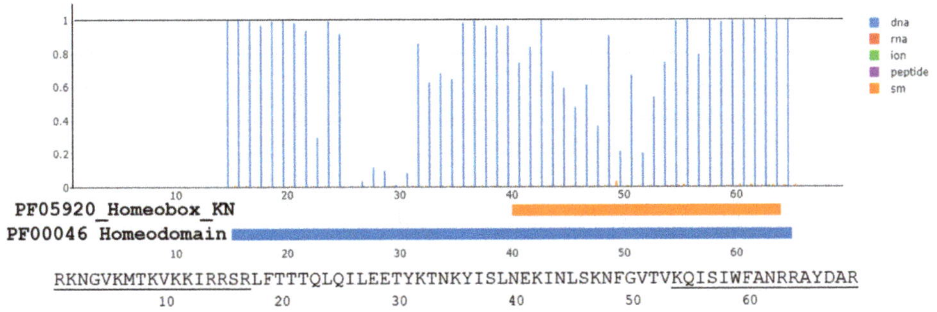

Figure 1. The dSPRINT server [47] prediction for DNA-binding probabilities (vertical axis, blue lines profile) of residues from a homeodomain found in a giant virus *Moumouvirus maliensis* protein QGR53678.1. Probabilities are negligible for binding residues to RNA, ions, other peptides, and small molecules (other colors for profile lines). See the main text for details on the Pfam domains PF05920 and PF00046. We added the query sequence below the graph produced by the dSPRINT server. The underlined residues are the predicted CPP segment (N-terminal) and the penetratin-like peptide (C-terminal).

There are many predicted CPP cryptides from giant viruses other than penetratin analogs. For example, the MLCPP and C2Pred servers predict with a high probability (0.94 and 0.96) that the RKNGVKMTKVKKIRRSR sequence (see Figure 1) should have the CPP activity. We can adopt a tentative name 9RK17 for that CPP cryptide, which is hidden in a putative homeodomain from the GenBank entry QGR53678.1 at a different sequence location from the penetratin analog KQISIWFANRRAY*DAR*K. We doubt that all CPP cryptides from giant viruses (such as 9RK17) have been examined in experiments for their cargo-transporting efficiency inside eukaryotic cells. For instance, the 21 amino acid long cryptide ALHARRRRARQRLCQHRVSIK is present in the hypothetical *Pandoravirus dulcis* (giant virus) protein YP_008318537.1. The predicted CPP probability is 0.95 (MLCPP server) and 0.90 (C2Pred server). A longer cryptide MTWRRSCWRLLRQRRRQPRSPKMMRKR is the N-terminal of hypothetical peptide YP_001425938.1 encoded by the *Paramecium bursaria Chlorella virus* FR483 genome (also a giant virus). The peptide has associated CPP probability predictions of 0.94 and 0.99 by MLCPP and C2Pred server.

Some bacteria and viruses tolerate the differences in the last four residues of natural penetratin analogs (such as W14 to D14 substitution). These residues are less critical for interaction with DNA. Examples of W14 to D14 substitution in penetratin-like peptides from the homeobox domain are found in human sequences, too (see Homeobox even-skipped homolog proteins 1 and 2 with the UniProt links P49640 and Q03828).

The penetratin's biological role in a homeodomain is to serve as a major aggregation site for DNA-binding residues. The same is likely to hold for all other presented Table 1 sequences. The dSPRINT server finds the same GO: 0003677 molecular function by which a gene product interacts selectively and non-covalently with DNA for these sequences. For corresponding proteins, the dSPRINT server finds PF00046_Homeodomain, PF05920_Homeobox_KN motif, or both motifs overlapping the penetratin analog. One example is the N-terminal part with 60 residues of the *Euryarchaeota archaeon* RYE98021.1 protein. For residues 11–40, the prediction for the PF05920_Homeobox_KN motif is associated with the E-value of 3.2×10^{-10}. For residues 25–54, the prediction with the E-value of 1.8×10^{-8} is for the PF00046_Homeodomain motif. The hexadecapeptide sequence RQVSVWFTNARKRIWL extends from Arg-18 to Leu-33, thus forming a part of both homeobox motifs. Extended sequence RQVSVWFTNARKRIWLPLRQKQARMRNKRAK, with residues 18–48, has a higher CPP probability score of 0.93. Therefore, CPP, DNA-binding ability, and the transcription factor DNA-binding function are frequently present in the same protein domains.

The UniProt database of all known and predicted proteins contains 85,650 sequences from 1394 species with the PF00046_Homeodomain annotation. While Table 1 is far from comprehensive, it still reports several additional species from Megaviricetes compared to the Brandes and Linial data analysis in 2019 [99]. It is, of course, due to the fast progress in genetic sequencing. An astonishing universality of that Pfam family motif in Animalia, Fungi, Protista, Eubacteria, Archaea, and Viruses indicates its conservation across almost all of life's superkingdoms and kingdoms.

The PF05920_Homeobox-KN Pfam domain (Figure 1, thick orange line below the x-axis) is also universal in all kingdoms of life. It belongs to the conserved homeobox transcription factor KN domain from TALE, KNOX, and MEIS genes [100]. Current Pfam taxonomy does not mention the presence of the PF05920_Homeobox-KN motif in bacteria and viruses.

A caveat to keep in mind for penetratin-like peptides from bacteria, archaea, and viruses is the hypothetical or predicted nature of some proteins containing them. Low annotation scores in public databases may lead to failed verification for claimed associated species.

3.3. *The Translocation Function of Homeobox Proteins, Homeobox, Penetratin, and Penetratin-like Peptides*

Homeodomain proteins fulfill many biological functions for which other segments in these proteins are also crucial. The unconventional transport mechanism for these proteins is an active research area [101]. Direct translocation of an identical protein in and out from eukaryotic cells is complex because eukaryotic plasma membranes are asymmetric. Their internal lipid layer has a different lipid composition from the external layer. Neutral polar lipids, such as phosphatidylcholine, prevail among phospholipids oriented (with their head groups) toward the cell exterior. Negatively charged phospholipids, such as phosphatidylserine, are plentiful only among polar lipids in contact with the cell cytoplasm. Moreover, fatty acids' unsaturation in the cytoplasmic plasma membrane leaflet is about twofold higher [102]. In the case of engrailed-2 homeoprotein transfer, the anionic phospholipid phosphatidylinositol-4,5-biphosphate is also involved [103]. It is a minor component of the plasma membrane inner leaflet [104] and even less frequent in the outer leaflet. Still, it is essential as a gatekeeper for cell signaling and molecular traffic among cells [105]. Moreover, cell surface carbohydrates are probably involved in the cellular uptake of homeoproteins from the external environment [106]. Therefore, the ability of such proteins for unconventional bidirectional transfer across the plasma membrane of some eukaryotic cells is likely to rely on distinct mechanisms for outside-directed and inside-directed transport.

Distinct mechanisms imply the existence of several dedicated protein motifs for targeting the plasma membrane from the cytoplasm and the cell outside. Specifically, the bidirectional transfer function must be in-built inside an extended penetratin-like region for each homeodomain segment. Dupont et al. [107] examined whether the penetratin extended in its N-terminal to encompass the turn region between the second and third helix is enough to ensure the peptide transport in and out of cells. Dupont et al. [107] named it the SecPen peptide QSLAQELGLNE**RQIKIWFQNRRMKWKK**, where the Sec peptide is underlined, and the penetratin domain is highlighted with bold font.

The QSLAQELGLNE Sec peptide is a cryptide in engrailed-2 proteins Q05917 (HME2_CHICK), P52730 (HME2B_XENLA), and P09015 (HME2A_DANRE), to mention only the reviewed Swiss-Prot proteins containing that peptide. The human analog of the QSLAQELGLNE peptide contains glycine to serine substitution. Sec and Pen allow for bidirectional membrane crossing [106]. These and other authors verified the validity of the signaling homeoproteins concept with far-reaching implications [108].

Homeoproteins are rich in multifunctional cryptides. For example, let us examine the UNIPROT Q05917 entry and structurally solved PDB 3ZOB sequence 3ZOB_1 with three α-helices [109] for chicken engrailed 2 homeoprotein. The GAG (glycosaminoglycans at the cell surface)-binding sequence **P**(186)**RSRKPKKKNPN**KEDKRPR(204) is located just before chicken engrailed 2 homeodomain (residues 200–259). That highly flexible protein region contains two CW BBXB quadruplets (Cardin-Weintraub motifs [110]) and one KKK triplet, all described as glycosaminoglycan or heparan sulfate binding motifs [111]. The bold font for the residues at the N-terminal highlight the motif, which is part of the putative nuclear localization signal (see Figure 1B from reference [111]). It is also a DNA-binding motif, which has a significant probability of penetrating cells (0.88, according to the MLCPP server). Thus, the multiplicity of functions for crucial motifs from engrailed proteins is more a rule than an exception.

Among other examples, the N-terminal hexapeptide QRRSRT for the Pax3 and Pax7 homeodomain is also a good starting point for the design of multifunctional peptides. We can ask what would be predicted activities for the sequence tandem peptide QRRSRT-GQRRSRT with inserted Gly residue as a middle flexible linker. That tridecapeptide is expected to be nontoxic by the Raghava ToxinPred server [38], highly cell-penetrating (the MLCPP server), and strongly DNA-binding (binding probability higher than 0.7 for all arginines according to the DP-BIND server [36]). However, predictions by the CAMP$_{R3}$ and AmpGram algorithms exclude its antimicrobial function. When we fuse the QRRSRT-GQRRSRT sequence with some antimicrobial peptide such as IKKIVSKIKKLLK (L-K6V1-temporin-1CEb) [112], it can gain multifunctional abilities without undesirable hemolytic and toxic effects. For instance, the hybrid peptide with the sequence KKLFKKILKYL-GG-QRRSRTGQRRSRT (BP100-CPP conjugate) is expected to have all six considered functions and lesser hemolytic activity compared to BP100. The same idea should work for N-terminal decapeptide GLNRRRKKRT from the homeobox domain of the pou2f1 transcription factor (Xenopus laevis African clawed frog, Uniprot entry P16143). The sequence tandem GLNRRRKKRTGLNRRRKKRT did not need middle Gly insertion, its cell-penetrating probability score of 0.98 is almost maximal, and all residues 3 to 19 of that 20 residues long peptide have DNA-binding probability higher than 0.8. Moreover, the tandem peptide may have antimicrobial activity against intracellular pathogens. The CAMP$_{R3}$ server SVM module result is 0.925 probability for the AMP activity, while the HAPPEN server predicts a negligible probability of 0.03 for the hemolytic activity.

The translocation function is the best researched for the homeobox protein engrailed-2 from chicken, which is 99% identical to human En2 [109,111]. However, for chick and human engrailed-2 protein, the hexadecapeptide analog of Drosophila antennapedia penetratin is different in underlined residues: SQIKIWFQNKRAKIKK (only one arginine instead of three). A decreased number of arginines opens the question about the importance of human and chick penetratin motifs for membrane translocation of corresponding homeodomain and intact engrailed proteins.

The previous paragraphs indicated that the translocation function might be mediated by protein motifs outside the homeobox domain acting in concert with the recognition helix from that domain. Suppose a minimal number of six consecutive arginines is needed for cell penetration [113]. In that case, the question is whether these residues are close in the 3D structure but not so close in sequence. Hence, we can speculate that CPP activity can be preserved after the number of arginines drops to the single one within the penetratin-like peptides during biological evolution with a compensatory increase in strategically placed arginines outside penetratin.

Firstly, it is easy to find cases when more arginines are in the homeodomain regions preceding the penetratin segment. Secondly, space separation may exist among negative and positive charges. Anionic residues (D and E) may be located only at the one homeodomain surface. The residues with positive charges dominate at the opposite homeodomain surface where the penetratin motif is situated. The spatial separation of anionic from cationic charges persists for the engrailed 2 protein when one examines only two last homeodomain helices with a turn between them. Thus, an electrostatic dipole moment and the corresponding electric field are more substantial for the whole homeodomain and the 2nd-helix-turn-3rd-helix compared to penetratin peptides, which are mostly devoid of negative charges.

We have recently published the observation that strong 3D electrostatic and 3D-hydrophobic moments are instrumental for better interaction between some flexible cationic peptides with helix-turn-helix secondary structures and membranes containing polar lipids with anionic head groups [114]. The calculated hydrophobic moment for an ideal α-helix rod (the 2D moment) is not relevant for the peptide–membrane interaction of highly plastic peptides such as penetratin [115]. Furthermore, a high degree of peptide helicity or amphipathicity is not required for penetratin internalization [116].

The helix-turn-helix motif of engrailed proteins is the ultrafast independently folding domain [117]. An additional internalization advantage for intact homeodomain is that its 20 times lower extracellular concentration of 5×10^{-8} M is enough to achieve substantial accumulation in the cell nuclei [118]. In contrast, micromolar penetratin concentrations must be added for efficient internalization [49].

Three arginines from the pAntp penetratin RQIKIWFQNRRMKWKK are not the only regulators of its translocation process. The substitution of two tryptophans with similarly bulky aromatic and hydrophobic phenylalanine residues inhibits penetration internalization [119]. The role of two tryptophans has been examined in the tryptophan fluorescence study after the first (Trp-6) or second Trp (Trp-14) has been substituted with the Phe residue [49]. The first Trp from the wild-type penetratin sequence motif WF inserts more deeply into the lipid bilayer than the second Trp. The WF motif is also better conserved across biological kingdoms (Table 1). Penetratin membrane incorporation is more profound in the presence of anionic polar lipids, such as phosphatidylserine.

To study the cell penetration mechanism, direct interaction with specific plasma membrane phospholipids is as essential for penetratin-like peptides as their binding to glycosaminoglycans at the cell surface. The mechanism and target molecules may differ among penetratin analogs, homeoboxes, and homeoproteins. We previously mentioned the involvement of phosphatidylinositol-4,5-biphosphate [103], a key lipid signaling molecule important for endocytosis, exocytosis, membrane fusion, and myriad other biological activities. In addition to cell-surface GAGs and heparan sulfate, polysialic acid is also the surface receptor for pAntp Drosophila homeobox peptide [118].

Lysines are less critical for penetratin uptake compared to arginines. When all lysines are replaced with arginines, a designed analog sequence RQIRIWFQNRRMRWRR-NH_2 exhibits almost 50% better internalization ability than wild-type penetratin [55]. Wild-type penetratin possesses moderate antimicrobial activity [50]. In comparison, Bahnsen et al. [55] found that the analog with seven arginines has about four times stronger antimicrobial activity against *E. coli*. However, the analog exhibits eight times greater toxicity to human cells. These activity changes are not predicted by the servers we used (compare results for pAntp peptide 1 from Table 2 and PenArg peptide 1 from Table 3). On the other hand, predictions and experimental validations agree that amphipathic antimicrobial peptides with high lysine content can have negligible hemolytic activity and low toxicity. One example is L-K6V1-Temporin-1CEb [112] (Table 3, peptide 40).

Electrostatic interactions are important for translocation into cells [120]. These interactions have been tuned during biological evolution by clustering positive charges near the C-terminal of penetratin-like peptides and by retaining lone arginine at the first or second N-terminal position in animals. The lengthwise charge asymmetry is accompanied by the hydrophobic interactions of peptide middle leading to the bend conformation parallel to the membrane surface.

Detailed molecular dynamics simulations and free energy calculations uncovered the role of Trp-6 interaction with Arg-1 and Arg-10 at the membrane surface [121]. In observed Trp-Arg stacking, the indol ring of W is positioned almost parallel to the guanidinium group of R. Trp-6 is more involved than Trp-14—the observation of the importance of WR cation–π interactions [122], which is in accordance with the better preservation of Trp−6 in penetratin-like peptides. We can safely assume that all of the presented penetratin-like sequences from Table 1 (and many more not present in that table) are membrane-active peptides. The membrane-activity terminology implies that peptide conformational plasticity and membrane curvature adaptation occurs after mostly disordered peptides from an aqueous solution reach the membrane surface [53,121,123,124]. The structural plasticity of penetratin (from random coil to beta-sheet and α-helix in different environments) is relatively high among other cell-penetrating peptides [125]. It contributes to its functional CPP versatility through clathrin-mediated endocytosis, caveolae-mediated endocytosis, macropinocytosis, and direct translocation by forming inverted micelles [53,126,127].

Clathrin-mediated endocytosis is an active transport process requiring GTP hydrolysis [128]. On the other hand, direct translocation is an energy-independent uptake. It is a self-initiated spontaneous process producing only transient perturbation of plasma membrane integrity [116]. Alves et al. [53] proclaimed: "penetratin usurps endocytotic cell processes but can also translocate into the cells." Translocation and uptake rates depend on CPP sequence and concentration, cell type, buffer, temperature, cargo (if any), and other experimental variables [56]. With such versatility, it is no wonder that penetratin can induce phase separation, de-packing of membrane lipids, negative curvature, and aggregation of lipid vesicles [123,129]. These macroscopic effects of penetratin are enhanced for cases of higher membrane fluidity and the presence of anionic phospholipids at the membrane surface.

One biological role of penetratin is the contribution to driving the translocation of its parent homeoprotein, but the translocation of intact homeoprotein is much more efficient (<1 nM [106]) in comparison with the penetratin uptake. Homeoproteins are natural cargoes for at least some penetratin-like peptides. Moreover, homeoproteins are active cargoes with non-penetratin protein regions participating in the synergetic amplification of specific translocations. The biological roles have not been examined for most of the natural penetratin-like peptides. That did not prevent widespread penetratin usage in life sciences and therapeutic applications.

3.4. Penetratin Sequence Optimization and Possible Applications

Penetratin sequence optimization by Kauffman et al. [56] resulted in considerably improved direct translocation (with different cargoes) by the RKKRWFRRRRPKWKK analog with six arginines, five lysines, and two tryptophans. Similarly designed penetratin analogs may be helpful delivery vehicles for biotechnological applications and systemic therapeutics (a fast-growing market). Older results on the vectorization strategies with penetratin are gathered in the book by Dupont et al. [130].

The mechanisms of CPP penetration and CPP-cargo transport across the blood–brain barrier are discussed this year by Zorko and Langel [131]. Penetratin is usually linked with a drug, protein, or nucleic acid cargo at its N-terminal. Škrlj et al. [132] used penetratin as the linker peptide connecting two antibody fragments specific for the pathological form of the prion protein. That vectorization strategy enabled efficient delivery across the blood–brain barrier. Liposomal formulation using penetratin molecules is an effective treatment strategy for delivering a therapeutic gene to the brain. The aim is, for instance, to reverse Alzheimer's disease pathophysiology [133]. Non-viral gene delivery for all therapeutic goals has advantages when penetratin or similar peptides are used as nontoxic vehicles that do not provoke an immune response.

In the proof of principle experiments, Liu et al. [134] demonstrated how penetratin-coated nanoparticles can reach the eye fundus, thus eliminating the need for invasive eye injection during the gene therapy treatment of diseases such as diabetic retinopathy and age-related macular degeneration. Needle-in-the-eye application is naturally associated with low patient compliance and increased infection risk.

The penetratin (PEN) and other cell-penetrating peptides have a promising potential for drug targeting and oncological pharmacotherapy [57,58]. Combating drug-resistant cancers by targeted delivery of drugs should facilitate the development of effective personalized therapies. The designed GEM-PEN conjugate improved the intracellular delivery and anticancer activity of gemcitabine (GEM) [135]. Anticancer peptides can also be covalently connected to penetratin. Kanovsky et al. [136] synthesized three p53 peptides PPLSQETFS, PPLSQETFSDLWKLL, and ETFSDLWKLL in peptide linkage to reversed penetratin analog sequence KKWKMRRNQFWVKVQRG. The authors did not explain their rationale for reversing the Antennapedia penetratin sequence G**RQIKIWFQNRRMKWKK** (in the bold font) or replacing isoleucines with valines with added terminal glycine. It is connected to the previous observation about the absence of chiral receptor requirement for the transduction ability of penetratin and its reversed analog (see the publication [137] cited by Kanovsky et al. [136]). The three p53 peptides are amino-terminal parts of that tumor suppressor protein, which can interact with oncogene-encoded ubiquitin-protein ligase mdm-2 (MDM2 [Q00987]), targeting p53 for degradation and accelerated proliferation of cancer cells.

Kanovsky et al. [136] reasoned that the blockage of p53-mdm-2 interactions could inhibit cell-transforming oncogenic events by competition of the peptides mentioned above to p53 for mdm-2 binding. Thus, these three peptides should be able to act as anticancer if they can reach intracellular mdm-2 target proteins. The attachment of reverse penetratin KKWKMRRNQFWVKVQRG sequence to the carboxy-terminal end of each peptide had a dual role—to enable transport of the peptides across the plasma membrane and to stabilize the α-helical conformation of each peptide for maximal interaction with mdm-2 proteins. NMR experiments subsequently confirmed the helical conformation [138] (see the PDB entry 1Q2F). Increased helical content of the peptide was not achieved when the penetratin leader sequence was attached to the amino-terminal end of the PPLSQETFSDLWKLL sequence. It resulted in considerably lower helical probabilities of reverse penetratin carboxy-terminal part (with added Gly residue) and bioactive peptide amino-terminal segment containing the Pro pair. Therefore, the N-terminal or C-terminal conjugation of a bioactive peptide to CPP is not arbitrary. It should be guided by the maximization of the interaction with internal targets of chimeric peptides. Chosen peptide conjugates by Kanovsky et al. [136] were highly cytotoxic on various tumor cells and did not affect normal cells in culture.

Interestingly, amino-terminal p53 peptides induce cell death in malignant cells without inducing apoptosis and independently of p53 protein activation, arguing for a general antiproliferative effect on these cells. The software tools ACPred and mACPred failed to predict the high probability of anticancer function for reverse VV–penetratin hybrid with N-terminal p53 peptide PPLSQETFS (see Table 2, peptide 11). Hence, the p53 peptide conjugated to penetratin was erroneously classified as noncancer (NACP).

Selivanova et al. [139] examined the option for C-terminal p53 peptides conjugated to penetratin. The importance of the p53 gene stems from observations that more than half of human tumors have mutations in that gene. Transcribed protein has several DNA binding domains. The G(361)SRAHSSHLKSKKGQSTSRHKK(382) sequence is the most highly charged cationic domain near the C-terminal (see P04637 UniProt entry), which regulates DNA binding. Selivanova et al. [139] investigated whether the C-terminal peptide can restore the growth suppressor function of mutant p53 proteins. The authors used the peptide **GSRAHSSHLKSKKGQSTSRHKK**WKMRRNQFWVKVQRG (named fusion peptide 46; see peptide 19 predictions in Table 2). By bold font and underlining, we highlighted the C-terminal p53 peptide and reversed penetratin to emphasize that CPP is ligated to the carboxy-terminal end of the bioactive peptide without its KK pair at the amino-terminal end because the KK pair is already present at the C-terminal of the fusion peptide.

Subekti and Kamagata [140] proposed the role of the flexible and disordered C-terminal p53 domain. It enables p53 to land on and twin around DNA, forming the encounter complex at lower salt concentrations. The flexibility facilitated the protein jumping along DNA at higher salt concentrations. Selivanova et al. [139] proved that the growth suppressor function of mutant p53 could be restored by an excess of the fusion peptide 46.

The authors proposed that the peptide can displace the C-terminal domain from its binding site to the core p53 domain.

Restoring the ability to bind DNA worked for Ala-143, His-175, Trp-248, Ser-249, His-273, and Lys-280 mutant forms of p53 [141]. Activated p53 induced apoptosis in Ew36 and BL41 Burkitt lymphoma cells, SW480 colon carcinoma cells, and breast cancer cells MCF-7, MDA-MB-468, and MDA-MB-231, despite mutant p53 forms being present in these cells [141]. Normal breast and colon cell lines were not affected. The corresponding peptide 19 from Table 2 has predicted DNA-binding, cell-penetrating, antimicrobial, antiviral, and antifungal activity combined with toxicity absence by some of the algorithms we used. However, peptide 19 is associated with modest probabilities of 0.61 and 0.65 for anticancer activity as calculated by the ACPred [26] and mACPpred [27] servers. Of course, experimental results should prevail in our minds over any theoretical predictions. We can anticipate the therapeutic benefits of anticancer-peptide-CPP conjugates when their pharmacokinetic parameters are improved for medical applications.

3.5. Multifunctional or Hybrid Penetratin-like Peptides

Table 2 results belong to three peptide classes. The first class contains natural sequences 1 (pAntp), and 3 (TriPaxB). Listed examples of longer natural peptides 4–6 with additional four residues at each peptide terminal contain the TriPaxB penetratin and belong to the second class. The first sequence (peptide 4 in Table 2) is from an uncharacterized cnidarian protein with 445 AA from medusa Clytia hemisphaerica (jellyfish). The following peptide (peptide 5) is found in the T2M9B9 UniProt entry for an unreviewed protein named LIM homeobox transcription factor 1-alpha (LMX1A). The protein LMX1A is from the fresh-water polyp Hydra vulgaris, claimed to be immortal [142,143]. The sequence for peptide 6 (A0A183IGD8) is from the parasitic stomach-dwelling worm of American martens Soboliphyme baturini and Loa loa eye worm. These three natural sequences were submitted to the dSPRINT server http://protdomain.princeton.edu/dsprint (accessed on 7 August 2022) [47]. They have a common PF00046_Homeodomain motif for the first 20 residues and the GO: 0003677 molecular functions by which a gene product interacts selectively and non-covalently with DNA. Rationally designed peptides 2 and 7–22 are the third class. Peptide 2 is the VV-penetratin sequence RQVKVWFQNRRMKWKK. It is present in the predicted homeobox proteins of some birds and fishes (UniProt entries A0A7K7IKL9, A0A7K9GUV0, and A0A1A8LZ63). The designed sequences validated in experiments have the "/E" extension in their abbreviated name. In silico design by this author is associated with the "/DJ" extension.

Regarding possible penetratin involvement in antimicrobial defense, Drosophila pAntp penetratin RQIKIWFQNRRMKWKK-NH_2 is fungicidal for the clinical isolates of *Cryptococcus neoformans* [51]. It exhibits moderate antibacterial activity against *Escherichia coli* and *Staphylococcus aureus* with MIC values from 32 to 64 μM [55]. Some of penetratin's natural analogs from Table 1 may have stronger antimicrobial potency or better therapeutic index. Our goal was to find or design multifunctional peptides with low predicted toxicity to healthy human cells. All Table 2 peptides have predicted cell-penetrating and DNA-binding activity combined with a considerably lower prediction for the hemolytic activity compared to pAntp penetratin. In addition, most Table 2 peptides have predicted antimicrobial, anticancer, antiviral, antifungal, and anti-inflammatory activity. For sequences 4–6, 11, and 14–15, the ACPred server does not predict anticancer activity. Some of them have been designed and validated as ACP (peptide 11).

It is not easy to achieve strongly predicted antifungal (probability higher than 0.7) along with other activities and low toxicity to red blood cells. At the end of Chapter 2, we explain our reasons for choosing the higher limit of 0.83 for hemolytic activity probability, which can still ensure good selectivity. The peptides 2–11, 13–18, and 20–22 from Table 2 satisfy that criterion. Three of them are constructs involving parts of the pexiganan antibiotic and TriPaxB or VV-penetratin (peptides 7–9). Peptide 10 is fused TriPaxB with the antifungal sequence BP16 studied by Badosa et al. [144]. Peptide 13 is reversed VV-penetratin [136] fused to the anticancer TPR peptide [145]. The Gly residue is a flexible linker between two bioactive peptides in both cases. The N-terminal part of peptide 15 is reversed amoebae penetratin (peptide 14 from Table 2), which we singled out in Table 1 as a natural penetratin-like peptide with the highest number of arginines (six). Short C-terminal sequence CGIKRTK is similar to tumor-homing peptide tLyp-1 with the sequence CGNKRTR [146]. The tLyp-1 and CGIKRTK are nontoxic but also not associated with other predicted activities except cell penetration (see peptide 1 from Table 5).

The optimization for better anti-inflammatory activity led to the best multifunctional peptides 20 (with underlined activity scores) and 21 from Table 2. They consist of a reverse penetratin analog [56] (see peptides 16 and 17) with two amino acid substitutions (A8 and I15) and analogs to the tumor-homing peptide [146]. The predicted toxicity to red blood cells is very low (0.01) for peptides 20 and 21. Another advantage of these peptides is their short length (22 residues). Their overall rank among all 176 sequences from Tables 2–5 is 6th and 22nd. Peptide 21 is an example of when increasing the number of substitutions to increase the anti-inflammatory activity impairs other functionalities. The peptide 22 is an analog of reversed optimized penetratin [56] (see Chapter 4 for details of its design). Its overall rank is 31st (Table 6). Still, its short length (18 residues) and predicted lack of hemolytic activity and toxicity argue for experimental validation of cell-penetrating, antibacterial, anticancer, and antiviral activity.

The tentative conclusions from Table 2 are the following. Searching through natural cryptides from biological databases is always a promising initial approach. Using the rational design may be more successful in widening the activity spectrum of bioactive-CPP conjugates. In vitro and in vivo tests can confirm whether some of Table 2 peptides remain viable candidates for drug development. For a hybrid pAntp–TPR anticancer sequence (peptide 12), predicted hemolytic activity slightly decreases in comparison with pAntp alone. The observed toxicity of peptide 12 to normal cell lines is significantly smaller than its toxicity to cancer cell lines [145].

If confirmed, the antifungal activity might be the most interesting for several reasons. Firstly, nature's design for penetratins gives these peptides the specialized ability to easily pass through the eukaryotic cell membrane and for DNA binding. Secondly, there are precious few drugs toxic to fungal cells causing different diseases but are nontoxic to human cells. One example is the urgent need for compounds inhibiting the growth of *C. neoformans* yeasts in patients who had organ transplantation and are immunocompromised. Thirdly, the conjugated antifungal–CPP hybrid peptide may gain additional activities, as predicted in Table 2 (see peptide 10). The rational design option for creating antifungal hybrid peptides targeting intracellular molecules is to conjugate penetratin or some penetratin analog with known antifungal peptides such as LKLFKKILKVL or KKLFKKILKKL [144]. They are active against pathogenic fungi Fusarium oxysporum. The probability for antifungal activity increased from 0.22 for the TriPaxB penetratin sequence RVVQVWFQNQRAKLKK (see Table 2, peptide 3) to 0.54 or higher for the constructs RVVQVWFQNQRAKLKK-G-LKLFKKILKVL or RVVQVWFQNQRAKLKK-G-KKLFKKILKKL (see Table 2, peptide 10 for the second construct predictions). The sequence should be submitted to other predictive algorithms (besides iAMPpred [31] and AntiFungal [32]) for serious consideration of experimental confirmations.

Confusingly, a dedicated server for the classification of peptides according to predicted antifungal activity—the http://webs.iiitd.edu.in/raghava/antifp (accessed on 7 August 2022) server, predicts as non-antifungal the peptides LKLFKKILKVL (BP33; [144]), KKLFKKILKKL (BP16; [144]), LKLFKKILKVLG, together with hybrid peptides LKLFKKILKVL-G-RVVQVWFQNQRAKLKK, RVVQVWFQNQRAKLKK-G-LKLFKKILKVL, and sequence 10 from Table 2.

Table 2. Hybrid penetratin-like peptides with predicted DNA binding, CPP, antimicrobial, anticancer, antiviral, antifungal, anti-inflammatory, hemolytic, and toxic activity.

No.	Peptide/Gene/Origin *	Extended TriPaxB or Reverse Penetratin/Sequence Number *	DNA-Bind. **	CPP $	Anti-Microbial ‡	Anti-Cancer $$	Anti-Viral &	Anti-Fungal ⁋	Anti-Inflamm. Activity §	Hemo-lytic ¥	Toxicity/Score †
1	P02833/*D. melanogaster* penetratin/E	**RQIKIWFQNRRMKWKK** /339–254/pAntp	+	0.998/H	0.97/0.42	0.812/0.985	1.0/0.70/0.77	0.28/0.95	0.57/0.68	0.94/+	−0.66
2	Rev. VV-pen. [136]/E	**KKWKMRRNQFWVKVQR**	+	0.956/H	0.96/0.53	0.649/0.981	0.10/0.44/0.28	0.15/0.68	0.52/0.66	0.19/−	−0.81
3	TriPaxB penetratin	**RVVQVWFQNQRAKLKK**	+	0.807/L	0.74/0.42	0.036/0.971	0.00/0.40/0.01	0.22/0.21	0.52/0.61	0.02/−	−1.42
4	A0A7M5V8Y3/N/A /*Clytia hemisphaerica*	GLSV**RVVQVWFQNQRAKLKK**IQKK/227–250	+	0.642/L	0.96/0.32	0.189/0.980	0.44/0.47/0.82	0.56/0.59	0.65/0.62	0.03/−	−1.45
5	T2M9B9/UP && /*Hydra vulgaris*	GLSV**RVVQVWFQNQRAKLKK**LHFK/227–250 and 108–131	+	0.761/L	0.93/0.37	0.065/0.983	0.66/0.46/0.97	0.58/0.45	0.66/0.61	0.03/−	−1.16
6	A0A1S0TPC1/UP &&/ *Loa loa*	NLSV**RVVQVWFQNQRAKLKK**IQRK/118–141	+	0.715/L	0.91/0.29	0.049/0.769	0.21/0.57/1.0	0.28/0.59	0.67/0.63	0.04/−	−1.47
7	PexNC-TriPaxB-I/DJ	GIGK-**RVVQVWFQNQRAKLKK**-ILKK	+	0.731/L	0.99/0.67	0.968/0.980	0.93/0.75/1.0	0.97/0.59	0.61/0.58	0.09/−	−1.51
8	PexShort-TriPaxB-II (PexT)/DJ	GIGKLKKAKKFGKKILKK-G-**RVVQVWFQNQRAKLKK**	+	0.792/L	1.0/0.98	0.995/0.951	0.98/0.76/0.52	1.0/0.61	0.64/0.58	0.13/−	−1.17
9	PexNC-rev. VV-pen./DJ	GIGK-G-**KKWKMRRNQFWVKVQR**-ILKK	+	0.849/H	1.0/0.58	0.919/0.982	1.0/0.65/0.95	0.94/0.93	0.55/0.67	0.26/−	−1.17
10	TriPaxB–antifungal BP16 [144]/DJ	**RVVQVWFQNQRAKLKK-G-**KKLFKKILKKL	+	0.816/L	0.98/0.95	0.992/0.981	1.0/0.70/0.93	0.98/0.54	0.54/0.64	0.62/+	−1.46
11	Anti-cancer-I-Rev. VV-pen. [136]/E	PPLSQETFS-**KKWKMRRNQFWVKVQRG**	+	0.503/H	0.41/0.53	NACP/NACP	0.40/0.90/1.0	0.15/0.05	0.62/0.62	0.13/−	−1.09
12	pAntp-TPR [145]/E	**RQIKIWFQNRRMKWKK-**KAYARIGNSYFK	+	0.834/H	0.91/0.50	0.923/0.939	1.0/0.80/0.54	0.83/0.65	0.59/0.62	0.91/+	−1.09
13	Rev.-VV-pen. [136]-TPR/DJ	**KKWKMRRNQFWVKVQR**-G-KAYARIGNSYFK	+	0.766/H	0.83/0.48	0.766/0.952	1.0/0.79/1.0	0.87/0.40	0.60/0.63	0.59/+	−1.13
14	Rev. amoeba (*Filasterea*) pen. with added N-term-Arg/DJ	**RRQKARRNQFWIRIVRR**	+	0.958/H	1.0/0.46	0.110/0.984	0.01/0.27/0.73	0.44/0.71	0.59/0.62	0.07/−	−0.58
15	Rev. R-am.pen.-tLyP-1 [146]/DJ	**RRQKARRNQFWIRIVRR-CGIKRTK**	+	0.962/H	0.98/0.51	0.259/0.984	0.78/0.91/0.93	0.88/0.43	0.68/0.62	0.02/−	−0.88
16	Optimal penetratin (o-pen P14 [56]/E	**RKKRWFRRRRPKWKK**	+	0.992/H	1.0/1.0	0.767/0.978	0.97/0.57/1.0	0.32/1.0	0.47/0.56	0.02/−	−0.89
17	Rev. opt. penetratin (r-o-p)/DJ	**KKWKPRRRRFWRKKR**	+	0.992/H	1.0/0.99	0.767/0.980	1.0/0.92/1.0	0.32/1.0	0.48/0.49	0.01/−	−1.11
18	Rev.opt.pen. (r-o-p)-tLyP-1 [146]/DJ	**KKWKPRRRRFWRKKR-CGIKRTK**	+	0.987/H	0.94/1.0	0.854/0.979	1.0/0.82/0.59	0.71/0.96	0.65/0.68	0.006/−	−1.30

Table 2. *Cont.*

No.	Peptide/Gene/Origin *	Extended TriPaxB or Reverse Penetratin/Sequence Number *	DNA-Bind. **	CPP $	Anti-Microbial ‡	Anti-Cancer $$	Anti-Viral &	Anti-Fungal ⁋	Anti-Inflamm. Activity §	Hemo-lytic ¥	Toxicity/Score †
19	Fusion peptide 46 [139]/E	GSRAHSSHLKSKKGQSTSRH-**KKWKMRRNQFWVKVQRG**	+	0.741/L	0.76/0.87	0.61/0.65	0.98/0.48/0.15	0.81/0.44	0.67/0.59	ND	−0.89
20	**Rev.opt.pen. (r-o-p A_8I_{15})-tLyP-1 [146]-analog1/DJ**	**KKWKPRRARFWRKKI-CGIKRTK**	+	0.987/H	0.96/0.993	0.972/0.98	1.0/0.8183/0.77	0.89/0.922	0.6674/0.647/1.397	0.007/−	−1.39
21	Rev.opt.pen. A_8I_{15}—tLyPA_3-1-analog2/DJ	**KKWKPRRARFWRKKI-CGAKRTK**	+	0.985/H	0.97/0.99	0.943/0.981	1.0/0.78/0.27	0.86/0.96	0.66/0.66/1.56083	0.006/−	−1.22
22	Rev. optimized penetratin analog/DJ	**GKRIGKKWKPRRRRFWRK**	+	0.991/H	1.0/1.0	0.944/0.979	1.0/0.96/0.95	0.59/1.0	0.61/0.61	0.003/−	−1.26

* Highlighted peptides (bold name) with underlined activity scores are our selection for the designed peptides with the best overall score (see Table 6). All peptides are assumed to be amidated at their C-terminal. Letter 'E' after peptide name means that the sequence has been synthesized and tested in experiments. DJ abbreviation means that according to our knowledge, we were the first to find or design that peptide. Bold sequence segments have predicted or verified CPP activity. Underlined residues are optimal substitutions for increasing anti-inflammatory activity or decreasing peptide toxicity. ** The results of DP-Bind server http://lcg.rit.albany.edu/dp-bind/ (accessed on 7 August 2022) by Hwang et al. [36] for sequence-based prediction of DNA-binding residues in DNA-binding proteins. The "+" sign means that the server found several DNA-binding residues. $ The probability that the peptide is cell-penetrating peptide (CPP) or non-CPP (NCPP) with the MLCPP server http://www.thegleelab.org/MLCPP/ [22]. Predicted high and low uptake efficiency is denoted with, respectively, letters 'H' and 'L'. ‡ Antimicrobial peptide probabilities with $CAMP_{R3}$ Support Vector Machine algorithm of the server http://www.camp.bicnirrh.res.in/predict (accessed on 7 August 2022) [24] and with AmpGram (http://biongram.biotech.uni.wroc.pl/AmpGram/ [25]. $$ The ACPred server (http://codes.bio/acpred/ [26] is used to classify peptides as anticancer (ACP) or non-anticancer (NACP) with a given probability. The mACPred server (http://thegleelab.org/mACPpred/ [27] results for the probability of anticancer activity are added after the '/' symbol. & Results of peptide antiviral prediction with servers ENNAVIA (https://research.timmons.eu/ennavia [28], sequence length restricted between 7 and 40 residues)/FIRM-AVP (https://msc-viz.emsl.pnnl.gov/AVPR/ (accessed on 7 August 2022) [29]/Meta-iAVP (http://codes.bio/meta-iavp/ (accessed on 7 August 2022) [30]. ⁋ Results of iAMPpred peptide antifungal prediction by Meher et al. [31] (http://cabgrid.res.in:8080/amppred/server.php, (accessed on 7 August 2022)) and Zhang et al. [32] (https://www.chemoinfolab.com/antifungal/, (accessed on 7 August 2022)). § Results for the prediction of anti-inflammatory activity (Anti-inf.) by the AIPpred (first number; http://www.thegleelab.org/AIPpred/ (accessed on 7 August 2022) [33], PreAIP (second number; http://kurata14.bio.kyutech.ac.jp/PreAIP/ (accessed on) [34] server, and the score output of the AntiInflam server (http://metagenomics.iiserb.ac.in/antiinflam/ (accessed on 7 August 2022) [35] server when it predicts the anti-inflammatory activity. ¥ The probability that the peptide has hemolytic activity by the HAPPENN server [40] https://research.timmons.eu/happenn (accessed on 7 ugust 2022). After the peptide name, we introduced the |lcl|cTer term to obtain the prediction for the amidated C-terminal. Symbols '+' and '−' are used for peptide classification as hemolytic or not. † Toxicity prediction by the ToxinPred server https://webs.iiitd.edu.in/raghava/toxinpred/ (accessed on 7 August 2022) [37–39]. We used batch submission for peptides [37]. The design module of that server was used when we wished to optimize the peptide for decreased toxicity after several amino acid substitutions. && UP = Uncharacterized protein.

Table 3. CPP bioactive peptide conjugates for intracellular targets I. Activity probabilities.

No.	Peptide or Parent Protein/ Gene/Origin/Reference *	CPP Constructs/Sequence Number *	CPP	Anti-Microbial	Anti-Cancer	Anti-Viral	Anti-Fungal	Anti-Inflamm.	Hemo-lytic	Toxicity/ Score
1	PenArg (Bahnsen-2013 [55])/E	**RQIRIWFQNRRMRWRR**	0.99/H	0.99/0.57	0.32/0.98	1.0/0.7/0.4	0.24/0.96	0.60/0.66	0.94	–1.12
2	DiR$_6$WF OLQ14316.1/ *S. microadriaticum*	**RRRRRRWFRRRRRRWFRKI** /603–621 DiR$_6$WF	0.99/H	1.00/0.97	0.92/0.91	1.0/0.3/1.0	0.43/0.82	0.57/0.59	0.68	–0.97
3	WFR$_8$ from CellPPD [$] scan of DiR$_6$WF/DJ	**RRWFRRRRRR**	0.99/H	1.00/0.99	0.95/0.98	0.9/0.6/0.9	0.42/ND	0.53/0.53	0.21	–0.92
4	Reverse WFR$_8$ (R$_8$FW)/DJ	**RRRRRRFWRR**	0.99/H	1.00/0.89	0.95/0.98	0.9/0.4/0.9	0.42/ND	0.56/0.53	0.08	–0.93
5	Ribos.-hom.-pept. (RHP)-pAntp/ [54]/E	YKWYYRGAA- **RQIKIWFQNRRMKWKK**	0.90/H	0.74/0.46	0.95/0.98	1.0/0.9/0.8	0.49/0.68	0.64/0.62	0.97	–0.63
6	HK2-WFR$_8$ [147]/DJ	MIASHLLAYFFTELN-GG- **RRWFRRRRRR**	0.80/H	0.62/0.19	0.15/0.99	1.0/0.8/1.0	0.17/0.45	0.62/0.59	0.30	–1.28
7	RHP [54] -WFR$_8$/DJ	YKWYYRGAA-**RRWFRRRRRR**	0.97/H	1.0/0.97	0.85/0.98	1.0/0.8/1.0	0.63/0.93	0.60/0.63	0.12	–1.10
8	RtLyp-1-G-VV-pen. [&]/DJ	**RCGNKRTR**-G- RQVKVWFQNRRMKWKK	0.94/H	0.78/0.49	0.12/0.98	1.0/0.5/1.0	0.57/0.83	0.58/0.61	0.24	–0.67
9	**L-K6V1 temporin 1CEb [112]-GG-WFR$_8$/DJ**	IKKIVSKIKKLLK-GG- **RRWFRRRRRR**	0.97/H	0.98/1.00	0.97/0.98	1.0/1.0/1.0	0.97/1.00	0.54/0.67/1.0796	0.17	–1.35
10	CAMEL [148]-WFR$_8$/DJ	KWKLFKKIGAVLKVL- **RRWFRRRRRR**	0.96/H	1.00/1.00	0.81/0.98	1.0/1.0/1.0	0.82/1.00	0.61/0.66	0.98	–1.33
11	Rev. WFR$_8$–CAMEL [148]/DJ	**RRRRRRFWRR**-GG- KWKLFKKIGAVLKVL	0.96/H	1.00/1.00	0.73/0.98	1.0/0.9/1.0	0.92/0.98	0.60/0.63	0.71	–1.33
12	[R4, R10]-chensinin-1b [149]- WFR$_8$/DJ	VWRRWRRFWRR-GG- **RRWFRRRRRR**	0.99/H	1.00/0.95	0.93/0.98	1.0/0.7/0.1	0.41/0.99	0.58/0.71	0.72	–1.02
13	ZY4 [150]-GG-WFR$_8$/DJ	VCKRWKKWKRKWKKWCV-GG- **RRWFRRRRRR**	0.98/H	0.99/1.00	0.91/0.98	1.0/0.9/0.8	0.40/1.00	0.53/0.68	0.60	–0.50
14	Puroindoline [151]-WFR$_8$/DJ	FPVTWRWWKWWKG-G- **RRWFRRRRRR**	0.99/H	1.00/1.00	0.87/0.98	1.0/0.9/1.0	0.21/0.99	0.61/0.66	0.85	–0.99
15	Rev. WFR$_8$_puroindoline/DJ	**RRRRRRFWRR**-GG- FPVTWRWWKWWKG	0.98/H	1.00/0.95	0.85/0.98	1.0/0.9/1.0	0.23/0.99	0.61/0.62	0.49	–1.01
16	Novispirin [152] -WFR$_8$/DJ	KNLRIIRKGIHIIKKY-GG- **RRWFRRRRRR**	0.95/H	1.00/1.00	0.95/0.98	1.0/1.0/1.0	0.94/0.99	0.63/0.62	0.53	–1.14
17	BP33 antifungal [144]/E	LKLFKKILKVL	0.85/H	0.84/1.00	1.0/0.98	1.0/0.5/1.0	0.98/1.00	0.48/0.65	0.57	–1.30
18	BP33 antif. [144]-pAntp/DJ	LKLFKKILKVL-G- **RQIKIWFQNRRMKWKK**	0.86/H	1.00/0.92	0.98/0.98	1.0/1.0/1.0	0.98/1.00	0.54/0.66	1.0	–1.09

Table 3. *Cont.*

No.	Peptide or Parent Protein/ Gene/Origin/Reference *	CPP Constructs/Sequence Number *	CPP	Anti-Microbial	Anti-Cancer	Anti-Viral	Anti-Fungal	Anti-Inflamm.	Hemo-lytic	Toxicity/ Score
19	TriPaxB-antifungal-BP33 [144]-with-GGG-tag/DJ	**RVVQVWFQNQRAKLKK**-LKLFKKILKVL-GGG	0.62/H	0.96/0.95	0.84/0.84	0.9/0.9/1.0	0.98/0.23	0.64/0.65	0.63	−1.58
20	rWFR$_8$-antif-BP16 [144]/DJ	**RRRRRRFWRR**-GG-KKLFKKILKKL	0.982/H	1.00/1.00	0.97/0.98	1.0/0.7/1.0	0.90/1.00	0.57/0.68	0.57	−1.40
21	T2R1 [88]-WFR$_8$/DJ	RHHWRRYARIGFRAVRTVIGK-G-**RRWFRRRRRR**	0.901/H	1.00/1.00	0.73/0.97	1.0/1.0/0.9	0.70/0.90	0.71/0.64	0.30	−1.18
22	WFR$_8$-DiPGLa-H [153]/DJ	**RRRRRRFWRR**-G-KIAKVALKALKIAKVALKAL	0.970/H	1.00/1.00	0.57/0.97	1.0/0.9/1.0	0.91/0.99	0.64/0.66	0.80	−1.09
23	WFR$_8$-TPR [145] with G_4 link/DJ	**RRWFRRRRRR**-GGGG-KAYARIGNSYFK	0.893/H	1.00/0.73	0.71/0.98	1.0/0.6/1.0	0.90/0.76	0.59/0.57	0.16	−1.38
24	GV1001 vaccine [154]-WFR$_8$/DJ	EARPALLTSRLRFIPK-GG-**RRWFRRRRRR**	0.951/H	1.00/0.59	0.95/0.98	1.0/1.0/1.0	0.66/0.95	0.69/0.74	0.05	−1.35
25	BP100 [155]-WFR$_8$/DJ	KKLFKKILKYL-GG-**RRWFRRRRRR**	0.981/H	1.00/1.00	0.45/0.98	1.0/1.0/1.0	0.92/0.97	0.60/0.69	0.71	−1.39
26	RWBP100 [156]-WFR$_8$/DJ	RRLFRRILRWL-GG-**RRWFRRRRRR**	0.994/H	1.00/0.97	0.84/0.98	1.0/0.8/1.0	0.53/0.99	0.61/0.70	0.65	−1.23
27	Mitochondrial targeting [157]-WFR$_8$/DJ	KLLNLISKLF-GGG-**RRWFRRRRRR**	0.938/L	1.00/0.98	0.43/0.98	1.0/0.9/0.8	0.81/0.99	0.62/0.67	0.82	−1.31
28	Nosangiotide [158]-WFR$_8$/DJ	RKKTFKEVANAVKISA-GG-**RRWFRRRRRR**	0.917/H	0.98/0.96	0.25/0.97	0.9/0.9/0.9	0.79/0.95	0.67/0.58	0.08	−1.09
29	Buforin [159] -WFR$_8$/DJ	TRSSRAGLQFPVGRVHRLLRK-GGG-**RRWFRRRRRR**	0.945/H	0.99/0.87	0.05/0.98	1.0/0.9/0.4	0.91/0.99	0.68/0.60	0.04	−0.89
30	Buforin-BR2 [160]/E	RAGLQFPVGRLLRRLLR	0.879/L	1.00/0.71	0.42/0.98	0.8/0.9/1.0	0.20/1.00	0.53/0.63	0.01	−1.12
31	BR2-WFR$_8$/DJ	RAGLQFPVGRLLRRLLR-GG-**RRWFRRRRRR**	0.960/H	1.00/0.97	0.43/0.98	1.0/0.9/1.0	0.68/1.00	0.53/0.63	0.25	−1.23
32	WFR$_8$-Zp3a [161]/DJ	**RRWFRRRRRR**-GIKAKIGIKIKK	0.98/H	0.99/1.00	0.84/0.98	1.0/0.8/1.0	0.89/0.98	0.53/0.66	0.07	−1.25
33	RHP [54]-rev. WFR$_8$/DJ	YKWYYRGAA-**RRRRRRFWRR**	0.97/H	1.00/0.80	0.85/0.98	1.0/0.9/1.0	0.63/0.95	0.61/0.62	0.04	−1.03
34	T2R3G3/DJ	RRRHHWRRYARIGFRAVRTVIGK-GGG	0.87/H	0.99/0.84	0.85/0.97	1.0/0.9/1.0	0.85/0.54	0.67/0.66	0.06	−1.19
35	**Temporin-asparagutin analog1/DJ**	IKKIVSKILKLLKV-G-**RRWFRRRRRR**	0.96/H	0.998/1.00	0.96/0.98	1.0/1.0/1.0	0.96/1.0	0.60/0.71/1.625	0.76	−1.47
36	**Temporin-asparagutin analog2/DJ**	IKKIVSKIRKLLK-GG-**RRWFRSRRRR**	0.96/H	0.92/0.99	0.96/0.98	1.0/1.0/1.0	0.97/0.99	0.62/0.66/1.5	0.18	−1.30
37	**Temporin-asparagutin analog3/DJ**	VKKIVSKIRKLLK-GG-**RRWFRSRRRR**	0.97/H	0.92/0.99	0.95/0.98	1.0/1.0/1.0	0.96/0.99	0.63/0.64/1.72	0.13	−1.27

Table 3. *Cont.*

No.	Peptide or Parent Protein/ Gene/Origin/Reference *	CPP Constructs/Sequence Number *	CPP	Anti-Microbial	Anti-Cancer	Anti-Viral	Anti-Fungal	Anti-Inflamm.	Hemo-lytic	Toxicity/ Score
38	Novispirin [152]-WFR$_8$-analog1/DJ	KNLRLIRKGIHIILKY-GG-**RRWFLRRRRR**	0.938/H	1.0/1.0	0.768/ 0.981	1.0/0.9854/1.0	0.96/0.995	0.5814/0.648/1.5622	0.551	−1.17
39	Temporin-1CEb [162]/E	ILPILSLIGGLLGK	0.453	0.789/1.0	0.991/ 0.984	0.101/0.083/0.68	0.98/0.97	0.47/0.62	0.959	−1.08
40	L-K6V1-Temporin-1CEb [112]/E	IKKIVSKIKKLLK	0.880/L	0.930/1.0	1.0/0.982	0.991/0.589/0.40	0.87/1.0	0.53/0.64	0.009	−1.20
41	T2R1 [88]/E	RHHWRRYARIGFRAVRTVIGK	0.907/H	0.973/0.617	0.96/0.984	0.999/0.901/0.89	0.67/0.764	0.63/0.63	0.017	−1.06
42	Rev. WFR$_8$-hinge-aurein 1.2 [3]/DJ	**RRRRRRFWRR**-GGGPPK-GLFDIIKKIAESF	0.817/H	0.941/0.994	0.897/0.916	1.0/0.874/1.0	0.94/0.988	0.609/ 0.575	0.082	−1.02
43	SVS-1 [163]/E	KVKVKVKVDPLPTKVKVKVK	0.817/L	0.96/0.746	0.962/0.973	0.0/0.4/0.344	0.48/0.978	0.43/0.41	0.003	−0.84
44	HPRP-A1-TAT [6,164]/E	FKKLKLFSKLWNW-**KRKKRQRRR**	0.975/H	0.997/0.997	0.527/0.984	1.0/0.928/0.972	0.69/0.987	0.586/0.669	0.043	−0.98
45	Beclin-1-R11 [165]/E	TNVFNATFEIWHDGEFGT-**RRRRRRRRRRR**	0.814/H	0.987/0.034	0.516/0.846	0.83/0.834/0.36	0.26/0.268	0.565/0.552	0.005	−0.92
46	Mapegin [88]/E	KIGKKILKALKGALKELA	0.707/H	0.588/1.0	1.0/0.982	0.783/0.589/0.988	0.98/1.0	0.59/0.67/1.55745	0.079	−1.32
47	MAP [166]/E	**KLALKLALKALKAALKLA**	0.998/H	0.794/1.0	0.979/0.986	0.345/0.096/0.918	0.42/1.0	0.54/0.73/0.69540	0.973	−1.13
48	Mapegin-TAT/DJ	KIGKKILKALKGALKELA-**GRKKRRQRRRPPQ**	0.878/H	0.929/0.997	0.764/0.981	0.998/0.975/0.506	0.96/1.0	0.65/0.65/1.52487	0.026	−1.04
49	Mapegin-a1-TAT/DJ	KIGKKILKALKLALKLLA-**GRKKRRQRRRPPQ**	0.958/H	0.980/1.0	0.613/0.983	0.998/0.975/0.630	0.94/1.0	0.67/0.76/2.13612	0.717	−1.09
50	**Mapegin-a2-TAT/DJ**	KITKKILKALKGALKELA-**GRKKRRQRRRMPQ**	0.881/L	0.518/0.994	0.717/0.942	0.998/0.93/0.972	0.97/0.996	0.68/0.65/1.53687	0.077	−1.81

* We used the servers listed in Table 2 and applied them in the same order for columns CPP to Toxicity. Highlighted peptides (bold name) with underlined activity scores are our selection for the designed peptides with the best overall score (see Table 6). Bold sequence segments have predicted or verified CPP activity. Underlined residues are optimal substitutions for increasing anti-inflammatory activity or decreasing peptide toxicity. $ The best CPP candidates from longer peptides were found by using the protein scanning CellPPD (http://crdd.osdd.net/raghava/cellppd/ (accessed on 7 August 2022) [167]. & See peptides 1 and 2 from Table 5 for the origin, references, and abbreviations of cancer-homing tLyP-1 peptides and their analogs.

Table 4. CPP bioactive peptide conjugates for intracellular targets II. Activity probabilities *.

No.	Peptide Name/Ref.	Extended CPP at the N or C-terminal *	CPP	Anti-Microbial	Anti-Cancer	Anti-Viral	Anti-Fungal	Anti-Inflamm.	Hemo-lytic	Toxicity/ Score
1	KW [168]/E	**KRKRWHW**	0.99/H	1.00/ND	0.98/0.98	0.8/0.4/1.0	0.38/ND	0.62/0.54	0.01	−0.93
2	Ribosomal-homing-peptide (RHP)-KW [54]/DJ	YKWYYRGAA-**KRKRWHW**	0.93/H	0.97/1.00	0.99/0.98	1.0/0.9/0.8	0.62/0.74	0.51/0.61	0.02	−0.58
3	L-K6V1 temp [112]-KW/DJ	IKKIVSKIKKLLK-GG-**KRKRWHW**	0.89/H	0.98/1.00	1.0/0.98	1.0/1.0/0.2	0.95/1.00	0.59/0.66	0.02	−1.35
4	CAMEL [148]-KW/DJ	KWKLFKKIGAVLKVL-**KRKRWHW**	0.92/H	1.00/1.00	0.99/0.98	1.0/1.0/1.0	0.78/0.99	0.61/0.67	0.94	−0.90
5	R_2-chensenin [149]-KW/DJ	VWRRWRRFWRR-GG-**KRKRWHW**	0.99/H	1.00/0.99	0.95/0.98	1.0/0.9/1.0	0.27/1.00	0.66/0.70	0.15	−1.03
6	ZY4 [150]-KW/DJ	VCKRWKKWKRKWKKWCV-GG-**KRKRWHW**	0.95/H	1.00/1.00	0.99/0.98	1.0/0.9/1.0	0.34/1.00	0.58/0.68	0.23	−0.36
7	Puroindoline [151]-KW/DJ	FPVTWRWWKWWKG-G-**KRKRWHW**	0.88/H	1.00/0.99	0.98/0.98	1.0/0.9/1.0	0.46/0.99	0.64/0.65	0.67	−0.83
8	Novispirin [152]-KW/DJ	KNLRIIRKGIHIIKKY-GG-**KRKRWHW**	0.90/L	0.98/1.00	0.99/0.98	1.0/1.0/1.0	0.96/1.00	0.63/0.63	0.43	−0.90
9	BP33 [144]-KW/DJ	LKLFKKILKVL-G-**KRKRWHW**	0.93/H	1.00/1.00	0.99/0.98	1.0/1.0/1.0	0.92/1.00	0.62/0.70	0.82	−1.19
10	T2R1 [88]-KW/DJ	RHHWRRYARIGFRAVRTVIGK-**KRKRWHW**	0.94/H	0.99/0.94	0.92/0.98	1.0/1.0/0.8	0.71/0.86	0.66/0.62	0.12	−1.09
11	DiPGLa-H [153]-KW peptide/DJ	KIAKVALKALKIAKVALKAL-**KRKRWHW**	0.92/L	0.98/1.00	0.99/0.98	1.0/1.0/1.0	0.97/0.99	0.49/0.63	0.94	−0.92
12	Neoepitope4-WFR_8 [169]/DJ	VLSHGSFVM-GG-**RRWFRRRRRR**	0.89/H	0.89/0.93	0.59/0.98	1.0/0.8/0.1	0.62/0.76	0.62/0.62	0.43	−1.22
13	WFR_8 -tumor homing [170]/DJ	**RRWFRRRRRR**-GG-IFLLWQR	0.99/H	1.00/0.78	0.48/0.98	1.0/0.5/0.8	0.46/0.96	0.63/0.63	0.07	−1.26
14	BP100 [155]-KW/DJ	KKLFKKILKYL-GG-**KRKRWHW**	0.93/H	1.00/1.00	1.0/0.98	1.0/1.0/1.0	0.94/0.99	0.58/0.65	0.61	−1.35
15	Mitoch. target. [157]-KW/DJ	KLLNLISKLF-GGG-**KRKRWHW**	0.80/L	0.97/1.00	0.74/0.98	1.0/1.0/0.9	0.91/0.98	0.63/0.67	0.41	−1.29
16	Nosangiotide [158]-KW/DJ	RKKTFKEVANAVKISA-GG-**KRKRWHW**	0.69/L	0.85/0.93	0.87/0.97	0.5/0.9/0.9	0.88/0.84	0.69/0.59	0.01	−1.03
17	Adepantin-1A [88]-WFR_8/DJ	GIKKAVGKALKGLKGLLKALGES -GG-**RRWFRRRRRR**	0.80/L	1.00/0.99	0.95/0.98	1.0/1.0/1.0	0.98/1.00	0.60/0.66/1.30566	0.66	−1.46
18	**WFR_8-adepantin-1A/DJ**	**RRWFRRRRRR**-GIKKAVGKALKGLKGLLKALGES	0.86/L	1.00/1.00	0.95/0.96	1.0/1.0/1.0	0.97/0.99	0.62/0.62/1.36028	0.63	−1.56
19	KW-pexiganan-L18 [88]/DJ	**KRKRWHW**-GIGKFLKKAKKFGKAFVLILKK	0.87/H	0.99/1.00	1.0/0.98	1.0/0.9/1.0	0.99/0.99	0.53/0.64	0.81	−1.04
20	RtLyp-1-flexampin [114]/DJ	RCGN**KRTR**-GIKKWVKGVAKGVAKDLAKKIL	0.59/L	0.92/1.00	1.0/0.97	1.0/1.0/1.0	1.00/1.00	0.44/0.63	0.68	−0.74

Table 4. *Cont.*

No.	Peptide Name/Ref.	Extended CPP at the N or C-terminal *	CPP	Anti-Microbial	Anti-Cancer	Anti-Viral	Anti-Fungal	Anti-Inflamm.	Hemo-lytic	Toxicity/ Score
21	Zyk-1- [88]-WFR$_8$/DJ	GIGREIIKKIIKKIGKKIGRII -GG-**RRWFRRRRRR**	0.89/H	1.00/1.00	0.99/0.98	1.0/1.0/1.0	0.96/0.99	0.60/0.66	0.88	−1.18
22	MG2-bombesin [171]/E	GIGKFLHSAKKFGKAFVGEIMNS-GG-QRLGNQWAVGHLM	0.30	0.83/0.85	0.86/0.54	1.0/0.9/0.9	0.97/0.41	0.53/0.55	ND	−0.97
23	MG2-pAntp [172]/E	GIGKFLHSAKKFGKAFVGEIMNS-GG-**KKWKMRRNQFWVKVQRG**	0.52/L	0.95/1.00	0.93/0.81	1.0/1.0/1.0	0.99/0.81	0.56/0.52	ND	−0.68
24	DP1 [173]/E	RRQRRTSKLMKR-GG-KLAKLAKKLAKLAK	0.95/L	0.84/1.00	0.91/0.98	0.7/0.7/0.2	0.95/0.55	0.50/0.65	0.03	−0.36
25	**KW-BMAP-18** [174]**/DJ**	**KRKRWHW**-GGLRSLGRKILRAWKKYG	0.90/H	1.00/1.00	0.98/0.98	1.0/1.0/1.0	0.88/0.98	0.58/0.68/1.3653	0.09	−1.01
26	Chrysophin-1-KW [175]/DJ	FFGWLIKGAIHAGKAIHGLI-GG-**KRKRWHW**	0.59/L	0.99/1.00	0.98/0.98	1.0/1.0/1.0	0.96/0.97	0.52/0.55	0.97	−1.03
27	KW-mastoparan [176]/DJ	**KRKRWHW**-GG-INLKALAALAKKIL	0.90/L	0.87/1.00	0.75/0.98	1.0/0.9/1.0	0.92/0.96	0.62/0.66	0.42	−1.11
28	KW-pleuricidin [177]/DJ	**KRKRWHW**-GWGSFFKKAAHVGKHVGKAALTHYL	0.66/L	0.89/1.00	0.99/0.98	1.0/0.9/0.9	0.96/1.00	0.60/0.65	0.37	−0.95
29	MTD [178]/E	**RRRRRRRRGRQ**-KLLNLISKLF	0.98/H	0.28/0.60	0.58/0.96	1.0/0.6/0.9	0.73/0.97	0.67/0.70	0.06	−1.06
30	**L-K6V1 temp** [112]**-KW-analog/DJ**	IKKIVSKIRKLLKR-G-**KRKRWHW**	0.95/H	0.98/1.00	1.0/0.98	1.0/1.0/0.8	0.92/1.0	0.65/0.66/1.678	0.07	−1.12
31	T2R1 [88]-KW-analog1/DJ	RHHWRRYARIGFRAVRSVIGK-**KTKRWHW**	0.92/H	0.93/0.94	0.98/0.98	1.0/1.0/1.0	0.69/0.97	0.66/0.62/1.36406	0.03	−1.09
32	T2R1 [88]-KW-analog2/DJ	RHHWRRLARIGFRAVRSVIGK-**KTKRWHW**	0.93/H	0.96/0.87	0.97/0.98	1.0/1.0/1.0	0.60/0.97	0.67/0.62/1.5722	0.05	−1.30
33	**KW-BMAP-18** [174]**-analog1/DJ**	**KRKRWHW**-GGLRSLGRKLLRAWKKYG	0.91/H	1.00/0.99	0.96/0.98	1.0/1.0/1.0	0.84/0.97	0.63/0.71/1.62236	0.08	−1.05
34	BP100 [155]-KW-analog/DJ	LKLFKKILKYLN-G-**KRKRWHW**	0.93/H	0.996/0.999	0.966/0.981	1.0/0.961/1.0	0.87/1.0	0.635/0.687/1.80571	0.894	−1.32
35	Zyk-1 [88]-WFR$_8$-analog/DJ	GIGLEIVKKIILKIGKKIGRII-GG-**RRWFRRRRRR**	0.83/L	0.999/0.998	0.986/0.977	1.0/0.985/0.964	0.98/0.99	0.60/0.614/1.599	0.938	−1.33
36	**KW-BMAP-18** [174]**-analog2/DJ**	**KRKRWHW**-GGLASLGRKLLRAWKKYG	0.85/H	0.988/0.986	0.951/0.982	1.0/0.971/1.0	0.85/0.97	0.684/0.708/1.85648	0.399	−1.09
37	**R$_8$FW-GGGPPKG-temp** [112] **R$_9$R$_{14}$/DJ**	**RRRRRRFWRR**-GGGPPKG-IKKIVSKIRKLLKR	0.95/H	0.997/1.0	0.954/0.968	1.0/0.958/0.822	0.97/0.99	0.71/0.60/1.25133	0.032	−1.18
38	**R$_8$FW-GGEPPKG-temp** [112] **R$_9$R$_{14}$/DJ**	**RRRRRRFWRR**-GGEPPKG-IKKIVSKIRKLLKR	0.94/H	0.998/0.988	0.926/0.973	1.0/0.96/0.996	0.96/0.944	0.70/0.596/1.51442	0.028	−1.20
39	**R$_7$A$_5$FW-GGEPPKG temp** [112]**/DJ**	**RRRRARFWRR**-GGEPPKG-IKKIVSKIRKLLKR	0.92/H	0.998/0.968	0.916/0.973	1.0/0.9654/0.95	0.97/0.927	0.72/0.597/1.80807	0.010	−1.25

Table 4. *Cont.*

No.	Peptide Name/Ref.	Extended CPP at the N or C-terminal *	CPP	Anti-Microbial	Anti-Cancer	Anti-Viral	Anti-Fungal	Anti-Inflamm.	Hemo-lytic	Toxicity/Score
40	L-K6V1 temp. [112]-GGEPPKG-KW/DJ	IKKIVSKIKKLLK-GGEPPKG-**KRKRWHW**	0.72/L	0.971/0.986	0.996/0.955	0.994/0.985/0.97	0.94/0.839	0.50/0.624	0.007	−1.15
41	R_8FW-GGGPPKG-IDR-1002 [9]/DJ	**RRRRRRFWRR**-GGGPPKG-VQRWLIVWRIRK	0.97/H	1.0/0.944	0.181/0.979	1.0/0.862/0.854	0.71/0.40	0.633/0.606	0.064	−1.17
42	R_8FW-GGGPPKG-IDR-1018 [9]/DJ	**RRRRRRFWRR**-GGGPPKG-VRLIVAVRIWRR	0.95/H	1.0/0.978	0.344/0.980	1.0/0.863/0.982	0.79/0.33	0.612/0.602	0.039	−1.17
43	R_8FW-GGGPPKG-IDR-1018-R_6/DJ	**RRRRRRFWRR**-GGGPPKG-VRLIV**R**VRIWRR	0.96/H	1.0/0.929	0.406/0.980	1.0/0.832/0.354	0.81/0.59	0.626/0.605	0.027	−1.21
44	R_8FW-GGEPPKG-IDR-1018-R_6/DJ	**RRRRRRFWRR**-GGEPPKG-VRLIV**R**VRIWRR	0.96/H	1.0/0.702	0.356/0.983	1.0/0.854/0.99	0.78/0.21	0.612/0.607/1.16498	0.026	−1.23
45	R_8FW-GGEPPKG-IDR-1018-L_1R_6/DJ	**RRRRRRFWRR**-GGEPPKG-LRLIV**R**VRIWRR	0.96/H	1.0/0.939	0.277/0.983	1.0/0.86/0.04	0.77/0.338	0.623/0.622/1.43256	0.025	−1.20
46	Pexiganan-L18 [88]/E	GIGKFLKKAKKFGKAFVLILKK	0.75/L	0.997/1.0	1.0/0.976	0.46/0.299/0.22	1.0/1.0	0.598/0.661	0.892	−0.94
47	Flexampin [114]/E	GIKKWVKGVAKGVAKDLAKKIL	0.56/L	0.990/1.0	1.0/0.977	0.993/0.937/0.544	0.99/1.0	0.423/0.531	0.817	−0.78
48	Zyk-1 [88]/E	GIGREIIKKIIKKIGKKIGRII	0.65/L	0.978/0.998	0.998/0.97	1.0/0.933/0.946	0.88/1.0	0.526/0.662	0.583	−0.86
49	Adepantin-1A [88]/E	GIKKAVGKALKGLKGLLKALGES	0.39	0.980/1.0	1.0/0.977	1.0/0.972/0.398	0.99/1.0	0.554/0.659/1.35587	0.17	−1.51
50	**Novispirin** [152]-**KW-analog2/DJ**	KNLRIFRKGIHIHKKY-GG-**KRKRWHW**	0.903/H	0.972/0.946	0.994/0.983	1.0/0.939/0.822	0.96/0.989	0.5884/0.6	0.195	−1.63
51	**WFR$_8$-adepantin-1A-analog2/DJ**	**RRWFRRRRRR**-GIKKAVGKALKGLKLLLKALGES	0.878/L	0.999/1.0	0.923/0.9485	1.0/0.987/0.908	0.96/0.983	0.616/0.622/1.62411	0.826	−1.63
52	KW-second-bovine-BMAP-18 [179]/DJ	**KRKRWHW**-GRFKRFRKKFKKLFKKIS	0.961/H	0.999/1.0	0.995/0.981	1.0/0.845/1.0	0.91/1.0	0.565/0.698	0.176	−1.09

* We used the servers listed in Table 2 and applied them in the same order. Highlighted peptides (bold name) with underlined activity scores are our selection for the designed peptides with the best overall score (see Table 6). Bold sequence segments have predicted or verified CPP activity. Underlined residues are optimal substitutions for increasing anti-inflammatory activity or decreasing peptide toxicity.

Table 5. Activity probabilities for CPP conjugated magainin analogs, MF constructs, and Arg-Pro rich peptides *.

No.	Parent-Protein/Gene/ Origin/Reference *	Extended CPP at the N or C-terminal *	CPP	Anti-Microbial	Anti-Cancer	Anti-Viral	Anti-Fungal	Anti-Inflamm.	Hemo -lytic	Tox./Score
1	Tumor-homing-tLyP-1 peptide [146]/E	**CGNKRTR**	0.91/L	0.00/ND	N/0.88	N/N/N	ND/ND	0.38/0.47	0.01	−0.42
2	A7RG57 C-term. from *N. vectensis*	**RCGIKRTK**	0.93/L	0.03/ND	0.93/0.95	0.6/0.5/0.5	0.92/ND	0.47/0.62	0.00	−0.88
3	MFC/DJ	RCGNKRFRWHW	0.94/H	0.43/0.91	0.97/0.98	1.0/0.8/1.0	0.38/0.98	0.47/0.63	0.01	−0.92
4	NLS-CE [180]/E	WRFVWMNPKKKRKV	0.92/H	0.99/0.54	0.46/0.98	0.8/0.5/0.8	0.13/0.76	0.47/0.59	0.11	−1.11
5	Zp3a [161]/E	GIKAKIGIKIKK	0.77/L	0.94/1.00	1.0/0.97	0.2/0.1/0.3	0.86/1.00	0.48/0.63	0.03	−0.68
6	Magainin 2 (MG2) [181]/E	GIGKFLHSAKKFGKAFVGEIMNS	0.22	0.95/1.00	1.0/0.98	1.0/1.0/1.0	0.99/0.98	0.56/0.55	0.83	−0.58
7	MG2-tLyP-1 [146]/DJ	GIGKFLHSAKKFGKAFVGEIMNS-GG-**CGNKRTR**	0.26	0.88/0.99	0.99/0.93	1.0/1.0/1.0	0.99/0.94	0.53/0.52	0.76	−0.35
8	MG2-KW [168]/DJ	GIGKFLHSAKKFGKAFVGEIMNS-GG-**KRKRWHW**	0.43	0.94/1.00	0.99/0.96	1.0/1.0/1.0	0.99/0.92	0.57/0.52	0.63	−0.68
9	MG2-WFR$_8$/DJ	GIGKFLHSAKKFGKAFVGEIMNS-GG-**RRWFRRRRRR**	0.74/L	0.93/1.00	0.95/0.97	1.0/1.0/1.0	0.98/0.99	0.61/0.52	0.72	−0.90
10	9P0-1 [182]/E	GIKKWLHSAKKFGKKFVKKIMNS	0.72/L	0.99/1.00	1.0/0.98	0.8/0.9/1.0	0.99/0.98	0.61/0.64	0.96	−0.42
11	MFC-9P0-1-analog [182]/DJ	**RCGNKRFRWHW**-GIKKWLHSAKKFGKKFVKKIMNS	0.76/H	0.92/1.00	1.0/0.93	1.0/1.0/0.9	0.95/0.96	0.63/0.70	0.86	−0.59
12	MFC-Zp3a [161]/DJ	**RCGNKRFRWHW**-GIKAKIGIKIKK	0.89/H	0.98/0.99	0.98/0.98	1.0/0.7/0.9	0.97/1.00	0.57/0.68	0.01	−1.05
13	9P1-3 [182]/E	GIKKWLHSAKKFPKKFVKKIMNS	0.73/L	0.99/1.00	1.0/0.98	0.9/0.9/0.6	0.97/0.98	0.63/0.64	0.94	−0.30
14	MFC-9P1-3 [182]/DJ	**RCGNKRFRWHW**-GIKKWLHSAKKFPKKFVKKIMNS	0.78/H	0.88/1.00	1.0/0.92	1.0/1.0/0.8	0.93/0.96	0.64/0.69	0.77	−0.49
15	MFC-PexShort/DJ	**RCGNKRFRWHW**-GIGKLKKAKKFGKKILKK	0.86/H	0.99/1.00	1.0/0.98	1.0/0.9/1.0	0.99/1.00	0.52/0.64	0.03	−1.19
16	MFC-PexNC/DJ	GIGK-G-**RCGNKRFRWHW**-ILKK	0.83/H	0.99/0.99	0.92/0.98	1.0/0.5/1.0	0.94/0.99	0.61/0.61	0.01	−0.65
17	MG2-$I_6V_9W_{12}T_{15}I_{17}$ [183]/E	GIGKFIHSVKKWGKTFIGEIMNS	0.26	0.97/0.99	1.0/0.85	1.0/0.9/1.0	0.93/0.99	0.55/0.57	0.93	−0.64
18	tLyP-1-MG2-$I_6V_9W_{12}T_{15}I_{17}$ [183]/DJ	**CGNKRTR**-GIGKFIHSVKKWGKTFIGEIMNS	0.33	0.87/1.00	1.0/0.27	1.0/0.9/1.0	0.95/0.97	0.50/0.63	0.78	−0.52
19	KW-MG2-$I_6V_9W_{12}T_{15}I_{17}$ [183]/DJ	**KRKRWHW**-GIGKFIHSVKKWGKTFIGEIMNS	0.46	0.80/1.00	1.0/0.50	1.0/1.0/1.0	0.85/0.98	0.55/0.64	0.57	−0.75
20	WFR$_8$ -MG2-$I_6V_9W_{12}T_{15}I_{17}$ [183]/DJ	**RRWFRRRRRR**-GIGKFIHSVKKWGKTFIGEIMNS	0.82/H	0.97/1.00	0.97/0.98	1.0/1.0/1.0	0.91/0.98	0.68/0.63	0.84	−1.08
21	MG2-Q_{19} [184]/E	GIGKFLHSAKKFGKAFVGQIMNS	0.48	0.99/1.00	1.0/0.98	1.0/1.0/1.0	1.00/1.00	0.54/0.58	0.89	−0.50
22	MG2-Q_{19}-tLyP-1 [184]/DJ	GIGKFLHSAKKFGKAFVGQIMNS-GC-**CGNKRTR**	0.32	0.93/1.00	0.97/0.96	1.0/1.0/0.9	1.00/0.99	0.51/0.57	0.82	−0.23

Table 5. *Cont.*

No.	Parent-Protein/Gene/ Origin/Reference *	Extended CPP at the N or C-terminal *	CPP	Anti-Microbial	Anti-Cancer	Anti-Viral	Anti-Fungal	Anti-Inflamm.	Hemo -lytic	Tox./Score
23	MG2-Q_{19}-KW [184]/DJ	GIGKFLHSAKKFGKAFVGQIMNS-GG-**KRKRWHW**	0.61/L	0.96/1.00	0.99/0.97	1.0/1.0/0.5	0.99/0.99	0.56/0.54	0.72	−0.58
24	MG2-Q_{19}-WFR$_8$ [184]/DJ	GIGKFLHSAKKFGKAFVGQIMNS-GG-**RRWFRRRRRR**	0.77/L	0.93/1.00	0.94/0.98	1.0/1.0/1.0	0.99/0.99	0.60/0.58	0.83	−0.82
25	Max-TI-MG2/DJ &&	GIAKFLDSAKKFGKKFVKTIMQL	0.31	0.99/1.00	1.0/0.98	0.8/0.9/1.0	1.00/0.98	0.57/0.59	0.97	−0.56
26	Max-TI-MG2-tLyP-1/DJ	GIAKFLDSAKKFGKKFVKTIMQL-GG-**CGNKRTR**	0.44	0.95/1.00	1.0/0.99	1.0/1.0/1.0	1.00/0.87	0.61/0.57	0.98	−0.38
27	RtLyP-1-Max-TI-MG2/DJ	**RCGNKRTR**-GIAKFLDSAKKFGKKFVKTIMQL	0.51/L	0.86/1.00	1.0/0.92	1.0/0.9/1.0	1.00/0.97	0.64/0.63	0.86	−0.41
28	Max-TI-MG2-KW/DJ	GIAKFLDSAKKFGKKFVKTIMQL-GG-**KRKRWHW**	0.55/L	0.98/1.00	1.0/0.98	1.0/1.0/0.5	1.00/0.95	0.69/0.57	0.98	−0.75
29	Max-TI-MG2-WFR$_8$/ DJ	GIAKFLDSAKKFGKKFVKTIMQL-GG-**RRWFRRRRRR**	0.77/H	0.97/1.00	0.97/0.98	1.0/1.0/1.0	0.99/0.97	0.64/0.58	0.98	−1.00
30	KAF5879953.1 36–47 MFCA	**RCNRKRFRWQWK**	0.97/H	1.00/0.64	0.86/0.98	0.1/0.6/1.0	0.14/0.75	0.56/0.66	0.01	−0.43
31	tLyp-1-RHP [54]/DJ	**CGNKRTR**-YKWYYRGAA	0.78/H	0.21/0.57	0.94/0.96	0.8/0.2/0.7	0.88/0.21	0.47/0.62	0.01	0.07
32	R-tLyP-1-RHP/DJ	**RCGNKRTR**-YKWYYRGAA	0.83/L	0.76/0.65	0.87/0.98	1.0/0.3/0.9	0.89/0.14	0.57/0.63	0.01	0.12
33	MFC-RHP/DJ	**RCGNKRFRWHW**-YKWYYRGAA	0.84/H	0.96/0.86	0.96/0.98	1.0/0.7/0.8	0.72/0.46	0.64/0.62	0.04	−0.51
34	MFC2/DJ	**RCGNKRFRWHW**-GG-RRAKWRR	0.97/H	1.00/0.97	0.60/0.98	1.0/0.9/1.0	0.37/0.91	0.64/0.64	0.01	−0.69
35	**MFC-PexSa/DJ**	**RCGNKRFRWHW**-GIGKLLKRKKFGKKILKK	0.90/H	0.99/1.00	1.0/0.97	1.0/1.0/0.5	0.99/1.00	0.58/0.65/1.60059	0.054	−1.34
36	MFC2-analog/DJ	**RCGNKRLIWHW**-GG-RRAKTRR	0.95/H	0.97/0.93	0.22/0.98	1.0/0.9/0.9	0.50/0.84	0.65/0.64/1.61375	0.005	−0.43
37	MG2-analog/DJ	GIGKLLKSALKFGKAFVGEIMNS	0.177	0.986/1.0	0.998/0.988	0.982/0.9643/0.926	1.0/0.994	0.6163/0.627/1.76783	0.98	−1.28
38	WFR$_8$-MG2-analog/DJ	**RRWFRRRRRR**-GIGKLLKSALKFGKAFVGEIMNS	0.783/H	0.99/1.0	0.839/0.971	1.0/0.99/1.0	0.96/0.98	0.723/0.646/1.5622	0.952	−1.44
39	CA-MA2 [185]/E	KWKLFKKI-P-KFLHSAKKF	0.895/L	0.997/1.0	1.0/0.98	0.983/0.73/0.56	0.94/0.996	0.62/0.645	0.008	−0.09
40	K6L9 [186]/E	LKLLKKLLKKLLKLL	0.958/H	0.918/1.0	0.996/0.92	0.999/0.927/0.71	0.13/1.0	0.62/0.607	0.907	−1.00
41	PR-39 pig P80054	RRRPRPPYLPRPRPPPFFPPRLPP RIPPGFPPRFPPRFP	0.760/L	1.00/1.0	0.993/0.92	1.0/0.857/0.064	0.82/0.965	0.50/0.550	ND	−0.71
42	Pyrrhocoricin [187]/E	VDKGSYLPRPTPPRPIYNRN	0.48	0.35/1.0	0.12/0.576	0.248/0.175/0.064	0.20/0.965	0.481/0.488	0.004	−1.25
43	R$_8$FW-Pyrrhocoricin/DJ	**RRWFRRRRRR**-GVDKGSYLPRPTPPRPIYNRN	0.864/L	0.964/1.0	0.41/0.98	1.0/0.61/0.984	0.80/0.96	0.561/0.588	0.064	−1.31
44	PR-35/E	RRRPRPPYLPRPRPPPFFPPRLPPRIPPGFPPRFP	0.762/L	1.0/1.0	0.978/0.9198	1.0/0.805/0.0	0.81/0.925	0.512/0.55	0.001	−0.66
45	**PR-35-analog/DJ**	RRRVRPPYLPR**V**RP**Q**PFFPLRL**LK**RISPGFPPRFP	0.821/L	0.993/0.995	0.481/0.854	1.0/0.984/0.962	0.90/0.919	0.637/0.581/2.18407	0.012	−1.44
46	CA-MA2-analog1/DJ	KWKLFKKI**L**K**L**LHSVKKF	0.895/H	0.996/1.0	1.0/0.9786	0.999/0.875/0.184	0.96/1.0	0.6326/0.735/1.8861	0.848	−0.84
47	L-K6V1-temp [112]-revP9 [188]/DJ	IKKIVSKIKKLLK-**PPWWRRRRR**	0.972/H	0.984/1.0	0.956/0.983	0.998/0.953/0.828	0.75/1.0	0.591/0.664	0.017	−1.17

Table 5. *Cont.*

No.	Parent-Protein/Gene/ Origin/Reference *	Extended CPP at the N or C-terminal *	CPP	Anti-Microbial	Anti-Cancer	Anti-Viral	Anti-Fungal	Anti-Inflamm.	Hemo -lytic	Tox./Score
48	**L-K4V1-temp-revP9-analog/DJ**	IKKIVSLILKLLK-**LPWWRRRRR**	0.959/H	0.999/1.0	0.451/0.982	0.999/0.959/1.0	0.65/1.0	0.74/0.764/1.965	0.190	−1.30
49	CA-MA2-analog2/DJ	KWRLFKKI-P-RFLRSARRF	0.954/H	1.0/0.948	0.977/0.980	1.0/0.935/0.758	0.87/0.992	0.605/0.625	0.054	−1.11
50	Sub-5 [189]/E	**RRWKIVVIRWRR**	0.932/H	1.0/0.994	0.935/0.975	0.784/0.579/0.762	0.30/1.0	0.516/0.643	0.037	−0.76
51	Sub-5-G-nuclear-loc.-signal [190]/DJ	**RRWKIVVIRWRR-G**-PKKKRKV	0.973/H	1.0/0.999	0.494/0.984	0.999/0.930/0.998	0.57/0.993	0.656/0.603	0.007	−0.93
52	**temp V_1R_9 (analog-3)-Sub-5/DJ**	VKKIVSKIRKLLK-GG-**RRWKIVVIRWRR**	0.940/H	0.983/1.0	0.972/0.976	0.999/0.974/0.916	0.92/1.0	0.528/0.641/1.49473	0.098	−0.94

* We used the servers listed in Table 2 and applied them in the same order. All peptides are assumed to be amidated at their C-terminal. MF abbreviation stands for multifunctional. Highlighted peptides (bold name) with underlined activity scores are our selection for the designed peptides with the best overall score (see Table 6). Bold sequence segments have predicted or verified CPP activity. Underlined residues are substitutions for increasing anti-inflammatory activity or decreasing peptide toxicity. && Repeated applications or our "Mutator" algorithm (http://split4.pmfst.hr/mutator/ (accessed on 7 August 2022); Kamech et al. [46] suggested amino acid substitutions (underlined) for predicted maximal therapeutic index of the magainin analog Max-TI-MG2.

Table 6. Ranking of predictions for the best multifunctional peptide constructs with the reward for a predicted negative mean of hemolytic and toxic activity.

Length-Amph-AMP *	Table-Peptide #	CPP	Anti-Microbial &	Anti-Cancer &	Anti-Viral &	Anti-Fung &	Anti-Inflamm. $	Sum/6	Rank †	Hemol. Probab.	Tox. Score	Reward Low tox.	Total Score §	Overall Rank	CPP Part
25-αd-temp V_1R_9	T3-37	0.97/H	0.955	0.965	1.00	0.975	0.997	0.9869	1	0.130	−1.27	0.570	0.92734	1st	WFS_6R_7
31-αtαd-temp R_9R_{14}	T4-39	0.92/H	0.983	0.9445	0.972	0.949	1.0412	0.9682	6	0.010	−1.25	0.620	0.91846	2nd	WFA_5R_7
25-αd-temp R_9	T3-36	0.96/H	0.955	0.97	1.00	0.98	0.927	0.9670	7	0.180	−1.30	0.560	0.90886	3rd	WFS_6R_7
31-αtαd-temp R_9R_{14}	T4-38	0.94/H	0.993	0.9495	0.985	0.952	0.9368	0.9594	10	0.028	−1.20	0.586	0.90606	4th	**WFR_8**
22-αd-temp	T4-30	0.95/H	0.99	0.99	0.927	0.96	0.996	0.9688	5	0.070	−1.12	0.525	0.90540	5th	KW
22-αd-r-o-p A_8I_{15}	T2-20	0.987/H	0.977	0.976	0.863	0.906	0.9038	0.9353		0.007	−1.39	0.692	0.90047	6th	tLyP-1
29-β αd-PexS	T5-35	0.90/H	0.995	0.985	0.83	0.995	0.9435	0.9414	21	0.054	−1.34	0.643	0.89877	7th	MFC
25-αd-temp	T3-9	0.97/H	0.99	0.975	1.00	0.985	0.757	0.9461	19	0.170	−1.35	0.590	0.89523	8th	WFR_8
31-αtαd-temp R_9R_{14}	T4-37	0.95/H	0.9985	0.961	0.927	0.98	0.8538	0.9450	20	0.032	−1.18	0.574	0.89200	9th	**WFR_8**
22-αtαd-temp	T5-48	0.959/H	1.00	0.7156	0.986	0.825	1.1563	0.9472	18	0.190	−1.30	0.555	0.89119	10th	rP9a
31-αtαd-mapegin-a2	T3-50	0.881/L	0.756	0.8295	0.967	0.983	0.9556	0.8953		0.077	−1.81	0.867	0.89118	11th	TATa
25-αd-BMAP	T4-33	0.905/H	0.991	0.9715	0.993	0.905	0.9868	0.9567	12	0.080	−1.05	0.485	0.88931	12th	KW
35-βtαd- PR-35a	T5-45	0.821/L	0.994	0.6675	0.982	0.910	1.134	0.9180		0.012	−1.44	0.714	0.88886	13th	whole

Table 6. *Cont.*

Length-Amph-AMP *	Table-Peptide #	CPP	Anti-Microbial &	Anti-Cancer &	Anti-Viral &	Anti-Fung &	Anti-Inflamm. $	Sum/6	Rank †	Hemol. Probab.	Tox. Score	Reward Low tox.	Total Score §	Overall Rank	CPP Part
25-αd- **temp L_9V_{14}**	**T3-35**	0.96/H	0.999	0.97	**1.00**	0.98	0.978	0.9738	4	0.760	−1.47	0.355	0.88540	14th	WFR_8
28-αd-**T2R1-L_7S_{17}-a2**	**T4-32**	0.93/H	0.914	0.974	0.997	0.785	0.9557	0.9260		0.050	−1.30	0.625	0.88300	15th	KT_2W
25-αd-**BMAP-18**	**T4-25**	0.90/H	1.00	0.98	1.00	0.930	0.875	0.9475	17	0.090	−1.01	0.460	0.87787	16th	KW
27-αtβd-temp V_1R_9	**T5-52**	0.940/H	0.992	0.974	0.963	0.960	0.888	0.9528	14	0.098	−0.94	0.421	0.87684	17th	Sub 5
25-β αd-**BMAP-a2**	**T4-36**	0.849/H	0.987	0.9665	0.990	0.912	1.0828	0.9646	8	0.399	−1.09	0.346	0.87616	18th	KW
33-αd-**adepantin-1A**	**T4-18**	0.86/L	**1.00**	0.955	**1.00**	0.98	0.8668	0.9436		0.630	−1.56	0.465	0.87525	19th	WFR_8
25-αtβd-**novispirin-a1**	**T4-50**	0.903/H	0.959	0.9885	0.920	0.975	0.5942	0.8899		0.195	−1.63	0.7175	0.87307	20th	KW
33-αd adep-1a-L_{15}	T4-51	0.878/L	0.9995	0.9358	0.965	0.972	0.954	0.9506	16	0.826	−1.63	0.402	0.87225	21	WFR_8
22-r-o-pA_8I_{15}	T2-21	0.985/H	0.98	0.962	0.683	0.91	0.960	0.9134		0.006	−1.22	0.607	0.86963	22	$tLyPA_3$-1
20-αβ BP100	T4-34	0.927/H	0.9975	0.9735	0.987	0.935	1.0426	0.9772	3	0.894	−1.32	0.213	0.86803	23	KW
19-αβ BP33	T4-9	0.93/H	**1.00**	0.985	**1.00**	0.96	1.001	0.9793	2	0.820	−1.19	0.185	0.86583	25	KW
28-αtα-novispirin-a1	T3-38	0.94/H	**1.00**	0.8745	0.995	0.978	0.9305	0.9526	15	0.551	−1.17	0.310	0.86073	26	WFL_5R_7
35-α adep1a	T4-17	0.80/L	0.995	0.965	**1.00**	0.99	0.8552	0.9342		0.660	−1.46	0.400	0.85789	29	WFR_8
31-αtα mapegin-a1	T3-49	0.958/H	0.990	0.798	0.868	0.97	1.1887	0.9621	9	0.717	−1.09	0.187	0.85127	30	TAT
18-αtα r-o-p-analog	T2-22	0.991/H	1.00	0.962	0.97	0.795	0.61	0.8879		0.003	−1.26	0.629	0.85091	31	whole
25-α-BMAP2-18	T4-52	0.961/H	0.9995	0.988	0.948	0.955	0.6315	0.9139		0.176	−1.09	0.457	0.84862	32	KW
34-αtα-Zyk1a	T4-35	0.833/L	0.9985	0.9815	0.983	0.987	0.9377	0.9534	13	0.938	−1.33	0.196	0.84520	33	WFR_8

* The amphiphilic character of the peptide was assessed by the SPLIT 3.5 server (http://split.djpept.com/split/ accessed on 7 August 2022 [42]). Bold or normal font α, β, and t symbols are stronger or weaker predicted profiles of hydrophobic moments for helix, beta-strand, and turn secondary structure. The "d" symbol is for predominantly disordered structure when indicated by the flDPnn server [191] for the first 20 peptides. The same server predicts DNA and RNA binding sites for all 20 best peptides from 41% to 100% of their residues. Peptide's abbreviations are in Tables 2–5. For instance, the temp abbreviation stands for the L-K6V1 temporin 1CEb with the sequence IKKIVSKIKKLLK [112]. The a1 or a2 abbreviation is for analog1 or analog2. The single code letter with the subscript for the residue sequence position is used for substituted amino acids. In the asparagutin case (WFR_8), R_7 or R_8 means the total number of arginines. # The peptide code number is "Tn-m" for "n" = 2,3,4,5, referring to the corresponding Table, and "m" for the peptide number in Table n. & Mean values of predicted probabilities for antimicrobial, anticancer, antiviral, and antifungal activity. See Table 2 for server addresses and corresponding references. We used the gray background to highlight cases among 20 best peptides when the probability for anticancer and antiviral activity is close to 1.0 (>0.95). $ Mean value of predicted scores by AIPpred, PreAIP, and AntiInflam servers. See Table 2 for server addresses and corresponding references. The AntiInflam server was included in the calculated mean for the cases when three or fewer amino acid substitutions were enough to raise the predicted score above 1.0 (except for the PR-35 analog with seven substitutions). † Peptides are first ranked (yellow background) regardless of their predicted hemolytic activity and toxicity. § Total score is calculated as: (CPP probability + mean antimicrobial probability + mean anti-cancer probability + mean antiviral probability + mean antifungal probability + mean anti-inflammatory score)/6 − (hemolytic activity probability + toxicity score)/2. The subtracted number is a positive reward for low toxicity. We used the blue and green background to rank the 20 best peptides according to their total score.

4. Design of Cell-Penetrating Multifunctional Peptides

4.1. Advantages of Cell-Penetrating Antimicrobial Peptides

Conventional antibiotics often have difficulties reaching pathogens in mammalian cells. The challenge of eliminating intracellular pathogens reflects in the persistence of related diseases, rising antibiotic resistance, and severe side effects [192,193]. Fortunately, many different drug delivery systems have been developed in recent years. One such delivery mechanism is covalently connecting a bioactive molecule to some cell-penetrating peptide that can target specific cell types, malignant cells, or intracellular pathogens [54]. In this chapter, we shall consider peptide–CPP hybrids. Noninvasive applications of therapeutic peptides conjugated to CPP offer new solutions to the problem of how to overcome the barriers in a body such as the plasma membrane, blood–brain barrier, intestinal lumen, skin barrier, air–lung barrier, blood–lung barrier, nasal cavity, or the posterior segment of the eye [194]. The CPP choice must consider the cell-penetrating ability or probability, uptake efficiency, toxicity, stability, half-life, immunogenicity, and other features that can all change depending on the attached cargo molecule. A short-length CPP conjugate has the practical advantage of being less expensive for synthesis and testing. For a peptide as bioactive cargo, we mainly chose among known antimicrobial or anticancer peptides. Homing peptides are a good choice for targeting specific populations of cells or intracellular organelles.

Peptide–CPP hybrids designed by other authors and us are in Tables 3–5. Our primary design goal was to have a broad spectrum of highly predicted functional activities (cell-penetrating, antibacterial, anticancer, antiviral, antifungal, and anti-inflammatory) and as low toxicity as possible. The short conjugate length was the secondary goal because combining many different functions in a short hybrid peptide is difficult.

4.2. Potential for Clearing Intracellular Drug-Resistant Bacteria

Besides cancer cells as targets for CPP-cargo molecules, there is a pressing need to discover nontoxic last-resort drugs to eliminate intracellular multidrug or pan-resistant bacteria [195]. Colistin is a peptide-fatty acid conjugate that belongs to the last-resort class of antibiotics against hard-to-treat bacteria. For several decades it was abandoned in medical practice due to its nephrotoxicity. Its toxicity and additional resistance induction are obstacles to clinical usage [196,197]. After multidrug resistance proliferated, medical doctors are again treating endangered patients with colistin by carefully balancing positives (saving patient's life) and negatives (a certain degree of damage to some organs).

It would be better to widen the availability of nontoxic peptides capable of clearing resistant intracellular bacterial targets [198]. Fortunately, some bacteriocins are highly specific bactericides for their target bacteria and nontoxic to eukaryotic cells. Among them, peptidoglycan hydrolases induce bacterial lysis by cleaving specific conserved bonds within the peptidoglycan (PG) of the bacterial cell wall. PG target bonds are well conserved, making it difficult for bacteria to develop resistance against PG hydrolases. These advantages are enhanced when PG hydrolases are fused to penetratin or some other cell-penetrating peptide. Such constructs eradicate intracellular drug-resistant *Staphylococcus aureus* [199]. These authors used the bacteriocin enzyme lysostaphin fused to penetratin or TAT peptide from HIV. Both constructs were equally efficient in clearing intracellular antibiotic-resistant strains of *S. aureus* responsible for recurrent infections. Therefore, CPP-fused PG hydrolases are promising therapeutic applications of penetratin and other cell-penetrating peptides.

Some cationic antimicrobial peptides (AMPs) are selective and refractory to resistance mechanisms developed by microbial pathogens and cancer cells [171]. Ribosomally synthesized peptides are more costly than small molecular weight drugs but less expensive compared to recently developed immunotherapy. As host defense peptides, AMPs are an essential component of our immune system, with some able to translocate across membranes without the need to design artificial AMP–CPP hybrids. There should be no undesired immune response to peptides recognized as innate by the human body, even if some slight modifications are introduced to enhance their stability.

Unfortunately, the research about AMPs is underfunded by pharmaceutical companies and governmental agencies charged with supporting health-oriented innovations. There was an initial failure of AMPs to achieve clinical applications, which resulted in a widespread bias against them, despite all evidence that AMPs can be used as multifunctional agents effective against bacteria, fungi, viruses, drug-resistant biofilms, and cancer [200–205]. Nevertheless, the promise of multifunctional AMPs will eventually come to fruition [206].

4.3. Short Cell-Penetrating Peptides and Their Conjugates

Optimized penetratin analog RKKRWFRRRRPKWKK [56] has six arginines, five lysines, and two tryptophans. Besides its high cell-penetrating ability, *in silico* predictions make a case for antibacterial, anticancer, and antiviral activity with considerably lower hemolytic activity than the pAnp penetratin (see prediction results for peptide 16 from Table 2). In known homeoproteins, there is no natural penetratin-like peptide of similar length (15–16 residues) with such a large number of positive charges ($\geq$+10). However, the hypothetical protein OLQ14316.1 from coral dinoflagellate symbiont *Symbiodinium microadriaticum* [207] contains a similar sequence R(603)RRRRRWFRRRRRRWFRKI(621), named DiR_6WF (Table 3, peptide 2), with an even higher number of arginines.

The decapeptide RRWFRRRRRR (abbreviation WFR_8) from that domain has the best chance of being a short CPP peptide, according to the CellPPD server [167]. Both peptides have a high CPP probability (0.99) and are predicted as nontoxic with antimicrobial, antiviral, and anticancer activity (see prediction results for peptides 2 and 3 from Table 3). Identical decapeptide R(122)RWFRRRRRR(131) from the asparagus plant (*Asparagus officinalis*) uncharacterized protein A0A5P1FK94 with 142 residues is also the best predicted CPP in that protein. We shall name it asparagutin. The natural function of asparagutin is unknown. The WF doublet from asparagutin is conserved in all penetratin-like peptides from homeodomains (see Table 1).

In Table 3, we mostly use pAntp penetratin and short CPP candidates—the decapeptide RRWFRRRRRR and its reversed version RRRRRRFWRR (peptides 3 and 4 from Table 3), which to our knowledge, have never been synthesized and tested. Asparagutin is considerably shorter than penetratin, but it may be more difficult for solid-state synthesis. Wender et al. [208] proposed a better pathway for synthesizing polyarginine peptides. We assume that difficulties synthesizing the RRWFRRRRRR sequence or its reversed analog should no longer be a serious issue. According to the VaxiJen server by Doytchinova and Flower [209] for the immunogenicity prediction (http://www.ddg-pharmfac.net/vaxijen/VaxiJen/VaxiJen.html, (accessed on 7 August 2022)), the asparagutin is the probable antigen for parasites and fungi and probable non-antigen for bacterial, viral, and tumor cell targets. The predicted cleavage site for different proteases is after the Phe residue (the result of Song et al. [210] server analysis at the link: https://prosper.erc.monash.edu.au/, (accessed on 7 August 2022)). Six terminal arginines after protease cleavage should still have the CPP ability, with somewhat lesser uptake efficiency than the widely used eight arginine CPP [211]. The hemolytic activity is negligible for the reversed sequence RRRRRRFWRR (0.08 probability).

Wei et al. [168] used molecular simulations to design the KRKRWHW peptide (named KW), which exhibited little cytotoxicity and high penetrating efficiency into mammalian cells. For that peptide and its 30 conjugates (see Table 4 peptides 1–11, 14–16, 19, 25–28, 30, 33, 34, 36, 40, 50, and 52 and Table 5 peptides 8, 19, 23, and 28), we obtained variable predictions for the hemolytic activity. Due to the importance given to low toxicity estimates, five KW-containing peptides with a low probability of harming red blood cells (0.4 or lesser probability) and low toxicity score (-1.01 or less) entered among the 20 best multifunctional constructs with a high overall score (see Table 6). These are hybrid peptides 25, 30, 33, 36, and 50 from Table 4. Despite different bioactive cargo (temporin, novispirin, or BMAP antimicrobial peptides), an excellent multifunctional activity is possible for all of them.

Identical septapeptide KRKRWHW is present in the C-terminal segment GQEQR **KRKRWHW**RKFHKK of bacterial protein A0A1G1FKX2 from Nitrospiraceae bacterium named the PSP1 C-terminal domain-containing protein (preliminary data). The segment is also predicted with a high uptake efficiency (CPP probability of 0.91) and increased antibacterial and antifungal activity compared to its KRKRWHW fragment. Its binding affinity for bacterial or eukaryotic mRNA may be more important according to the PROSITE pattern https://prosite.expasy.org/doc/PS51411 (accessed on 7 August 2022) for the PSP1 C-terminal domain profile. The DP-Bind server predicts DNA-binding sites for all but the first three residues: QRKRKRWHWRKFHKK. When the whole A0A1G1FKX2 protein (preliminary data) is examined with the RNABindRPlus web server http://ailab1.ist.psu.edu/RNABindRPlus/ (accessed on 7 August 2022), thirty binding sites to RNA are predicted, but none of them are even close to the C-terminal sequence GQEQR**KRKRWHW**RKFHKK.

The biological significance of the PSP1 C-terminal domain for cell cycle regulation is still under investigation [212]. Anyway, it is possible that rationally optimized molecular docking and dynamics simulations by Wei et al. [168] rediscovered short nontoxic CPP, which nature has already developed as a protein motif in some bacteria. The KRKRWHW peptide (KW) exhibits non-covalent binding to disaccharide trehalose. Trehalose provides an exceptional stabilization of proteins during the desiccation procedure for extended storage [213,214]. Loading trehalose in mammalian cells is considerably more efficient in combination with the KW peptide and less damaging than other procedures for introducing that disaccharide into cells [168].

Anticancer and antiviral activities are well predicted for the KW peptide fused to BMAP-18 cathelicidin fragment GGLRSLGRKILRAWKKYG of BMAP-28 antimicrobial peptide, which targets mitochondria [174] (peptide 25, Table 4). BMAP antibiotics cause mitochondrial depolarization and cytochrome c release by opening the mitochondrial permeability transition pore.

We used peptides CGIKRTK, CGAKRTK, CGNKRTR, RCGNKRTR, and RCGIKRTK as short CPPs for designing multifunctional constructs (see Table 2 peptides 15, 18, 20, and 21; Table 3 peptide 8; Table 4 peptide 20; Table 5 peptides 1, 2, 7, 18, 22, 26, 27, 31, and 32). The tLyP-1 tumor-homing peptide CGNKRTR [146] is found in predicted helicases from *Ferroplasma* species (Archaea) HII82410.1, A0A1V0N279, and A0A7K4FM37. *Ferroplasma* sp. loves a hot acid, heavy-metal rich environment (pH from 0 to 2 and temperatures from 35 to 55 °C. The archeon exhibits strange ancient bioenergetics dependent on oxidizing ferrous iron (Fe^{2+}) to ferric iron (Fe^{3+}). Helicases containing the CGNKRTR motif from *Ferroplasma* sp. are classified as DEAD/DEAH-box helicases—the essential enzymes for the survival of advanced invasive melanomas [215], lung adenocarcinoma [216], and renal cell carcinoma [217]. Hence, a connection may exist spanning billions of years of biological evolution with the evolution of invasive cancer cells.

Unsurprisingly, helicases have been popular study subjects from 1976 onward due to their ability to unwind duplex DNA [218]. The CGNKRTR peptide is also present in the unchanged or slightly changed form at the C-terminal of integral membrane protein for sodium-dependent phosphate transport from *Actinia tenebrosa* and *Nematostella vectensis* (sea anemones): respectively, XP_031563687.1, and XP_032222729.1 (A7RG57). Septapeptides are too short of having solid evidence about their biological significance in the absence of broad conservation. Octapeptide RCGIKRTK from the C-terminal of *N. vectensis* predicted protein A7RG57 has higher probabilities for multifunctional activity than CGNKRTR (see peptide 2 prediction results in Table 5). All conjugates mentioned above with the CGNKRTR or its analogs are interesting for synthesis and testing. All have a well-predicted broad activity spectrum, and only two (peptides 26 and 27 from Table 5) have higher predicted toxicity to healthy mammalian red blood cells than magainin-2.

The predicted probability for anticancer activity is high for some hybrid peptides. It is 0.92 or higher as the output of both ACP servers for peptides 20 and 21 from Table 2, 20 from Table 4, and peptides 2, 7, 22, 26, 27, and 31 from Table 5 containing tLyP-1 or its analogs. The IFLLWQR septapeptide (IF7, see peptide 13 from Table 4) binds to the annexin-1 protein, which is over-expressed on the endothelial caveolae surfaces of different tumors [219]. Through endocytosis, annexin family proteins are internalized, allowing IF7 conjugates with anticancer drugs (such as anticancer peptides) to penetrate tumor cells freely. Many other short tumor-homing peptides are described in the literature [170].

Xia Xu developed with collaborators several additional short CPP for helping anticancer drugs enter tumor cells. These are RRRRRWW [220], RRRRQWWQW [221], and RRRRRWWPP [188]. Employed servers suggest an antibacterial, antiviral, and antifungal activity for the IKKIVSKIKKLLK-PPWWRRRRR conjugate, good cell-penetrating ability, and low toxicity (see peptide 47, Table 5). The reversed sequence of the RRRRRWWPP positioned the proline residues near the peptide middle due to expectations of increased selectivity [185,222].

The high electric field of energized mitochondria attracts arginine-rich CPPs after they pass through the plasma membrane. Peptide 13 from Table 4 may have multiple means for internalizing tumor cells and reaching mitochondria due to its asparagutin moiety. Peptide 6 from Table 3 is an example of how attached asparagutin RRWFRRRRRR can promote the uptake of mitochondrial-homing peptide MIASHLLAYFFTELN (dubbed pHK). Woldetsadik et al. [147] fused the homing peptide with the penetration-accelerating sequence GKPILFF [223]. The hybrid peptide MIASHLLAYFFTELN-GKPILFF-amide (pHK-PAS) disrupted the association of hexokinase II (HK2) with mitochondria in cancer cells. It led to mitochondrial dysfunction and apoptosis of cancer cells without substantially increased cytotoxicity to normal cells [147]. Thus, the hybrid peptide containing pHK and either RRWFRRRRRR or GKPILFF can be the artificial death signal for malignant mitochondria with potential therapeutic applications (see peptide 6, Table 3). The pHK-PAS peptide is predicted as non-ACP by both servers for anticancer peptides illustrating difficulties in constructing such servers.

Malignant mitochondria and their protein–protein interactions contributing to cancer phenotype are key targets for chemotherapy because the respiratory metabolism of mitochondria is crucial for cancer survival despite the Warburg effect. Mitochondrial structure and function are different between normal cells and cancer cells. These differences offer a potential for the design of anticancer compounds acting on mitochondria for the selective killing of cancer cells [224]. The peptide pHK prevents the hexokinase II association with outer mitochondrial membrane VDAC porin [225]. The pentadecapeptide M(1)IASHLLAYFFTELN(15) is the VDAC-binding N-terminal domain of human HK2 (Uniprot entry P52789), acting as a surrogate peptide for HK2. HK2-VDAC association helps keep mitochondrial permeability transition pores in closed conformation when bound to the ATP–synthasome complex [226]. Mitochondria die together with the cell containing mitochondria when transition pores are continuously open due to the inhibition of the HK2-VDAC association. HK2 enzymes are gatekeepers of life and death [227].

There are, of course, many other possibilities to fuse the pHK peptide with some cell-penetrating peptide for easier access to malignant mitochondria. One such option for targeting cancer cells with a designed artificial death signal has been explored by Chiara et al. [225]. These authors used the HIV-1 TAT CPP peptide to create the MIASHLLA YFFTELN(β-Ala)-GYGRKKRRQRRRG-amide hybrid, called HK2-TAT. Unfortunately, subsequent experiments revealed that a low concentration of that hybrid peptide (1 μM HK2-TAT) causes rat heart ischemia [228]. Hence, additional study is needed with different pHK-CPP conjugates. One possibility is the MIASHLLAYFFTELN-GG-RCGNKRTK construct that uses the tLyp-1 analog for the penetration acceleration of pHK. Its advantage would be considerably lower toxicity (0.09 probability for hemolytic activity) in comparison with HK2-asparagutin (0.44), HK2-TAT (0.34), and HK2-PAS (0.29).

Designed short tumor-homing peptides KW and tLyP-1 (peptide 1 from Table 4 and peptide 1 from Table 5) are similar in N-terminal and C-terminal parts. The hybrid construct CGNKRFRWHW may have a good combination of CPP and other multifunctional activities for its short length. We added the Arg residue at its N-terminal because it is present as a natural tLyP-1 analog RCGIKRTK. Central KRFR motif is present in some cathelicidin antimicrobial peptides. The resulting RCGNKRFRWHW conjugate (peptide 3 from Table 5) will be named MFC for the Multi-Functional Construct. A likely membrane-stabilized structure of the MFC is an amphipathic beta-strand for residues 5–11 (SPLIT prediction). The DP-Bind server predicts DNA binding for all RCGNKRFRWHW residues. The most interesting expected features are low toxicity and the absence of any hemolysis combined with high cell-penetrating, anticancer, and antiviral activity of that undecapeptide. Two C-terminal tryptophans are natural fluorescence probes for examining the location and microenvironment of MFC added to membrane vesicles, organelles, or living cells. A high density of positive charges and hydrophobic residues should help MFC accumulation by topologically closed membranes with active bioenergetics. Histidine presence should make it sensitive to pH changes. The presence of reactive cysteine facilitates chemical modification for fine-tuning desired effects.

BLASTP search discovered only one natural MFC analog (peptide 30 from Table 5 named MFCA) with a similar sequence RCNRKRFRWQWK. The MFCA peptide is found as the 36–47 segment of the uncharacterized protein (partial) KAF5879953.1 during a recent genome analysis of walking catfish Clarias magur. Its predicted CPP probability is promising 0.97 with a high score of 0.76 for uptake efficiency, but other predicted multifunctional activities are not enhanced compared to MFC. The equally low likelihood for the hemolytic activity of 0.01 leaves enough space for fine-tuning that peptide without making it toxic to healthy human cells. Hybrid peptides 11, 12, 14–16, and 33–35 from Table 5 illustrate how adding bioactive cargo sequences to MFC can result in widely different hemolytic activity predictions. Seven conjugates are associated with predicted hemolytic activity of 0.06 or less (peptides 12, 15, 16, and 33–35 from Table 5). For three of them (peptides 15, 16, and 35), we used the same design approach as before by adding a shorter pexiganan sequence (PexShort) or pexiganan's N and C terminal tetrapeptides (PexNC) (see peptides 8–10 from Table 2) to respective MFC terminals.

The peptides 15 and 35 from Table 5 with sequences RCGNKRFRWHW-GIGKLKKAKK FGKKILKK and RCGNKRFRWHW-GIGKL**L**K**R**KKFGKKILKK have a maximal probability (between 0.97 and 1.0) for clearing antibacterial, antifungal, and anticancer intracellular targets. Peptide 35 is optimized for anti-inflammatory activity after two amino acid substitutions (bold and underlined residues), and its overall rank is seventh among all of the considered peptides from Tables 2–5. An unexpected finding is a high probability (0.93 or higher) for the antifungal activity of MFC conjugates 11, 12, 14–16, and 35. The pexiganan analog cargo of these peptides may have a similar capability of depolarizing mitochondria and killing fungi and parasitic intracellular protozoans as the pexiganan but must be stabilized against proteolytic degradation [229].

For peptide 12 from Table 5, the bioactive cargo is Zp3a sequence GIKAKIGIKIKK (see also peptide 32 from Table 3). That peptide was recently designed by Zeng et al. [161] to eradicate the resistant Vibrio species pathogens, a frequent cause of disease outbreaks related to seafood consumption. When combined with our MFC construct, or asparagutin, a good compromise is achieved for Zp3a hybrids for predicted toxicity absence and broad-spectrum multifunctional activity. These molecules are more likely than Zp3a to enter the cytoplasm and disrupt mitochondrial membranes.

Mitochondrial-targeting peptide KLLNLISKLF is the prodeath domain MTD of the Noxa, the BH3-only Bcl-2 family protein [157,178,230]. It causes cellular death by opening the mitochondrial permeability transition pore and needs some cytosolic factor to become toxic. Moreover, the peptide requires help to penetrate the cytoplasmic membrane to reach mitochondria. Seo et al. [178] used the CPP-MTD sequence RRRRRRRRGRQ-KLLNLISKLF (peptide 29, Table 4) to study MTD killing mechanism. Jeong et al. [157] used the cationic RIMRILRILKLAR segment from the S5 subunit of a voltage-gated potassium channel (Kv2.1) connected to KLLNLISKLFCSGT via glycine triplet. We fused it with the asparagutin (peptide 27, Table 3) or the KRKRWHW CPP sequence (peptide 15, Table 4). All multifunctional predictions are pretty good for these three hybrid peptides. Low toxicity predictions are, however, questionable because all cell types can be penetrated, and the selectivity for cancer cells is not expected without some tumor-homing mechanism.

There are tumor-homing peptides that can be fused to the MTD. Seo et al. [178] used CGNKRTRGC and CNGRCVSGCAGRC tumor vascular-targeting motifs discovered by Arap et al. [231] to design selective MTD–CPP hybrids. The C2Pred server by Tang et al. [23] predicts that the hybrid peptide CGNKRTRGCGGKLLNLISKLF (named TU3: MTD) gains the CPP ability. That was verified in experiments by Seo et al. [178]. The Chosun University from South Korea patented TU3: MTD and similar peptides in 2012 (US patent 2012/0165269 A1).

Pfeiffer et al. [176] discovered that the antimicrobial peptide mastoparan (INLKALAA LAKKIL-amide) facilitates the mitochondrial permeability transition. Mastoparan peptide from wasp venom has a broad spectrum of activities. Among others, it causes cell death of malignant melanoma cells by activating the mitochondrial apoptosis pathway [232]. The hybrid peptide KW–mastoparan (peptide 27 from Table 4) has promising multifunctional potential too.

Peptide 24 from Table 4 is the DP1 pro-apoptotic peptide constructed by Mai et al. [173] with the sequence: RRQRRTSKLMKR-GG-KLAKLAKKLAKLAK. The N-terminal half is the protein transduction domain PTD-5 [233], which is connected via Gly-Gly linker to the C-terminal antimicrobial peptide (KLAKLAK)2 [234]. The DP1 is an efficient killer of tumor cells from accessible solid tumors both in vitro and in vivo. The probable mechanism is disrupting the mitochondrial membranes from these cells [173].

4.4. Magainin-2 Analogs Fused to Cell-Penetrating Peptides

Our Mutator server for predicting the therapeutic index TI [46] results in the maximal possible TI = 94.9 for the magainin analog GIAKFLDSAKKFGKKFVKTIMQL (peptide 25 from Table 5). We underlined substituted residues regarding magainin-2. Maximal TI is the best compromise between low hemolytic and robust antimicrobial activity. That magainin analog entered before or after CGNKRTR CPP into constructs 26 and 27, which we designed for the present paper. The HAPPENN server by Timmons and Hewage [40] rejects both magainin conjugates after a probability prediction of 0.98 and 0.86 for their hemolytic activity. It illustrates how different algorithms for predicting the same functionality can produce contrasting results.

Some examples when predictions agree with experimental results are magainin-2-pAntp [172] and magainin-2-bombesin conjugate [171,235] (see prediction results for peptides 22 and 23 from Table 4). Magainin-2 and bombesin were both isolated from frog skin. Bombesin is a cancer-homing peptide apt to recognize various human cancer cells. The magainins exhibit a modest anticancer activity (see peptide 6 from Table 5 and references [236–238]. Liu et al. [235] provided a positive answer to whether the conjugation of magainin 2 (MG2) to the bombesin could enhance the selectivity and cytotoxicity of hybrid peptide MG2B against tumor cells. It induced apoptosis of tumor cells in vivo and in vitro. The killing mechanism involves increased binding to cancer cell membranes and increased translocation into these cells. Cellular uptake of MG2B was confirmed by Liu et al. [235] after using fluorescein-labeled MG2B and fluorescence-activated cell sorting. Hence, we have the experimental confirmation for the CPP activity of MG2B despite Table 4 (peptide 22) prediction of the smallest CPP probability (0.30) for MG2B among all 52 peptides from that table. Unconfirmed MG2B ability is for treating polymicrobial co-infections (bacterial, viral, and fungal) and cancer. Immunocompromised persons receiving common anticancer drugs, patients with organ transplants exposed to immunosuppressants, or patients with a partially destroyed immune system (after HIV infection, for instance) are prone to co-infections. They can benefit from antimicrobial peptide conjugates with the unique potential to fight such infections [171].

Liu et al. [172] also examined magainin-2-penetratin conjugate (MG2A abbreviation, peptide 23 from Table 4) for its selective anticancer activity. They observed that penetratin binds to chondroitin sulfate (CS), which is overexpressed on the surface of some tumor cells.

Thus, penetratin should be able to act as a tumor-homing and cell-penetrating peptide at the same time while enhancing the anticancer activity of magainin 2. Achieved selectivity was not outstanding because the therapeutic index was not higher than three to five, meaning that cytotoxicity to normal cells was only five times lower. Still, MG2A performed better than MG2B, according to predictions for all beneficial activities (Table 4). Liu et al. [172,235] did not examine these peptides' antiviral and antifungal efficacy.

Magainin analogs coupled to shorter CPP are in Table 5 (peptides 7–9, 18–20, 22–24, 26–29, and 38). Some of them have better predicted overall performance than MG2A. In the absence of experimental confirmation, there is no way to ensure their therapeutic index is also better, but we have some reasons to expect so. Tumor-homing peptide CGNKRTR and other short CPPs, such as KRKRWHW, RCGIKRTK, RCGNKRFRWHW, RRWFRRRRRR, and RRRRRRFWRR may be able to provide good selectivity. Little cytotoxicity to mammalian cells and high penetrating efficiency was confirmed for the KRKRWHW peptide [168] (peptide 1 from Table 4). However, the predicted hemolytic activity for hybrids 7–9, 18–20, 22–24, 26–29, and 38 is spread around the probability for magainin 2 (0.83) with no value lower than 0.57 for peptide 19 (the conjugate with KRKRWHW).

One can find in the literature multiple confirmations for the broad-spectrum activity of magainin 2, its analogs and hybrids. It includes antibacterial [182,239], antiviral [240], antiprotozoal [241], and antifungal activity [242] in addition to antitumoral properties. To lower production costs, recombinant expressing systems have been developed to obtain large amounts of biologically active peptides [239]. Certain magainin analogs from Table 5 also have confirmed antimicrobial activity (peptides 10 and 13 [182]; peptide 17 [183]; peptide 21 [184]). Peptides 10 (9P0-1) and 13 (9P1-3) exhibited, respectively, 8 to 125 and 4 to 65 times stronger antibacterial activity than their parent peptide 6 (magainin-2) in Azuma et al. [182] experiments with *Escherichia coli* ATCC25922 and *Staphylococcus epidermidis* ATCC12228 strain. That would be difficult to anticipate based on a slight probability increase (from 0.95 to 0.99) for antimicrobial activity of analogs 10 and 13 by the $CAMP_{R3}$ algorithms (the SVM module) reported in Table 5. The $CAMP_{R3}$ Discriminant Analysis (DA) classifier obtains the same (correct) ranking for the antimicrobial potency, that is, 9P0-1 > 9P1-3 > MG2.

Older designed MG2 analogs are peptide 17 [183] and peptide 21 [184] from Table 5. Predicted SVM probabilities by the $CAMP_{R3}$ server are 0.965 and 0.985 for the antimicrobial activity of these peptides. The peptide 17 has confirmed antibacterial potency is from 6 to 40 times more potent in comparison to MG2 against, respectively, *Pseudomonas aeruginosa* and *Escherichia coli*. A slight increase from 0.946 (for MG2) to 0.965 (for peptide 17) for the probability of AMP activity cannot be easily interpreted as confirmation of the server's accuracy in predicting an order of magnitude stronger antibacterial activity detected in experiments. Instead, it is a possible indication that the applied design principles of Dathe et al. [183] are a good choice. For peptide 21, one amino acid substitution (Q19) was enough for Matsuzaki et al. [184] to observe 4 to 8 times stronger antibacterial activity against the *Acinetobacter calcoaceticus* ATCC 14987 and *Escherichia coli* ATCC 8739 strains. That significant improvement also corresponded to a slight increase in predicted SVM probability, from 0.946 for MG2 to 0.985 for Q19MG2. Attached asparagutin to peptide 17 significantly increased the probability for the CPP activity of the hybrid peptide 20 (also from Table 5) without any apparent decrease in its potential for other MF activities. Two CPP hybrids with peptide 21 with similar predicted features are peptides 23 and 24.

4.5. Imperfect and Perfect Activity-Enhancing Palindromes

The palindromic motifs RLLRRLLR and RWQWR enhance the antibacterial activity against Gram-negative and Gram-positive strains [243] when chimeric peptides are constructed based on buforin 2 sequence TRSSRAGLQFPVGRVHRLLRK [159] and lactoferricin fragment RRWQWRMKKLG [244]. Both buforin 2 and lactoferricin have confirmed strong antibacterial, anticancer, antifungal, anti-endotoxin, DNA-binding, and cell-penetrating properties (see [8,159,245–247] for validated activities of buforin-like peptides, and [248–251] for lactoferricin-like peptides). Those and similar palindromic motifs can be employed as LEGO pieces to achieve the desired fine-tuning of desired specificity and selectivity. Asparagutin decapeptides RRWFRRRRRR and RRRRRFWRR are imperfect arginine-rich palindromes with an excellent CPP potential (peptides 3 and 4 from Table 3).

In silico tests were performed with 48 asparagutin hybrids, including some analogs with one amino acid substitution, which decreased the number of arginines to seven. These are peptides 3, 4, 6, 7, 9–16, 20–29, 31–33, 35–38 and 42 from Table 3, peptides 12, 13, 17, 18, 21, 35, 37–39, 41–45, and 51 from Table 4, and peptides 9, 20, 24, 29, 38, and 43 from Table 5. Summary Table 6 lists 8 asparagutin hybrids among the best 20 multifunctional peptides according to the overall score. All magainin analogs fused to asparagutin retained the hemolytic activity and toxicity predictions similar to or worse than magainins. That eliminated them from the ranks of the 20 best peptides (Table 6) due to the strict requirements of the overall score for significantly lower hemolytic activity and toxicity predictions.

Some authors concluded that the guanidino groups from arginines play a crucial role in the membrane permeability of various molecules having different structures [211,252]. Designed penetratin analogs underlined the importance of the cell-penetrating role of the last seven residues of *Drosophila* pAntp penetratin [253,254], namely, residues R(10)RM KWKK(16). It is the motif BBXBXBB when B stands for cationic residues (R, K) and X stands for hydrophobic residues. Alanine substitutions at each sequence position of that septapeptide destroyed the cell-penetrating function of penetratin analogs except for position 12 (Met-12 to Ala-12 substitution). Table 1 illustrates that natural evolution during the last billion years also tolerated alanine substitution at the twelfth position of all penetratin analogs. Examples of penetratin-like peptides from all animals (including sponges and Placozoa) contain the same BBXBXBB palindromic motif. Exceptions from that septapeptide palindromic rule are easier to find in homeotic proteins from other kingdoms of life. Degenerate peptidic palindrome would probably be a better description [255] because palindromic BB sides are connected with an asymmetric linker region (XBX is usually MKW or AKW).

Binding to palindromic DNA sequences with perfect dyad symmetry does not require an equally ideal arrangement of the recognition helix from a transcription factor. The DNA-binding proteins often contain imperfect palindromic motifs, which mediate interaction with the DNA palindromic sequence. For instance, the RRSRARK septapeptide from DNA-recognition helix L(230)KRARNTEAARRSRARKLQRMKQL(253) or A(229)LKRARNTEAARRSRARKLQRMKQ(252) [256] of yeast transcriptional activator GCN4 (2DGC PBD identification for the P03069 protein) is anchored inside the major groove of the palindromic ATF/CREB site and conforms to the same BBXBXBB peptide palindrome with an asymmetric linker [257,258].

The BBXB is the simpler of two Cardin–Weintraub motifs [110] for heparin sulfate proteoglycan recognition [259], indicating that penetratin-like peptides can first bind to negatively charged glycosaminoglycans before they enter eukaryotic cells. Most cationic CPP conform to this motif due to the high density of positively charged residues [260]. Cell surface proteoglycans promote the uptake of arginine-rich penetratin-like peptides [261], but the uptake mechanism is still disputed [53,262]. Peptide-phospholipid interaction at the plasma membrane surface may mediate internalization at low, while accumulated peptide-glycosaminoglycan clusters activate endocytosis at higher, peptide concentrations [263]. By the way, both choices for the recognition helix (see above) from the GCN4 master regulator of gene expression (which activates more than 500 genes [264]) also have a high probability (0.95 to 0.96 according to the MLCPP server) to act as cell-penetrating peptides. So does the recognition helix ERKRLRNRLAATKCRKRKLERIAR [256] from the JunB prokaryotic transcription factor (CPP probability 0.96), which contains shorter BBXB and longer BBBXXB CW motifs (underlined). A dual role of CW motifs is essential for exported morphogens such as Sonic hedgehog protein and growth factors midkine and pleiotrophin, which bind to heparan sulfate in the form of monomers or multimers and show bactericidal activity [265,266].

4.6. Construction of Chimeras Containing Bacterial Pheromones or Ribosomal-Homing Peptide

Almost all chimeric peptides from Tables 3–5 are predicted to exhibit antibacterial, antiviral, and anticancer activity. Homing peptides often gain multifunctional abilities when fused to CPP sequences. Adding the N-terminal ribosomal-homing peptide YKWYYRGAA (RHP) to penetratin produces peptide 5 from Table 3 with the sequence YKWYYRGAARQIKIWFQNRRMKWKK, which readily enters into and kills all eukaryotic cells, whether healthy or malignant [54]. A killing mechanism involves binding to the ribosomal protein RPL29 and disrupting ribosomal function. Both algorithms for predicting anticancer activity, the ACPred [26] and mACPred [27], agree on predicting high ACP probability (respectively, 0.95 and 0.98). Antiviral activity for that peptide is also possible (probabilities equal to or higher than 0.8). In vivo usefulness is doubtful due to the peptide's nonselective cytotoxicity, which agrees with the probability of 0.97 for its hemolytic activity.

Sequence 7 from Table 3 contains the same ribosomal-homing motif, but its CPP part is our WFR_8 peptide. Predictions are better for almost all activities calculated in that Table than the peptide 5 results. The most encouraging is the prediction by the HAPPENN server for hemolytic activity. The peptide YKWYYRGAARRWFRRRRRR is expected to be non-hemolytic (with a small probability of 0.12 for the hemolytic activity). The predicted absence of hemolytic activity is even better for peptide 2 from Table 4 (0.02 probability), which we constructed as fused ribosomal-homing peptide YKWYYRGAA and short cell-penetrating sequence KRKRWHW designed by Wei et al. [168]. Hexadecapeptides YKWYYRGAAKRKRWHW and KRKRWHWGYKWYYRGAA (also 0.02 probability for hemolytic activity) look like promising lead compounds for selective anticancer activity (probability range from 0.97 to 0.99). Cell-penetrating peptide-based anticancer therapies provide the advantage of rapid delivery to intracellular targets and low toxicity compared to other drugs [267,268].

We can also consider designed hybrids when ribosomal-homing peptide YKWYYRGAA is fused with other shorter CPPs of minimal toxicity, such as reverse-WFR_8, CGNKRTR, RCGIKRTK, and RCGNKRFRWHW (respectively, peptides 4 from Table 3, and 1–3 from Table 5). These are sequences YKWYYRGAARRRRRRFWRR (peptide 33 from Table 3), CGNKRTRYKWYYRGAA, RCGIKRTKYKWYYRGAA, and RCGNKRFRWHWYKWYYRGAA (peptides 31–33 from Table 5). All of them should have good cell-penetrating activity (probability range from 0.78 to 0.97) without any hemolytic activity (probability predictions of 0.04 or less). If some other well-predicted activities are confirmed (anticancer, antiviral, or antifungal) among these four MF candidates, this would be an additional motivation for drug development.

The significant achievement in using pheromones for targeting specific pathogenic bacteria is the construction of the C16G2 peptide <u>TFFRLFNRSFTQALGK</u>GGG<u>KNLRIIRKGIHIIKKY</u>, which is specifically targeted toward dental caries causing *Streptococcus mutans* [269,270]. The underlined domains in the peptide's tripartite structure have different functions. The N-terminal part is the targeting sequence TFFRLFNRSFTQALGK derived from *S. mutans* competence-stimulating peptide, quorum-sensing bacterial pheromone. By itself, this domain has weak antibacterial activity. The GGG triplet is introduced next to provide a flexible linker. Underlined C-terminal domain KNLRIIRKGIHIIKKY is well-known broad-spectrum peptide antibiotic novispirin G10 [152,271] derived from sheep AMP ovispirin-1 by glycine for isoleucine substitution at the sequence position 10 to decrease ovispirin toxicity to human cells. It is the "killing domain" forming kinked amphipathic alpha helix in a membrane with resulting high hydrophobic moment. The HAPPENN and ToxinPred offer conflicting predictions. Expected hemolytic activity is very high (0.986 probability), while toxicity is low (−0.98 score).

Just-described discoveries opened a new field of specifically targeted chimeric antimicrobial peptides with a bright perspective of being used daily as a mouth rinse or as an essential ingredient in toothpaste to prevent caries. The importance of research in the case of C16G2 is illustrated by many clinical NIH-funded trials involving voluntary participants, with seven already completed: https://clinicaltrials.gov/ct2/results?term=C16G2&Search=Search (accessed on 26 July 2022).

One can use the same principle to construct other chimeric antimicrobial peptides with a flexible linker connecting the AMP region and the pheromone for targeted bacteria. One possibility to test is combining the S. mutants UA 159 mature pheromone GLDWWSL [272,273] with short but powerful broad-spectrum antimicrobial peptide RRLFRRILRWL [156]. With the same GGG linker, we designed specifically targeted chimeric AMP: GLDWWSLGGGRRLFRRILRWL, which is considerably shorter (21 amino acid residues) and cheaper to synthesize than the C16G2 peptide (35 amino acid residues). It has a very high hydrophobic moment for an amphipathic helix in the second half of its sequence. The hemolytic activity prediction for that peptide decreased to an acceptable magainin 2 probability (0.823). The predicted toxicity score is substantially lower (−1.52).

For gangrene-causing *Streptococci* sp., some other Streptococci-specific pheromones can be helpful, either alone [274], or when combined with a broad-spectrum AMP. For instance, it may be interesting to test the SilCR competence-stimulating peptide DIFKLVIDHISMKARKK linked with GGG triplet to RRLFRRILRWL or KNLRIIRKGIHIIKKY AMP when *Streptococcus pyogenes* or *Streptococcus dysgalactiae* is detected in necrotizing tissue. In the case of *Streptococcus oralis*, implicated in throat infection or dental plaque formation, the pheromone choice can be DWRISETIRNLIFPRKK. For multi-drug-resistant Streptococcus strains, it would be advantageous to have an alternative option of antibiotics. The few examples we described for chimeric-targeted AMPs are only a minuscule portion of all possibilities. Still, the critical point here is that we can perform the rational design of promising chimeric peptides in silico before testing in the laboratory.

4.7. The Optimization of Multifunctional Constructs

Table 5 peptides 31–52 represent in silico attempts to answer different questions about the design of multifunctional peptides. A rational approach toward better anti-inflammatory activity increased the overall score of MFC (peptide 3) fused with short pexiganan analog (peptide 35) enough to classify it among the best 20 multifunctional peptide constructs (seventh). The same approach was successful with the PR-35 analog (peptide 45), the 13th peptide in the overall rank (Table 6). The parent peptide for the PR-35 analog is the antimicrobial PR-39 cathelicidin from the pig (the P80054 UniProt entry). Interestingly, all seven automatic substitutions replaced prolines to increase the predicted anti-inflammatory activity without decreasing the potential for CPP and most other PR-39 and PR-35 functionalities (compare peptides 41, 44, and 45 from Table 5).

Cecropin-magainin-2 hybrid peptide 39 (dubbed P18 by Shin et al. [185]) is the opposite example when suggested amino acid substitutions by the Anti-inflammatory server by Gupta et al. [35] produced its analog (peptide 46) with a high probability for hemolytic activity and no toxicity decrease. Substitution of central Pro residues with Leu eliminated low hemolytic activity predicted and observed for P18. However, substitutions suggested by the ToxinPred server by Gupta et al. [37,38] and the HeliQuest server by Gautier et al. [275] decreased the predicted hemolytic and toxic activity. In the optimized sequence KW**R**LFKKI-P-**R**FL**R**SA**RR**F (peptide 49 from Table 5), we selected substitutions that replaced all but the first cationic residue with Arg. We rejected all substitutions for central proline residue to maintain the high selectivity [222]. The other five servers predicted better multifunctional activities for that highly amphipathic helical peptide CA-MA2-analog2, including its cell-penetrating ability.

The amphipathic peptide LKLLKKLLKKLLKLL-NH_2 (peptide 40, named K6L9) does not look promising due to observed and predicted potent hemolytic activity [186]. Still, its good antimicrobial and anticancer properties [276] stimulated the search for non-hemolytic analogs. For helical peptides with a continuous hydrophobic face, the selectivity can be increased together with the reduction in the hemolytic activity by inserting charged or D-amino acid residues into that helix face [277,278]. The LKlLKkLlkKLLkLL-NH_2 analog of

K6L9, named D-K6L9, has five D-amino acid residues (lower case letters indicate D-amino acids). It does not show any hemolytic activity, and it is better protected from in vivo cleavage by proteases [186]. Another ingenious chemical modification is the introduction of the site-specific isopeptide bond switch in K6L9. One such peptide, Amp1EP9 [279], is a stable and non-toxic antimicrobial peptide with other possible beneficial functions, such as anticancer and cell-penetrating. Unfortunately, the servers used in this review work only for the proteinogenic amino acids interconnected with peptide bonds. We can, however, imitate the D-K6L9 peptide by Gly and Arg substitutions into sequence locations 3 and 8 (Gly substitutions) and 6, 9, and 13 (Arg substitutions). The resulting LKGLKRLGRKLLRLL-NH_2 peptide has a considerably lower probability of hemolytic activity (0.153 instead of 0.907) with similar predictions for all other functionalities.

Like PR-39, pyrrhocoricin is also a proline-rich antibacterial peptide (peptide 42 from Table 5). That host defense peptide from insects is devoid of in vitro or in vivo toxicity and has confirmed low hemolytic activity [187,280] (probability of 0.004 according to the HAPPENN server). Akin to other proline-rich peptides, pyrrhocoricin can enter a cell's cytoplasm and exhibits multiple functions [280]. A recent finding is that the PRP repeat from pyrrhocoricin blocks the exit tunnel of 70S bacterial ribosome, which is essential for synthesizing all proteins [281,282]. Together with its cell-penetrating ability, this would explain the very high selectivity index and nanomolar concentration of pyrrhocoricin, which is enough to kill *E. coli* D22 and *Agrobacterium tumefaciens* [187]. It may be possible to broaden and strengthen the activity spectrum of pyrrhocoricin by fusing it with asparagutin (see Table 5 results for peptide 43).

4.8. Antimicrobial Peptides with Anticancer Activity Fused to Cell-Penetrating Peptides

A common theme in research about cancer and multidrug-resistant bacteria is the toxic side effects of last-resort drugs and natural obstacles impeding them from reaching their targets. Multifunctional peptides have the potential to overcome both hindrances. Besides magainins, many other natural peptides have verified antimicrobial and anticancer activity. Antibacterial AMPs with anticancer activity (ACP) are often cytotoxic to healthy human cells, but some are highly potent against bacteria and cancer cells while harmless to normal mammalian cells. Hoskin and Ramamoorthy [1] introduced classifications based on two general modes of AMP anticancer activity and several structural features in their influential review.

The structure of BMAP peptides, cecropins, LL-37, hCAP-18, magainins, temporins, fowlicidins, gaegurins, aureins, citropins, brevinins, ranatuerins, melittins, and their analogs is predominantly amphipathic α-helical in the membrane environment. Melittins are cytotoxic to all cells. Defensins, lactoferricins, and tachyplexins form amphiphilic β-sheet structure, while Pro-Arg-rich cathelicidin PR-39 and pyrrhocoricin lack the secondary structure. Some ACPs have a cyclic structure usually formed by disulfide bonds. Gomesin, tachyplexin I, and defensins are well-known examples. Our DADP database of anuran defense peptides ([283]; http://split4.pmfst.hr/dadp/, accessed on 7 August 2022) contains 108 peptides with dual AMP and ACP functions.

Gaspar et al. [2] enlisted 18 primary sequences for peptides with published data about their anticancer activity toward solid and hematological tumors. They concluded that the remaining challenges are delivery to tumor cells and lowering toxicity profile against healthy cells. The review of Deslouches and Di [171] lists 18 representative AMPs exhibiting anticancer activity as promising targets for drug development. The ADP database version 3 ([284]; https://aps.unmc.edu/AP/, accessed on 7 August 2022) contains 266 AMPs with anticancer activity. That is close to 8% of all their entries for antimicrobial peptides (a total of 3425 peptides). A richer $CAMP_{R3}$ database with more than ten thousand antimicrobial peptides contains even more ACPs. The CancerPPD database [285] encompasses more than 600 experimentally confirmed anticancer peptides. Felício et al. [3] concluded their review of dual AMP and ACP activities with a statement that at least 10 of these peptides can be approved for clinical applications during the next five years. Low selectivity, high production costs, and low resistance to proteolytic cleavage slowed down the progress in the drug delivery pipeline. Still, some peptide candidates exhibited cytotoxic activity and good selectivity against multidrug-resistant cancer cells.

A more recent review by Tornesello et al. [286] mentions only one natural dual-action peptide (AMP and ACP), which reached phase II of clinical trial steps for the melanoma target. It is the LL-37 peptide with the primary structure: LLGDFFRKSKEKIGKE-FKRIVQRIKDFLRNLVPRTES.

The LL-37 is one of the best-known multifunctional peptides and the only cathelicidin expressed in humans. Nijnik and Hancock [287] enumerated 12 different experimentally confirmed functions for LL-37, including immune modulation, wound healing, and angiogenesis, besides its antimicrobial and inhibition of biofilm formation activity. They did not discuss early indications of its anticancer, antiviral, antifungal, DNA binding, and cell-penetrating activity. Two LL-37 weaknesses are its weak potential for cell penetration (probabilities 0.68 and 0.45 for, respectively, CPP activity and uptake efficiency according to the MLCPP server) and low therapeutic index between 3 to 5 due to its toxicity to eukaryotic cells at slightly higher concentrations [1]. The selectivity index measured by hemolysis and minimal inhibitory concentration for bacterial growth is about 20 [288]. Regarding anticancer activity, LL-37 suppresses tumorigenesis in gastric cancer, but there is a perplexing implication for LL-37 in promoting breast, ovarian, and lung cancers [289].

Efforts to minimize the cost of peptide synthesis identified the LL-37 central helical region as the most important for its antibacterial, antibiofilm, and antiviral activity [290]. The same author (Guangshun Wang) subsequently added glycine at the N-terminal of their peptide GF-17 with the primary structure FKRIVQRIKDFLRNLV, which retained some antimicrobial and anticancer activity. To make it more resistant to proteases and more potent against multidrug-resistant ESKAPE bacterial species, Wang et al. [291] substituted two L-isoleucines and one L-leucine with three D-leucines. They also introduced several chemical modifications to make it more hydrophobic [291]. In the most active stable version of the GF-17 peptide, these authors replaced both phenylalanines with biphenylalanines. Substitution of Phe for biphenylalanine residues increases peptide hydrophobicity and self-assembly propensity. The resulting GF-17 analog, named 17BIPHE2 by Wang et al. [291], was equally potent against the *S. aureus* USA300 MRSA strain and the Gram-negative multidrug-resistant strains (MIC = 3.1 μM) with considerably higher SI = 73 compared to its parent peptide LL-37.

In our studies on how peptide antibacterial performance changes between Gram-negative and Gram-positive species [292], we have seen that high selectivity is more difficult to achieve against Gram-positive species such as *Staphylococcus aureus*. One possible reason is that more active peptides against *S. aureus* strains are more hydrophobic and more toxic to human cells. This makes it challenging to find the best compromise between low toxicity to healthy human cells and high wide-spectrum potency against most pathogenic bacteria and cancer cell types. Nevertheless, the 17BIPHE2 peptide exhibits 16 times better performance PE = SI/MIC than pexiganan's performance against *S. aureus* strains (see reference [292] for antibacterial performance definition and estimates). Still shorter LL-37 dodecapeptide with one D-Leu residue in its primary structure KRIVK*L*ILKWLR, named KR-12-a5(6-DL) by Kim et al. [293], had a mean MIC = 3.4 μM, and SI = 61.2 (D-Leu at 6th location is in italic font).

In our experience, the majority of natural or designed peptide antibiotics with an excellent performance against a broad spectrum of Gram-negative and Gram-positive bacteria (including some multidrug clinical isolates) are likely to exhibit some degree of selective anticancer activity too. Good examples are the peptides we designed and named trichoplaxin-2a, pexiganan-L18, flexampin, zyk-1, adepantin-1a, and mapegin [88]. Their respective sequences are: RHHWRRYARIGFRAVRTVIGK (T2R1), GIGKFLKKAKKFGKAFVLILKK (PEXA), GIKKWVKGVAKGVAKDLAKKIL (FLEX), GIGREIIKKIIKKIGKKIGRII (ZYK1), GIKKAVGKALKGLKGLLKALGES (A1A), and KIGKKILKALKGALKELA (MAPA). For prostate cancer PC-3 cells, the IC50 concentrations ranged from 1.5 (Zyk-1) to 12 μM (A1A), which is 40 to 5 times stronger anticancer activity compared to the Polybia-MP1 anticancer peptide IDWKKLLDAAKQIL-NH2 [88,294].

There are other examples when experimental confirmations exist for the conjugates to target cancer cells or their organelles [146,147,158,160,295]. Conjugates with reversed optimal penetratin (peptides 17, 18, 20, and 21 from Table 2) belong to the same category. Their cancer-homing C-terminals are tLyP-1 peptides or their analogs (see peptide 1 from Table 5). Such peptides can be the artificial death signal for malignant mitochondria and tumors. The associated probability for hemolytic activity is negligible (see the HAPPENN server results from Table 2). Thus, therapeutic applications are possible for nontoxic or weakly toxic anticancer peptide conjugates with tLyP-1, even when one of the two servers we used does not predict anticancer activity.

A particular class of anticancer peptides can elicit tumor eradication through cytotoxic T-cell responses. For instance, cancer vaccination is performed with telomerase peptide EARPALLTSRLRFIPK named GV1001 [296]. The peptide can internalize into the cell cytoplasm [154]. Uptake efficiency prediction is boosted from low to high when the GG linker is introduced, and asparagutin is attached to construct the hybrid peptide 24 from Table 3.

Transforming dual-function (antimicrobial and anticancer) into a multiple-function peptide is easy in silico. One example is the asparagutin–adepantin hybrid sequence (peptide 18 from Table 4), which ranks 19th without substitutions (see overall rank from Table 6). This would not be possible if the conjugate did not excel at all six predicted activities in combination with low toxicity. One amino acid substitution in the adepantin 1A (Gly15 replacement with Leu15) increased the anti-inflammatory activity score from 1.36 to 1.62, according to the AntiInflam server. Still, the overall score decreased from 19th to 21st (see peptide 51 in Tables 4 and 6). It illustrates how easily optimizing anti-inflammatory activity can increase hemolytic activity and decrease other beneficial functions.

4.9. Design Examples for Low Toxicity and Multiple Activities

The design for common antimicrobial, anticancer, and cell-penetrating ability can start with known AMP to which CPP is fused to increase the cell-penetrating efficiency of a hybrid peptide. It can also begin with known CPP by introducing amino acid substitutions to widen its activity spectrum. Let us first describe how we achieved the goal of in vitro antibacterial and anticancer activity for a modified CPP named mapegin [88]. Its parent CPP is well-known MAP sequence KLALKLALKALKAALKLA [166]. Rational design by Juretić et al. [88] resulted in the mapegin sequence K**IGK**K**I**LKALK**G**ALK**E**LA (named MAPA). It differs from the MAP sequence in highlighted and underlined amino acid residues I2, G3, K4, I6, G12, and E16, which increased flexibility (due to two glycines) but did not decrease the high amphipathicity feature of the parent peptide. We confirmed the predicted decrease in hemolytic activity and good antibacterial and anticancer activity. Minimal inhibitory concentrations of mapegin against *E. coli* and *S. aureus* bacteria (including drug-resistant strains) ranged from 0.5 to 8 μM, while IC50 against PC-3 prostate cancer cells was 8 μM [88].

Selectivity (toxicity absence) was not so good. For healthy human fibroblasts, the therapeutic index was about three. Regarding the hemolysis of human erythrocytes, the selectivity index was variable for different bacterial strains but more often on the low side. For *E. coli* and *S. aureus* the SI range was $10 < SI < 40$. The 50% hemolysis after mapegin application was reached already with the peptide concentration of 20 μM. It is still an improvement in the hemolytic activity of the parent peptide (MAP), which is toxic to red blood cells. Moreover, mapegin is at least two times stronger antibacterial compound than MAP. The probability of hemolytic activity is low for mapegin, according to the HAPPENN server (0.079). Predicted cell-penetrating, antifungal, and anti-inflammatory activity of the mapegin await experimental confirmation. The cell-penetrating activity is expected to decrease due to six amino acid substitutions introduced into already excellent MAP CPP.

If we want to regain an excellent CPP function, the mapegin can be fused to some known CPP, such as the TAT peptide. We formed hybrid peptides mapegin–TAT (T3-

48), mapegin–TAT analog1 optimized for higher anti-inflammatory activity (T3-49), and mapegin–TAT analog2 optimized for lower toxicity (T3-50). These are peptides 48–50 from Table 3. Their good overall rank (27th, 30th, and 11th, Table 6) makes all of them interesting for various applications. The disadvantage of hybrid peptides is their longer length and the increased cost to synthesize them.

We performed the rational design to obtain wide-spectrum antibacterial compounds before any tests on cancer cell lines [88]. Some dual-function peptides (PEXA, FLEX, ZYK1, A1A, and T2R1) are as good initial choices for creating hybrid peptides as the mapegin (see predictions for peptides 17–21, 35, 46–49, and 51 from Table 4). Observed MIC concentration values against *E. coli* ATCC 25922 and *S. aureus* ATCC 29213 were around one micromolar for all these peptides. The activity and the therapeutic index TI were surprisingly good against human prostate PC-3 cancer cells. After comparing peptide toxicity toward healthy human fibroblasts, we observed that the TI range was from about 3 (for mapegin and pexiganan-L18) to 10 (trichoplaxin-2a) [88]. Thus, for these six peptides, the therapeutic index tested on PC-3 cancer cells is not as high as the selectivity index for bacteria, which ranges from about 10 to more than 1000. Nevertheless, it is better than the TI for the anticancer peptide MP1 [294,297], which we used as a control. Since MP1 exhibits a moderate anticancer activity on tumor cell lines (around IC50 = 50 μM), our peptide antibiotics also have considerably better activity against cancer cells. There are, of course, other examples of how one can modify CPP or AMP templates for designing their anticancer or multifunctional analogs [1,3,5,6,12,166,298–301].

Our choice of online servers, mACPpred and ACPred, for anticancer activity is subjective and subject to flaws. There are some contradictory predictions for the anticancer activity (peptides 3–6, 14, and 15 from Table 2; peptides 6, 8, 28, and 29 from Table 3; peptide 41 from Table 4; and peptide 36 from Table 5). The reader can notice that the ACPred server frequently gives the ACP probability of around 0.98. This would be difficult to falsify in experiments because there is always the possibility that the peptide is active against a particular cancer cell line but inactive against other malignant cell types.

The lack of toxicity for proliferating human cells is questionable if a permanent blockage occurs for selected transcription sites in human DNA. On the other hand, a surrogate peptide that inhibits DNA binding of transcription factors needed for cancer cell proliferation may be useful in cancer treatments. It would be a welcome outcome for our hybrid peptides to directly prove their worth as anticancer peptides. Novel short CPP can serve as penetratin to import anticancer cargo drugs to desired internal targets in tumor cells. There are many other DNA/RNA-binding cryptides that can be used directly or in a modified form to increase libraries of multifunctional peptide assets. All transcription factors (TF) are prospective parent proteins for such peptides.

5. Summary Comments about Peptide Constructs

All the 20 best peptides (1st to 20th in the overall rank) have a high probability of intrinsic disorder throughout their length (see Table 6 legend). Due to their plasticity, there is no conflict with assuming a partially ordered structure in a suitable microenvironment. They often obtain an amphipathic secondary structure consisting of two arms with a flexible linker between them (α-helix or β-strand-hinge-α-helix or β-strand) when bound to an anionic membrane surface. After cell penetration and interaction with internal macromolecules, the peptides can change their conformation again. There is a high probability of forming DNA or RNA contacts, but it differs in the extent and sequence location among different peptides and their segments. For the best 20 peptides, the predicted binding sites with nucleic acids encompass 41% (sixth) to 100% (first and third) of their length (see Table 6 legend). Predicted protein binding residues make up from 10% to 70% of their length.

The spectrum of the most disordered and malleable structures adapting the conformation to different targets is not reserved for the listed Table 6 sequences of two-arm peptides. From the remaining nine Table 6 peptides and other Tables 2–5 sequences, there are also examples when all of their residues are predicted with disordered conformation and high binding probability to nucleic acids. This is the case for the 22nd peptide, which is the conjugate of reversed optimal penetratin analog with the tLyp-1 analog (see peptide 21 Table 2), and the T2R3G3 construct with an overall score of 0.7981 (see peptide 34 from Table 3). The T2R3G3 is a modified trichoplaxin 2 analog sequence after adding two N-terminal and three C-terminal residues. It is a highly amphipathic α-helix membrane-binding structure for its central 6–21 segment (SPLIT algorithm prediction). The only outstanding feature of the first peptide (temporin analog fused to asparagutin analog) is its absence of predicted protein-binding contacts and the perfect separation between DNA-binding (1–11) and RNA-binding segment (residues 12–25).

We verified that with different scoring methods, temporin-CPP hybrids with a central bend interrupting helical structure are still top-ranking multifunctional peptides. Glycine, as a single or double linker in the central position, allows for a greater freedom of movement and better exploration of targets for the hybrid peptides. Increased flexibility contributes to better selectivity and lesser toxicity of hybrid peptides containing such a linker. Higher selectivity is the outcome for some of the designed peptides when central proline residue or proline doublet introduces the hinge between bioactive and cell-penetrating peptide segments.

Temporins were described and named by Simmaco et al. [302] as the smallest natural antibacterial peptides known at that time. They were first found from the skin secretion of *Rana esculenta* [303] and *Rana temporaria* [302], amphibian species widely distributed in Western and Central Europe. The top-listed in silico-designed candidates (Table 6) are certain temporin analogs fused to the RRWKIVVIRWRR, RRWFRRRRRR, or KRKRWHW cell-penetrating peptides. Natural temporins are amidated at their C-terminal, have a low net charge (from −1 to +3), and have a short length of between 8 and 17 amino acid residues [304,305]. Typically, they exhibit an amphipathic α-helical conformation in a nonpolar environment. Low toxicity to healthy mammalian cells, low cost for their synthesis, and multifunctional activity against bacteria, viruses, filamentous fungi, yeasts, protozoa, and cancer cells are well-known advantages of some natural temporins [304]. Temporin L, with the highest net charge (+3), has the broadest activity spectrum [306].

The therapeutically promising ability of temporins is that they do not harm macrophages at concentrations lethal to these cells' intracellular parasites [304]. Anti-protozoa activity was not considered in our review, but neither were the anti-endotoxin, chemotactic, synergistic, and anti-biofilm formation activities attributed to temporins [307,308]. Of special interest are anticancer, antiviral, and fungicidal abilities of some temporins [304,309,310].

Synthetic analogs are often better than their "parent" peptides for desired activity. Shang et al. [112,311] examined highly charged analogs of temporin 1CEb starting from its sequence ILPILSLIGGLLGK-NH_2 [162]. One of these analogs with six lysines and the sequence IKKIVSKIKKLLK-NH_2 was named L-K6V1 [112]. It forms considerably less hydrophobic and more amphipathic helix in a membrane environment. Regarding their functionality spectrum, the analog gained better cell-penetrating and antimicrobial ability while losing its hemolytic activity (compare peptides 39 and 40 from Table 3). These improvements are much more apparent in experimental validations [112]. The L-K6V1 peptide (peptide 40, Table 3) still does not enter among the 20 best peptides from Tables 2–5 (Table 6). It, however, served in turn as the "parent "peptide for fusing it with short and powerful CPP, such as the KW peptide (peptide 1, Table 4) or asparagutin (peptide 3, Table 3).

The broadest spectrum of best predictions is with the asparagutin analog RRWFR**S**RRRR, Gly-Gly linker, and L-K6V1 analogs. One of these sequences, the temporin-asparagutin analog 3 (peptide 37, Table 3) with the sequence **V**KKIVSKI**R**KLLK-GG-RRWFR**S**RRRR, ranked as the best one. The preliminary score (when toxic and hemolytic activity is not considered) and the overall score (when low toxicity is also considered in the overall mean score) agree on the highest ranking for that hybrid peptide.

Other temporin-asparagutin analogs with the G, GG, GGEPPKG, or GGGPPKG linker (Table 4, peptide 39; Table 3 peptide 36; Table 4, peptides 38 and 30; Table 3 peptide 9; Table 4 peptide 37; Table 3, peptide 35) ranked 2nd to 5th, 8th, 9th, and 14th, respectively, in the overall multifunctional score. The TA peptide 9 from Table 3 is already predicted with potent anti-inflammatory activity without needing any amino acid substitution. Sequences 30 from Table 4 (5th) and 48 from Table 5 (10th) are the shortest temporin-CPP conjugates with only 22 residues. To construct the 10th best peptide (peptide 48, Table 5), we used the novel P9 CPP carrier, RRRRRWWPP [188], as the reversed version (revP9) and added it to the C-terminal of L-K6V1 temporin [112]. One Pro residue remained near the central position after optimizing a hybrid peptide with the AntiInflam server. These nine temporin analogs are predicted with a nearly perfect score for antiviral activity. All of them enter among the 15 multifunctional peptides with the best overall score. The design of the 17th best peptide consisted in adding the N-terminal part of the first best peptide (**V**KKIVSKI**R**KLLKGG) to the CPP construct RRWKIVVIRWRR without any additional optimization. Among many possible applications, we can mention treating skin ulcers caused by the herpes virus. In any case, it is encouraging that in silico search for sequences with the best combination of multifunctional activities, intracellular targeting, and low toxicity zeroed on the class of temporin–CPP hybrids as 60% of the 15 best and 50% of the 20 best peptides. In contrast, ten temporin construct "winners" make up only about 6% of all peptides (176) we considered.

The second class of predicted top performers encompasses optimized penetratins and their analogs fused to the tumor-homing peptide tLyP-1. Optimal penetratin sequence GKRIGKKWKPRRRRFWRK with 18 residues (Table 2, peptide 22) ranks 31st among the best multifunctional peptides. We used the reversed optimal penetratin [56] as the parent peptide. The design consisted in increasing its alpha hydrophobic moment and applying several methods for improving its therapeutic index: locating the proline in the sequence middle, forming a hydrophobic sector interrupted with a charged residue, and introducing the small GXXXG motif at its N-terminal for stimulating peptides association in membrane environment [312]. We removed two C-terminal residues from the parent sequence KKWKPRRRRFWRKKR and added the pentapeptide GKRIG to its N-terminal to achieve these goals. A different approach is additional optimization for better anti-inflammatory activity and adding the tumor-homing peptide tLyp-1 [146] or its analog CGAKRTK to the C-terminal. The overall rank increased for hybrids 20 and 21 from Table 2 (6th and 22nd).

Our multifunctional construct RCGNKRFRWHW (peptide 3, Table 5) was useful when conjugated with the pexiganan analog optimized with two substitutions for better anti-inflammatory activity (T5-35). It ranked as the seventh best peptide. The predicted membrane-associated structure of MFC-PexS has a low profile of alpha and beta hydrophobic moments, distinguishing it from most other top-ranking peptides.

When fused mapegin and TAT CPP are optimized for low toxicity, the 11th peptide is obtained with 31 residues (Table 3, peptide 50). It has the lowest toxicity score of −1.81 and the highest reward score of 0.867 for the mean of low hemolytic probability and toxicity score. Any remaining confirmed activity (antiviral, antifungal, and anti-inflammatory) would be beneficial.

BMAP peptide analogs target mitochondria and cause apoptosis [174,313]. The most active peptide part (the 18 residues cathelicidin fragment from bovine) is fused to short CPP (the KW peptide). The top-scoring conjugates are peptide 33 from Table 4 (12th), and peptides 25 and 36 from Table 4 (16th and 18th). Optimizing peptide 25 from Table 4 for higher anti-inflammatory activity (with conservative substitution Leu for Ile) did not impair other beneficial functionalities of the peptide 33 sequence KRKRWHW-GGLRSLGRK**L**LRAWKKYG (Table 4).

Recently, experimentalists confirmed broad activity against enveloped viruses by the second bovine cathelicidin fragment with the sequence GRFKRFRKKFKKLFKKIS [179]. It was derived from BMAP-27 [314]. Its variant GRFKRFRKKFKKLFKKLS exhibited anti-parasitic activity [315]. We verified in silico that the hybrid peptide KRKRWHW-GRFKRFRKKFKKLFKKIS (peptide 52 from Table 4) is nontoxic for mammalian cells. Adding KW peptide conferred high multifunctional activities (32nd in the overall rank) without optimization. Thus, cathelicidin-CPP constructs are also promising lead compounds for multifunctionality.

We optimized only the best peptide candidates for higher anti-inflammatory activity. As a rule, we limited substitutions to three. One exception is the proline-arginine-rich peptide PR-35 (peptide 44 from Table 5). The optimized sequence RRR**V**RPPYLPR**V**RP**Q**PFFP **L**RL**LK**RI**S**PGFPPRFP has seven substituted residues (peptide 45 from Table 5). Its predicted toxicity to mammalian cells is low, and the overall rank is high (13th). There is, however, a decrease in expected cell-penetrating and anticancer activity compared to parent peptide PR-35.

Novispirin analogs also deserve several comments. The novispirin analog sequence KNLRIIRKGIHIIKKY (dubbed G2) lacks arginine at the fifth sequence location of novispirin-G10. It is used for anti-biofilm and anti-caries applications [269,270,316,317]. This was our starting peptide for creating and optimizing CPP chimeras. With KW CPP linked via Gly doublet after the G2 peptide, the optimization for lower toxicity resulted in the sequence KNLRI**F**RKGIHI**H**KKY-GG-KRKRWHW (T4-50), which scored 20th in the overall rank.

Intriguingly, 11 out of 20 best multifunctional peptides exhibit anticancer and antiviral probability close to 1.0 (>0.95, see Table 6 results from columns 5 and 6 highlighted in the gray background). A common feature of cancer phenotype and cell transformation into the viral factory is intensive bioenergetics [227], which is likely to be inhibited by antimicrobial peptides, such as temporin, BMAP, adepantin-1, and trichoplaxin-2 analogs.

6. Conclusions

Nature endowed host defense peptides with multifaceted activity. Natural AMPs with CPP activity, or CPP fragments, can interact with multiple sites of bacterial or fungal cells. There are hundreds of internal protein targets for penetratin, lactoferricin B, and PR-39, to name just a few well-known peptides explored with the protein microarray technique [318–320]. Thus, we should not constrain rational design to the "magic bullet" goal. Some short synthetic CPP, such as Sub 5 [189] (see last rows of Table 5), have remarkably diverse internal protein targets [321]. Multiple targeting and rapid action minimize the chance of resistance development in targeted microorganisms or cancer cells. Marketed single-target drugs are frequently unable to reach internal targets and are prone to mistargeting with associated side effects. Fast-evolving microbes or malignant cells quickly develop resistance to such drugs. Deleterious effects then predominate benefits. However, targeting sequences conjugated to CPP offer a precision medicine tool for acting on well-protected organelles [322], intracellular pathogens, hijacked processes in pathological conditions, and foreign molecules in our cells.

Advanced prediction tools combined with expert design allow the construction of about 20 nontoxic CPP-hybrids with a high score for anti-inflammatory activity and a high probability ($\geq$0.7) for the intrinsic disorder, cell-penetrating, antibacterial, antifungal, antiviral, and anticancer activity. Such flexible peptides with a high cationic charge often adapt the two arms structure after coming into contact with anionic molecules. For instance, an amphipathic helix-hinge-helix conformation can bridge different molecules and exhibit complex functionality. Designed peptides should pass easily through the plasma membrane in the eukaryotic cells. Their likely internal targets are respiring mitochondria, unprotected parts of nucleic acids, or negatively charged molecules in the cell wall and cytoplasmic membrane of bacterial cells. Multiple protein targets are also possible due to the wide range of predicted functions. In conclusion, the review is the argument for exploring wide-spectrum multifunctionality *in silico*, *in vitro*, and *in vivo*. Let us hope pharmaceutical companies and governmental regulations become less refractory to the multifunctional drug potential of cell-penetrating antimicrobial peptides and their conjugates.

Funding: This research received no external funding.

Institutional Review Board Statement: Not applicable.

Informed Consent Statement: Not applicable.

Data Availability Statement: Data is contained within the article.

Conflicts of Interest: The author declares no conflict of interest.

References

1. Hoskin, D.W.; Ramamoorthy, A. Studies on anticancer activities of antimicrobial peptides. *Biochim. Biophys. Acta* **2008**, *1778*, 357–375. [CrossRef] [PubMed]
2. Gaspar, D.; Veiga, A.S.; Castanho, M.A.R.B. From antimicrobial to anticancer peptides. A review. *Front. Microbiol.* **2013**, *4*, 294. [CrossRef] [PubMed]
3. Felício, M.R.; Silva, O.N.; Gonçalves, S.; Santos, N.C.; Franco, O.L. Peptides with Dual Antimicrobial and Anticancer Activities. *Front. Chem.* **2017**, *5*, 5. [CrossRef]
4. Henriques, S.T.; Lawrence, N.; Chaousis, S.; Ravipati, A.S.; Cheneval, O.; Benfield, A.H.; Elliott, A.G.; Kavanagh, A.M.; Cooper, M.A.; Chan, L.Y.; et al. Redesigned Spider Peptide with Improved Antimicrobial and Anticancer Properties. *ACS Chem. Biol.* **2017**, *12*, 2324–2334. [CrossRef] [PubMed]
5. Zhang, C.; Yang, M.; Ericsson, A.C. Antimicrobial Peptides: Potential Application in Liver Cancer. *Front. Microbiol.* **2019**, *10*, 1257. [CrossRef]
6. Liscano, Y.; Oñate-Garzón, J.; Delgado, J.P. Peptides with Dual Antimicrobial–Anticancer Activity: Strategies to Overcome Peptide Limitations and Rational Design of Anticancer Peptides. *Molecules* **2020**, *25*, 4245. [CrossRef]
7. Rozek, T.; Wegener, K.T.; Bowie, J.H.; Olver, I.N.; Carver, J.A.; Wallace, J.C.; Tyler, M.J. The antibiotic and anticancer active aurein peptides from the Australian Bell Frogs Litoria aurea and Litoria raniformis. The solution structure of aurein 1.2. *Eur. J. Biochem.* **2000**, *267*, 5330–5341. [CrossRef]
8. Lee, H.S.; Park, C.B.; Kim, J.M.; Jang, S.A.; Park, I.Y.; Kim, M.S.; Cho, J.H.; Kim, S.C. Mechanism of anticancer activity of buforin IIb, a histone H2A-derived peptide. *Cancer Lett.* **2008**, *271*, 47–55. [CrossRef]
9. Hilchie, A.L.; Wuerth, K.; Hancock, R.E.W. Immune modulation by multifaceted cationic host defense (antimicrobial) peptides. *Nat. Chem. Biol.* **2013**, *9*, 761–768. [CrossRef]
10. Drayton, M.; Deisinger, J.P.; Ludwig, K.C.; Raheem, N.; Müller, A.; Schneider, T.; Straus, S.K. Host Defense Peptides: Dual Antimicrobial and Immunomodulatory Action. *Int. J. Mol. Sci.* **2021**, *22*, 11172. [CrossRef]
11. Shin, M.K.; Lee, B.; Kim, S.T.; Yoo, J.S.; Sung, J.S. Designing a Novel Functional Peptide With Dual Antimicrobial and Anti-inflammatory Activities via in Silico. *Methods Front. Immunol.* **2022**, *13*, 821070. [CrossRef] [PubMed]
12. Hilchie, A.L.; Hoskin, D.W.; Power Coombs, M.R. Anticancer Activities of Natural and Synthetic Peptides. *Adv. Exp. Med. Biol.* **2019**, *1117*, 131–147. [CrossRef]
13. Ajesh, K.; Sreejith, K. Peptide antibiotics: An alternative and effective antimicrobial strategy to circumvent fungal infections. *Peptides* **2009**, *30*, 999–1006. [CrossRef] [PubMed]
14. Duncan, V.M.S.; O'Neil, D.A. Commercialization of antifungal peptides. *Fungal Biol. Rev.* **2013**, *26*, 156–165. [CrossRef]
15. Ciociola, T.; Giovati, L.; Conti, S.; Magliani, W.; Santinoli, C.; Polonelli, L. Natural and synthetic peptides with antifungal activity. *Future Med. Chem.* **2016**, *8*, 1413–1433. [CrossRef]
16. Hoffmann, A.R.; Guha, S.; Wu, E.; Ghimire, J.; Wang, Y.; He, J.; Garry, R.F.; Wimley, W.C. Broadspectrum antiviral entry inhibition by interfacially active peptides. *J. Virol.* **2020**, *94*, e01682-20. [CrossRef]
17. Hollmann, A.; Cardoso, N.P.; Espeche, J.C.; Maffía, P.C. Review of antiviral peptides for use against zoonotic and selected non-zoonotic viruses. *Peptides* **2021**, *142*, 170570. [CrossRef]
18. Henriques, S.T.; Melo, M.N.; Castanho, M.A.R.B. Cell-penetrating peptides and antimicrobial peptides: How different are they? *Biochem. J.* **2006**, *399*, 1–7. [CrossRef]
19. Pärn, K.; Eriste, E.; Langel, Ü. The Antimicrobial and Antiviral Applications of Cell-Penetrating Peptides. *Methods Mol. Biol.* **2015**, *1324*, 223–245. [CrossRef]
20. Brasseur, R.; Divita, G. Happy birthday cell penetrating peptides: Already 20 years. *Biochim. Biophys. Acta* **2010**, *1798*, 2177–2181. [CrossRef]
21. Gallo, M.; Defaus, S.; Andreu, D. 1988-2018, Thirty years of drug smuggling at the nano scale. Challenges and opportunities of cell-penetrating peptides in biomedical research. *Arch. Biochem. Biophys.* **2019**, *661*, 74–86. [CrossRef]
22. Manavalan, B.; Subramaniyam, S.; Shin, T.H.; Kim, M.O.; Lee, G. Machine-learning-based prediction of cell-penetrating peptides and their uptake efficiency with improved accuracy. *J. Proteome Res.* **2018**, *17*, 2715–2726. [CrossRef]
23. Tang, H.; Su, Z.D.; Wei, H.H.; Chen, W.; Lin, H. Prediction of cell-penetrating peptides using feature selection techniques. *Biochem. Biophys. Res. Commun.* **2016**, *477*, 150–154. [CrossRef] [PubMed]
24. Waghu, F.H.; Barai, R.S.; Gurung, P.; Idicula-Thomas, S. CAMP$_{R3,}$ A database on sequences, structures and signatures of antimicrobial peptides. *Nucleic Acids Res.* **2016**, *44*, D1094–D1097. [CrossRef] [PubMed]
25. Burdukiewicz, M.; Sidorczuk, K.; Rafacz, D.; Pietluch, F.; Chilimoniuk, J.; Rödiger, S.; Gagat, P. AmpGram: A proteome screening tool for prediction and design of antimicrobial peptides. *Int. J. Mol. Sci.* **2020**, *21*, 4310. [CrossRef] [PubMed]
26. Schaduangrat, N.; Nantasenamat, C.; Prachayasittikul, V.; Shoombuatong, W. ACPred: A computational tool for the prediction and analysis of anticancer peptides. *Molecules* **2019**, *24*, 1973. [CrossRef]

27. Boopathi, V.; Subramaniyam, S.; Malik, A.; Lee, G.; Manavalan, B.; Yang, D.C. mACPpred: A support vector machine-based meta-predictor for identification of anticancer peptides. *Int. J. Mol. Sci.* **2019**, *20*, 1964. [CrossRef]
28. Timmons, P.B.; Hewage, C.H. ENNAVIA is a novel method which employs neural networks for antiviral and anti-coronavirus activity prediction for therapeutic peptides. *Brief. Bioinform.* **2021**, *22*, bbab258. [CrossRef]
29. Chowdhury, A.S.; Reehl, S.M.; Kehn-Hall, K.; Bishop, B.; Webb-Robertson, B.J.M. Better understanding and prediction of antiviral peptides through primary and secondary structure feature importance. *Sci. Rep.* **2020**, *10*, 19260. [CrossRef]
30. Schaduangrat, N.; Nantasenamat, C.; Prachayasittikul, V.; Shoombuatong, W. Meta-iAVP: A sequence-based meta-predictor for improving the prediction of antiviral peptides using effective feature representation. *Int. J. Mol. Sci.* **2019**, *20*, 5743. [CrossRef]
31. Meher, P.K.; Sahu, T.K.; Saini, V.; Rao, A.R. Predicting antimicrobial peptides with improved accuracy by incorporating the compositional, physico-chemical and structural features into Chou's general PseAAC. *Sci. Rep.* **2017**, *7*, 42362. [CrossRef] [PubMed]
32. Zhang, J.; Yang, L.; Tian, Z.; Zhao, W.; Sun, C.; Zhu, L.; Huang, M.; Guo, G.; Liang, G. Large-Scale Screening of Antifungal Peptides Based on Quantitative Structure-Activity Relationship. *ACS Med Chem Lett.* **2021**, *13*, 99–104. [CrossRef]
33. Manavalan, B.; Shin, T.H.; Kim, M.O.; Lee, G. AIPpred: Sequence-Based Prediction of Anti-inflammatory Peptides Using Random Forest. *Front. Pharmacol.* **2018**, *9*, 276. [CrossRef] [PubMed]
34. Khatun, M.S.; Hasan, M.M.; Kurata, H. PreAIP: Computational Prediction of Anti-inflammatory Peptides by Integrating Multiple Complementary Features. *Front. Genet.* **2019**, *10*, 129. [CrossRef] [PubMed]
35. Gupta, S.; Sharma, A.K.; Shastri, V.; Madhu, M.K.; Sharma, V.K. Prediction of anti-inflammatory proteins/peptides: An in silico approach. *J. Transl. Med.* **2017**, *15*, 7. [CrossRef] [PubMed]
36. Hwang, S.; Gou, Z.; Kuznetsov, I.B. DP-Bind: A web server for sequence-based prediction of DNA-binding residues in DNA-binding proteins. *Bioinformatics* **2007**, *23*, 634–636. [CrossRef] [PubMed]
37. Gupta, S.; Kapoor, P.; Chaudhary, K.; Gautam, A.; Kumar, R.; Raghava, G.P. Peptide toxicity prediction. *Methods Mol. Biol.* **2015**, *1268*, 143–157. [CrossRef]
38. Gupta, S.; Kapoor, P.; Chaudhary, K.; Gautam, A.; Kumar, R.; Open Source Drug Discovery Consortium; Raghava, G.P.S. In silico approach for predicting toxicity of peptides and proteins. *PLoS ONE* **2013**, *8*, e73957. [CrossRef]
39. Usmani, S.S.; Kumar, R.; Bhalla, S.; Kumar, V.; Raghava, G.P.S. In Silico Tools and Databases for Designing Peptide-Based Vaccine and Drugs. *Adv. Protein Chem. Struct. Biol.* **2018**, *112*, 221–263. [CrossRef]
40. Timmons, P.B.; Hewage, C.M. HAPPENN is a novel tool for hemolytic activity prediction for therapeutic peptides which employs neural networks. *Sci. Rep.* **2020**, *10*, 10869. [CrossRef]
41. Wei, L.; Ye, X.; Sakurai, T.; Mu, Z.; Wei, L. ToxIBTL: Prediction of peptide toxicity based on information bottleneck and transfer learning. *Bioinformatics* **2022**, *38*, 1514–1524. [CrossRef] [PubMed]
42. Juretić, D.; Lučin, A. The preference functions method for predicting protein helical turns with membrane propensity. *J. Chem. Inf. Comput. Sci.* **1998**, *38*, 575–585. [CrossRef]
43. Juretić, D.; Zoranić, L.; Zucić, D. Basic charge clusters and predictions of membrane protein topology. *J. Chem. Inf. Comput. Sci.* **2002**, *42*, 620–632. [CrossRef]
44. Juretić, D.; Vukičević, D.; Ilić, N.; Antcheva, N.; Tossi, A. Computational Design of Highly Selective Antimicrobial Peptides. *J. Chem. Inf. Model.* **2009**, *49*, 2873–2882. [CrossRef] [PubMed]
45. Juretić, D.; Vukičević, D.; Petrov, D.; Novković, M.; Bojović, V.; Lučić, B.; Ilić, I.; Tossi, A. Knowledge-based computational methods for identifying or designing novel, non-homologous antimicrobial peptides. *Eur. Biophys. J.* **2011**, *40*, 371–385. [CrossRef] [PubMed]
46. Kamech, N.; Vukičević, D.; Ladram, A.; Piesse, C.; Vasseur, J.; Bojović, V.; Simunić, J.; Juretić, D. Improving the selectivity of antimicrobial peptides from anuran skin. *J. Chem. Inf. Model.* **2012**, *52*, 3341–3351. [CrossRef]
47. Etzion-Fuchs, A.; Todd, D.A.; Singh, M. dSPRINT: Predicting DNA, RNA, ion, peptide and smallmolecule interaction sites within protein domains. *Nucleic Acids Res.* **2021**, *49*, e78. [CrossRef]
48. Le Roux, I.; Joliot, A.H.; Bloch-Gallego, E.; Prochiantz, A.; Volovitch, M. Neurotrophic activity of the Antennapedia homeodomain depends on its specific DNA-binding properties. *Proc. Natl. Acad. Sci. USA* **1993**, *90*, 9120–9124. [CrossRef]
49. Christiaens, B.; Symoens, S.; Vanderheyden, S.; Engelborghs, Y.; Joliot, A.; Prochiantz, A.; Vandekerckhove, J.; Rosseneu, M.; Vanloo, B. Tryptophan fluorescence study of the interaction of penetratin peptides with model membranes. *Eur. J. Biochem.* **2002**, *269*, 2918–2926. [CrossRef]
50. Palm, C.; Netzereab, S.; Hällbrink, M. Quantitatively determined uptake of cell-penetrating peptides in non-mammalian cells with an evaluation of degradation and antimicrobial effects. *Peptides* **2006**, *27*, 1710–1716. [CrossRef]
51. Masman, M.F.; Rodriguez, A.M.; Raimondi, M.; Zacchino, S.A.; Luiten, P.G.M.; Somlai, C.; Kortvelyesi, T.; Penke, B.; Enriz, R.D. Penetratin and derivatives acting as antifungal agents. *Eur. J. Med. Chem.* **2009**, *44*, 212–228. [CrossRef] [PubMed]
52. Zhu, W.L.; Shin, S.Y. Antimicrobial and cytolytic activities and plausible mode of bactericidal action of the cell penetrating peptide penetratin and its Lys-linked two-stranded peptide. *Chem. Biol. Drug Des.* **2009**, *73*, 209–215. [CrossRef] [PubMed]
53. Alves, I.D.; Jiao, C.Y.; Aubry, S.; Aussedat, B.; Burlina, F.; Chassaing, G.; Sagan, S. Cell biology meets biophysics to unveil the different mechanisms of penetratin internalization in cells. *Biochim. Biophys. Acta* **2010**, *1798*, 2231–2239. [CrossRef] [PubMed]

54. Rangel, R.; Guzman-Rojas, L.; le Roux, L.G.; Staquicini, F.I.; Hosoya, H.; Barbu, E.M.; Ozawa, M.G.; Nie, J.; Dunner, K., Jr.; Langley, R.R.; et al. Combinatorial targeting and discovery of ligand-receptors in organelles of mammalian cells. *Nat. Commun.* **2012**, *3*, 788. [CrossRef] [PubMed]
55. Bahnsen, J.S.; Franzyk, H.; Sandberg-Schaal, A.; Nielsen, H.M. Antimicrobial and cell-penetrating properties of penetratin analogs: Effect of sequence and secondary structure. *Biochim. Biophys. Acta* **2013**, *1828*, 223–232. [CrossRef]
56. Kauffman, W.B.; Guha, S.; Wimley, W.C. Synthetic molecular evolution of hybrid cell penetrating peptides. *Nat. Commun.* **2018**, *9*, 2568. [CrossRef]
57. Vale, N.; Duarte, D.; Silva, S.; Correia, A.S.; Costa, B.; Gouveia, M.J.; Ferreira, A. Cell-Penetrating Peptides in Oncologic Pharmacotherapy: A Review. *Pharmacol. Res.* **2020**, *162*, 105231. [CrossRef]
58. Shoari, A.; Tooyserkani, R.; Tahmasebi, M.; Löwik, D.W. Delivery of Various Cargos into Cancer Cells and Tissues via Cell-Penetrating Peptides: A Review of the Last Decade. *Pharmaceutics* **2021**, *13*, 1391. [CrossRef]
59. Bellen, H.J.; Wilson, C.; Gehring, W.J. Dissecting the complexity of the nervous system by enhancer detection. *Bioessays* **1990**, *12*, 199–204. [CrossRef]
60. Quiring, R.; Walldorf, U.; Kloter, U.; Gehring, W.J. Homology of the eyeless gene of Drosophila to the Small eye gene in mice and Aniridia in humans. *Science* **1994**, *265*, 785–789. [CrossRef]
61. Halder, G.; Callaerts, P.; Gehring, W.J. Induction of ectopic eyes by targeted expression of the eyeless gene in Drosophila. *Science* **1995**, *267*, 1788–1792. [CrossRef] [PubMed]
62. Gehring, W.J.; Ikeo, K. Pax 6, mastering eye morphogenesis and eye evolution. *Trends Genet.* **1999**, *15*, 371–377. [CrossRef]
63. Punzo, C.; Seimiya, M.; Flister, S.; Gehring, W.J.; Plaza, S. Differential interactions of eyeless and twin of eyeless with the sine oculis enhancer. *Development* **2002**, *129*, 625–634. [CrossRef] [PubMed]
64. Gehring, W.J. New Perspectives on Eye Development and the Evolution of Eyes and Photoreceptors. *J. Hered.* **2005**, *96*, 171–184. [CrossRef]
65. Kozmik, Z. The role of Pax genes in eye evolution. *Brain Res. Bull.* **2008**, *75*, 335–339. [CrossRef]
66. Gehring, W.J. The evolution of vision. *WIREs Dev. Biol.* **2014**, *3*, 1–40. [CrossRef]
67. Chi, N.; Epstein, J.A. Getting your Pax straight: Pax proteins in development and disease. *Trends Genet.* **2002**, *18*, 41–47. [CrossRef]
68. Gruschus, J.M.; Tsao, D.H.H.; Wang, L.H.; Nirenberg, M.; Ferretti, J.A. The three-dimensional structure of the vnd/NK-2 homeodomain-DNA complex by NMR spectroscopy. *J. Mol. Biol.* **1999**, *289*, 529–545. [CrossRef]
69. Birrane, G.; Soni, A.; Ladias, J.A. Structural Basis for DNA Recognition by the Human PAX3 Homeodomain. *Biochemistry* **2009**, *48*, 1148–1155. [CrossRef]
70. Gehring, W.J.; Qian, Y.Q.; Billeter, M.; Furukubo-Tokunaga, K.; Schier, A.F.; Resendez-Perez, D.; Affolter, M.; Otting, G.; Wüthrich, K. Homeodomain-DNA recognition. *Cell* **1994**, *78*, 211–223. [CrossRef]
71. Dupont, E.; Prochiantz, A.; Joliot, A. Penetratin Story: An Overview. In *Cell-Penetrating Peptides*; Methods in Molecular Biology; Humana Press: Totowa, NJ, USA, 2011; Volume 683, pp. 21–29. [CrossRef]
72. Holland, P.W. Evolution of homeobox genes. *Wiley Interdiscip. Rev. Dev. Biol.* **2013**, *2*, 31–45. [CrossRef] [PubMed]
73. Arslan, D.; Legendre, M.; Seltzer, V.; Abergel, C.; Claverie, J.-M. Distant Mimivirus relative with a larger genome highlights the fundamental features of Megaviridae. *Proc. Natl. Acad. Sci. USA* **2011**, *108*, 17486–17491. [CrossRef] [PubMed]
74. Jeudy, S.; Bertaux, L.; Alempic, J.-M.; Lartigue, A.; Legendre, M.; Belmudes, L.; Santini, S.; Philippe, N.; Beucher, L.; Biondi, E.G.; et al. Exploration of the propagation of transpovirons within Mimiviridae reveals a unique example of commensalism in the viral world. *ISME J.* **2020**, *14*, 727–739. [CrossRef] [PubMed]
75. Havrilak, J.A.; Al-Shaer, L.; Baban, N.; Akinci, N.; Layden, M.J. Characterization of the dynamics and variability of neuronal subtype responses during growth, degrowth, and regeneration of *Nematostella vectensis*. *BMC Biol.* **2021**, *19*, 104. [CrossRef] [PubMed]
76. Leach, W.B.; Reitzel, A.M. Decoupling behavioral and transcriptional responses to color in an eyeless cnidarian. *BMC Genom.* **2020**, *21*, 361. [CrossRef]
77. Kaniewska, P.; Alon, S.; Karako-Lampert, S.; Hoegh-Guldberg, O.; Levy, O. Signaling cascades and the importance of moonlight in coral broadcast mass spawning. *eLife* **2015**, *4*, e09991. [CrossRef]
78. Sharma, S.; Wang, W.; Stolfi, A. Single-cell transcriptome profiling of the *Ciona* larval brain. *Dev. Biol.* **2019**, *448*, 226–236. [CrossRef]
79. Oonuma, K.; Tanaka, M.; Nishitsuji, K.; Kato, Y.; Shimai, K.; Kusakabe, T.G. Revised lineage of larval photoreceptor cells in Ciona reveals archetypal collaboration between neural tube and neural crest in sensory organ formation. *Dev. Biol.* **2016**, *420*, 178–185. [CrossRef]
80. Kusakabe, T.; Kusakabe, R.; Kawakami, I.; Satou, Y.; Satoh, N.; Tsuda, M. Ci-opsin1, a vertebrate-type opsin gene, expressed in the larval ocellus of the ascidian *Ciona intestinalis*. *FEBS Lett.* **2001**, *506*, 69–72. [CrossRef]
81. Hadrys, T.; DeSalle, R.; Sagasser, S.; Fischer, N.; Schierwater, B. The Trichoplax PaxB gene: A putative Proto-PaxA/B/C gene predating the origin of nerve and sensory cells. *Mol. Biol. Evol.* **2005**, *22*, 1569–1578. [CrossRef]
82. Monteiro, A.S.; Schierwater, B.; Dellaporta, S.L.; Holland, P.W.H. A low diversity of ANTP class homeobox genes in Placozoa. *Evol. Dev.* **2006**, *8*, 174–182. [CrossRef] [PubMed]
83. Srivastava, M.; Larroux, C.; Lu, D.R.; Mohanty, K.; Chapman, J.; Degnan, B.M.; Rokhsar, D.S. Early evolution of the LIM homeobox gene family. *BMC Biol.* **2010**, *8*, 4. [CrossRef] [PubMed]

84. Sebé-Pedrós, A.; de Mendoza, A.; Lang, B.F.; Degnan, B.M.; Ruiz-Trillo, I. Unexpected repertoire of metazoan transcription factors in the unicellular holozoan *Capsaspora owczarzaki*. *Mol. Biol. Evol.* **2011**, *28*, 1241–1254. [CrossRef] [PubMed]
85. Simunić, J.; Petrov, D.; Bouceba, T.; Kamech, N.; Benincasa, M.; Juretić, D. Trichoplaxin—A new membrane-active antimicrobial peptide from placozoan cDNA. *Biochim. Biophys. Acta* **2014**, *1838*, 1430–1438. [CrossRef]
86. Majzoub, K.; Wrensch, F.; Baumert, T.F. The Innate Antiviral Response in Animals: An Evolutionary Perspective from Flagellates to Humans. *Viruses* **2019**, *11*, 758. [CrossRef]
87. Kamm, K.; Schierwater, B.; DeSalle, R. Innate immunity in the simplest animals–placozoans. *BMC Genom.* **2019**, *20*, 5. [CrossRef]
88. Juretić, D.; Golemac, A.; Strand, D.E.; Chung, K.; Ilić, N.; Goić-Barišić, I.; Pellay, F.-X. The spectrum of design solutions for improving the activity-selectivity product of peptide antibiotics against multidrug-resistant bacteria and prostate cancer PC-3 cells. *Molecules* **2020**, *25*, 3526. [CrossRef]
89. Mayorova, T.D.; Hammar, K.; Jung, J.H.; Aronova, M.A.; Zhang, G.; Winters, C.A.; Reese, T.S.; Smith, C.L. Placozoan fiber cells: Mediators of innate immunity and participants in wound healing. *Sci. Rep.* **2021**, *11*, 23343. [CrossRef]
90. Romanova, D.Y.; Nikitin, M.A.; Shchenkov, S.V.; Moroz, L.L. Expanding of Life Strategies in Placozoa: Insights From Long-Term Culturing of Trichoplax and Hoilungia. *Front. Cell Dev. Biol.* **2022**, *10*, 823283. [CrossRef]
91. Prakash, V.N.; Bull, M.S.; Prakash, M. Motility-induced fracture reveals a ductile-to-brittle crossover in a simple animal's epithelia. *Nat. Phys.* **2021**, *17*, 504–511. [CrossRef]
92. Martinelli, C.; Spring, J. Expression pattern of the homeobox gene Not in the basal metazoan *Trichoplax adhaerens*. *Gene Expr. Patterns* **2004**, *4*, 443–447. [CrossRef] [PubMed]
93. Green, M.; Loewenstein, P.M. Autonomous Functional Domains of Chemically Synthesized Human lmmunodeficiency Virus Tat Trans-Activator Protein. *Cell* **1988**, *55*, 1179–1188. [CrossRef]
94. Galdiero, S.; Falanga, A.; Vitiello, M.; Grieco, P.; Caraglia, M.; Morelli, G.; Galdiero, M. Exploitation of viral properties for intracellular delivery. *J. Pept. Sci.* **2014**, *20*, 468–478. [CrossRef]
95. van den Berg, A.; Dowdy, S.F. Protein transduction domain delivery of therapeutic macromolecules. *Curr. Opin. Biotechnol.* **2011**, *22*, 888–893. [CrossRef] [PubMed]
96. Shen, Y.; Yu, W.; Hay, J.G.; Sauthoff, H. Expressed cell-penetrating peptides can induce a bystander effect, but passage through the secretory pathway reduces protein transduction activity. *Mol. Ther.* **2011**, *19*, 903–912. [CrossRef] [PubMed]
97. Hemmati, S.; Behzadipour, Y.; Haddad, M. Decoding the proteome of severe acute respiratory syndrome coronavirus 2 (SARS-CoV-2) for cell-penetrating peptides involved in pathogenesis or applicable as drug delivery vectors. *Infect. Genet. Evol.* **2020**, *85*, 104474. [CrossRef]
98. Krüger, D.M.; Neubacher, S.; Grossmann, T.N. Protein-RNA interactions: Structural characteristics and hotspot amino acids. *RNA* **2018**, *24*, 1457–1465. [CrossRef]
99. Brandes, N.; Linial, M. Giant Viruses—Big Surprises. *Viruses* **2019**, *11*, 404. [CrossRef]
100. Bürglin, T.R.; Affolter, M. Homeodomain proteins: An update. *Chromosoma* **2016**, *125*, 497–521. [CrossRef]
101. Rabouille, C. Pathways of Unconventional Protein Secretion. *Trends Cell Biol.* **2017**, *27*, 230–240. [CrossRef]
102. Lorent, J.H.; Levental, K.R.; Ganesan, L.; Rivera-Longsworth, G.; Sezgin, E.; Doktorova, M.D.; Lyman, E.; Levental, I. Plasma membranes are asymmetric in lipid unsaturation, packing, and protein shape. *Nat. Chem. Biol.* **2020**, *16*, 644–652. [CrossRef] [PubMed]
103. Amblard, I.; Dupont, E.; Alves, I.; Miralvès, J.; Queguiner, I.; Joliot, A. Bidirectional transfer of homeoprotein EN2 across the plasma membrane requires PIP_2. *J. Cell Sci.* **2020**, *133*, jcs211327. [CrossRef] [PubMed]
104. Hammond, G.R.V.; Fischer, M.J.; Anderson, K.E.; Holdich, J.; Koteci, A.; Balla, T.; Irvine, R.F. PI4P And PI(4,5)P_2 Are Essential But Independent Lipid Determinants Of Membrane Identity. *Science* **2012**, *337*, 727–730. [CrossRef] [PubMed]
105. Di Paolo, G.; De Camilli, P. Phosphoinositides in cell regulation and membrane dynamics. *Nature* **2006**, *443*, 651–657. [CrossRef]
106. Joliot, A.; Prochiantz, A. Homeoproteins as natural Penetratin cargoes with signaling properties. *Adv. Drug Deliv. Rev.* **2008**, *60*, 608–613. [CrossRef]
107. Dupont, E.; Prochiantz, A.; Joliot, A. Identification of a signal peptide for unconventional secretion. *J. Biol. Chem.* **2007**, *282*, 8994–9000. [CrossRef]
108. Prochiantz, A.; Di Nardo, A.A. Homeoprotein signaling in the developing and adult nervous system. *Neuron* **2015**, *85*, 911–925. [CrossRef]
109. Carlier, L.; Balayssac, S.; Cantrelle, F.-X.; Khemtémourian, L.; Chassaing, G.; Joliot, A.; Lequin, O. Investigation of Homeodomain Membrane Translocation Properties: Insights from the Structure Determination of Engrailed-2 Homeodomain in Aqueous and Membrane-Mimetic Environments. *Biophys. J.* **2013**, *105*, 667–678. [CrossRef]
110. Cardin, A.D.; Weintraub, H.J. Molecular modeling of protein-glycosaminoglycan interactions. *Arteriosclerosis* **1989**, *9*, 21–32. [CrossRef]
111. Cardon, S.; Bolbach, G.; Hervis, Y.P.; Lopin-Bon, C.; Jacquinet, J.; Illien, F.; Walrant, A.; Ravault, D.; He, B.; Molina, L.; et al. A cationic motif in Engrailed-2 homeoprotein controls its internalization via selective cell-surface glycosaminoglycans interactions. *bioRxiv* **2021**. [CrossRef]
112. Shang, D.; Li, X.; Sun, Y.; Wang, C.; Sun, L.; Wei, S.; Gou, M. Design of Potent, Non-Toxic Antimicrobial Agents Based upon the Structure of the Frog Skin Peptide, Temporin-1CEb from Chinese Brown Frog, *Rana chensinensis*. *Chem. Biol. Drug Des.* **2012**, *79*, 653–662. [CrossRef]

113. Tünnemann, G.; Cardoso, M.C. Cell-Penetrating Peptides—Uptake, Toxicity, and Applications. In *Membrane-Active Peptides: Methods and Results on Structure and Function*; Castanho, M.A.R.B., Ed.; International University Line: La Jolla, CA, USA, 2009; Chapter 14; pp. 330–362.
114. Juretić, D.; Sonavane, Y.; Ilić, N.; Gajski, G.; Goić-Barišić, I.; Tonkić, M.; Kozic, M.; Maravić, A.; Pellay, F.-X.; Zoranić, L. Designed peptide with a flexible central motif from ranatuerins adapts its conformation to bacterial membranes. *Biochim. Biophys. Acta* **2018**, *1860*, 2655–2668. [CrossRef]
115. Kozić, M.; Vukičević, D.; Simunić, J.; Rončević, T.; Antcheva, N.; Tossi, A.; Juretić, D. Predicting the Minimal Inhibitory Concentration for Antimicrobial Peptides with Rana-box Domain. *J. Chem. Inf. Model.* **2015**, *55*, 2275–2287. [CrossRef]
116. Dupont, E.; Prochiantz, A.; Joliot, A. Penetratin Story: An Overview. In *Cell-Penetrating Peptides*; Methods in Molecular Biology; Humana Press: Totowa, NJ, USA, 2015; Volume 1324, pp. 29–37. [CrossRef]
117. Religa, T.L.; Johnson, C.M.; Vu, D.M.; Brewer, S.H.; Dyer, R.B.; Fersht, A.R. The helix–turn– helix motif as an ultrafast independently folding domain: The pathway of folding of Engrailed homeodomain. *Proc. Natl. Acad. Sci. USA* **2007**, *104*, 9272–9277. [CrossRef] [PubMed]
118. Joliot, A.H.; Triller, A.; Volovitch, M.; Pernelle, C.; Prochiantz, A. Alpha-2,8-Polysialic acid is the neuronal surface receptor of antennapedia homeobox peptide. *New Biol.* **1991**, *3*, 1121–1134. [PubMed]
119. Derossi, D.; Joliot, A.H.; Chassaing, G.; Prochiantz, A. The third helix of the Antennapedia homeodomain translocates through biological membranes. *J. Biol. Chem.* **1994**, *269*, 10444–10450. [CrossRef]
120. Balayssac, S.; Burlina, F.; Convert, O.; Bolbach, G.; Chassaing, G.; Lequin, O. Comparison of Penetratin and Other Homeodomain-Derived Cell-Penetrating Peptides: Interaction in a Membrane-Mimicking Environment and Cellular Uptake Efficiency. *Biochemistry* **2006**, *45*, 1408–1420. [CrossRef]
121. Polyansky, A.A.; Volynsky, P.E.; Arseniev, A.S.; Efremov, R.G. Adaptation of a Membrane-active Peptide to Heterogeneous Environment. I. Structural Plasticity of the Peptide. *J. Phys. Chem. B* **2009**, *113*, 1107–1119. [CrossRef]
122. Chan, D.I.; Prenner, E.J.; Vogel, H.J. Tryptophan- and arginine-rich antimicrobial peptides: Structures and mechanisms of action. *Biochim. Biophys. Acta* **2006**, *1758*, 1184–1202. [CrossRef] [PubMed]
123. Lamazière, A.; Wolf, C.; Lambert, O.; Chassaing, G.; Trugnan, G.; Ayala-Sanmartin, J. The Homeodomain Derived Peptide Penetratin Induces Curvature of Fluid Membrane Domains. *PLoS ONE* **2008**, *3*, e1938. [CrossRef] [PubMed]
124. Fleissner, F.; Pütz, S.; Schwendy, M.; Bonn, M.; Parekh, S.H. Measuring Intracellular Secondary Structure of a Cell-Penetrating Peptide in Situ. *Anal. Chem.* **2017**, *89*, 11310–11317. [CrossRef] [PubMed]
125. Eiríksdóttir, E.; Konate, K.; Langel, Ü.; Divita, G.; Deshayes, S. Secondary structure of cell-penetrating peptides controls membrane interaction and insertion. *Biochim. Biophys. Acta* **2010**, *1798*, 1119–1128. [CrossRef]
126. Derossi, D.; Calvet, S.; Trembleau, A.; Brunissen, A.; Chassaing, G.; Prochiantz, A. Cell Internalization of the Third Helix of the Antennapedia Homeodomain Is Receptor-independent. *J. Biol. Chem.* **1996**, *271*, 18188–18193. [CrossRef] [PubMed]
127. Duchardt, F.; Fotin-Mleczek, M.; Schwarz, H.; Fischer, R.; Brock, R. A Comprehensive Model for the Cellular Uptake of Cationic Cell-penetrating Peptides. *Traffic* **2007**, *8*, 848–866. [CrossRef] [PubMed]
128. Kaksonen, M.; Roux, A. Mechanisms of clathrin-mediated endocytosis. *Nat. Rev. Mol. Cell Biol.* **2018**, *19*, 313–326. [CrossRef]
129. Almeida, C.; Lamazière, A.; Filleau, A.; Corvis, Y.; Espeau, P.; Ayala-Sanmartin, J. Membrane re-arrangements and rippled phase stabilisation by the cell penetrating peptide penetratin. *Biochim. Biophy. Acta* **2016**, *1858*, 2584–2591. [CrossRef]
130. Dupont, E.; Prochiantz, A.; Joliot, A. *Penetratins*; CRC: Boca Raton, FL, USA, 2006.
131. Zorko, M.; Langel, Ü. Cell-Penetrating Peptides. *Methods Mol. Biol.* **2022**, *2383*, 3–32. [CrossRef]
132. Škrlj, N.; Drevenšek, G.; Hudoklin, S.; Romih, R.; Čurin Šerbec, V.; Dolinar, M. Recombinant Single-Chain Antibody with the Trojan Peptide Penetratin Positioned in the Linker Region Enables Cargo Transfer Across the Blood–Brain Barrier. *Appl. Biochem. Biotechnol.* **2013**, *169*, 159–169. [CrossRef]
133. Arora, S.; Sharma, D.; Singh, J. GLUT-1, An Effective Target To Deliver Brain-Derived Neurotrophic Factor Gene across the Blood Brain Barrier. *ACS Chem. Neurosci.* **2020**, *11*, 1620–1633. [CrossRef]
134. Liu, C.; Jiang, K.; Tai, L.; Liu, Y.; Wei, G.; Lu, W.; Pan, W. Facile Noninvasive Retinal Gene Delivery Enabled by Penetratin. *ACS Appl. Mater Interfaces* **2016**, *8*, 19256–19267. [CrossRef]
135. Vale, N.; Ferreira, A.; Fernandes, I.; Alves, C.; Araújo, M.J.; Mateus, N.; Gomes, P. Gemcitabine anti-proliferative activity significantly enhanced upon conjugation with cell-penetrating peptides. *Bioorg Med. Chem. Lett.* **2017**, *27*, 2898–2901. [CrossRef]
136. Kanovsky, M.; Raffo, A.; Drew, L.; Rosal, R.; Do, T.; Friedman, F.K.; Rubinsteini, P.; Visseri, J.; Robinson, R.; Brandt-Rauf, P.W.; et al. Peptides from the amino terminal mdm-2-binding domain of p53, designed from conformational analysis, are selectively cytotoxic to transformed cells. *Proc. Natl. Acad. Sci. USA* **2001**, *98*, 12438–12443. [CrossRef]
137. Derossi, D.; Chassaing, G.; Prochiantz, A. Trojan peptides: The penetratin system for intracellular delivery. *Trends Cell Biol.* **1998**, *8*, 84–87. [CrossRef] [PubMed]
138. Rosal, R.; Pincus, M.R.; Brandt-Rauf, P.W.; Fine, R.L.; Michl, J.; Wang, H. NMR Solution Structure of a Peptide from the mdm-2 Binding Domain of the p53 Protein that Is Selectively Cytotoxic to Cancer Cells. *Biochemistry* **2004**, *43*, 1854–1861. [CrossRef] [PubMed]
139. Selivanova, G.; Iotsova, V.; Okan, I.; Fritsche, M.; Ström, M.; Groner, B.; Grafström, R.C.; Wiman, K.G. Restoration of the growth suppression function of mutant p53 by a synthetic peptide derived from the p53 C-terminal domain. *Nat. Med.* **1997**, *3*, 632–638. [CrossRef] [PubMed]

140. Subekti, D.R.G.; Kamagata, K. The disordered DNA-binding domain of p53 is indispensable for forming an encounter complex to and jumping along DNA. *Biochem. Biophys. Res. Commun.* **2021**, *534*, 21–26. [CrossRef]
141. Bidwell, G.L., 3rd; Raucher, D. Therapeutic peptides for cancer therapy. Part I peptide inhibitors of signal transduction cascades. *Expert Opin. Drug Deliv.* **2009**, *6*, 1033–1047. [CrossRef]
142. Martínez, D.E. Mortality patterns suggest lack of senescence in hydra. *Exp. Gerontol.* **1998**, *33*, 217–225. [CrossRef]
143. Vogg, M.C.; Buzgariu, W.; Suknovic, N.S.; Galliot, B. Cellular, Metabolic, and Developmental Dimensions of Whole-Body Regeneration in Hydra. *Cold Spring Harb. Perspect. Biol.* **2021**, *13*, a040725. [CrossRef]
144. Badosa, E.; Ferré, R.; Francés, J.; Bardají, E.; Feliu, L.; Planas, M.; Montesinos, E. Sporicidal activity of synthetic antifungal undecapeptides and control of *Penicillium* rot of apples. *Appl. Environ. Microbiol.* **2009**, *75*, 5563–5569. [CrossRef]
145. Horibe, T.; Kohno, M.; Haramoto, M.; Ohara, K.; Kawakami, K. Designed hybrid TPR peptide targeting Hsp90 as a novel anticancer agent. *J. Transl. Med.* **2011**, *9*, 8. [CrossRef] [PubMed]
146. Roth, L.; Agemy, L.; Kotamraju, V.R.; Braun, G.; Teesalu, T.; Sugahara, K.N.; Hamzah, J.; Ruoslahti, E. Transtumoral targeting enabled by a novel neuropilin-binding peptide. *Oncogene* **2012**, *31*, 3754–3763. [CrossRef]
147. Woldetsadik, A.D.; Vogel, M.C.; Rabeh, W.M.; Magzoub, M. Hexokinase II–derived cell-penetrating peptide targets mitochondria and triggers apoptosis in cancer cells. *FASEB J.* **2017**, *31*, 2168–2184. [CrossRef] [PubMed]
148. Andreu, D.; Ubach, J.; Boman, A.; Wåhlin, B.; Wade, D.; Merrifield, R.B.; Boman, H.G. Shortened cecropin A-melittin hybrids. Significant size reduction retains potent antibiotic activity. *FEBS Lett.* **1992**, *296*, 190–194. [CrossRef]
149. Dong, W.; Dong, Z.; Mao, X.; Sun, Y.; Li, F.; Shang, D. Structure-activity analysis and biological studies of chensinin-1b analogues. *Acta Biomater.* **2016**, *37*, 59–68. [CrossRef]
150. Mwangi, J.; Yin, Y.; Wang, G.; Yang, M.; Li, Y.; Zhang, Z.; Lai, R. The antimicrobial peptide ZY4 combats multidrug-resistant *Pseudomonas aeruginosa* and *Acinetobacter baumannii* infection. *Proc. Natl. Acad Sci. USA* **2019**, *116*, 26516–26522. [CrossRef]
151. Jing, W.; Demcoe, A.R.; Vogel, H.J. Conformation of a bactericidal domain of puroindoline A: Structure and mechanism of action of a 13-residue antimicrobial peptide. *J. Bacteriol.* **2003**, *185*, 4938–4947. [CrossRef]
152. Sawai, M.V.; Waring, A.J.; Kearney, W.R.; McCray, P.B., Jr.; Forsyth, W.R.; Lehrer, R.I.; Tack, B.F. Impact of single-residue mutations on the structure and function of ovispirin/novispirin antimicrobial peptides. *Protein Eng.* **2002**, *15*, 225–232. [CrossRef] [PubMed]
153. Rončević, T.; Gajski, G.; Ilić, N.; Goić-Barišić, I.; Tonkić, M.; Zoranić, L.; Simunić, J.; Benincasa, M.; Mijaković, M.; Tossi, A.; et al. PGLa-H tandem-repeat peptides active against multidrug resistant clinical bacterial isolates. *Biochim. Biophys. Acta Biomembr.* **2017**, *1859*, 228–237. [CrossRef]
154. Lee, S.A.; Kim, B.R.; Kim, B.K.; Kim, D.W.; Shon, W.J.; Lee, N.R.; Inn, K.S.; Kim, B.J. Heat shock protein-mediated cell penetration and cytosolic delivery of macromolecules by a telomerase-derived peptide vaccine. *Biomaterials* **2013**, *34*, 7495–7505. [CrossRef] [PubMed]
155. Mink, C.; Strandberg, E.; Wadhwani, P.; Melo, M.N.; Reichert, J.; Wacker, I.; Castanho, M.A.R.B.; Ulrich, A.S. Overlapping Properties of the Short Membrane-Active Peptide BP100 With (i) Polycationic TAT and (ii) α-helical Magainin Family Peptides. *Front. Cell. Infect. Microbiol.* **2021**, *11*, 609542. [CrossRef] [PubMed]
156. Torcato, I.M.; Huang, Y.H.; Franquelim, H.G.; Gaspar, D.; Craik, D.J.; Castanho, M.A.R.B.; Henriques, S.T. Design and characterization of novel antimicrobial peptides, R-BP100 and RW-BP100, with activity against Gram-negative and Gram-positive bacteria. *Biochim. Biophys. Acta* **2013**, *1828*, 944–955. [CrossRef]
157. Jeong, J.H.; Kim, K.; Lim, D.; Jeong, K.; Hong, Y.; Nguyen, V.H.; Kim, T.H.; Ryu, S.; Lim, J.A.; Kim, J.I.; et al. Anti-tumoral effect of the mitochondrial target domain of Noxa delivered by an engineered *Salmonella typhimurium*. *PLoS ONE* **2014**, *9*, e80050. [CrossRef] [PubMed]
158. Howl, J.; Matou-Nasri, S.; West, D.C.; Farquhar, M.; Slaninová, J.; Ostenson, C.-G.; Zorko, M.; Ostlund, P.; Kumar, S.; Langel, U.; et al. Bioportide: An emergent concept of bioactive cell-penetrating peptides. *Cell Mol. Life Sci.* **2012**, *69*, 2951–2966. [CrossRef] [PubMed]
159. Park, C.B.; Yi, K.-S.; Matsuzaki, K.; Kim, M.S.; Kim, S.C. Structure-activity analysis of buforin II, a histone H2A-derived antimicrobial peptide: The proline hinge is responsible for the cell-penetrating ability of buforin II. *Proc. Natl. Acad. Sci. USA* **2000**, *97*, 8245–8250. [CrossRef]
160. Lim, K.J.; Sung, B.H.; Shin, J.R.; Lee, Y.W.; Kim, D.J.; Yang, S.Y.; Kim, S.C. A Cancer Specific Cell-Penetrating Peptide, BR2, for the Efficient Delivery of an scFv into Cancer Cells. *PLoS ONE* **2013**, *8*, e66084. [CrossRef]
161. Zeng, P.; Cheng, Q.; Xu, J.; Xu, Q.; Xu, Y.; Gao, W.; Wong, K.Y.; Chan, K.F.; Chen, S.; Yi, L. Membrane-disruptive engineered peptide amphiphiles restrain the proliferation of penicillins and cephalosporins resistant *Vibrio alginolyticus* and *Vibrio parahaemolyticus* in instant jellyfish. *Food Control* **2022**, *135*, 108827. [CrossRef]
162. Shang, D.; Yu, F.; Li, J.; Zheng, J.; Zhang, L.; Li, Y. Molecular Cloning of cDNAs Encoding Antimicrobial Peptide Precursors from the Skin of the Chinese Brown Frog, *Rana chensinensis*. *Zoolog. Sci.* **2009**, *26*, 220–226. [CrossRef]
163. Sinthuvanich, C.; Veiga, A.S.; Gupta, K.; Diana Gaspar, D.; Blumenthal, R.; Schneider, J.P. Anticancer β-hairpin peptides: Membrane-induced folding triggers activity. *J. Am. Chem. Soc.* **2012**, *134*, 6210–6217. [CrossRef]
164. Hao, X.; Yan, Q.; Zhao, J.; Wang, W.; Huang, Y.; Chen, Y. TAT Modification of Alpha-Helical Anticancer Peptides to Improve Specificity and Efficacy. *PLoS ONE* **2015**, *10*, e0138911. [CrossRef]
165. Hakata, Y.; Tsuchiya, S.; Michiue, H.; Ohtsuki, T.; Matsui, H.; Miyazawa, M.; Kitamatsu, M. A novel leucine zipper motif-based hybrid peptide delivers a functional peptide cargo inside cells. *Chem. Commun.* **2015**, *51*, 413–416. [CrossRef] [PubMed]

166. Oehlke, J.; Scheller, A.; Wiesner, B.; Krause, E.; Beyermann, M.; Klauschenz, E.; Melzig, M.; Bienert, M. Cellular uptake of an alpha-helical amphipathic model peptide with the potential to deliver polar compounds into the cell interior non-endocytically. *Biochim. Biophys. Acta* **1998**, *1414*, 127–139. [CrossRef]
167. Gautam, A.; Chaudhary, K.; Kumar, R.; Raghava, G.P. Computer-Aided Virtual Screening and Designing of Cell-Penetrating Peptides. *Methods Mol. Biol.* **2015**, *1324*, 59–69. [CrossRef] [PubMed]
168. Wei, Y.; Li, C.; Zhang, L.; Xu, X. Design of novel cell penetrating peptides for the delivery of trehalose into mammalian cells. *Biochim. Biophys. Acta* **2014**, *1838*, 1911–1920. [CrossRef]
169. Radvanyi, L.G. Targeting the cancer mutanome of breast cancer. *Nat. Med.* **2018**, *24*, 703–704. [CrossRef] [PubMed]
170. Gautam, A.; Kapoor, P.; Chaudhary, K.; Kumar, R.; Open Source Drug Discovery Consortium; Raghava, G.P.S. Tumor homing peptides as molecular probes for cancer therapeutics, diagnostics and theranostics. *Curr. Med. Chem.* **2014**, *21*, 2367–2391. [CrossRef] [PubMed]
171. Deslouches, B.; Di, Y.P. Antimicrobial peptides with selective antitumor mechanisms: Prospect for anticancer applications. *Oncotarget* **2017**, *8*, 46635–46651. [CrossRef] [PubMed]
172. Liu, S.; Yang, H.; Wan, L.; Cheng, J.; Lu, X. Penetratin-mediated delivery enhances the antitumor activity of the cationic antimicrobial peptide Magainin II. *Cancer Biother. Radiopharm.* **2013**, *28*, 289–297. [CrossRef] [PubMed]
173. Mai, J.C.; Mi, Z.; Kim, S.H.; Ng, B.; Robbins, P.D. A proapoptotic peptide for the treatment of solid tumors. *Cancer Res.* **2001**, *61*, 7709–7712. [PubMed]
174. Risso, A.; Braidot, E.; Sordano, M.C.; Vianello, A.; Macrì, F.; Skerlavaj, B.; Zanetti, M.; Gennaro, R.; Bernardi, P. BMAP-28, an antibiotic peptide of innate immunity, induces cell death through opening of the mitochondrial permeability transition pore. *Mol. Cell Biol.* **2002**, *22*, 1926–1935. [CrossRef]
175. Hsu, J.C.; Lin, L.C.; Tzen, J.T.C.; Chen, J.Y. Characteristics of the antitumor activities in tumor cells and modulation of the inflammatory response in RAW264.7 cells of a novel antimicrobial peptide, chrysophsin-1, from the red sea bream (*Chrysophrys major*). *Peptides* **2011**, *32*, 900–910. [CrossRef] [PubMed]
176. Pfeiffer, D.R.; Gudz, T.I.; Novgorodov, S.A.; Erdahl, W.L. The peptide mastoparan is a potent facilitator of the mitochondrial permeability transition. *J. Biol. Chem.* **1995**, *270*, 4923–4932. [CrossRef]
177. Cole, A.M.; Weis, P.; Diamond, G. Isolation and characterization of pleurocidin, an antimicrobial peptide in the skin secretions of winter flounder. *J. Biol. Chem.* **1997**, *272*, 12008–12013. [CrossRef]
178. Seo, Y.W.; Woo, H.N.; Piya, S.; Moon, A.R.; Oh, J.W.; Yun, C.W.; Kim, K.K.; Min, J.Y.; Jeong, S.Y.; Chung, S.; et al. The Cell Death–Inducing Activity of the Peptide Containing Noxa Mitochondrial-Targeting Domain Is Associated with Calcium Release. *Cancer Res.* **2009**, *69*, 8356–8365. [CrossRef] [PubMed]
179. Liu, R.; Liu, Z.; Peng, H.; Lv, Y.; Feng, Y.; Kang, J.; Lu, N.; Ma, R.; Hou, S.; Sun, W.; et al. Bomidin: An Optimized Antimicrobial Peptide With Broad Antiviral Activity Against Enveloped Viruses. *Front. Immunol.* **2022**, *13*, 851642. [CrossRef] [PubMed]
180. Diener, C.; Martínez, G.G.R.; Blas, D.M.; Castillo, G.D.A.; Corzo, G.; Castro-Obregon, S.; Del Rio, G.D. Effective Design of Multifunctional Peptides by Combining Compatible Functions. *PLoS Comput. Biol.* **2016**, *12*, e1004786. [CrossRef]
181. Zasloff, M. Magainins, a class of antimicrobial peptides from Xenopus skin: Isolation, characterization of two active forms, and partial cDNA sequence of a precursor. *Proc. Natl. Acad. Sci. USA* **1987**, *84*, 5449–5453. [CrossRef] [PubMed]
182. Azuma, E.; Choda, N.; Odaki, M.; Yano, Y.; Matsuzaki, K. Improvement of Therapeutic Index by the Combination of Enhanced Peptide Cationicity and Proline Introduction. *ACS Infect. Dis.* **2020**, *6*, 2271–2278. [CrossRef]
183. Dathe, M.; Wieprecht, T.; Nikolenko, H.; Handel, L.; Maloy, W.L.; MacDonald, D.L.; Beyermann, M.; Bienert, M. Hydrophobicity, hydrophobic moment and angle subtended by charged residues modulate antibacterial and haemolytic activity of amphipathic helical peptides. *FEBS Lett.* **1997**, *403*, 208–212. [CrossRef]
184. Matsuzaki, K.; Sugishita, K.; Harada, M.; Fujii, N.; Miyajima, K. Interactions of an antimicrobial peptide, magainin 2, with outer and inner membranes of Gram-negative bacteria. *Biochim. Biophys. Acta* **1997**, *1327*, 119–130. [CrossRef]
185. Shin, S.Y.; Lee, S.H.; Yand, S.T.; Park, E.J.; Lee, D.G.; Lee, M.K.; Eom, S.H.; Song, W.K.; Kim, Y.; Hahm, K.-S.; et al. Antibacterial, antitumor and hemolytic activities of α-helical antibiotic peptide, P18 and its analogs. *J. Pept. Res.* **2001**, *58*, 504–514. [CrossRef] [PubMed]
186. Braunstein, A.; Papo, N.; Shai, Y. In vitro activity and potency of an intravenously injected antimicrobial peptide and its DL amino acid analog in mice infected with bacteria. *Antimicrob. Agents Chemother.* **2004**, *48*, 3127–3129. [CrossRef]
187. Otvos, L., Jr.; Bokonyi, K.; Varga, I.; Otvos, B.I.; Hoffmann, H.; Ertl, H.C.; Wade, J.D.; McManus, A.M.; Craik, D.J.; Bulet, B. Insect peptides with improved protease-resistance protect mice against bacterial infection. *Protein Sci.* **2000**, *9*, 742–749. [CrossRef] [PubMed]
188. Wei, Y.; Zhang, M.; Jiao, P.; Zhang, X.; Yang, G.; Xu, X. Intracellular Paclitaxel Delivery Facilitated by a Dual-Functional CPP with a Hydrophobic Hairpin Tail. *ACS Appl. Mater. Interfaces* **2021**, *13*, 4853–4860. [CrossRef]
189. Hilpert, K.; Volkmer-Engert, R.; Walter, T.; Hancock, R.E. High-throughput generation of small antibacterial peptides with improved activity. *Nat. Biotechnol.* **2005**, *23*, 1008–1012. [CrossRef] [PubMed]
190. Cerrato, C.P.; Künnapuu, K.; Langel, Ü. Cell-penetrating peptides with intracellular organelle targeting. *Expert Opin. Drug Deliv.* **2017**, *14*, 245–255. [CrossRef]
191. Hu, G.; Katuwawala, A.; Wang, K.; Wu, Z.; Ghadermarzi, S.; Gao, J.; Kurgan, L. flDPnn: Accurate intrinsic disorder prediction with putative propensities of disorder functions. *Nat. Commun.* **2021**, *12*, 4438. [CrossRef]

192. Tucker, A.N.; Carlson, T.J.; Sarkar, A. Challenges in Drug Discovery for Intracellular Bacteria. *Pathogens* **2021**, *10*, 1172. [CrossRef] [PubMed]
193. Rüter, R. Delivery of Antibiotics by Cell-Penetrating Peptides to Kill Intracellular Pathogens. *Methods Mol. Biol.* **2022**, *2383*, 335–345. [CrossRef] [PubMed]
194. Kamei, N.; Nielsen, E.J.B.; Khafagy, E.-S.; Takeda-Morishita, M. Noninvasive insulin delivery: The great potential of cell-penetrating peptides. *Ther. Deliv.* **2013**, *4*, 315–326. [CrossRef]
195. Liu, Y.; Jia, Y.; Yang, K.; Wang, Z. Heterogeneous Strategies to Eliminate Intracellular Bacterial Pathogens. *Front. Microbiol.* **2020**, *11*, 563. [CrossRef] [PubMed]
196. El-Sayed, M.A.E.G.; Zhong, L.L.; Shen, C.; Yang, Y.; Doi, Y.; Tian, G.B. Colistin and its role in the era of antibiotic resistance: An extended review (2000–2019). *Emerg. Microbes Infect.* **2020**, *9*, 868–885. [CrossRef] [PubMed]
197. Főldes, A.; Székely, E.; Voidăzan, S.T.; Dobreanu, M. Comparison of Six Phenotypic Assays with Reference Methods for Assessing Colistin Resistance in Clinical Isolates of Carbapenemase-Producing Enterobacterales: Challenges and Opportunities. *Antibiotics* **2022**, *11*, 377. [CrossRef] [PubMed]
198. Upert, G.; Luther, A.; Obrecht, D.; Ermert, P. Emerging peptide antibiotics with therapeutic potential. *Med. Drug Discov.* **2021**, *9*, 100078. [CrossRef]
199. Röhrig, C.; Huemer, M.; Lorgé, D.; Luterbacher, S.; Phothaworn, P.; Schefer, C.; Sobieraj, A.M.; Zinsli, L.V.; Mairpady Shambat, S.; Leimer, N.; et al. Targeting hidden pathogens: Cell-penetrating enzybiotics eradicate intracellular drug-resistant *Staphylococcus aureus*. *mBio* **2020**, *11*, e00209-20. [CrossRef]
200. Hu, J.; Chen, C.; Zhang, S.; Zhao, X.; Xu, H.; Zhao, X.; Lu, J.R. Designed antimicrobial and antitumor peptides with high selectivity. *Biomacromolecules* **2011**, *12*, 3839–3843. [CrossRef]
201. Boohaker, R.J.; Lee, M.W.; Vishnubhotla, P.; Perez, J.M.; Khaled, A.R. The use of therapeutic peptides to target and to kill cancer cells. *Curr. Med. Chem.* **2012**, *19*, 3794–3804. [CrossRef]
202. Harris, F.; Dennison, S.R.; Singh, J.; Phoenix, D.A. On the selectivity and efficacy of defense peptides with respect to cancer cells. *Med. Res. Rev.* **2013**, *33*, 190–234. [CrossRef]
203. Freire, J.M.; Gaspar, D.; Veiga, A.S.; Castanho, M.A.R.B. Shifting gear in antimicrobial and anticancer peptides biophysical studies: From vesicles to cells. *J. Pept. Sci.* **2015**, *21*, 178–185. [CrossRef]
204. Melvin, J.A.; Montelaro, R.C.; Bomberger, J.M. Clinical potential of engineered cationic antimicrobial peptides against drug resistant biofilms. *Expert Rev. Anti Infect. Ther.* **2016**, *14*, 989–991. [CrossRef]
205. Hilchie, A.L.; Sharon, A.J.; Haney, E.F.; Hoskin, D.W.; Bally, M.B.; Franco, O.L.; Corcoran, J.A.; Hancock, R.E.W. Mastoparan is a membranolytic anti-cancer peptide that works synergistically with gemcitabine in a mouse model of mammary carcinoma. *Biochim. Biophys. Acta* **2016**, *1858*, 3195–3204. [CrossRef] [PubMed]
206. Fox, J.L. Antimicrobial peptides stage a comeback. *Nat. Biotechnol.* **2013**, *31*, 379–382. [CrossRef] [PubMed]
207. Aranda, M.; Li, Y.; Liew, Y.J.; Baumgarten, S.; Simakov, O.; Wilson, M.C.; Piel, J.; Ashoor, H.; Bougouffa, S.; Bajic, V.B.; et al. Genomes of coral dinoflagellate symbionts highlight evolutionary adaptations conducive to a symbiotic lifestyle. *Sci. Rep.* **2016**, *6*, 39734. [CrossRef] [PubMed]
208. Wender, P.A.; Jessop, T.C.; Pattabiraman, K.; Pelkey, E.T.; VanDeusen, C.L. An efficient, scalable synthesis of the molecular transporter octaarginine via a segment doubling strategy. *Org. Lett.* **2001**, *3*, 3229–3232. [CrossRef]
209. Doytchinova, I.A.; Flower, D.R. VaxiJen: A server for prediction of protective antigens, tumour antigens and subunit vaccines. *BMC Bioinform.* **2007**, *8*, 4. [CrossRef]
210. Song, J.; Tan, H.; Perry, A.J.; Akutsu, T.; Webb, G.I.; Whisstock, J.C.; Pike, R.N. PROSPER: An integrated feature-based tool for predicting protease substrate cleavage sites. *PLoS ONE* **2012**, *7*, e50300. [CrossRef]
211. Futaki, S.; Nakase, I. Cell-Surface Interactions on Arginine-Rich Cell-Penetrating Peptides Allow for Multiplex Modes of Internalization. *Acc. Chem. Res.* **2017**, *50*, 2449–2456. [CrossRef]
212. Benz, C.; Urbaniak, M.D. Organising the cell cycle in the absence of transcriptional control: Dynamic phosphorylation co-ordinates the *Trypanosoma brucei* cell cycle posttranscriptionally. *PLoS Pathog.* **2019**, *15*, e1008129. [CrossRef]
213. Kaushik, J.K.; Bhat, R. Why is trehalose an exceptional protein stabilizer? An analysis of the thermal stability of proteins in the presence of the compatible osmolyte trehalose. *J. Biol. Chem.* **2003**, *278*, 26458–26465. [CrossRef]
214. Comizzoli, P.; Loi, P.; Patrizio, P.; Hubel, A. Long-term storage of gametes and gonadal tissues at room temperatures: The end of the ice age? *J. Assist. Reprod. Genet.* **2022**, *39*, 321–325. [CrossRef]
215. Bhattacharya, C.; Wang, X.; Becker, D. The DEAD/DEAH box helicase, DDX11, is essential for the survival of advanced melanomas. *Mol. Cancer* **2012**, *11*, 82. [CrossRef] [PubMed]
216. Li, J.; Liu, L.; Liu, X.; Xu, P.; Hu, Q.; Yu, Y. The Role of Upregulated *DDX11* as A Potential Prognostic and Diagnostic Biomarker in Lung Adenocarcinoma. *J. Cancer* **2019**, *10*, 4208–4216. [CrossRef] [PubMed]
217. Park, J.S.; Lee, M.E.; Jang, W.S.; Rha, K.H.; Lee, S.H.; Lee, J.; Ham, W.S. The DEAD/DEAH Box Helicase, DDX11, Is Essential for the Survival of Advanced Clear Cell Renal Cell Carcinoma and Is a Determinant of PARP Inhibitor Sensitivity. *Cancers* **2021**, *13*, 2574. [CrossRef]
218. Brosh, R.M., Jr.; Matson, S.W. History of DNA Helicases. *Genes* **2020**, *11*, 255. [CrossRef] [PubMed]

219. Hatakeyama, S.; Sugihara, K.; Shibata, T.K.; Nakayama, J.; Akama, T.O.; Tamura, N.; Wong, S.-M.; Bobkov, A.A.; Takano, Y.; Ohyama, C.; et al. Targeted drug delivery to tumor vasculature by a carbohydrate mimetic peptide. *Proc. Natl. Acad. Sci. USA* **2011**, *108*, 19587–19592. [CrossRef] [PubMed]
220. Wei, Y.; Zhang, L.; Fu, Y.; Xu, X. Rapid delivery of paclitaxel with an organic solvent-free system based on a novel cell penetrating peptide for suppression of tumor growth. *J. Mater. Chem. B* **2017**, *5*, 7768–7774. [CrossRef]
221. Wei, Y.; Ma, L.; Zhang, L.; Xu, X. Noncovalent interaction-assisted drug delivery system with highly efficient uptake and release of paclitaxel for anticancer therapy. *Int. J. Nanomed.* **2017**, *12*, 7039–7051. [CrossRef]
222. Bobone, S.; Bocchinfuso, G.; Park, Y.; Palleschi, A.; Hahm, K.S.; Stella, L. The importance of being kinked: Role of Pro residues in the selectivity of the helical antimicrobial peptide P5. *J. Pept. Sci.* **2013**, *19*, 758–769. [CrossRef]
223. Takayama, K.; Nakase, I.; Michiue, H.; Takeuchi, T.; Tomizawa, K.; Matsui, H.; Futaki, S. Enhanced intracellular delivery using arginine-rich peptides by the addition of penetration accelerating sequences (Pas). *J. Control. Release* **2009**, *138*, 128–133. [CrossRef]
224. Armstrong, J.S. Mitochondria: A target for cancer therapy. *Br. J. Pharmacol.* **2006**, *147*, 239–248. [CrossRef]
225. Chiara, F.; Castellaro, D.; Marin, O.; Petronilli, V.; Brusilow, W.S.; Juhaszova, M.; Sollott, S.J.; Forte, M.; Bernardi, P.; Rasola, A. Hexokinase II detachment from mitochondria triggers apoptosis through the permeability transition pore independent of voltage-dependent anion channels. *PLoS ONE* **2008**, *3*, e1852. [CrossRef]
226. Bernardi, P.; Rasola, A.; Forte, M.; Lippe, G. The mitochondrial permeability transition pore: Channel formation by F-ATP synthase, integration in signal transduction, and role in pathophysiology. *Physiol. Rev.* **2015**, *95*, 1111–1155. [CrossRef] [PubMed]
227. Juretić, D. *Bioenergetics: A Bridge Across Life and Universe*; CRC Press: Boca Raton, FL, USA, 2022. [CrossRef]
228. Nederlof, R.; Gürel-Gurevin, E.; Eerbeek, O.; Xie, C.; Deijs, G.S.; Konkel, M.; Hu, J.; Weber, N.C.; Schumacher, C.A.; Baartscheer, A.; et al. Reducing mitochondrial bound hexokinase II mediates transition from non-injurious into injurious ischemia/reperfusion of the intact heart. *J. Physiol. Biochem.* **2017**, *73*, 323–333. [CrossRef] [PubMed]
229. Kulkarni, M.M.; McMaster, W.R.; Kamysz, E.; Kamysz, W.; Engman, D.M.; McGwire, B.S. The major surface-metalloprotease of the parasitic protozoan, *Leishmania*, protects against antimicrobial peptide-induced apoptotic killing. *Mol. Microbiol.* **2006**, *62*, 1484–1497. [CrossRef]
230. Seo, Y.W.; Shin, J.N.; Ko, K.H.; Cha, J.H.; Park, J.Y.; Lee, B.R.; Yun, C.W.; Kim, Y.M.; Seol, D.W.; Kim, D.W.; et al. The molecular mechanism of Noxa-induced mitochondrial dysfunction in p53-mediated cell death. *J. Biol. Chem.* **2003**, *278*, 48292–48299. [CrossRef] [PubMed]
231. Arap, W.; Pasqualini, R.; Ruoslahti, E. Cancer treatment by targeted drug delivery to tumor vasculature in a mouse model. *Science* **1998**, *279*, 377–380. [CrossRef] [PubMed]
232. de Azevedo, R.A.; Figueiredo, C.R.; Ferreira, A.K.; Matsuo, A.L.; Massaoka, M.H.; Girola, N.; Auada, A.V.V.; Farias, C.F.; Pasqualoto, K.F.M.; Rodrigues, C.P.; et al. Mastoparan induces apoptosis in B16F10-Nex2 melanoma cells via the intrinsic mitochondrial pathway and displays antitumor activity in vivo. *Peptides* **2015**, *68*, 113–119. [CrossRef]
233. Mi, Z.; Mai, J.; Lu, X.; Robbins, P.D. Characterization of a class of cationic peptides able to facilitate efficient protein transduction in vitro and in vivo. *Mol. Ther.* **2000**, *2*, 339–347. [CrossRef]
234. Javadpour, M.M.; Juban, M.M.; Lo, W.C.; Bishop, S.M.; Alberty, J.B.; Cowell, S.M.; Becker, C.L.; McLaughlin, M.L. De novo antimicrobial peptides with low mammalian cell toxicity. *J. Med. Chem.* **1996**, *39*, 3107–3113. [CrossRef]
235. Liu, S.; Yang, H.; Wan, L.; Cai, H.W.; Li, S.L.; Li, Y.P.; Cheng, J.Q.; Lu, X.F. Enhancement of cytotoxicity of antimicrobial peptide magainin II in tumor cells by bombesin-targeted delivery. *Acta Pharmacol. Sin.* **2011**, *32*, 79–88. [CrossRef]
236. Ohsaki, Y.; Gazdar, A.F.; Chen, H.C.; Johnson, B.E. Antitumor activity of magainin analogues against human lung cancer cell lines. *Cancer Res.* **1992**, *52*, 3534–3538. [PubMed]
237. Baker, M.A.; Maloy, W.L.; Zasloff, M.; Jacob, L.S. Anticancer efficacy of Magainin2 and analogue peptides. *Cancer Res.* **1993**, *53*, 3052–3057. [PubMed]
238. Cruz-Chamorro, L.; Puertollano, M.A.; Puertollano, E.; de Cienfuegos, G.A.; de Pablo, M.A. In vitro biological activities of magainin alone or in combination with nisin. *Peptides* **2006**, *27*, 1201–1209. [CrossRef]
239. Ramos, R.; Moreira, S.; Rodrigues, A.; Gama, M.; Domingues, L. Recombinant expression and purification of the antimicrobial peptide magainin-2. *Biotechnol. Prog.* **2013**, *29*, 17–22. [CrossRef]
240. Lee, D.G.; Park, Y.; Jin, I.; Hahm, K.S.; Lee, H.H.; Moon, Y.H.; Woo, E.R. Structure-antiviral activity relationships of cecropin A-magainin 2 hybrid peptide and its analogues. *J. Pept. Sci.* **2004**, *10*, 298–303. [CrossRef]
241. Jacob, L.; Zasloff, M. Potential therapeutic applications of magainins and other antimicrobial agents of animal origin. *Ciba Found. Symp.* **1994**, *186*, 197–223. [CrossRef] [PubMed]
242. Fernández de Ullivarri, M.; Arbulu, S.; Garcia-Gutierrez, E.; Cotter, P.D. Antifungal Peptides as Therapeutic Agents. *Front. Cell. Infect. Microbiol.* **2020**, *10*, 105. [CrossRef]
243. Pineda-Castañeda, H.M.; Huertas-Ortiz, K.A.; Leal-Castro, A.L.; Vargas-Casanova, Y.; Parra-Giraldo, C.M.; García-Castañeda, J.E.; Rivera-Monroy, Z.J. Designing Chimeric Peptides: A Powerful Tool for Enhancing Antibacterial Activity. *Chem. Biodivers.* **2021**, *18*, e2000885. [CrossRef]
244. Théolier, J.; Fliss, I.; Jean, J.; Hammami, R. MilkAMP: A comprehensive database of antimicrobial peptides of dairy origin. *Dairy Sci. Technol.* **2014**, *94*, 181–193. [CrossRef]
245. Kobayashi, S.; Chikushi, A.; Tougu, S.; Imura, Y.; Nishida, M.; Yano, Y.; Matsuzaki, K. Membrane Translocation Mechanism of the Antimicrobial Peptide Buforin 2. *Biochemistry* **2004**, *43*, 15610–15616. [CrossRef]

246. Cho, J.H.; Sung, B.H.; Kim, S.C. Buforins: Histone H2A-derived antimicrobial peptides from toad stomach. *Biochim. Biophys. Acta* **2009**, *1788*, 1564–1569. [CrossRef] [PubMed]
247. Jang, S.A.; Kim, H.; Lee, J.Y.; Shin, J.R.; Kim, D.J.; Cho, J.H.; Kim, S.C. Mechanism of action and specificity of antimicrobial peptides designed based on buforin IIb. *Peptides* **2012**, *34*, 283–289. [CrossRef]
248. Schibli, D.J.; Hwang, P.M.; Vogel, H.J. The structure of the antimicrobial active center of lactoferricin B bound to sodium dodecyl sulfate micelles. *FEBS Lett.* **1999**, *446*, 213–217. [CrossRef]
249. Strøm, M.B.; Rekdal, Ø.; Svendsen, J.S. The effects of charge and lipophilicity on the antibacterial activity of undecapeptides derived from bovine lactoferricin. *J. Peptide Sci.* **2002**, *7*, 36–43. [CrossRef] [PubMed]
250. Strøm, M.B.; Haug, B.E.; Rekdal, Ø.; Skar, M.L.; Stensen, W.; Svendsen, J.S. Important structural features of 15-residue lactoferricin derivatives and methods for improvement of antimicrobial activity. *Biochem. Cell Biol.* **2002**, *80*, 65–74. [CrossRef] [PubMed]
251. Gifford, J.L.; Hunter, H.N.; Vogel, H.J. Lactoferricin: A lactoferrin-derived peptide with antimicrobial, antiviral, antitumor and immunological properties. *Cell Mol. Life Sci.* **2005**, *62*, 2588–2598. [CrossRef]
252. Wender, P.A.; Galliher, W.C.; Goun, E.A.; Jones, L.R.; Pillow, T.H. The design of guanidinium-rich transporters and their internalization mechanisms. *Adv. Drug Deliv. Rev.* **2008**, *60*, 452–472. [CrossRef]
253. Fischer, P.M.; Zhelev, N.Z.; Wang, S.; Melville, J.E.; Fåhraeus, R.; Lane, D.P. Structure-activity relationship of truncated and substituted analogues of the intracellular delivery vector Penetratin. *J. Peptide Res.* **2000**, *55*, 163–172. [CrossRef]
254. Fischer, P.M.; Krausz, E.; Lane, D.P. Cellular delivery of impermeable effector molecules in the form of conjugates with peptides capable of mediating membrane translocation. *Bioconjug. Chem.* **2001**, *12*, 825–841. [CrossRef]
255. Ohno, S. Of palindromes and peptides. *Hum. Genet.* **1992**, *90*, 342–345. [CrossRef]
256. O'Neil, K.T.; Hoess, R.H.; DeGrado, W. F Design of DNA-binding peptides based on the leucine zipper motif. *Science* **1990**, *249*, 774–778. [CrossRef] [PubMed]
257. Keller, W.; König, P.; Richmond, T.J. Crystal Structure of a bZIP/DNA Complex at 2.2 Å: Determinants of DNA Specific Recognition. *J. Mol. Biol.* **1995**, *254*, 657–667. [CrossRef] [PubMed]
258. Suckow, M.; Lopata, M.; Seydel, A.; Kisters-Woike, B.; von Wilcken-Bergmann, B.; Muller-Hill, B. Mutant bZip-DNA complexes with four quasi-identical protein-DNA interfaces. *EMBO J.* **1996**, *15*, 598–606. [CrossRef]
259. Ohlig, S.; Pickhinke, U.; Sirko, S.; Bandari, S.; Hoffmann, D.; Dreier, R.; Farshi, P.; Götz, M.; Grobe, K. An emerging role of Sonic hedgehog shedding as a modulator of heparan sulfate interactions. *J. Biol. Chem.* **2012**, *287*, 43708–43719. [CrossRef]
260. Wallbrecher, R.; Verdurmen, W.P.R.; Schmidt, S.; Bovee-Geurts, P.H.; Broecker, F.; Reinhardt, A.; van Kuppevelt, T.H.; Seeberger, P.H.; Brock, R. The stoichiometry of peptide-heparan sulfate binding as a determinant of uptake efficiency of cell-penetrating peptides. *Cell. Mol. Life Sci.* **2014**, *71*, 2717–2729. [CrossRef]
261. Åmand, H.L.; Rydberg, H.A.; Fornander, L.H.; Lincoln, P.; Nordén, B.; Esbjörner, E.K. Cell surface binding and uptake of arginine- and lysine-rich penetratin peptides in absence and presence of proteoglycans. *Biochim. Biophys. Acta* **2012**, *1818*, 2669–2678. [CrossRef]
262. Ramsey, J.D.; Flynn, N.H. Cell-penetrating peptides transport therapeutics into cells. *Pharmacol. Ther.* **2015**, *154*, 78–86. [CrossRef]
263. Alves, I.D.; Bechara, C.; Walrant, A.; Zaltsman, Y.; Jiao, C.-Y.; Sagan, S. Relationships between Membrane Binding, Affinity and Cell Internalization Efficacy of a Cell-Penetrating Peptide: Penetratin as a Case Study. *PLoS ONE* **2011**, *6*, e24096. [CrossRef]
264. Natarajan, K.; Meyer, M.R.; Jackson, B.M.; Slade, D.; Roberts, C.; Hinnebusch, A.G.; Marton, M.J. Transcriptional profiling shows that Gcn4p is a master regulator of gene expression during amino acid starvation in yeast. *Mol. Cell Biol.* **2001**, *21*, 4347–4368. [CrossRef] [PubMed]
265. Svensson, S.L.; Pasupuleti, M.; Walse, B.; Malmsten, M.; Mörgelin, M.; Sjögren, C.; Olin, A.I.; Collin, M.; Schmidtchen, A.; Palmer, R.; et al. Midkine and pleiotrophin have bactericidal properties: Preserved antibacterial activity in a family of heparin-binding growth factors during evolution. *J. Biol. Chem.* **2010**, *285*, 16105–16115. [CrossRef]
266. Farshi, P.; Ohlig, S.; Pickhinke, U.; Höing, S.; Jochmann, K.; Lawrence, R.; Dreier, R.; Dierker, T.; Grobe, K. Dual Roles of the Cardin-Weintraub Motif in Multimeric Sonic Hedgehog. *J. Biol. Chem.* **2011**, *286*, 23608–23619. [CrossRef] [PubMed]
267. Farsinejad, S.; Gheisary, Z.; Samani, S.E.; Alizadeh, A.M. Mitochondrial targeted peptides for cancer therapy. *Tumor Biol.* **2015**, *36*, 5715–5725. [CrossRef] [PubMed]
268. Habault, J.; Poyet, J.-L. Recent Advances in Cell Penetrating Peptide-Based Anticancer Therapies. *Molecules* **2019**, *24*, 927. [CrossRef]
269. Eckert, R.; He, J.; Yarbrough, D.K.; Qi, F.; Anderson, M.H.; Shi, W. Targeted killing of *Streptococcus mutans* by a pheromone-guided "smart" antimicrobial peptide. *Antimicrob. Agents Chemother.* **2006**, *50*, 3651–3657. [CrossRef]
270. Guo, L.; McLean, J.S.; Yang, Y.; Eckert, R.; Kaplan, C.W.; Kyme, P.; Sheikh, O.; Varnum, B.; Lux, R.; Shi, W.; et al. Precision-guided antimicrobial peptide as a targeted modulator of human microbial ecology. *Proc. Natl. Acad. Sci. USA* **2015**, *112*, 7569–7574. [CrossRef] [PubMed]
271. Steinstraesser, L.; Tack, B.F.; Waring, A.J.; Hong, T.; Boo, L.M.; Fan, M.F.; Remick, D.I.; Su, G.L.; Lehrer, R.I.; Wang, S.C. Activity of novispirin G10 against *Pseudomonas aeruginosa* in vitro and in infected burns. Antimicrob. *Agents Chemother.* **2002**, *46*, 1837–1844. [CrossRef] [PubMed]
272. Shanker, E.; Morrison, D.A.; Talagas, A.; Nessler, S.; Federle, M.J.; Prehna, G. Pheromone Recognition and Selectivity by ComR Proteins among *Streptococcus* Species. *PloS Pathog.* **2016**, *12*, e1005979. [CrossRef]
273. Chang, J.C.; Federle, M.J. PptAB Exports Rgg Quorum-Sensing Peptides in *Streptococcus*. *PLoS ONE* **2016**, *11*, e0168461. [CrossRef]

274. Hidalgo-Grass, C.; Dan-Goor, M.; Maly, A.; Eran, Y.; Kwinn, L.A.; Nizet, V.; Ravins, M.; Jaffe, J.; Peyser, A.; Moses, A.E.; et al. Effect of a bacterial pheromone peptide on host chemokine degradation in group A streptococcal necrotising soft-tissue infections. *Lancet* **2004**, *363*, 696–703. [CrossRef]
275. Gautier, R.; Douguet, D.; Antonny, B.; Drin, G. HELIQUEST: A web server to screen sequences with specific α-helical properties. *Bioinformatics* **2008**, *24*, 2101–2102. [CrossRef]
276. Papo, N.; Braunstein, A.; Eshhar, Z.; Shai, Y. Suppression of Human Prostate Tumor Growth in Mice by a Cytolytic D-, L-Amino Acid Peptide: Membrane Lysis, Increased Necrosis, and Inhibition of Prostate Specific Antigen Secretion. *Cancer Res.* **2004**, *64*, 5779–5786. [CrossRef] [PubMed]
277. Matsuzaki, K. Control of cell selectivity of antimicrobial peptides. *Biochim. Biophys. Acta* **2009**, *1788*, 1687–1692. [CrossRef] [PubMed]
278. Jiang, Z.; Vasil, A.I.; Vasil, M.L.; Hodges, R.S. "Specificity determinants" improve therapeutic indices of two antimicrobial peptides piscidin 1 and dermaseptin S4 against the Gram-negative pathogens *Acinetobacter baumannii* and *Pseudomonas aeruginosa*. *Pharmaceuticals* **2014**, *7*, 366–391. [CrossRef] [PubMed]
279. Wani, N.A.; Stolovicki, E.; Hur, D.B.; Shai, Y. Site-Specific Isopeptide Bond Formation: A Powerful Tool for the Generation of Potent and Nontoxic Antimicrobial Peptides. *J. Med. Chem.* **2022**, *65*, 5085–5094. [CrossRef]
280. Kragol, G.; Hoffmann, R.; Chattergoon, M.A.; Lovas, S.; Cudic, M.; Bulet, P.; Condie, B.A.; Rosengren, K.J.; Montaner, L.J.; Otvos, L., Jr. Identification of crucial residues for the antibacterial activity of the proline-rich peptide, pyrrhocoricin. *Eur. J. Biochem.* **2002**, *269*, 4226–4437. [CrossRef] [PubMed]
281. Loveland, A.B.; Svidritskiy, E.; Susorov, D.; Lee, S.; Park, A.; Zvornicanin, S.; Demo, G.; Gao, F.B.; Korostelev, A.A. Ribosome inhibition by C9ORF72-ALS/FTD-associated poly-PR and poly-GR proteins revealed by cryo-EM. *Nat. Commun.* **2022**, *13*, 2776. [CrossRef] [PubMed]
282. Brakel, A.; Krizsan, A.; Itzenga, R.; Kraus, C.N.; Otvos, L., Jr.; Hoffmann, R. Influence of Substitutions in the Binding Motif of Proline-Rich Antimicrobial Peptide ARV-1502 on 70S Ribosome Binding and Antimicrobial Activity. *Int. J. Mol. Sci.* **2022**, *23*, 3150. [CrossRef]
283. Novković, M.; Simunić, J.; Bojović, V.; Tossi, A.; Juretić, D. DADP: The Database of Anuran Defense Peptides. *Bioinformatics* **2012**, *28*, 1406–1407. [CrossRef]
284. Wang, G.; Li, X.; Wang, Z. APD3, the antimicrobial peptide database as a tool for research and education. *Nucleic Acids Res.* **2016**, *44*, D1087–D1093. [CrossRef]
285. Tyagi, A.; Tuknait, A.; Anand, P.; Gupta, S.; Sharma, M.; Mathur, D.; Joshi, A.; Singh, S.; Gautam, A.; Raghava, G.P. CancerPPD: A database of anticancer peptides and proteins. *Nucleic Acids Res.* **2015**, *43*, D837–D843. [CrossRef]
286. Tornesello, A.L.; Borrelli, A.; Buonaguro, L.; Buonaguro, F.M.; Tornesello, M.L. Antimicrobial Peptides as Anticancer Agents: Functional Properties and Biological Activities. *Molecules* **2020**, *25*, 2850. [CrossRef] [PubMed]
287. Nijnik, A.; Hancock, R.E.W. The roles of cathelicidin LL-37 in immune defences and novel clinical applications. *Curr. Opin. Hematol.* **2009**, *16*, 41–47. [CrossRef] [PubMed]
288. Rajasekaran, G.; Kim, E.Y.; Shin, S.Y. LL-37-derived membrane-active FK-13 analogs possessing cell selectivity, anti-biofilm activity and synergy with chloramphenicol and anti-inflammatory activity. *Biochim. Biophys. Acta Biomembr.* **2017**, *1859*, 722–733. [CrossRef] [PubMed]
289. Wu, W.K.K.; Wang, G.; Coffelt, S.B.; Betancourt, A.M.; Lee, C.W.; Fan, D.; Wu, K.; Yu, J.; Sung, J.J.Y.; Cho, C.H. Emerging Roles of the Host Defense Peptide LL-37 in Human Cancer and its Potential Therapeutic Applications. *Int. J. Cancer* **2010**, *127*, 1741–1747. [CrossRef]
290. Wang, G.; Mishra, B.; Epand, R.F.; Epand, R.M. High-quality 3D structures shine light on antibacterial, anti-biofilm and antiviral activities of human cathelicidin LL-37 and its fragments. *Biochim. Biophys. Acta* **2014**, *1838*, 2160–2172. [CrossRef]
291. Wang, G.; Hanke, M.L.; Mishra, B.; Lushnikova, T.; Heim, C.E.; Thomas, V.C.; Bayles, K.W.; Kielian, T. Transformation of human cathelicidin LL-37 into selective, stable, and potent antimicrobial compounds. *ACS Chem. Biol.* **2014**, *9*, 1997–2002. [CrossRef]
292. Juretić, D.; Simunić, J. Design of α-helical antimicrobial peptides with a high selectivity index. *Expert Opin. Drug Discov.* **2019**, *14*, 1053–1063. [CrossRef]
293. Kim, E.Y.; Rajasekaran, G.; Shin, S.Y. LL-37-derived short antimicrobial peptide KR-12-a5 and its d-amino acid substituted analogs with cell selectivity, anti-biofilm activity, synergistic effect with conventional antibiotics, and anti-inflammatory activity. *Eur. J. Med. Chem.* **2017**, *136*, 428–441. [CrossRef]
294. Souza, B.M.; Mendes, M.A.; Santos, L.D.; Marques, M.R.; César, L.M.; Almeida, R.N.; Pagnocca, F.C.; Konno, K.; Palma, M.S. Structural and functional characterization of two novel peptide toxins isolated from the venom of the social wasp Polybia paulista. *Peptides* **2005**, *26*, 2157–2164. [CrossRef]
295. Kerkis, I.; de Brandão Prieto da Silva, A.R.; Pompeia, C.; Tytgat, J.; de Sá Junior, P.L. Toxin bioportides: Exploring toxin biological activity and multifunctionality. *Cell Mol. Life Sci.* **2017**, *74*, 647–661. [CrossRef]
296. Kyte, J.A. Cancer vaccination with telomerase peptide GV1001. *Expert Opin. Investig. Drugs.* **2009**, *18*, 687–694. [CrossRef] [PubMed]
297. Wang, K.R.; Zhang, B.Z.; Zhang, W.; Yan, J.X.; Li, J.; Wang, R. Antitumor effects, cell selectivity and structure-activity relationship of a novel antimicrobial peptide polybia-MP1. *Peptides* **2008**, *29*, 963–968. [CrossRef] [PubMed]

298. Bitler, B.G.; Schroeder, J.A. Anti-Cancer Therapies that Utilize Cell Penetrating Peptides. *Recent Pat. Anticancer Drug Discov.* **2010**, *5*, 99–108. [CrossRef] [PubMed]
299. Riedl, S.; Zweytick, D.; Lohner, K. Membrane-active host defense peptides—Challenges and perspectives for the development of novel anticancer drugs. *Chem. Phys. Lipids* **2011**, *164*, 766–781. [CrossRef]
300. Chen, C.; Chen, Y.; Yang, C.; Zeng, P.; Xu, H.; Pan, F.; Lu, J.R. High Selective Performance of Designed Antibacterial and Anticancer Peptide Amphiphiles. *ACS Appl. Mater. Interfaces* **2015**, *7*, 17346–17355. [CrossRef]
301. Vernen, F.; Craik, D.J.; Lawrence, N.; Henriques, S.T. Cyclic Analogues of Horseshoe Crab Peptide Tachyplesin I with Anticancer and Cell Penetrating Properties. *ACS Chem. Biol.* **2019**, *14*, 2895–2908. [CrossRef]
302. Simmaco, M.; Mignogna, G.; Canofeni, S.; Miele, R.; Mangoni, M.L.; Barra, D. Temporins, antimicrobial peptides from the European red frog *Rana temporaria*. *Eur. J. Biochem.* **1996**, *242*, 788–792. [CrossRef]
303. Simmaco, M.; De Biase, D.; Severini, C.; Aita, M.; Erspamer, G.F.; Barra, D.; Bossa, F. Purification and characterization of bioactive peptides from skin extracts of *Rana esculenta*. *Biochim. Biophys. Acta* **1990**, *1033*, 318–323. [CrossRef]
304. Mangoni, M.L. Temporins, anti-infective peptides with expanding properties. *Cell. Mol. Life Sci.* **2006**, *63*, 1060–1069. [CrossRef]
305. Romero, S.M.; Cardillo, A.B.; Ceron, M.C.M.; Camperi, S.A.; Giudicessi, S.L. Temporins: An Approach of Potential Pharmaceutic Candidates. *Surg. Infect.* **2020**, *21*, 309–322. [CrossRef]
306. Rinaldi, A.C.; Mangoni, M.L.; Rufo, A.; Luzi, C.; Barra, D.; Zhao, H.; Kinnunen, P.K.J.; Bozzi, A.; Di Giulio, A.; Simmaco, M. Temporin L: Antimicrobial, haemolytic and cytotoxic activities, and effects on membrane permeabilization in lipid vesicles. *Biochem. J.* **2002**, *368 Pt 1*, 91–100. [CrossRef] [PubMed]
307. Mangoni, M.L.; Shai, Y. Temporins and their synergism against Gram-negative bacteria and in lipopolysaccharide detoxification. *Biochim. Biophys. Acta* **2009**, *1788*, 1610–1619. [CrossRef] [PubMed]
308. Oger, P.-C.; Piesse, C.; Ladram, A.; Humblot, V. Engineering of Antimicrobial Surfaces by Using Temporin Analogs to Tune the Biocidal/antiadhesive Effect. *Molecules* **2019**, *24*, 814. [CrossRef] [PubMed]
309. Marcocci, M.E.; Amatore, D.; Villa, S.; Casciaro, B.; Aimola, P.; Franci, G.; Grieco, P.; Galdiero, M.; Palamara, A.T.; Mangoni, M.L.; et al. The amphibian antimicrobial peptide temporin B inhibits in vitro herpes simplex virus 1 infection. *Antimicrob. Agents Chemother.* **2018**, *62*, e02367-17. [CrossRef]
310. Roy, M.; Lebeau, L.; Chessa, C.; Damour, A.; Ladram, A.; Oury, B.; Boutolleau, D.; Bodet, C.; Lévêque, N. Comparison of Anti-Viral Activity of Frog Skin Anti-Microbial Peptides Temporin-Sha and [K3]SHa to LL-37 and Temporin-Tb against Herpes Simplex Virus Type 1. *Viruses* **2019**, *11*, 77. [CrossRef]
311. Shang, D.; Liang, H.; Wei, S.; Yan, X.; Yang, Q.; Sun, Y. Effects of antimicrobial peptide L-K6, a temporin-1CEb analog on oral pathogen growth, Streptococcus mutans biofilm formation, and anti-inflammatory activity. *Appl. Microbiol. Biotechnol.* **2014**, *98*, 8685–8695. [CrossRef]
312. Russ, W.P.; Engelman, D.M. The GxxxG Motif: A Framework for Transmembrane Helix-Helix Association. *J. Mol. Biol.* **2000**, *296*, 911–919. [CrossRef]
313. Zanetti, M. The role of cathelicidins in the innate host defenses of mammals. *Curr. Issues Mol. Biol.* **2005**, *7*, 179–196. [CrossRef]
314. Wang, G.; Watson, K.M.; Buckheit, R.W., Jr. Anti-Human Immunodeficiency Virus Type 1 Activities of Antimicrobial Peptides Derived from Human and Bovine Cathelicidins. *Antimicrob. Agents Chemother.* **2008**, *52*, 3438–3440. [CrossRef]
315. Haines, L.R.; Thomas, J.M.; Jackson, A.M.; Eyford, B.A.; Razavi, M.; Watson, C.N.; Gowen, B.; Hancock, R.E.W.; Pearson, T.W. Killing of Trypanosomatid Parasites by a Modified Bovine Host Defense Peptide, BMAP-18. *PLoS Negl. Trop. Dis.* **2009**, *3*, e373. [CrossRef]
316. Eckert, R.; Qi, F.; Yarbrough, D.K.; He, J.; Anderson, M.H.; Shi, W. Adding selectivity to antimicrobial peptides: Rational design of a multidomain peptide against *Pseudomonas* spp. *Antimicrob. Agents Chemother.* **2006**, *50*, 1480–1488. [CrossRef] [PubMed]
317. Sullivan, R.; Santarpia, P.; Lavender, S.; Gittins, E.; Liu, Z.; Anderson, M.H.; He, J.; Shi, W.; Eckert, R. Clinical Efficacy of a Specifically Targeted Antimicrobial Peptide Mouth Rinse: Targeted Elimination of *Streptococcus mutans* and Prevention of Demineralization. *Caries Res.* **2011**, *45*, 415–428. [CrossRef] [PubMed]
318. Shah, P.; Hsiao, F.S.; Ho, Y.H.; Chen, C.S. The proteome targets of intracellular targeting antimicrobial peptides. *Proteomics* **2016**, *16*, 1225–1237. [CrossRef] [PubMed]
319. Le, C.F.; Fang, C.M.; Sekaran, S.D. Intracellular targeting mechanisms by antimicrobial peptides. *Antimicrob. Agents Chemother.* **2017**, *61*, e02340-16. [CrossRef]
320. Shah, P.; Chen, C.S. Systematic Screening of Penetratin's Protein Targets by Yeast Proteome Microarrays. *Int. J. Mol. Sci.* **2022**, *23*, 712. [CrossRef] [PubMed]
321. Shah, P.; Chen, C.S. Systematic Identification of Protein Targets of Sub5 Using *Saccharomyces cerevisiae* Proteome Microarrays. *Int. J. Mol. Sci.* **2021**, *22*, 760. [CrossRef]
322. Cerrato, C.P.; Langel, Ü. An update on cell-penetrating peptides with intracellular organelle targeting. *Expert Opin. Drug Deliv.* **2022**, *19*, 133–146. [CrossRef]

antibiotics

Article

Behind the Curtain: In Silico and In Vitro Experiments Brought to Light New Insights into the Anticryptococcal Action of Synthetic Peptides

Tawanny K. B. Aguiar [1], Nilton A. S. Neto [1], Romério R. S. Silva [1], Cleverson D. T. Freitas [1], Felipe P. Mesquita [2], Luciana M. R. Alencar [3], Ralph Santos-Oliveira [4,5], Gustavo H. Goldman [6] and Pedro F. N. Souza [1,2,*]

1 Department of Biochemistry and Molecular Biology, Federal University of Ceará, Fortaleza 60451-970, CE, Brazil
2 Drug Research and Development Center, Department of Physiology and Pharmacology, Federal University of Ceará, Fortaleza 60430-275, CE, Brazil
3 Department of Physics, Laboratory of Biophysics and Nanosystems, Federal University of Maranhão, São Luís 65080-805, MA, Brazil
4 Laboratory of Nanoradiopharmaceuticals and Radiopharmacy, Zona Oeste State University, Rio de Janeiro 23070-200, RJ, Brazil
5 Brazilian Nuclear Energy Commission, Nuclear Engineering Institute, Rio de Janeiro 21941-906, RJ, Brazil
6 Faculty of Pharmaceutical Sciences of Ribeirão Preto, University of São Paulo, São Paulo 14040-903, SP, Brazil
* Correspondence: pedrofilhobio@gmail.com or pedrofilhobio@ufc.br

Citation: Aguiar, T.K.B.; Neto, N.A.S.; Silva, R.R.S.; Freitas, C.D.T.; Mesquita, F.P.; Alencar, L.M.R.; Santos-Oliveira, R.; Goldman, G.H.; Souza, P.F.N. Behind the Curtain: In Silico and In Vitro Experiments Brought to Light New Insights into the Anticryptococcal Action of Synthetic Peptides. *Antibiotics* **2023**, *12*, 153. https://doi.org/10.3390/antibiotics12010153

Academic Editors: Agostinho Antunes, Guillermin Agüero-Chapin and Yovani Marrero-Ponce

Received: 16 December 2022
Revised: 8 January 2023
Accepted: 10 January 2023
Published: 11 January 2023

Copyright: © 2023 by the authors. Licensee MDPI, Basel, Switzerland. This article is an open access article distributed under the terms and conditions of the Creative Commons Attribution (CC BY) license (https://creativecommons.org/licenses/by/4.0/).

Abstract: *Cryptococcus neoformans* is the pathogen responsible for cryptococcal pneumonia and meningitis, mainly affecting patients with suppressed immune systems. We have previously revealed the mechanism of anticryptococcal action of synthetic antimicrobial peptides (SAMPs). In this study, computational and experimental analyses provide new insights into the mechanisms of action of SAMPs. Computational analysis revealed that peptides interacted with the PHO36 membrane receptor of *C. neoformans*. Additionally, ROS (reactive oxygen species) overproduction, the enzymes of ROS metabolism, interference in the ergosterol biosynthesis pathway, and decoupling of cytochrome c mitochondrial membrane were evaluated. Three of four peptides were able to interact with the PHO36 receptor, altering its function and leading to ROS overproduction. SAMPs-treated *C. neoformans* cells showed a decrease in scavenger enzyme activity, supporting ROS accumulation. In the presence of ascorbic acid, an antioxidant agent, SAMPs did not induce ROS accumulation in *C. neoformans* cells. Interestingly, two SAMPs maintained inhibitory activity and membrane pore formation in *C. neoformans* cells by a ROS-independent mechanism. Yet, the ergosterol biosynthesis and lactate dehydrogenase activity were affected by SAMPs. In addition, we noticed decoupling of Cyt *c* from the mitochondria, which led to apoptosis events in the cryptococcal cells. The results presented herein suggest multiple mechanisms imposed by SAMPs against *C. neoformans* interfering in the development of resistance, thus revealing the potential of SAMPs in treating infections caused by *C. neoformans*.

Keywords: redox system; *Cryptococcus neoformans*; ROS metabolism; ergosterol; synthetic antimicrobial peptides

1. Introduction

Currently, treatments against bacterial and fungal infections are limited due to the development of resistance to drugs by pathogens [1]. *C. neoformans* is a good example of a multidrug-resistant pathogen that causes dangerous infections worldwide [2]. Cryptococcosis and cryptococcal meningitis caused by *C. neoformans* mainly affect people with compromised immune systems. It is estimated 278,000 infections occur yearly in HIV-positive patients worldwide, leading to 181,000 deaths annually [3].

The high level of resistance presented by *C. neoformans* narrows down the number of drugs that can be used in treatments. For example, *C. neoformans* presents intrinsic resistance to caspofungin, which inhibits the enzyme (1→3)-β-D-glucan synthase and, nevertheless, perturbs the turnover of the fungal cell wall [1,3,4]. Therefore, combined treatment of amphotericin B (AmB) and flucytosine (FC) are commonly used to treat cryptococcosis infections [4]. However, prolonged exposure results in the emergence of cryptococcal populations resistant to this treatment, as well as to the toxicity of those drugs [5].

To cope with this problem imposed by *C. neoformans*, SAMPs have emerged as promising alternative molecules due to their mechanism of action, which is generally associated with membrane pore formation. This mechanism makes it difficult for microorganisms to acquire resistance, low toxicity, and allergenicity [6–8]. Recently, our research group reported the anti-cryptococcal potential of SAMPs PepGAT, PepKAA, *Rc*Alb-PepII, and *Rc*Alb-PepIII [7]. Studies on mechanisms of action revealed that SAMPs prompted membrane pore formation and apoptosis induced by DNA degradation in *C. neoformans* cells [7].

In this study, an in silico and in vitro approach provided new insight into the mechanism of action of SAMPs (PepGAT, PepKAA, *Rc*Alb-PepII, and *Rc*Alb-PepIII) against *C. neoformans*. In silico analysis revealed that three SAMPs bind to the PHO36 receptor of *C. neoformans,* inducing conformational alteration. In vitro analysis showed a high accumulation of ROSs in *C. neoformans* treated with SAMPs. In further experiments, it was determined that peptides cause a disbalance in redox enzymes and lactate dehydrogenase activity in *C. neoformans* cells. Additionally, SAMPs induced the decoupling of cytochrome *c* from the mitochondrion and inhibited ergosterol biosynthesis. Together, these findings strengthen the need for employment of these SAMPs against *C. neoformans* infections.

2. Results

2.1. ROS Accumulation in C. neoformans *Cells*

Recently, we showed that the SAMPs PepGAT, PepKAA, *Rc*Alb-PepII, and *Rc*Alb-PepIII presented an MIC_{50} against *C. neoformans* cells of 0.04, 0.04, 25, and 0.04 $\mu g\ mL^{-1}$, respectively [7]. In the same study, some mechanisms of action were evaluated. In this study, new information about the mechanism of action is presented. All of the experiments were performed at MIC_{50} for all peptides.

The first step analyzed whether the SAMPs were able to induce the accumulation of different types of ROS. The first analysis was conducted to evaluate the accumulation of anion superoxide ($O2^{\bullet-}$) (Figure 1). The experiment was designed using nitro blue tetrazolium (NBT), which is converted into formazan with a blue or cyan color in the presence of $O2^{\bullet-}$. As expected, the control cells of *C. neoformans* (Figure 1—DMSO panel) presented no blue or cyan dots, indicating no conversion of NBT in formazan and, thus, no accumulation of $O2^{\bullet-}$. In contrast, SAMPs-treated *C. neoformans* cells presented a blue or cyan color, suggesting the conversion of NBT by high levels of $O2^{\bullet-}$ into formazan (Figure 1: panel of peptides; blue or cyan dots—black arrow). Additionally, the quantification of formazan corroborated the data of light microscopy. All treatments presented the statistical significance of the control.

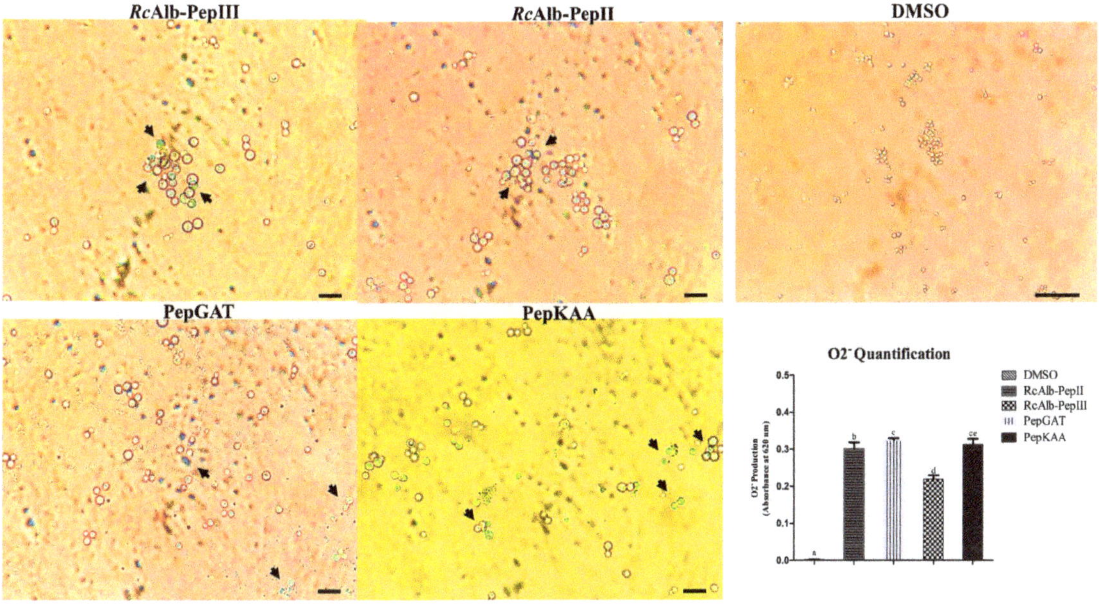

Figure 1. Qualitative and quantitative analysis of anion superoxide accumulation in *C. neoformans*. Light microscopy analysis of the conversion of NBT into formazan (blue or cyan dots–black arrows). The panel of DMSO represents the control cells, and other panels are treated *C. neoformans* cells with synthetic peptides. The inserted graphic represents the quantitative analysis of anion superoxide accumulation in *C. neoformans* cells. In control bar indicates 100 μm. In treated cells bar indicate 50 μm. The different lowercase letters indicate statistical significance at $p > 0.05$.

In further experiments, the accumulation of H_2O_2 was induced by SAMPs in *C. neoformans* cells (Figure 2). The control cells treated with DMSO solution presented no accumulation of H_2O_2 (Figure 2). In contrast, all peptides induced ROS accumulation in *C. neoformans* cells. Based on the brightness fluorescence, RcAlb-PepIII, PepGAT, and PepKAA presented a higher accumulation of ROSs than RcAlb-PepII. Interestingly, in Figure 2, the light field shows that cells treated with PepGAT presented a conformational alteration, leading them to assume an elongated shape. This was not observed in the control cells.

2.2. Synthetic Peptides Alter the Activity of Enzymes in ROS Metabolism

The detection of both $O2^{\bullet-}$ and H_2O_2 in *C. neoformans* cells treated with SAMPs led us to investigate the activity of the enzymes involved in redox metabolism. The first enzyme analyzed was the superoxide dismutase (SOD). As expected, control cells of *C. neoformans* presented the highest SOD activity (4.98 AU mgP^{-1}). In contrast, *C. neoformans* cells treated with RcAlb-PepII and RcAlb-PepIII presented no SOD activity. Cells of *C. neoformans* treated with PepGAT and PepKAA still presented SOD activity, but the activity values were three and four times lower than those of the control cells (Figure 3A).

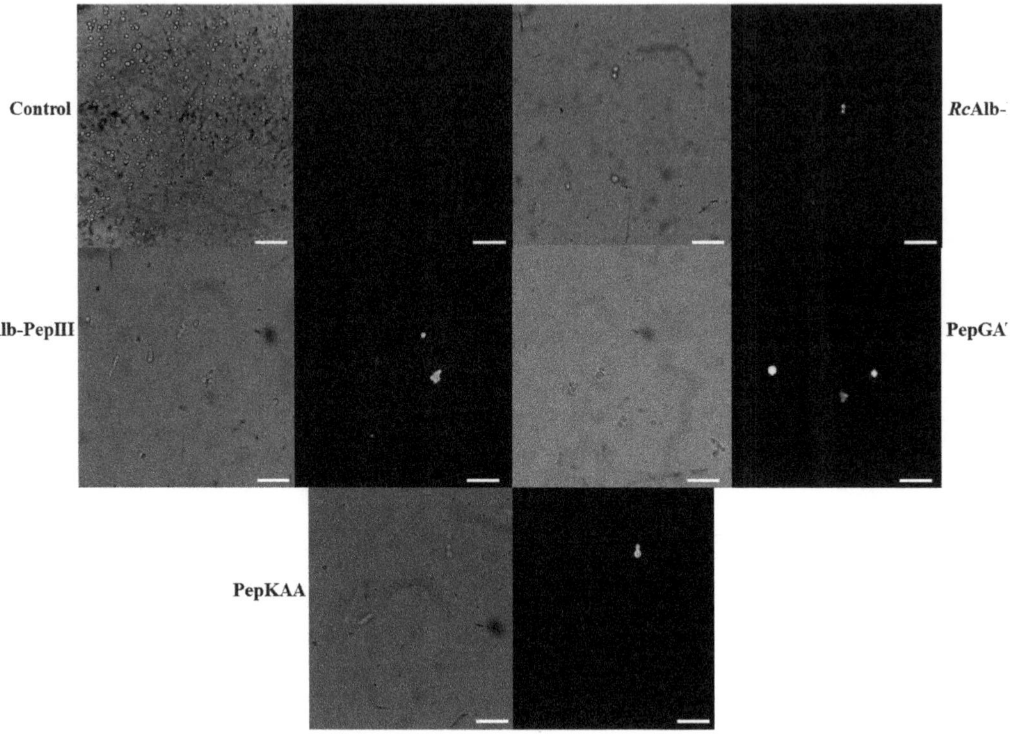

Figure 2. Hydrogen peroxide detection in *C. neoformans* cells. Green fluorescence revealed the overaccumulation of H_2O_2 in *C. neoformans* cells induced by synthetic peptides. Control cells were treated with 5% DMSO in 0.15 M NaCl. Bars indicate 100 μm.

Regarding the catalase activity (CAT), the control cells presented the highest levels of activity compared to the treated cells (Figure 3B). As with SOD, RcAlb-PepIII did not present CAT activity (Figure 3B). In this case, no CAT activity was detected for PepKAA. RcAlb-PepII and PepGAT presented CAT activity levels three and five times lower than those of the control cells (Figure 3B).

For ascorbate peroxidase (APX), only cells treated with PepGAT presented no APX activity (Figure 3C). The cells treated with DMSO (control) presented the highest activity (3.43 AU mgP^{-1}). In the case of the other SAMPs, RcAlb-PepIII, PepKAA, and RcAlb-PepII presented APX activity levels 7.4, 4, and 3.43 times lower, respectively, than *C. neoformans* cells treated with DMSO (Figure 3C).

2.3. *Anticryptococcal Activity of Peptides Is Affected by Ascorbic Acid*

To determine the role of ROSs ($O2^{\bullet -}$ and H_2O_2) in the activity of SAMPs against *C. neoformans*, the activity was observed in the presence of ascorbic acid (AsA, 10 mM) (Figure 4). As reported above, all of the experiments in this study were performed with MIC_{50} concentration. As shown in Figure 4A, in the absence of AsA, the SAMPs still presented MIC_{50} activity (Figure 4A white columns). However, in the presence of AsA, in which all ROSs ($O2^{\bullet -}$ and H_2O_2) were consumed, all SAMPs had affected activity levels. The most affected was RcAlb-PepII, which completely lost its activity (Figure 4A dashed columns). The other peptides still presented some activity, but the activity levels were below 20%. To prove the absence of ROS, a microscopic fluorescence analysis was conducted in the presence of AsA, which revealed that no ROSs were produced.

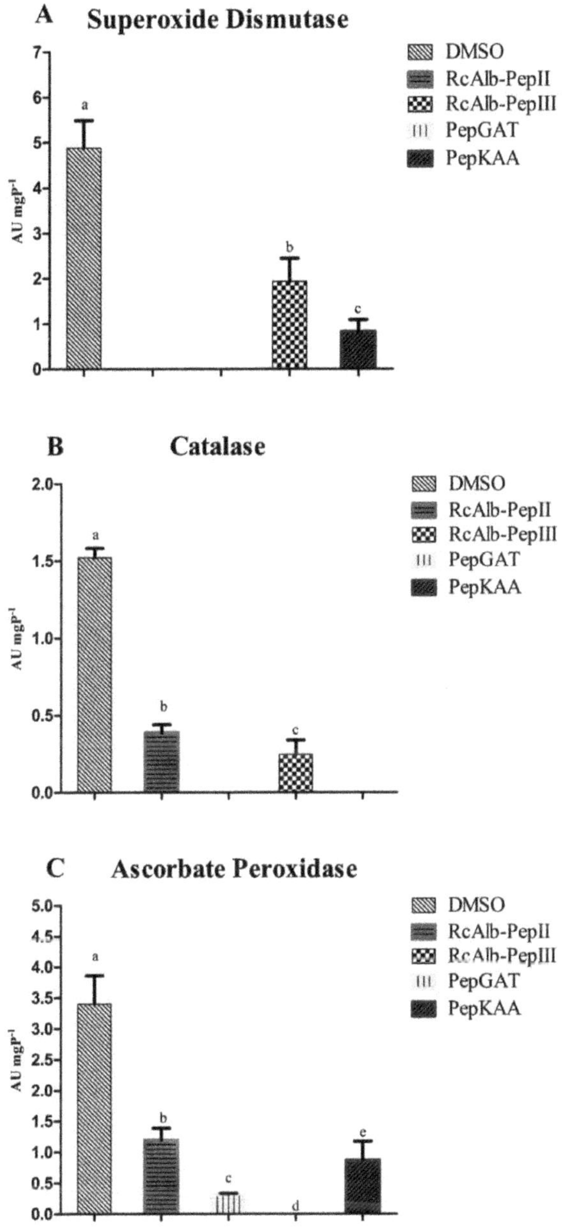

Figure 3. The activity of redox enzymes in *C. neoformans* cells. (**A**) SOD, (**B**) CAT, and (**C**) APX. All activities the enzymes were tested in *C. neoformans* cells treated and non-treated with synthetic peptides. SOD is an that enzyme that convert anion superoxide into hydrogen peroxide that is consumed by CAT and APX. The different lowercase letters indicate statistical significance at $p > 0.05$.

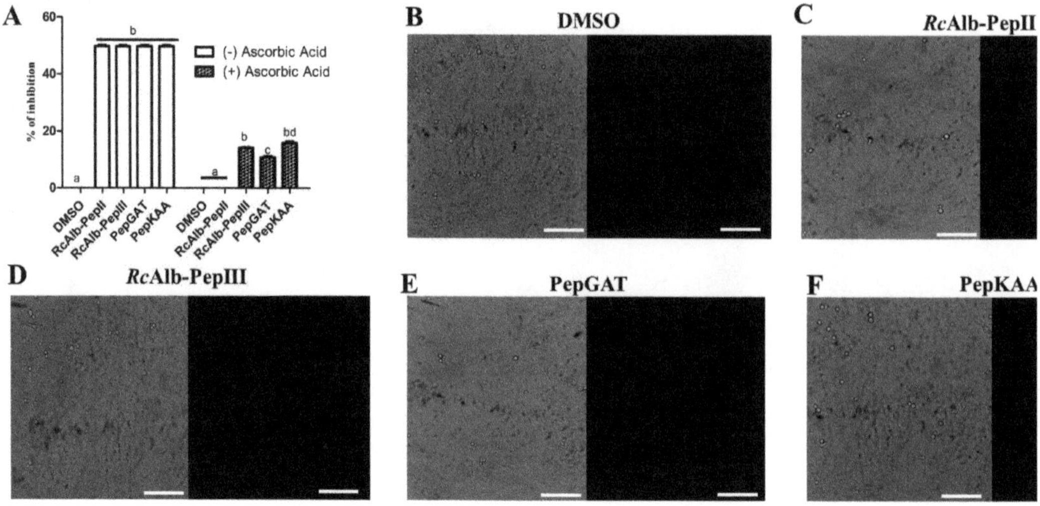

Figure 4. Effect of the antioxidant agent, ascorbic acid, in the activity of synthetic peptides against *C. neoformans*. (**A**) Inhibitory activity of synthetic peptides against *C. neoformans* in the presence of 10 mM of ascorbic acid. (**B–F**) Fluorescence microscopy analysis showed no detection of H_2O_2 in the cells of *C. neoformans* in the presence of 10 mM of ascorbic acid. Bars indicate 100 µm. The different lowercase letters in (**A**) indicates statistical significance at $p > 0.05$.

As Aguiar et al. [7] revealed, all SAMPs can induce pore formation. Herein, we aimed to evaluate whether this pore formation was ROS-dependent. The fluorescence microscopy of the propidium iodide uptake assay with AsA revealed that SAMPs did not induce pore formation. RcAlb-PepII entirely lost its activity in the presence of AsA (Figure 4A), and was unable to induce pore formation in *C. neoformans* cells (Figure 5). Likewise, PepGAT did not induce pore formation in *C. neoformans* cells in the presence of AsA (Figure 5). In contrast, RcAlb-PepIII and PepKAA still maintained some inhibitory activity and induced pore formation in *C. neoformans* cells in the presence of AsA, suggesting that this mechanism is not dependent on ROSs (Figure 5).

2.4. Synthetic Peptides Interfere in Other Metabolic Processes on *C. neoformans* Cells

Here, it was evaluated whether SAMPs could inhibit the biosynthesis of ergosterol in *C. neoformans* cells (Figure 6A). As expected, the control cells did not present any inhibition in ergosterol biosynthesis. In this assay, the control used for inhibition was itraconazole (ITR), inhibiting the biosynthesis of ergosterol at 47%. All tested SAMPs presented values of inhibition higher than those of ITR. RcAlb-PepII, RcAlb-PepIII, PepGAT, and PepKAA inhibited, respectively, 80%, 85%, 75%, and 89% of the biosynthesis of ergosterol in *C. neoformans* cells (Figure 6A).

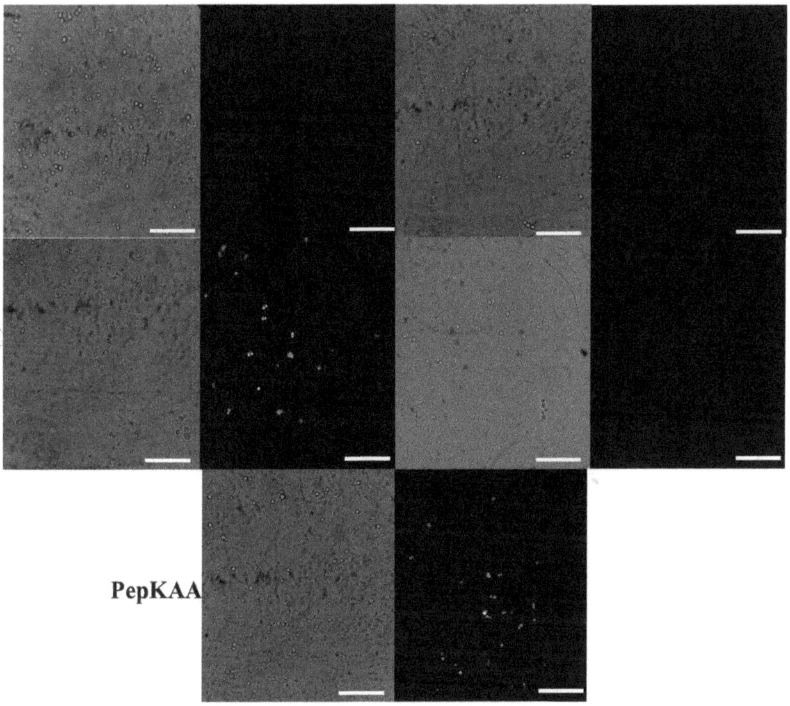

Figure 5. Effect of the antioxidant agent, ascorbic acid, in the membrane pore formation induced by synthetic peptides in *C. neoformans*. Propidium iodide uptake assay to evaluate the ability of synthetic peptides in induce pore formation in *C. neoformans* cells in the presence of 10 mM of ascorbic acid. Bars indicate 100 μm.

The energetic metabolism of *C. neoformans* was investigated after contact with SAMPs (Figure 6B,C). First, the ability of SAMPs to interfere with the activity of lactate dehydrogenase (LHD) in *C. neoformans* cells (Figure 6B) was analyzed. Control cells presented the highest activity of LDH (227.25 UA mgP^{-1}) (Figure 6B). Apart from RcAlb-PepII (24.21 UA mgP^{-1}), which presented LDH activity 10 times lower than the control cells, in the cells treated with RcAlb-PepIII, PepGAT, and PepKAA, no activity of LDH was detected (Figure 6B).

It was also analyzed whether peptides could induce the decoupling of Cyt c from the mitochondrial membranes of *C. neoformans* cells (Figure 6C). As expected, DSMO was unable to release Cyt c from the mitochondrial membranes of *C. neoformans*. In this experiment, the positive control that induced Cyt c from *C. neoformans* was H_2O_2, which presented the highest level of Cyt c decoupling of *C. neoformans* cells (Figure 6C). All SAMPs induced the decoupling of Cyt c from the mitochondrial membrane of *C. neoformans*. However, all of these values were below that of H_2O_2 (Figure 6C). Among SAMPs, the highest value for Cyt decoupling was presented by PepKAA.

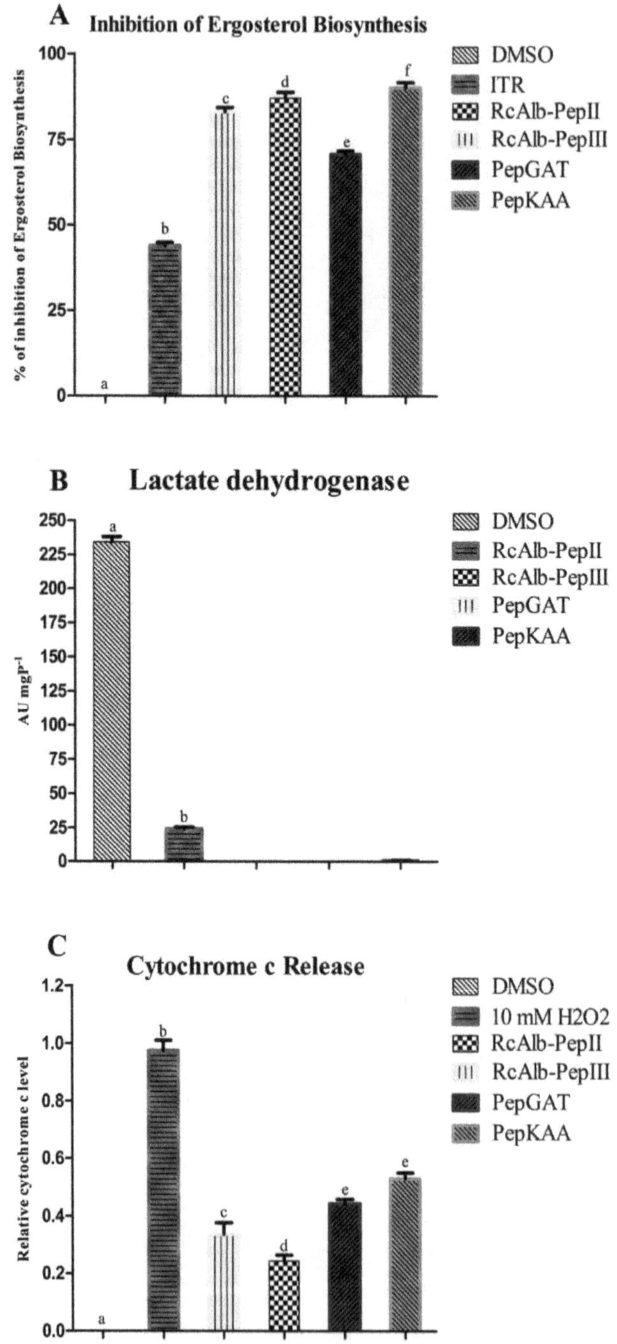

Figure 6. Effect of synthetic peptides in the cellular process of *C. neoformans*. (**A**) inhibition of the biosynthesis of ergosterol, (**B**) lactate dehydrogenase activity, and (**C**) release of Cytochrome c from the mitochondrial membrane. The different lowercase letters indicate statistical significance at $p > 0.05$.

2.5. Computational Simulations

Aiming to produce more information about the mechanisms of action of SAMPs, we performed a docking analysis to try to explain more about the action of peptides. The protein chosen was the membrane receptor PHO36 from *C. neoformans*. First, the sequence of PHO36 from *Saccharomyces cerevisiae* was employed to fish the sequence of PHO36 from *C. neoformans*. After finding the protein sequence, the Swiss model server was employed to construct a three-dimensional (3D) model. Then, ClusPro 2.0 Web Server was used to perform the docking analysis. PHO36 is a transmembrane protein. Based on that, the peptides that did not interact in the transmembrane domain were only considered for docking analysis, as shown in Figure 7 (red dashed lines). Among the tested SAMPs, RcAlb-PepIII was the only peptide that interacted in the transmembrane domain; thus, the result was not considered.

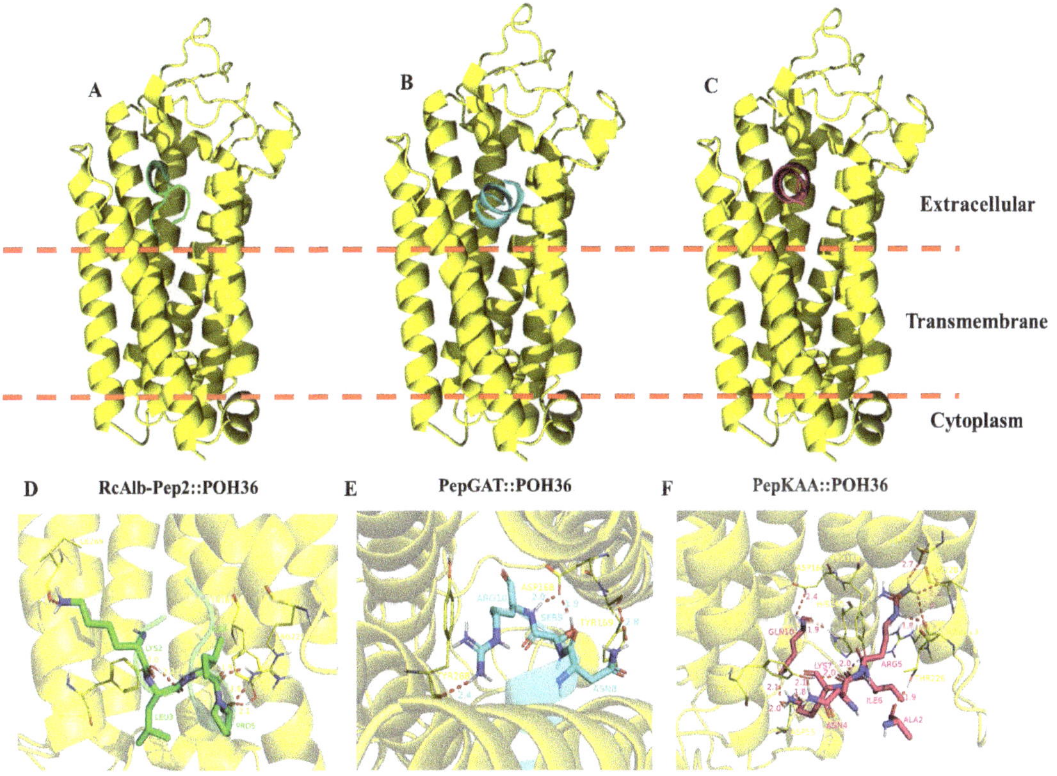

Figure 7. Molecular docking analysis of synthetic peptides and PHO36 receptor from *C. neoformans*. Overview of the interaction of peptides (**A**) RcAlb-PepII, (**B**) PepGAT, and (**C**) PepKAA with PHO36 from C. neoformans. Zoomed view of peptides (**D**) RcAlb-PepII, (**E**) PepGAT, and (**F**) PepKAA with PHO36 from *C. neoformans* showing amino acid residues involved in the interaction and distance.

Contrary to RcAlb-PepIII, all the other peptides interacted with PHO36 in the extracellular domain (Figure 7). The binding energy of peptides with PHO36 was −632.98, −678.98, and 578.12 kCal mol^{-1}, respectively, for RcAlb-PepIII, PepGAT, and PepKAA. An analysis of RMSD (root-mean-square deviation) indicated changes in the atomic position, and then in the 3D structure, of PHO36. The values of RMSD were 1.542, 0.876, and 1.247, respectively, for RcAlb-PepIII, PepGAT, and PepKAA. These values indicate that the interaction of peptides with PHO36 changed its structure and, thus, its functions in cells (Figure 7).

The peptides interacted with the PHO36 receptor from *C. neoformans*, which was supported by hydrogen bonds and salt bridge-type interactions.

3. Discussion

C. neoformans causes severe infections in immune-deficient patients, such as patients with transplanted organs and those in intensive care units [1,2,4]. As *C. neoformans* is resistant to several drugs used in its treatment, it becomes essential to search for bioactive molecules as an alternative to conventional treatment [9,10]. This study was developed based on this emergence to find new molecules in order to overcome the resistance of *C. neoformans* to drugs. Herein, we provide new mechanisms behind the activity of four synthetic peptides against *C. neoformans*.

Our SAMPs demonstrated inhibitory activity (MIC50) in a previous study at low concentrations [7]. The mechanisms evaluated at that time were pore formation, DNA damage, apoptosis induction, and damage caused by peptides to the cell wall and pores in the membrane [7]. Based on previously published results regarding DNA damage and apoptosis induction, we began the analysis by evaluating the redox metabolism in *C. neoformans* cells after contact with peptides (Figures 1–3). The induction of ROS overaccumulation in microorganisms by peptides was not a surprise, but it could explain how SAMPs act against *C. neoformans* [11–14].

In pathogenic fungi with controlled production, ROSs have many beneficial effects on pathogens, such as developmental process, increased virulence, biofilm formation, and infection [15]. On the other hand, ROSs are a byproduct of the natural metabolic process in cells. Without a proper scavenger system to balance their levels, ROSs could bring damage to cells by interaction with vital molecules such as DNA, lipids, and protein, leading to death [15].

Usually, H_2O_2 is the main molecule analyzed in experiments of ROS accumulation induced by peptides in cells because it is more stable and easy to evaluate [11–13]. Here, to better picture the redox state in *C. neoformans* cells, we analyzed the accumulation of $\bullet O_2^-$ (Figure 1), which is one of the most unstable ROSs and is rapidly converted into H_2O_2 [15]. Our results revealed a higher accumulation of $\bullet O_2^-$ in *C. neoformans* cells after treatment with peptides (Figure 1). Uncontrolled accumulation of $\bullet O_2^-$ accelerates the oxidative damage to DNA molecules caused by iron. The $\bullet O_2^-$ induces an increase in iron levels by releasing it from proteins and enzyme clusters. The free iron interacts with DNA molecules, oxidizing it and leading to fragmentation [16]. This result is in accordance with our previously published result that *C. neoformans* cells presented fragmented DNA after treatment with the same synthetic peptides [7]. To prevent the damage caused by $\bullet O_2^-$, cells use the SOD enzyme to produce H_2O_2, which is more stable than $\bullet O_2^-$, but still lethal [15]. Our results revealed a high accumulation of H_2O_2 in *C. neoformans* cells after incubation with peptides (Figure 2).

Although H_2O_2 induces damage to DNA molecules, as does $\bullet O_2^-$, it usually has other targets, such as proteins and lipids. In the case of lipids, H_2O_2 causes the oxidation of lipids in the membrane by a process known as lipid peroxidation. This process could lead to membrane destabilization and, consequently, pore formation, increasing membrane permeability [17,18]. In addition, H_2O_2 also interacts with proteins, damaging them and inhibiting their activity [19]. Recently, Branco et al. [19], using a proteomic approach, revealed that *Klebsiella pneumoniae* cells treated with a synthetic peptide presented a high accumulation of H_2O_2, followed by an increase in the accumulation of proteins involved in the recovery of proteins damaged by ROS. This result suggests that the higher levels of H_2O_2 are involved with protein damage, in agreement with our hypothesis.

It is clear that synthetic peptides cause a perturbation in redox homeostasis of $\bullet O_2^-$ and H_2O_2 (Figures 1 and 2). However, more information about how peptides accomplish this is necessary. Based on this, the activity of scavenger enzymes was evaluated in *C. neoformans* cells. The enzymes evaluated were SOD, CAT, and APX (Figure 3). First, it is necessary to understand the role of these enzymes in ROS metabolism. SOD enzymes are involved in the conversion of $\bullet O_2^-$ into H_2O_2; CAT and APX are responsible for converting H_2O_2 into H_2O and O_2 [15]. These enzymes are responsible for the delicate balance of ROS levels that distinguishes the beneficial from the harmful effects of ROSs.

As revealed in Figure 3A, SAMPs-treated *C. neoformans* cells presented reduced SOD activity. This reduced SOD activity is responsible for two problems: (1) the reduced activity of the SOD enzyme is responsible for low levels of conversion of $\bullet O_2^-$ into H_2O_2, leading to accumulation of $\bullet O_2^-$ (Figure 1 blue or cyan dots). (2) Low activity of SOD in *C. neoformans* cells treated with peptides is still associated with H_2O_2, even if it is at a low concentration. However, the activity of CAT and APX (Figure 3B,C), which are involved in scavenging of H_2O_2, is also reduced in cells treated with peptides, leading to the accumulation of H_2O_2 in *C. neoformans* cells (Figure 2 green fluorescence). Therefore, synthetic peptides, by an unknown mechanism, insult the balance between SOD (converts $\bullet O_2^-$ into H_2O_2), CAT, and APX (H_2O_2 in H_2O and O_2), producing a scenario wherein $\bullet O_2^-$ and H_2O_2 (Figures 1 and 2) accumulate at the same in *C. neoformans* cells, thus potentializing the damage caused by ROS. As far as we know, our study is the first to demonstrate ROS accumulation and propose how peptides induce it by negatively modulating the activity of redox enzymes involved in ROS metabolism.

There are few studies with similar results to ours regarding redox enzymes with peptides in yeasts, and even in *C. neoformans*. However, Neto et al. [20] reported that $MoCBP_3$ from *Moringa oleifera* seeds also caused perturbation in the redox enzymes, leading to the accumulation of ROSs. In that case, the authors only measured the accumulation of H_2O_2.

Our data revealed that ROSs are important to the anticryptococcal activity of SAMPs. However, one question arises: Is the antimicrobial action of peptides fully or partially dependent on ROSs? An experiment with the antioxidant AsA provided new clues for the answer to this question. In the presence of 10 mM of AsA, all peptides had affected activity (Figure 4A). The most affected peptide, RcAlb-PepII, completely lost its activity. Similar results were posted by Neto et al. [20] for an anticandidal protein that had its activity reduced by 60% in the presence of AsA. Fluorescence microscopy (Figure 4B–F) proved that there was no ROS accumulation in *C. neoformans* treated with peptides in the presence of AsA.

A common mechanism of action of peptides against pathogens is the induction of pore formation on the membrane, leading to the loss of internal content and, subsequently, death [21,22]. The pore formation process depends on many aspects. It could be driven directly by the binding of peptides with lipids in the membrane or an indirect process driven by ROS species [13,15,18]. In a previous work, Aguiar et al. [7] showed that all synthetic peptides induced pore formation in *C. neoformans*. Here, as shown, the same peptides had activity in the absence of ROS, which was consumed by AsA. Therefore, we attempted to understand whether the ability of peptides to form pores is dependent on ROS accumulation. To do so, peptides were incubated with *C. neoformans* cells and AsA. After incubation, an iodide propidium uptake assay was performed. The result was quite surprising and exciting (Figure 5). The peptides RcAlb-PepII and PepGAT lost the ability to induce pore formation in *C. neoformans* membranes (Figure 5). For RcAlb-PepII, the result corroborates the loss of activity in the AsA (Figure 4A).

The exciting results occurred with RcAlb-PepIII and PepKAA, which, even in AsA preventing ROS accumulation (Figure 4), induced pore formation in *C. neoformans* cells. This result suggests that the induction of pore formation by these peptides is ROS-dependent and might be driven by the direct interaction of peptides with the membrane. RcAlb-PepIII and PepKAA are cationic peptides with a net charge, respectively, of +1 and +3, and they have hydrophobic potential [8,23]. These features are important for pore formation in two ways: (1) positive charge is important to ionic interaction with the negative charge of lipid heads in the membrane, and (2) hydrophobic potential is critical for inserting peptides into the membrane's hydrophobic core [8].

In our previous study [7], we observed that the presence of exogenous ergosterol affected the activity of peptides against *C. neoformans*, suggesting that peptides can bind to sterol in fungal membranes [7]. Therefore, we experimented with verifying whether peptides also inhibited ergosterol biosynthesis. In this experiment, the control was the antifungal drug ITR (Figure 6A). All peptides presented inhibition higher than ITR. ITR is an antifungal drug belonging to the azole class, whose main mechanism is to inhibit the ergosterol synthesis pathway. Our results demonstrate that peptides are more effective in inhibiting biosynthesis than ITR. Recently, the antifungal $MoCBP_2$ protein, purified from *M. oleifera* seeds, could not inhibit the biosynthesis of ergosterol. New targets and different mechanisms in potential new drugs are important due to the resistance to the current antifungal [24].

All of our data suggest that synthetic peptides dysregulate the redox metabolism of *C. neoformans* cells. As we know, ROSs are natural byproducts of cell metabolism [15]. The energetic metabolism is essential to cell response to environmental insults because it provides energy, as NADPH and ATP are used to produce response proteins [25]. Even the regarding the importance of energetic metabolism to cells, studies reporting alterations caused by peptides in energetic metabolism are scarce. Herein, we attempted to understand whether peptides could cause perturbation in the production of energy by *C. neoformans*. First, the activity of the LDH enzyme in C. neoformans cells was analyzed after the treatment with peptides. All peptides dramatically reduced the activity of LDH (Figure 6B).

LDH is involved in the carbohydrate metabolic pathway, and it catalyzes the conversion of pyruvate into lactate, regenerating the NAD^+ from NADH [26]. This reaction is important to regenerate the NAD^+ in order to maintain the glycolytic pathway, and to produce ATP and pyruvate in order to run the Krebs cycle [26]. Another experiment suggested that peptides interfere in the energetic metabolism of *C. neoformans* cells. The analysis of Cyt c decoupling from the mitochondrial membrane induced by peptides indicates that peptides interfere with mitochondria's energy production.

Inducing the decoupling of Cyt c from mitochondrial membrane peptides causes two problems for *C. neoformans* cells. First, Cyt c is a key molecule in the electron transport chain (ETC) to support ATP synthesis [27]. Inducing the decoupling of Cyt c peptides to destabilize the ETC leads to a depletion in the ATP levels of the cell. Second, the release of the mitochondrial membrane by Cyt c acts as a stimulus for cells to begin apoptosis. Thus, peptides may be inducing this event. It is essential to note that all peptides induced apoptosis in *C. neoformans* cells, as revealed by our previously published study [7].

In an attempt to find possible protein targets for peptides to induce these damages in *C. neoformans* cells, computational simulations were employed. The target chosen was a transmembrane protein known as PHO36. PHO36 is a receptor adiponectin-like protein involved in lipid and phosphate metabolism in yeasts [28]. PHO36 works with RAS proteins in the same pathway that is involved in several cellular events essential for the life of yeasts, such as division, apoptosis, longevity, differentiation, nitrogen, and carbon nutrition [28].

Herein, molecular modeling analysis revealed that RcAlb-PepII, PepGAT, and PepKAA interact with PHO36 in the extracellular domain, resulting in conformational alterations to its structure. By interacting with PHO36 and changing its structures, peptides inhibit PHO36 function in cells, negatively affecting several cellular processes in yeasts. Additionally, misfunction is related to a stimulus for apoptosis in yeast cells. Lopes et al. [29] recently reported that a synthetic peptide interacting with PHO36 from *C. albicans* induced ROS accumulation, DNA fragmentation, and apoptosis. Our results revealed that RcAlb-PepII, PepGAT, and PepKAA interact with PHO36 and cause the same damage. These results suggest PHO36 as a new target for antimicrobial activity mediated by synthetic peptides.

4. Materials and Methods

4.1. Fungal Strains, Chemicals, and Synthetic Peptides

C. neoformans (ATCC 32045) was obtained from the Department of Biochemistry and Molecular Biology at the Federal University of Ceará (UFC), Fortaleza, Brazil. The high-grade chemicals were obtained from Sigma Aldrich (São Paulo, SP, Brazil). The SAMPs PepGAT (GATIRAVNSR), PepKAA (KAANRIKYFQ), *Rc*Alb-PepII (AKLIPTIAL), and *Rc*Alb-PepIII (SLRGCC) were synthesized and purchased from the Chempeptide company (Shanghai, China).

4.2. Antifungal Assay

The antifungal assay was performed following the methodology [7,30]. Yeasts were cultivated in YPD (yeast extract peptone dextrose) agar for fifteen days. After that, harvested in a YPD medium. Because the MIC50 found previously was 0.04 μg mL^{-1} [7] for all synthetic peptides, that was the concentration chosen at which to perform all studies of the mechanisms. Thus, 25 μL of YPD with cryptococcal cells (10^6 cells mL^{-1}) and 25 μL of SAMPs at their final concentrations (0.04 μg mL^{-1}) were added and incubated for 24 h at 30 °C before each assay. The activity of SAMPs was also tested in the presence of 10 mM AsA to verify whether the activity of SAMPs was dependent of ROS overproduction [20].

4.3. Detection of ROS Overproduction

To evaluate the peptide-induced ROS generation (H_2O_2), a fluorometric assay with DCFH-DA (2′,7′ dichlorofluorescein diacetate) was performed. Briefly, after the antifungal assay, the samples were washed with NaCl 0.15 M and centrifuged (5000× *g* for 10 min at 4°C). Next, 9 μL of DCFH-DA was added, and cells were incubated for 20 min at 22 ± 2°C in the dark. Then, the samples were washed two times with NaCl 0.15 mM and centrifuged as described. Finally, cryptococcal cells were transferred to slides and observed with a fluorescence microscope (Olympus System BX 41, Tokyo, Japan) with an excitation wavelength of 535 nm and an emission wavelength of 617 nm [31].

Qualitative and quantitative assays for anion superoxide followed the example of Choi et al. [32]. For the qualitative assay, *C. neoformans* cells were treated with SAMPs. Then, they were washed with 0.15 M NaCl to remove the excess media. Afterward, cells were incubated with 0.1 mM of nitroblue tetrazolium (NBT) for 3 h at room temperature (22 ± 2°C) in the dark. Cells were then visualized using a light microscope (Olympus System BX 41, Tokyo, Japan). The quantitative assay was placed in the same way as the qualitative. The difference was that the quantitative assay was performed in 96-well plates, and the conversion of NBT to formazan was quantified at 630 nm in a microplate reader (Epoch, Biotek, Santa Clara, CA, United States).

In addition, the same assay used to detect H_2O_2 was performed in the presence of 10 mM ascorbic acid (AsA) [20]. Moreover, the pore formation in the presence and absence of 10 mM AsA was assessed using the Propidium Iodide (PI) influx assay, following the methodology described in [7].

4.4. Redox System Enzyme Activity

4.4.1. Catalase (CAT)

The CAT activity was assessed according to [33] to evaluate the catalase activity. After the antifungal assay, conducted at the same conditions described previously, cells were washed three times with 0.15 M NaCl, resuspended in 0.05 M sodium acetate buffer pH 5.2, frozen for 24 h, sonicated for 30 min, and centrifuged for 10 min (10,000× *g* at 4 °C), and the supernatant was collected as described by [20]. A total of 200 μL of samples were incubated with 700 μL phosphate buffer with 50 mM potassium, pH 7.0, at 30 °C for 10 min. Subsequently, 100 μL of 112 mM H_2O_2 was added, starting the reaction. The mixture was placed into a quartz cuvette (1 cm^{-1}) and absorbance was assessed. The reduction in absorbance at 240 nm was measured at intervals of 10 s until reaching 1 min. A decrease of 1.0 absorbance unit per minute was assumed to represent 1 unit of catalase activity (AU).

4.4.2. Ascorbate Peroxidase (APX)

Ascorbate peroxidase activity was evaluated following the methodology previously described by Souza et al. [33]. After the antifungal assay, 800 μL tubes contained 50 mM potassium phosphate buffer, pH 6.0, which consisted of 0.5 mM of L-ascorbic acid and 100 µL of 2 mM hydrogen peroxide in 100 µL of either the treated sample or the control. Then, they were incubated at 30 °C for 10 min. The enzymatic activity was measured through ascorbate oxidation, indicating the action of the enzyme, for 1 min at 10 s intervals using the spectrophotometer at a length of wave of 290 nm. Ascorbate peroxidase activity was expressed (UA) by reducing absorbance by 0.01 at 290 nm, indicating the use of ascorbate to remove H_2O_2 by milligram of the protein (UA/mg).

4.4.3. Superoxide Dismutase (SOD)

Superoxide dismutase activity was measured according to Souza et al. [33] in 96-well microplates. In triplicate, 1 M potassium phosphate buffer, pH 7.8 (10 µL), 1 mM 2,2′,2″,2‴- ethylenediaminetetraacetic acid (EDTA) (20 µL), 10 µL of Triton × 0.25%, 20 µL of 130 mM L-Methionine, 100 µL of samples in deionized water in the presence and absence of peptides (MIC50), and 100 mM of riboflavin (20 µL) were homogenized and kept in the dark for 5 min. Then, the reactional mixture was placed in a 96-well microplate, exposed to fluorescent light (32 W), and read at 630 nm in intervals of 1 min until reaching 5 min. All reagents without yeast extract (replaced by ultrapure water) were used as controls. The enzyme activity was measured as the difference between the absorbance recorded for the light reaction and the corresponding dark reaction (estimated per min). This was expressed in activity units (AU). One unit of SOD activity (1 AU) corresponded to the amount of the sample needed to inhibit the photoreduction of NBT by 50%.

4.5. *Ergosterol Biosynthesis Inhibition*

The ergosterol biosynthesis inhibition was evaluated following the method described previously by Neto et al. [20]. Ergosterol content was calculated based on the following equations:

$$\%\ \text{ergosterol} + 24(28)\ [\text{DHE} = (\text{Abs}282/290) \times \text{F}]/\text{pellet weight} \tag{1}$$

$$\%\ 23(28)\ \text{DHE} = [(\text{Abs}230/518) \times \text{F}]/\text{pellet weight} \tag{2}$$

$$\%\ \text{ergosterol} = \%\ \text{ergosterol} + 24(28)\ \text{DHE} - \%\ 24(28)\ \text{DHE} \tag{3}$$

24(28) DHE refers to 24(28) dehydroergosterol, a class of sterol that presents an absorbance reading similar to that of ergosterol at 282 nm. F, in both equations, represents the factor for dilution in ethanol.

4.6. *Lactate Dehydrogenase Activity*

The LDH Liquiform™ kit (Labtest Diagnóstica, BR) was used to evaluate lactate dehydrogenase activity, following the manufacturer's instructions.

4.7. *Cytochrome c Release*

Because cytochrome *c* release is related to apoptotic events in cells, we evaluated the induction of cytochrome *c* release by peptides following the methodology described in Neto et al. [20]. The Cyt c was measured using a microtiter plate reader at 550 nm.

4.8. *Bioinformatics Assays*

4.8.1. Molecular Modeling of PHO36 Receptor from the *C. neoformans* Genome

The C. *neoformans* amino acid sequence for PHO36 was taken using homolog genes from the NCBI database (http://www.ncbi.nlm.nih.gov (accessed on 10 November 2022)) with the BLAST tool, using the sequence of *Saccharomyces cerevisiae*.

The 3D models of the PHO36 from C. *neoformans* were built by comparative modeling using the A chain of the revised crystals of the adiponectin receptors (PDB code: 5LXG and 5LWY) by means of the SWISS-MODEL (https://swissmodel.expasy.org/interactive (accessed on 10 November 2022)) [29]. All the checks and refinements in the models were performed following the protocol established by Lopes et al. [29]. The best 3D model was submitted to the simulation of interaction (receptor and each peptide).

4.8.2. Molecular Docking

Molecular docking studies between the synthetic peptides (ligands) and the plasma membrane receptor of *C. neoformans* were performed using the protein–protein ClusPro 2.0 docking server (https://cluspro.bu.edu/login.php (accessed on 12 November 2022)), and the output files were analyzed using the PyMol program.

4.9. Statistical Analysis

All experiments were performed three times, and the values are expressed as the mean ± standard error. GraphPad Prism 5.01 (GraphPad Software Company, Santa Clara, CA, USA) for Microsoft Windows was used to run the statistical analyses. All data obtained in the assays were compared using ANOVA followed by the Tukey test ($p < 0.05$).

5. Conclusions

The synthetic peptides evaluated in this study displayed anticryptococcal activity by multiple mechanisms of action. Synthetic peptides interfered with the redox enzymes, leading to the accumulation of ROSs, which are involved in cell death. It was also shown that some peptides induced pore formation in a ROS-dependent manner, while others did the same in a ROS-independent manner. All peptides caused perturbation in the energetic metabolism by inhibiting the activity of LDH and decoupling Cyt c from the mitochondrial membrane. Altogether, these results reinforce the potential of these synthetic peptides against *C. neoformans* and describe their activity along with a promise to develop new forms of treatment against *C. neoformans* infections.

Author Contributions: All authors made substantial contributions. The conception and design of the study and acquisition of data, analysis, and interpretation were performed by T.K.B.A., N.A.S.N., R.R.S.S., C.D.T.F., F.P.M., L.M.R.A., R.S.-O., G.H.G. and P.F.N.S. Microscopic analyses were carried out by T.K.B.A., N.A.S.N., and P.F.N.S. Writing and revision of the article were carried out by T.K.B.A. and P.F.N.S. Lastly, P.F.N.S. performed the final approval and submission. All authors have read and agreed to the published version of the manuscript.

Funding: Special thanks to CAPES for providing the postdoctoral grant to Pedro F. N. Souza (grant number 88887.318820/2019-00).

Institutional Review Board Statement: Not applicable.

Informed Consent Statement: Not applicable.

Data Availability Statement: The data supporting this study's findings are available upon request from the corresponding author.

Acknowledgments: We are grateful to the staff of the central analytical facilities of UFC, Brazil.

Conflicts of Interest: The authors report no conflicts of interest.

References

1. Qadri, H.; Shah, A.H.; Mir, M. Novel Strategies to Combat the Emerging Drug Resistance in Human Pathogenic Microbes. *Curr. Drug Targets* **2021**, *22*, 1424–1436. [CrossRef] [PubMed]
2. Nelson, B.N.; Hawkins, A.N.; Wozniak, K.L. Pulmonary Macrophage and Dendritic Cell Responses to *Cryptococcus neoformans*. *Front. Cell. Infect. Microbiol.* **2020**, *10*, 37. [CrossRef] [PubMed]
3. Moreira-Walsh, B.; Ragsdale, A.; Lam, W.; Upadhya, R.; Xu, E.; Lodge, J.K.; Donlin, M.J. Membrane Integrity Contributes to Resistance of *Cryptococcus neoformans* to the Cell Wall Inhibitor Caspofungin. *mSphere* **2022**, *7*, e00134-22. [CrossRef] [PubMed]
4. Mourad, A.; Perfect, J.R. The War on Cryptococcosis: A Review of the Antifungal Arsenal. *Mem. Inst. Oswaldo Cruz* **2018**, *113*. [CrossRef]
5. Laniado-Laborín, R.; Cabrales-Vargas, M.N. Amphotericin B: Side Effects and Toxicity. *Rev. Iberoam. Micol.* **2009**, *26*, 223–227. [CrossRef] [PubMed]

6. Grimaldi, M.; De Rosa, M.; Di Marino, S.; Scrima, M.; Posteraro, B.; Sanguinetti, M.; Fadda, G.; Soriente, A.; D'Ursi, A.M. Synthesis of New Antifungal Peptides Selective against *Cryptococcus neoformans*. *Bioorg. Med. Chem.* **2010**, *18*, 7985–7990. [CrossRef]
7. Aguiar, T.K.B.; Neto, N.A.S.; Freitas, C.D.T.; Silva, A.F.B.; Bezerra, L.P.; Malveira, E.A.; Branco, L.A.C.; Mesquita, F.P.; Goldman, G.H.; Alencar, L.M.R.; et al. Antifungal Potential of Synthetic Peptides against *Cryptococcus neoformans*: Mechanism of Action Studies Reveal Synthetic Peptides Induce Membrane–Pore Formation, DNA Degradation, and Apoptosis. *Pharmaceutics* **2022**, *14*, 1678. [CrossRef]
8. Souza, P.F.N.; Marques, L.S.M.; Oliveira, J.T.A.; Lima, P.G.; Dias, L.P.; Neto, N.A.S.; Lopes, F.E.S.; Sousa, J.S.; Silva, A.F.B.; Caneiro, R.F.; et al. Synthetic Antimicrobial Peptides: From Choice of the Best Sequences to Action Mechanisms. *Biochimie* **2020**, *175*, 132–145. [CrossRef]
9. Bermas, A.; Geddes-McAlister, J. Combatting the Evolution of Antifungal Resistance in *Cryptococcus neoformans*. *Mol. Microbiol.* **2020**, *114*, 721–734. [CrossRef]
10. Zafar, H.; Altamirano, S.; Ballou, E.R.; Nielsen, K. A Titanic Drug Resistance Threat in *Cryptococcus neoformans*. *Curr. Opin. Microbiol.* **2019**, *52*, 158. [CrossRef]
11. Seyedjavadi, S.S.; Khani, S.; Eslamifar, A.; Ajdary, S.; Goudarzi, M.; Halabian, R.; Akbari, R.; Zare-Zardini, H.; Imani Fooladi, A.A.; Amani, J.; et al. The Antifungal Peptide MCh-AMP1 Derived From Matricaria Chamomilla Inhibits Candida Albicans Growth via Inducing ROS Generation and Altering Fungal Cell Membrane Permeability. *Front. Microbiol.* **2020**, *10*, 3150. [CrossRef] [PubMed]
12. Kim, J.Y.; Park, S.C.; Noh, G.; Kim, H.; Yoo, S.H.; Kim, I.R.; Lee, J.R.; Jang, M.K. Antifungal Effect of A Chimeric Peptide Hn-Mc against Pathogenic Fungal Strains. *Antibiotics* **2020**, *9*, 454. [CrossRef] [PubMed]
13. Delattin, N.; Cammue, B.P.; Thevissen, K. Reactive Oxygen Species-Inducing Antifungal Agents and Their Activity against Fungal Biofilms. *Future Med. Chem.* **2014**, *6*, 77–90. [CrossRef]
14. Peng, C.; Liu, Y.; Shui, L.; Zhao, Z.; Mao, X.; Liu, Z. Mechanisms of Action of the Antimicrobial Peptide Cecropin in the Killing of Candida Albicans. *Life* **2022**, *12*, 1581. [CrossRef] [PubMed]
15. Zhang, Z.; Chen, Y.; Li, B.; Chen, T.; Tian, S. Reactive Oxygen Species: A Generalist in Regulating Development and Pathogenicity of Phytopathogenic Fungi. *Comput. Struct. Biotechnol. J.* **2020**, *18*, 3344. [CrossRef] [PubMed]
16. Keyer, K.; Imlay, J.A. Superoxide Accelerates DNA Damage by Elevating Free-Iron Levels. *Proc. Natl. Acad. Sci. USA* **1996**, *93*, 13635. [CrossRef] [PubMed]
17. Kang, K.A.; Piao, M.J.; Kim, K.C.; Cha, J.W.; Zheng, J.; Yao, C.W.; Chae, S.; Hyun, J.W. Fisetin Attenuates Hydrogen Peroxide-Induced Cell Damage by Scavenging Reactive Oxygen Species and Activating Protective Functions of Cellular Glutathione System. *In Vitro Cell. Dev. Biol. Anim.* **2014**, *50*, 66–74. [CrossRef]
18. Uhl, L.; Gerstel, A.; Chabalier, M.; Dukan, S. Hydrogen Peroxide Induced Cell Death: One or Two Modes of Action? *Heliyon* **2015**, *1*, e00049. [CrossRef]
19. Branco, L.A.C.; Souza, P.F.N.; Neto, N.A.S.; Aguiar, T.K.B.; Fernanda, M.; Carvalho, N.N.; Branco, L.A.C.; Souza, P.F.N.; Neto, N.A.S.; Aguiar, T.K.B.; et al. New Insights into the Mechanism of Antibacterial Action of Synthetic Peptide Mo-CBP3-PepI against Klebsiella Pneumoniae. *Antibiotics* **2022**, *11*, 1753. [CrossRef] [PubMed]
20. Da Silva Neto, J.X.; da Costa, H.P.S.; Vasconcelos, I.M.; Pereira, M.L.; Oliveira, J.T.A.; Lopes, T.D.P.; Dias, L.P.; Araújo, N.M.S.; Moura, L.F.W.G.; Van Tilburg, M.F.; et al. Role of Membrane Sterol and Redox System in the Anti-Candida Activity Reported for Mo-CBP2, a Protein from Moringa Oleifera Seeds. *Int. J. Biol. Macromol.* **2020**, *143*, 814–824. [CrossRef]
21. Cirac, A.D.; Moiset, G.; Mika, J.T.; Koçer, A.; Salvador, P.; Poolman, B.; Marrink, S.J.; Sengupta, D. The Molecular Basis for Antimicrobial Activity of Pore-Forming Cyclic Peptides. *Biophys. J.* **2011**, *100*, 2422. [CrossRef] [PubMed]
22. Lipkin, R.; Lazaridis, T. Computational Studies of Peptide-Induced Membrane Pore Formation. *Philos. Trans. R. Soc. B Biol. Sci.* **2017**, *372*, 20160219. [CrossRef] [PubMed]
23. Dias, L.P.; Souza, P.F.N.; Oliveira, J.T.A.; Vasconcelos, I.M.; Araújo, N.M.S.; Tilburg, M.F.V.; Guedes, M.I.F.; Carneiro, R.F.; Lopes, J.L.S.; Sousa, D.O.B. RcAlb-PepII, a Synthetic Small Peptide Bioinspired in the 2S Albumin from the Seed Cake of Ricinus Communis, Is a Potent Antimicrobial Agent against Klebsiella Pneumoniae and Candida Parapsilosis. *Biochim. Biophys. Acta Biomembr.* **2020**, *1862*, 183092. [CrossRef]
24. Bouz, G.; Doležal, M. Advances in Antifungal Drug Development: An Up-To-Date Mini Review. *Pharmaceuticals* **2021**, *14*, 1312. [CrossRef]
25. Wellen, K.E.; Thompson, C.B. Cellular Metabolic Stress: Considering How Cells Respond to Nutrient Excess. *Mol. Cell* **2010**, *40*, 323. [CrossRef] [PubMed]
26. Farhana, A.; Lappin, S.L. Biochemistry, Lactate Dehydrogenase. In *StatPearls*; StatPearls Publishing: Treasure Island, FL, USA, 2022.
27. Fontanesi, F.; Soto, I.C.; Barrientos, A. Cytochrome *c* Oxidase Biogenesis: New Levels of Regulation. *IUBMB Life* **2008**, *60*, 557–568. [CrossRef] [PubMed]
28. Narasimhan, M.L.; Coca, M.A.; Jin, J.; Yamauchi, T.; Ito, Y.; Kadowaki, T.; Kim, K.K.; Pardo, J.M.; Damsz, B.; Hasegawa, P.M.; et al. Osmotin Is a Homolog of Mammalian Adiponectin and Controls Apoptosis in Yeast through a Homolog of Mammalian Adiponectin Receptor. *Mol. Cell* **2005**, *17*, 171–180. [CrossRef] [PubMed]
29. Lopes, F.E.S.; da Costa, H.P.S.; Souza, P.F.N.; Oliveira, J.P.B.; Ramos, M.V.; Freire, J.E.C.; Jucá, T.L.; Freitas, C.D.T. Peptide from Thaumatin Plant Protein Exhibits Selective Anticandidal Activity by Inducing Apoptosis via Membrane Receptor. *Phytochemistry* **2019**, *159*, 46–55. [CrossRef]

30. *M27-A3*; Reference Method for Broth Dilution Antifungal Susceptibility Testing of Yeasts. Approved Standard—Third Edition; Clinical and Laboratory Standards Institute: Pittsburgh, PA, USA, 2008.
31. Lima, P.G.; Souza, P.F.N.; Freitas, C.D.T.; Bezerra, L.P.; Neto, N.A.S.; Silva, A.F.B.; Oliveira, J.T.A.; Sousa, D.O.B. Synthetic Peptides against Trichophyton Mentagrophytes and T. Rubrum: Mechanisms of Action and Efficiency Compared to Griseofulvin and Itraconazole. *Life Sci.* **2021**, *265*, 118803. [CrossRef]
32. Hyung, S.C.; Jun, W.K.; Cha, Y.N.; Kim, C. A Quantitative Nitroblue Tetrazolium Assay for Determining Intracellular Superoxide Anion Production in Phagocytic Cells. *J. Immunoass. Immunochem.* **2006**, *27*, 31–44. [CrossRef]
33. Souza, P.F.N.; Silva, F.D.A.; Carvalho, F.E.L.; Silveira, J.A.G.; Vasconcelos, I.M.; Oliveira, J.T.A. Photosynthetic and Biochemical Mechanisms of an EMS-Mutagenized Cowpea Associated with Its Resistance to Cowpea Severe Mosaic Virus. *Plant Cell Rep.* **2017**, *36*, 219–234. [CrossRef] [PubMed]

Disclaimer/Publisher's Note: The statements, opinions and data contained in all publications are solely those of the individual author(s) and contributor(s) and not of MDPI and/or the editor(s). MDPI and/or the editor(s) disclaim responsibility for any injury to people or property resulting from any ideas, methods, instructions or products referred to in the content.

MDPI
St. Alban-Anlage 66
4052 Basel
Switzerland
Tel. +41 61 683 77 34
Fax +41 61 302 89 18
www.mdpi.com

Antibiotics Editorial Office
E-mail: antibiotics@mdpi.com
www.mdpi.com/journal/antibiotics

www.ingramcontent.com/pod-product-compliance
Lightning Source LLC
LaVergne TN
LVHW070449100526
838202LV00014B/1691